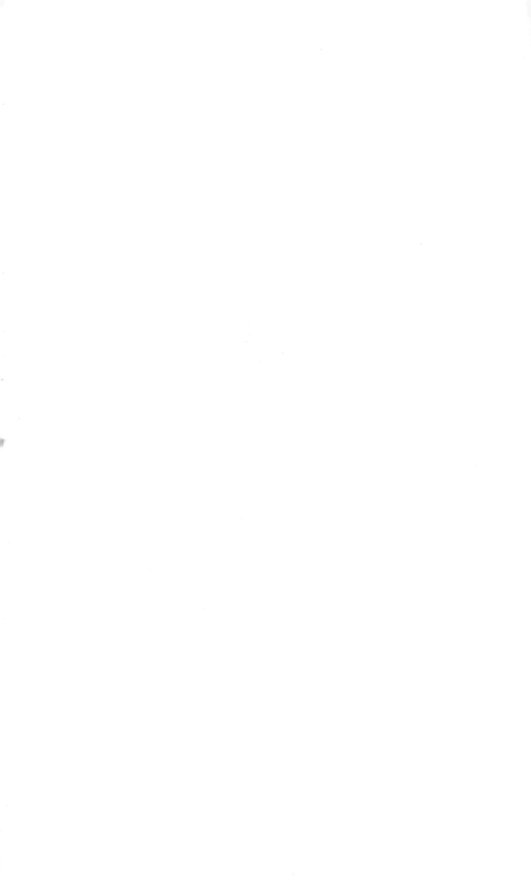

BIOLOGY OF PERSONALITY
AND INDIVIDUAL DIFFERENCES

Biology of Personality and Individual Differences

Edited by

TURHAN CANLI

THE GUILFORD PRESS
New York   London

Library of Congress Cataloging-in-Publication Data
Biology of personality and individual differences / edited by Turhan Canli.
   p. cm.
   Includes bibliographical references and index.
   ISBN 1-59385-252-5 (hardcover)
   1. Personality—Physiological aspects. 2. Neuropsychology. I. Canli, Turhan.
   [DNLM: 1. Psychophysiology—methods. 2. Personality—physiology.
3. Neuropsychology—methods. 4. Genetics, Behavioral. 5. Neurophysiology—methods. WL 103 B6159 2006]
   QP402.B56 2006
   612.8—dc22

                                                    2005016217

About the Editor

Turhan Canli, PhD, is Assistant Professor in the Department of Psychology at Stony Brook University and a member of the Graduate Program in Genetics. He holds degrees from Tufts University (BA, 1998) and from Yale University (PhD, 1993). Dr. Canli's research focuses on the neurogenetic basis of personality and emotion, using a combination of cognitive-behavioral paradigms, noninvasive brain imaging (functional magnetic resonance imaging) and stimulation (transcranial magnetic stimulation), and genotyping for gene polymorphisms related to personality traits.

Contributors

A. Leo Beem, PhD, Department of Biological Psychology, Vrije Universiteit, Amsterdam, The Netherlands

Jamil Bhanji, BS, Department of Psychology, Stanford University, Stanford, California

Dorret I. Boomsma, PhD, Department of Biological Psychology, Vrije Universiteit, Amsterdam, The Netherlands

Turhan Canli, PhD, Graduate Program in Genetics and Department of Psychology, Stony Brook University, Stony Brook, New York

Danielle C. Cath, MD, Department of Psychiatry, Vrije Universiteit, Amsterdam, The Netherlands

Silvana Chiavegatto, PhD, Department and Institute of Psychiatry and Laboratory of Genetics and Molecular Cardiology, Heart Institute, University of São Paulo Medical School, São Paulo, Brazil

Rebecca E. Cooney, BA, Department of Psychology, Stanford University, Stanford, California

Richard A. Depue, PhD, Laboratory of Neurobiology of Temperament and Personality, Department of Human Development, Cornell University, Ithaca, New York

Thalia C. Eley, PhD, Social, Genetic and Developmental Psychiatry Centre, Institute of Psychiatry, King's College London, London, United Kingdom

Don C. Fowles, PhD, Department of Psychology, University of Iowa, Iowa City, Iowa

Nathan A. Gillespie, PhD, Virginia Institute of Psychiatric and Behavioral Genetics, Richmond, Virginia

Samuel D. Gosling, PhD, Department of Psychology, University of Texas at Austin, Austin, Texas

Ian H. Gotlib, PhD, Department of Psychology, Stanford University, Stanford, California

Stephan Hamann, PhD, Department of Psychology, Emory University, Atlanta, Georgia

Ahmad R. Hariri, PhD, Department of Psychiatry, Western Psychiatric Institute and Clinic, University of Pittsburgh School of Medicine, Pittsburgh, Pennsylvania

Wendy Heller, PhD, Department of Psychology and Beckman Institute, University of Illinois at Urbana–Champaign, Champaign, Illinois

John D. Herrington, MPhil, Wisconsin Psychiatric Institute and Clinics, Madison, Wisconsin

Jutta Joormann, PhD, Department of Psychology, Stanford University, Stanford, California

James E. King, PhD, Department of Psychology, University of Arizona, Tucson, Arizona

Marisa Knight, BA, Department of Psychology, University of California, Santa Cruz, California

Brian Knutson, PhD, Department of Psychology, Stanford University, Stanford, California

Nancy S. Koven, PhD, Department of Psychology, University of Illinois at Urbana–Champaign, Champaign, Illinois

Jennifer Y. F. Lau, BSc, Social, Genetic and Developmental Psychiatry Centre, Institute of Psychiatry, King's College London, London, United Kingdom

Klaus-Peter Lesch, MD, Department of Psychiatry and Psychotherapy, University of Würzburg, Würzburg, Germany

Nicholas G. Martin, MD, Queensland Institute of Medical Research, Brisbane, Queensland, Australia

Mara Mather, PhD, Department of Psychology, University of California, Santa Cruz, California

Pranjal H. Mehta, BA, Department of Psychology, University of Texas at Austin, Austin, Texas

Christel M. Middeldorp, MD, Departments of Biological Psychology and Psychiatry, Vrije Universiteit, Amsterdam, The Netherlands

Gregory A. Miller, PhD, Departments of Psychology and Psychiatry and Beckman Institute, University of Illinois at Urbana–Champaign, Champaign, Illinois

Kelly L. Minor, PhD, Department of Psychology, Stanford University, Stanford, California

Robert Plomin, PhD, Social, Genetic and Developmental Psychiatry Centre, Institute of Psychiatry, King's College London, London, United Kingdom

Rajita Sinha, PhD, Department of Psychiatry, Yale University School of Medicine, New Haven, Connecticut

Mireille van den Berg, PhD, Department of Biological Psychology, Vrije Universiteit, Amsterdam, The Netherlands

Richard van Dyck, MD, Department of Psychiatry, Vrije Universiteit, Amsterdam, The Netherlands

Essi Viding, PhD, Social, Genetic and Developmental Psychiatry Centre, Institute of Psychiatry, King's College London, London, United Kingdom

Alexander Weiss, PhD, Department of Psychology, University of Edinburgh, Edinburgh, United Kingdom

Marvin Zuckerman, PhD, Department of Psychology, University of Delaware, Newark, Delaware

Acknowledgments

This book is the result of a conference held on the campus of Stony Brook University, August 13–15, 2004. I thank my department and the university (particularly Ann Brody and Berengaria Brine of the Office for Conferences and Special Events), as well as my assistant, Jezreel Otto. I also thank Anne E. Moyer for her continued and unwavering support in all I do, and her critical mind in all I think. The conference was funded by a grant from the National Institute of Mental Health (No. 1R13MH06783501A1). I am deeply grateful for the support I received. Finally, I want to thank Seymour Weingarten, Editor in Chief of The Guilford Press, for supporting the publication of this book.

I dedicate this book to my parents, whose love and support has been immeasurable.

TURHAN CANLI

Contents

1. Introduction   1
   Turhan Canli

I. OVERVIEW AND A HISTORICAL PERSPECTIVE

2. Jeffrey Gray's Contributions to Theories of Anxiety,   7
   Personality, and Psychopathology
   Don C. Fowles

II. STUDIES OF EXTRAVERSION AND RELATED TRAITS

3. Biosocial Bases of Sensation Seeking   37
   Marvin Zuckerman

4. Interpersonal Behavior and the Structure of Personality: 60
   Neurobehavioral Foundation of Agentic Extraversion
   and Affiliation
   Richard A. Depue

5. Genomic Imaging of Extraversion   93
   Turhan Canli

6. Neural Substrates for Emotional Traits?:   116
   The Case of Extraversion
   Brian Knutson and *Jamil Bhanji*

7. Mapping the Neural Correlates of Dimensions of Personality,   133
   Emotion, and Motivation
   John D. Herrington, Nancy S. Koven, Gregory A. Miller,
   and *Wendy Heller*

III. AGE AND SEX AS DETERMINANTS OF INDIVIDUAL DIFFERENCES

8. The Affective Neuroscience of Aging and Its Implications   159
for Cognition
Marisa Knight and Mara Mather

9. Sex Differences in Neural Responses to Sexual Stimuli   184
in Humans
Stephan Hamann

10. Sex Differences in Brain Functional Magnetic Resonance   203
Imaging Response to Stress
Rajita Sinha

IV. GENETIC AND NEURAL ANALYSES OF ANXIETY-RELATED TRAITS

11. Neuroticism as a Genetic Marker for Mood and Anxiety   225
Nathan A. Gillespie and Nicholas G. Martin

12. The Association of Personality with Anxious   251
and Depressive Psychopathology
*Christel M. Middeldorp, Danielle C. Cath, Mireille van den Berg,
A. Leo Beem, Richard van Dyck, and Dorret I. Boomsma*

13. 5-HT$_{1A}$ Receptor and Anxiety-Related Traits: 273
Pharmacology, Genetics, and Imaging
Klaus-Peter Lesch and Turhan Canli

14. Genetically Driven Variation in Serotonin Function: 295
Impact on Amygdala Reactivity and Individual Differences
in Fearful and Anxious Personality
Ahmad R. Hariri

V. INDIVIDUAL DIFFERENCES IN CHILDREN

15. Etiology of Psychopathic Tendencies in Children: 317
Distinguishing a Genetically Vulnerable Subgroup of
Children with Antisocial Behavior
Essi Viding and Robert Plomin

16. A Cognitive-Behavioral Genetic Approach to Emotional   335
Development in Childhood and Adolescence
Jennifer Y. F. Lau and Thalia C. Eley

Contents

17. Cognitive and Biological Functioning in Children at Risk   353
    for Depression
    Ian H. Gotlib, Jutta Joormann, Kelly L. Minor, and Rebecca E. Cooney

VI. PERSONALITY IN ANIMALS

18. Using Mouse Models to Unravel Aggressive Behavior   385
    Silvana Chiavegatto

19. Searching for Genetic and Environmental Contributions   407
    to Personality and Happiness in Chimpanzees
    (*Pan troglodytes*)
    Alexander Weiss and James E. King

20. How Can Animal Studies Contribute to Research   427
    on the Biological Bases of Personality?
    Pranjal H. Mehta and Samuel D. Gosling

    Index   449

BIOLOGY OF PERSONALITY
AND INDIVIDUAL DIFFERENCES

1

Introduction

Turhan Canli

Recent methodological advances in genetics and neuroscience have catalyzed work on the biological basis of personality and individual differences. Yet even active researchers rarely have the opportunity to learn about all of these developments, because geneticists, psychologists, and neuroscientists only rarely attend the same scientific meetings. This lack of communication motivated a remarkable conference that was held in August 2004 on the campus of Stony Brook University on Long Island, New York, entitled "The Biological Basis of Personality and Individual Differences." Funded by the National Institute of Mental Health, this conference brought together researchers from clinical psychology and psychiatry; cognitive, affective, and behavioral neuroscience; and comparative psychology. Presentations covered the structure of personality and its mapping onto biology; the biology of traits; genetic markers for individual differences and vulnerability toward psychopathology; functional neuroimaging approaches; and the correspondence between human and animal personality.

Until now, the reader who wanted to follow these exciting developments had to seek out scholarly journals from a vast array of scientific disciplines. This book represents an attempt to offer a current and cross-sectional overview of the field and is intended for a wide audience. Practicing clinicians; social, personality, and cognitive psychologists; neuroscientists working in neuroimaging; behavioral neuroscientists; and behavioral and molecular geneticists will all find new and exciting insights in this book. The book's major themes are divided into six sections. Starting in Part II, each chapter not only presents current empirical work placed in a larger scholarly context, but

1

also concludes with a section entitled "Looking Forward," in which the authors speculate on the future of their respective fields.

Part I is a historical perspective on broad questions regarding the mapping of personality onto the brain. Few investigators had a better grasp of these questions than Jeffrey Gray. He was the first to commit to be a speaker for the Stony Brook conference. His passing a few months before the meeting came as a great personal shock and as a tremendous loss to the field. Gray's contributions are thoughtfully represented and reviewed by Fowles (Chapter 2), to the extent that this is possible in one chapter. His summary makes for an appropriate starting point, because Gray's work transcended animal and human studies, and included both basic physiology and clinical applications; as such, it sets the stage for the diverse set of chapters that follows.

Part II narrows the focus by presenting different research approaches to extraversion and related traits. Zuckerman (Chapter 3) opens this section with a discussion of the biosocial bases of sensation seeking, a trait related to extraversion. Depue (Chapter 4) deconstructs positive interpersonal aspects of extraversion into two independent traits of agency and affiliation. He presents recent data on the neurobiology of these traits, discussing their phenotypic, neurobehavioral, and genetic aspects. I (Canli) then look at the positive affective characteristics of extraversion to show how brain reactivity to emotional stimuli correlates with individual differences in this trait, and, furthermore, how it is associated with variation within specific genes. I argue that this "genomic imaging" approach may eventually lead to the development of neurogenetic, causal models of personality. Knutson and Bhanji (Chapter 6) focus on the interplay of positive arousal and gain anticipation in extraversion; they show how newer neuroimaging methods, particularly event-related functional magnetic resonance imaging, can be utilized to obtain a better understanding of the temporal dynamics and function localization of these processes. Innovations in neuroimaging are also the topic of the chapter by Herrington, Koven, Miller, and Heller (Chapter 7), who highlight the importance of novel analytical strategies in revealing individual differences in brain laterality, as they relate to personality, emotion, and motivation.

Part III moves from traits to other determinants of individual differences. Knight and Mather (Chapter 8) focus on the exciting emerging field of the affective neuroscience of aging, and present work on the interaction between emotion and cognition across the adult life span. Hamann (Chapter 9) discusses sex differences in neural responses to sexual stimuli, presenting data on how men and women differ in activation of limbic structures that mediate emotion, motivation, and physiological responses. Sinha (Chapter 10) concludes the section with a chapter on gender differences in the context of brain responses to emotional stress. Her chapter also marks a transition toward clinical issues, which characterize the next two sections.

Part IV presents genetic and neural analyses related to anxiety and mood disorders, and to traits linked to these. The first two chapters demonstrate the utility of large-scale twin registries in behavioral genetics. Gillespie and Martin (Chapter 11) explore the genetic and environmental contributors to neuroticism; they make the point that this trait is an ideal phenotypic candidate to discover quantitative trait loci associated with negative mood and anxiety. Middeldorp, Cath, van den Berg, Beem, van Dyck, and Boomsma (Chapter 12) investigate the association of neuroticism, extraversion, and sensation seeking with anxious and depressive psychopathology, based on data from the Netherlands Twin Register of more than 45,000 twins. The last two chapters of this section demonstrate the power of molecular genetics in conjunction with an endophenotype approach to detect genetic effects in much smaller samples. Lesch and I (Chapter 13) discuss how variation within the serotonin 1A (5-HT_{1A}) receptor gene (*HTR1A*) is associated with anxiety and emotional brain reactivity, presenting data to suggest a nonlinear relationship between *HTR1A* genotype and its influence on cognitive and neural systems engaged in attention to negative emotional stimuli. Hariri (Chapter 14) closes the section with a discussion of genetic variation within the serotonin transporter gene–linked or promoter region (*5-HTTLPR*) and its effect on amygdala activation and individual differences in fearful and anxious personality traits.

Part V narrows the topic of mood and personality disorders to children. Viding and Plomin (Chapter 15) present data on children with psychopathic personality traits who are genetically vulnerable to antisocial behavior. Lau and Eley (Chapter 16) investigate two pathways by which genetic factors may contribute to the development of anxiety and depression in children and adolescents, using a cognitive-behavioral genetic approach. Gotlib, Joormann, Minor, and Cooney (Chapter 17) close the section with an examination of the cognitive and biological characteristics of children at high risk for depression. Their preliminary findings highlight the opportunity to develop better detection tools and thus to improve the odds for successful prevention of depression.

Part VI, the closing section, serves as a bridge between research on human and animal personality. Chiavegatto (Chapter 18) starts off the section with a discussion of studies on aggression in genetically altered mice. Weiss and King (Chapter 19) present data on personality, happiness, and genes in chimpanzees. They find evidence for genes that are common to trait dominance and to subjective well-being, but also find that each factor is uniquely associated with environmental variables. Mehta and Gosling (Chapter 20) close the section with a broader look at the study of human versus animal personality. They demonstrate that personality can indeed be studied in animals, and that there are five major benefits of animal studies for research on human personality; they suggest that a better understanding of the biological basis of personality will result from the integration of human and animal studies.

I

Overview and a Historical Perspective

2

Jeffrey Gray's Contributions to Theories of Anxiety, Personality, and Psychopathology

Don C. Fowles

To understand Jeffrey Gray's work, it is essential to understand the importance of (1) the anxiolytic drugs and (2) the theoretical framework provided by the tradition of animal learning theory, which had been a dominant force in psychology for much of the 20th century up to about the 1960s, when the "cognitive revolution" gained ascendancy. Gray reasoned that it ought to be possible to conceptualize the underlying processes by which the anxiolytic drugs exert their effects in terms of the constructs of animal learning theory. The anxiolytic drugs were fundamentally important in his work for two reasons other than their widespread use.

First, they provided a criterion for what constitutes "anxiety." As reviewed by Barlow (2002, Ch. 2), anxiety is a complex construct, and there still is not necessarily agreement as to its meaning. Over the years, different investigators have defined or inferred anxiety on the basis of numerous conceptualizations and/or operational definitions. In this context of ambiguity, it is no small matter to have a firm basis for defining and researching anxiety. Gray's ingenious approach was to define anxiety *as the process that is reduced by anxiolytic drugs*. Although other definitions are possible, Gray's was reasonable and defensible (Gray & McNaughton, 2000, pp. 3–4)—and, importantly, it provided a clear operational criterion.

Second, the effects of the anxiolytic drugs can be studied in animals. Gray's second goal—one that occupied most of his career—was to identify the neural substrate for anxiety. The only practicable way to achieve this is with experimental animals. The common strategy of studying anxiety by relying on introspective self-report does not lend itself to animal research and, in any case, suffers from the often poor validity of self-reports about internal processes.

Gray's use of the effects of anxiolytic drugs to define the processes associated with anxiety bridges this gap between the introspections of humans and animal work (Gray & McNaughton, 2000, p. 3), and it also bridges the gap between behavior and brain processes. This approach of using anxiolytic drugs in animal research inherently involves an emphasis on anxious *behavior* (as opposed to conscious *experience* in humans), consistent with Gray's interest in theories from animal learning. It also emphasizes internal neural processes that can be examined (e.g., via functional magnetic resonance imaging) in a way that conscious experience cannot.

GRAY'S EARLY WORK

The Effects of Anxiolytic Drugs

In a massive review of the literature, Gray (1977) attempted to identify the behavioral effects of anxiolytic drugs or "minor tranquilizers," the underlying psychological processes altered by these drugs, and the brain structures involved in these effects of minor tranquilizers. Although numerous other papers addressed the second and third questions, this publication provided the definitive answer to the first question. In order to conceptually organize this literature, Gray provided a brief summary of a theoretical context derived from animal learning, taken from his earlier book-length presentation (Gray, 1975). In this view, organisms are seen as maximizing exposure to rewarding ("appetitive") events and minimizing exposure to punishing ("aversive") events. Rewarding or appetitive events consist of presentation of a reward (Rew), termination of punishment (Pun!), or omission of an expected punishment (nonPun), while punishing or aversive events consist of presentation of punishment (Pun), termination of reward (Rew!), and omission of an expected reward (nonRew). Omission of an expected reward occurs in the early stages of extinction, in which a previously reliable response-contingent reward is omitted, producing frustration. Omission of an expected punishment occurs in the active avoidance paradigm, in which punishment (usually electric shock) reliably follows presentation of a tone until the animal learns to make an instrumental response that takes it into a safe area, producing relief. Through a process of classical conditioning, conditioned stimuli (CSs) paired with these events come to acquire some of their emotional and motivational properties.

Gray (1977) reviewed the effects of minor tranquilizers (barbiturates, alcohol, and benzodiazepines) in animal studies on behavior in the following paradigms: rewarded behavior; passive avoidance; classical conditioning of fear; escape behavior; one-way active avoidance; two-way active avoidance;

responses elicited by aversive stimuli; and frustrative nonreward (as seen in resistance to extinction, discrimination learning, intermittent schedules in the Skinner box, incomplete reduction of reward, and the aftereffects of non-reward). Based especially on the effects of sodium amytal, but with ample parallel effects for the other drugs, this review found the effects of the minor tranquilizers to be highly specific: They selectively antagonize or reduce the behavioral effects of *conditioned* stimuli for punishment (Pun-CSs), frustrative nonreward (nonRew-CSs), and, more tentatively, novel stimuli. The behavioral effects in question were the suppression of responses associated with these stimuli. Note that the minor tranquilizers did not alter the effects of the *unconditioned* punishment or reward stimuli described above, nor did they alter the effects of conditioned reward (Rew-CSs) in simple reward paradigms or conditioned nonpunishment (nonPun-CSs) in active avoidance paradigms.

The Behavioral Inhibition System and the Effects of Anxiolytic Drugs

Based on these and other considerations, Gray (1971, 1975, 1976a) had earlier proposed a "behavioral inhibition system" (BIS), the features of which he summarized again in 1977. The BIS responds especially to three types of input: Pun-CSs, nonRew-CSs, and novel features of the environment. Outputs from the BIS (1) suppress any ongoing operant behavior, (2) increase attention to the environment (especially to novel stimuli), and (3) increment the level of (nonspecific) arousal, with the result that the responses ultimately chosen will be characterized by greater behavioral vigor (e.g., running faster).

Although the effects of the BIS are seen in numerous paradigms, two easily understood prototypical paradigms are extinction and conflict or passive avoidance. In the early phases of extinction, the BIS processes input from CSs associated with the frustration due to the absence of expected reward, and it tends to suppress or inhibit the approach response. There is conflict between this inhibitory process and the tendency still to make a previously rewarded response. In the alley runway version of passive avoidance, or the conflict paradigm, the organism anticipates punishment (e.g., having to cross an electrified metal grid) as it approaches the goal box where it has learned to expect a reward. The BIS then processes the CSs associated with this punishment and tends to inhibit the approach response. There is conflict between the desire to approach the reward and the desire not to approach the punishment. Because punishment is avoided by not making a response, the avoidance is called "passive avoidance." Gray liked to note that the conditioned response (inhibition) to Pun-CSs is, in important respects, opposite to the unconditioned response (behavioral activation) to the unconditioned stimulus itself.

The effects of the anxiolytic drugs map nicely onto the stimuli that activate the BIS and the response-inhibitory effects of the BIS, allowing the elegantly simple proposal that *anxiolytic drugs antagonize the BIS.* Two experimental paradigms were important in showing that this effect was not just one of disinhibiting behavior, but rather included the emotional/arousing aspects of the BIS. The first had to do with the "partial reinforcement acquisition effect" (PRAE). In the alley runway, it is often found that at the end of training, animals receiving reward only 50% of the time (on a random schedule) run faster than animals receiving 100% reinforcement. This PRAE is abolished by anxiolytic drugs, which is noteworthy, because this reduced behavioral vigor is the opposite of the disinhibition seen in most of the paradigms affected by anxiolytic drugs. The PRAE can be understood, however, by attributing the increased running speed to the BIS-produced arousal associated with its processing of the nonRew-CSs in a partial reinforcement schedule. Thus the anxiolytic drugs antagonize the BIS itself and do not just block its inhibitory output.

The second phenomenon is called the "partial reinforcement extinction effect" (PREE). Animals trained on partial reinforcement are more resistant to extinction than those trained on 100% reinforcement. Administration of anxiolytic drugs during training reduces or even reverses this PREE (if the drugs are not administered during extinction); that is, *fewer* responses are seen during extinction as a result of drug administration during training. Again, this effect cannot be understood as due to simple response disinhibition, but it can be understood in terms of the emotional effects of the BIS. That is, the PREE can be attributed to activation of the BIS by nonRew-CSs that reflect the effects of the nonrewarded trials during acquisition with partial reinforcement. This experience with aversive arousal during acquisition reduces the effects of nonRew-CSs during extinction. Thus Gray was able to make the case that (1) a single system conceptualized as the BIS is involved in all the paradigms affected by anxiolytic drugs and (2) the anxiolytic drugs selectively antagonize the BIS.

Several aspects of Gray's concept of the BIS and the learning theory in which it was embedded are noteworthy, especially in comparison with Hullian theory that had dominated much of American psychology in earlier decades. First, in Hullian theory the concept of inhibition played a modest role. In contrast, inhibition of behavior was a primary function of the BIS and a direct consequence of response-contingent aversive outcomes, such as those seen in extinction and passive avoidance. This conceptualization is critical to explaining the antagonistic effects of anxiolytic drugs in these paradigms.

Second, Hullian theory passionately eschewed cognitive constructs in the form of expectancies, whereas they are central to Gray's tabulation of motivationally relevant events. Viewing expectancies as critical to organizing behavior even for rodents is strikingly different from Hullian and Skinnerian approaches to animal learning, and it considerably counters the perception that animal learning theory and cognitive theories are inherently incompatible.

Third, as a result of invoking expectancies, the active avoidance paradigm—in which punishment is avoided by making an active response that takes the organism to safety—is viewed as parallel to a *simple reward* paradigm, rather than as an aversive paradigm. In both paradigms, an active response provides relief from an aversive state. In addition, punishment and omission of reward elicit similar behaviors (e.g., aggression). Although this parallelism is obvious once one thinks about it, many investigators have viewed active avoidance as an aversive paradigm, unlike the positive aspects of simple reward. As already noted, the anxiolytic drugs do not antagonize active avoidance, but do antagonize passive avoidance. Without this sharp conceptual distinction between active and passive avoidance, it would be difficult to understand the effects of anxiolytic drugs.

The BIS and the Neural Substrate for an Anxiety System (circa 1976)

During the 1970s, Gray published several papers proposing that the BIS is the anxiety system—that is, with titles such as "The Neuropsychology of Anxiety" or "A Neuropsychological Theory of Anxiety" (Gray, 1976b, 1978, 1979) and "The Behavioural Inhibition System: A Possible Substrate for Anxiety" (Gray, 1976a). The compelling logic of calling the BIS the anxiety system was that (1) he had demonstrated that a behavioral system largely conceptualized on the basis of the animal learning literature was antagonized by the anxiolytic drugs; and (2) the function of the BIS is to process CSs for aversive outcomes (punishment, frustrative nonreward), as would be expected for an anxiety system. Gray had then proceeded to map the BIS and the effects of anxiolytic drugs onto structures in the central nervous system (CNS). On the basis of a similarity between the behavioral effects of lesions and the behavioral effects of anxiolytic drugs, the septal area and the hippocampus had emerged as key structures in the functioning of the BIS and the effects of anxiolytic drugs on behavior. Additional early results showed a remarkable convergence of numerous experimental approaches in support of the theory, and they more precisely identified key neural correlates of the BIS.

Hippocampal theta—high-voltage (500- to 1000-μV) waves in the 6- to 10-Hz range in rodents—played a central role in these studies. The pacemaker cells controlling hippocampal theta lie in the medial septal area and can be driven by applying brief electrical pulses at the appropriate frequencies (a process named "theta driving") or blocked at high (>100-Hz) frequencies. In some paradigms, recordings from the hippocampus in free-responding animals revealed that theta centered on 7.7 Hz was associated with being exposed to frustrative nonreward (e.g., the alley runway) or exploring a novel environment. Theta at 6–7 Hz was observed in connection with eating, drinking, grooming, and the like, which Gray called "fixed action patterns," whereas theta at 9–10 Hz was observed when an animal was moving down the runway toward a well-learned goal. Thus theta centered on 7.7 Hz was found in some studies to be associated with conditions that presumably activated the BIS. Based on this finding, the theory predicted that enhancing 7.7-Hz theta through theta driving should facilitate the effects of the BIS, while high-frequency stimulation should block BIS activity.

To understand the first series of studies in this context, recall the PREE, in which BIS activation during partial reinforcement was presumed to account

for the greater resistance to extinction following partial than continuous reinforcement. Anxiolytic drugs during acquisition reduce this effect, presumably
by attenuating the BIS response to nonRew stimuli. Of course, the BIS was
assumed to facilitate normal extinction following continuous reinforcement.
The following results were obtained:

- Extinction following continuous reinforcement was facilitated by enhancing theta in the 7.7-Hz range through septal driving.
- The PREE effect could be induced by septal driving of theta in the 7.7-
  Hz range on half the trials during acquisition with continuous reinforcement. That is (by theory), activating the BIS on half the acquisition trials mimicked the BIS-activating effects of nonreward, and it
  produced the same resistance to extinction seen with partial reinforcement during acquisition.
- High-frequency septal blocking of the theta that would have occurred
  with partial reinforcement during acquisition reduced the expected
  resistance to extinction associated with the PREE.
- Medial septal area lesions (which presumably prevent BIS activation)
  increased resistance to extinction under continuous reinforcement conditions and reduced resistance to extinction under partial reinforcement conditions, both findings being consistent with the assumed effect
  of the BIS.

All but the last of these findings depend on the hypothesis that theta in the
7.7-Hz range reflects BIS activity, increasing the precision of the theory and
providing a new domain of supporting electrophysiological evidence beyond
lesion studies.

Another series of studies examined the effect of the anxiolytic drugs on
the septal theta driving, providing additional support for the association
between the BIS and 7.7-Hz theta. If one plots the minimum voltage required
to drive theta in the free-moving rat as a function of frequency of stimulation,
the voltage is at a minimum at 7.7 Hz, with a U-shaped dip in the threshold
being formed by points plotted for 6.9, 7.7, and 9.1 Hz. Several anxiolytic
(but not nonanxiolytic) drugs were found to selectively raise the threshold at
7.7 Hz, having a lesser effect at higher and lower frequencies, and eliminating
the U-shaped dip.

The research then turned to considering what input to the septal area
might be involved in the effects of anxiolytic drugs on the septal area and hippocampus. Numerous pharmacological manipulations of various transmitters
suggested that inputs from noradrenergic and perhaps serotonergic neurons—
and not dopaminergic or cholinergic neurons—are involved. The picture was
more straightforward for noradrenergic pathways. Drugs (haloperidol, alpha-
methyl-*p*-tyrosine) that block the effects of both dopamine and noradrenaline
eliminated the U-shaped dip in the theta-driving curve. Further manipulations
indicated that blockage of noradrenaline and not dopamine was responsible

for this effect. The obvious candidate was the pathway consisting of nor-adrenergic neurons that originate in the locus coeruleus (a small nucleus in the brainstem) and ascend via the dorsal bundle to innervate the hippocampus, cerebellum, and neocortex. Existing evidence already indicated a reduction in neuronal activity and noradrenergic turnover in this pathway by the barbitu-rates and benzodiazepines. Selective destruction of the dorsal bundle by a neurotoxin reduced by 98% the levels of noradrenaline in the hippocampus and eliminated the U-shaped dip in the theta-driving curve. These data sug-gested that this ascending noradrenergic projection from the locus coeruleus to the hippocampus selectively facilitates septal driving of the hippocampus in the 7.7-Hz range. Gray (1976a) proposed that the anxiolytic drugs exert their behavioral effects through a reduction of activity in this noradrenergic path-way. Somewhat later, McNaughton and Mason (1980) confirmed the general parallelism between lesions of this dorsal ascending noradrenergic bundle (DANB) and the effects of anxiolytic drugs and lesions of the hippocampus and septal area. However, these authors also noted a number tasks for which DANB lesions did not produce the expected effects, suggesting that additional mechanisms must be responsible for some of the effects of anxiolytic drugs (see also Gray & McNaughton, 2000, p. 13).

The effects of serotonin (implicated by pharmacological studies in the control of behavioral inhibition) appeared to be rather different. Parachloro-phenylalanine (PCPA) prevents synthesis of serotonin and eliminates the 7.7-Hz theta dip, but it does so by *lowering* the threshold at frequencies other than 7.7 Hz. 5-Hydroxytryptamine (5-HTP) restores serotonin and restores the 7.7-Hz theta dip. Gray concluded that the shape of the theta-driving curve in the undrugged animal depends on both neurotransmitters—with serotonin inhibiting (or raising the threshold of) frequencies other than 7.7 Hz, and noradrenaline facilitating (or lowering the threshold of) septal driving at 7.7 Hz—and that it is the shape of the curve that is important.

A variety of evidence suggested that serotonergic neurons are important in behavioral inhibition and pointed to the major bundle of serotonergic neu-rons originating in the midbrain raphe nuclei. These neurons ascend from the raphe nuclei to the septal area by way of the medial forebrain bundle. The hippocampus also receives serotonergic input via fibers that pass through the septum and that normally would be cut by medial septal lesions. Thus Gray (1976a) proposed that ascending noradrenergic and serotonergic pathways exert an important influence on a BIS involving the medial septal area and the hippocampus (see also Gray & McNaughton, 2000, p. 13).

Selective Breeding and the Theta-Driving Curve

The discovery of the 7.7-Hz theta-driving dip and its association with the BIS led to another, very interesting set of experiments with the Maudsley Reactive (MR) and Maudsley Nonreactive (MNR) strains of rats. These strains were selectively bred using defecation in a brightly lit open field, on the dual assumption (1) that the open field is aversive to rats in the original Wistar population, and (2) that defecation is an index of the fear response. A variety of evidence suggested that the MR rats (high defecators) are more fearful than the MNR rats. When male MR and MNR rats were studied, the results were exactly as predicted: The MR rats showed normal theta-driving curves, whereas the MNR rats were completely without the 7.7-Hz dip. (The results for females are too complicated to describe here.) Gray concluded that the absence of the 7.7-Hz dip in the MNR rats was a consequence of selective breeding, and that this finding strongly supported the inference of a functional link between the level of fearfulness and shape of the theta-driving curve.

GRAY'S LATER THEORY OF ANXIETY

In the interest of saving space, we can now skip forward to the last comprehensive summary of this work on anxiety (Gray & McNaughton, 2000), entitled *The Neuropsychology of Anxiety: An Enquiry into the Functions of the Septo-Hippocampal System* (2nd ed.). This work was published with Gray's one-time student Neil McNaughton, who was for many years his colleague/collaborator and now is the heir apparent to this approach to anxiety and anxiety disorders. Although McNaughton was a major contributor to this 2000 revision of the earlier book (Gray, 1982), their collective effort constitutes an excellent statement of the evolution of Gray's contributions. A more recent review of the theory with revisions by McNaughton and Corr (2004) is highly recommended, but it is not included here because Gray was not involved. The first part of the present summary describes the continuity and change with respect to the core theory already described, while the second part describes the expansion of the theory into the questions of what the BIS is, how it functions, and how it articulates with the septo-hippocampal system (SHS) and other brain structures.

The Effects of Anxiolytic Drugs

Gray and McNaughton were able to report a major success of the theory presented above, having to do with new anxiolytic drugs. In order to appreciate these findings, one must note that in addition to the effects of anxiolytic drugs on the 7.7-Hz dip in the theta-driving curve already described, McNaughton (e.g., Coop, McNaughton, Warnock, & Laverty, 1990; McNaughton & Coop, 1991; McNaughton & Sedgwick, 1978) later found a second universal effect. This research was in part a response to the failure of the DANB lesions to account for all of the effects of anxiolytic drugs. Stimulation of the reticular formation elicits hippocampal theta, with the frequency of theta increasing in linear fashion with increasing stimulating *voltage* (not frequency). The anxiolytic drugs lower theta frequency for a given level of stimulation (Gray & McNaughton, 2000, pp. 12, 205–207). Over the years, this lowering of reticular-elicited theta rhythm held up across the classic anxiolytic drugs discussed above, becoming a second cornerstone of the original theory.

In 2000 Gray and McNaughton emphasized that these two crucial effects—raising the 7.7 Hz dip and lowering the frequency of reticularly elicited theta—had been found for "novel" anxiolytics, of which buspirone and the anxiolytic antidepressant imipramine are the exemplars (pp. 1–2, 4–5, 12). By this time it had been established that the classic anxiolytic drugs all enhance the functioning of the inhibitory neurotransmitter gamma-aminobutyric acid (GABA), albeit by different *primary* mechanisms of action (p. 63). In contrast, the novel anxiolytics operate by way of qualitatively different mechanisms. For example, the anxiolytic effects of buspirone are believed to be associated with its agonistic effects on the serotonin receptor 5-HT_{1A} and subsequent 5-HT_{1A} receptor down-regulation, with no effect on GABA (pp. 65–66).

Another development by the time of the Gray and McNaughton (2000) review was a greater emphasis on generalized anxiety (and generalized anxiety disorder, or GAD), in contrast to panic attacks and responses to phobic stimuli. Consistent with the emphasis of others (e.g., Barlow, 2000, 2002; Bouton, Mineka, & Barlow, 2001) on this distinction between anxiety and fear/panic, Gray and McNaughton noted that on average, there is specificity in drug effects: The anxiolytic drugs reduce generalized or anticipatory anxiety and not panic attacks or simple phobic responses, whereas drugs that attenuate panic tend not to ameliorate generalized anxiety (e.g., pp. 3, 7, 68, 70)—a phenomenon termed "a pharmacological double dissociation" (p. 7). The authors concluded that generalized anxiety reflects excessive activity of the BIS, whereas panic and the phobic response reflect activation of a fight–flight or fight–flight–freeze system involved in fear that is separate from the BIS (pp. 2–3, 7, 41–45, 52, 292, 322–324). This conclusion is not surprising, but it does provide greater theoretical precision and a sharper distinction between fear and anxiety than in the early work.

Over time, the hypotheses above that the anxiolytic drugs exerted their effects in part by a reduction in activity (and therefore a reduction in the release of the neurotransmitter in the SHS) in the ascending noradrenergic and serotonergic pathways projecting from the locus coeruleus and the median raphe nucleus, respectively, continued to receive support (Gray & McNaughton, 2000, pp. 13, 118–119, 229–231). The noradrenergic pathway is more strongly associated with behavioral tasks involving CSs for frustrative nonreward, whereas the serotonergic pathway is more strongly associated with disinhibition in tasks involving CSs for punishment (painful stimuli). In addition, injections of a benzodiazepine into a structure (in the posterior hypothalamus) known as the supramammillary nucleus, which projects to the medial septum, reduced the frequency of reticular-elicited control of theta. The authors concluded, "Our theory now holds that anxiolytic drugs directly reduce the release of noradrenaline and serotonin into the septo-hippocampal system and directly alter the encoding of theta frequency via areas such as the supramammillary nucleus" (p. 13). Parenthetically, it should be noted that se-rotonergic activity originating in the raphe nucleus exerts an inhibitory effect on the fight–flight–panic system associated especially with the periaqueductal grey (pp. 3, 7, 44–45, 110–113, 292, 297–302). This effect is distinct from its effect on the BIS and potentially accounts for the broader spectrum of clinical action of serotonergic drugs as compared to classical anxiolytics.

The Behavioral Inhibition System

Gray and McNaughton (2000) reaffirmed the earlier conclusions regarding the pattern of behavioral effects of anxiolytic drugs (pp. 72–82), including the novel anxiolytics; however, the conclusions were based on far fewer studies for the latter drugs, and the effects were clearer when chronic administration or other means of preventing short-term interaction with the pituitary–adrenal system was used (McNaughton, Panickar, & Logan, 1996; Zhu & McNaughton, 1995). These effects included the familiar passive avoidance and extinction paradigms, as well as the conceptually similar tasks involving successive discrimination, fixed-interval reward schedules, and differential reinforcement of low rates of response. In addition, the authors included approach–approach conflict tasks, in which correct performance requires inhibiting a response that was previously correct but currently is incorrect. As in earlier writings, these effects can be understood as inhibiting prepotent or at least competing responses that, by virtue of context or altered contingen-cies, interfere with correct acquisition (pp. 76, 80).

A similar analysis applies to tasks involving memory. Many investigators have seen the hippocampus as centrally involved in memory per se (or spatial cognition per se for some authors), but Gray and McNaughton rebutted that view (pp. 2, 15–18, 158–203). Rather, they assimilated the ostensible demon-strations of memory deficits following hippocampal lesions to the more basic processes already identified as components of the BIS: a reduced ability to increase the negative valence of strongly competing but incorrect alternatives, resulting in a lessened ability to inhibit these incorrect competing memories (pp. 17–18, 202–203). According to their analysis, memory per se is not impaired. Memory appears to be impaired in some tasks, because investiga-tors have not realized that the deficits associated with hippocampal lesions reflect the intrusion of incorrect information. The theoretical parsimony of subsuming deficits in both memorial tasks and simple conflict situations to an effect on a single underlying process is obvious (p. 202), especially when both classical and novel anxiolytics impair the quintessential test of hippocampal function, the Morris water maze (pp. 77–78).

The conceptualization of the inputs to and outputs from the BIS changed somewhat over the years. Rather than listing the inputs described above (Pun-CSs, nonRew-CSs, novelty, and some innate "fear" stimuli) that activate the BIS, Gray and McNaughton (2000, pp. 39, 52–53, 55, 83) derived this list from a more fundamental property. Ethoexperimental analysis (Blanchard &

Blanchard, 1990) emphasized that some stimuli, such as the odor of a cat for a rat, indicate "potential threat" rather than an actual threat. Gray and McNaughton conceptualized such stimuli as innate *anxiety* stimuli. However, Gray and McNaughton (p. 84), driven by the previous distinction between active and passive avoidance, proposed that "defensive direction" is the fundamental distinction rather than actual versus potential threat. The BIS is activated when the animal approaches a dangerous situation, whereas the fight–flight system is activated when an animal leaves a dangerous situation (see also comments below regarding the hierarchical defense system).

As in earlier presentations, the output from the BIS consists of behavioral inhibition and increments in arousal and attention (p. 54). Behavioral inhibition is achieved via projections from the subiculum (described as the hippocampal "main output station") to the nucleus accumbens and other goal-processing structures—projections from which can produce inhibition of behavior (via, e.g., the basal ganglia) on the one hand, and increased attention to the environment (via the thalamocortical sensory processing system) on the other hand (pp. 32–33). Increments in arousal are effected through projections to the amygdala (p. 8), as discussed below.

Gray and McNaughton's (2000) conceptualization of the BIS restricts the nature of this behavioral inhibition: "All inputs to the hippocampus represent goals," allowing the hippocampus to detect "when there is a conflict between concurrently active goals" (p. 23; see also pp. 27–29, 32, 84, 225, 240–241). Thus the input stimuli activate the BIS only when "*they must be approached*" (p. 84; emphasis in original) and only when input is such as to produce "a genuine conflict between incompatible goals" (p. 86). As a contrasting example, a mirror drawing task produces motor conflict but does not involve motivational conflict (pp. 24, 32, 241), because there is no conflict about the goal of good performance. This emphasis on goal conflict maps nicely onto ethological research focused on the reactions of prey to their predators when faced with the need to forage for food in potentially dangerous places—a clear instance of a conflict between approach and avoidance goals. Consistent with this ethological perspective, Gray and McNaughton comment that the BIS "controls behavior whenever the animal's primary purpose is to achieve some goal which requires it to move towards a source of danger" (p. 84).

The Septo-Hippocampal System

The results above constitute core findings regarding the effects of anxiolytic drugs and the nature of inputs to and outputs from the BIS. They were, however, only a beginning for Gray's efforts to understand the structure and functioning of the neural substrate for the BIS, beginning with the SHS. This attempt constituted a major part of his research and evolved throughout his career. Helpful references to track this evolution of theory are two book-length reviews of his own and others' research in their original versions (Gray, 1971, 1982) and in second editions (Gray, 1987; Gray & McNaughton,

2000). His theorizing later extended to a more global view, including an attempt to tackle the problem of consciousness in a book published just after his death (Gray, 2004). As above, the current summary is taken from Gray and McNaughton (2000). A much more detailed explication of the summary below, including especially an analysis of the various brain structures involved in these processes and what they contribute, can be found in Chapter 10 of the Gray and McNaughton book.

The hippocampus is described as a structure with relatively simple fundamental computational properties. As a result (unlike an earlier version of the theory in which the SHS itself performed the complex functions), the complex functions of the SHS are seen as resulting from the interaction of the SHS with other structures (p. 19): temporal lobe memory stores, complex motor programs (basal ganglia, frontal cortex), "fixed action patterns" (amygdala, hypothalamus), and thalamo-cortical perceptual systems (p. 27). The computational abilities serve primarily to suppress undesirable computations in other structures, rather than to carry out some desirable computation (p. 18).

All of the hippocampal inputs represent goals, and the computational properties allow the SHS to act as a "comparator," detecting when there is conflict between currently highly activated goals. As long as no goal conflict is detected (a match with expectations), the comparator operates in a "just checking" mode. If goal conflict is detected (a mismatch), the comparator shifts to a "control" mode and generates output with an affectively negative bias—in other words, output that selectively increases the valence of affectively negative stimuli (stimuli associated with adverse outcomes) and associated memories, promoting avoidance over approach motivation (pp. 23–29, 233–235, 241–247). Through recursive networks, this output progressively increases bias over time until one goal dominates and implements a behavioral response. In the meantime (during failure to resolve conflict), the SHS produces output that activates exploratory mechanisms seeking new input from the environment that helps to resolve the conflict. The affectively negative bias directly affects motor output in the present, and it promotes learning of negative biases that affect future motor behavior.

The Amygdala

Gray and McNaughton (2000, p. 1) began their book by commenting that current orthodoxy views the amygdala rather than the SHS as the "key brain structure underlying anxiety." This comment refers to a large and elegant literature on the neural pathways involved in classical aversive *fear* conditioning—especially the work of Davis (e.g., Davis, Walker, & Lee, 1999; Lang, Davis, & Öhman, 2000) and LeDoux (e.g., 1996; 2000; and 2002, pp. 212–229), which emerged in parallel with Gray's own work. The impact of this literature on their theory is seen in the following statement from the Preface:

neither in the first edition nor here do we equate anxiety with hippocampal function [emphasis in original]. Rather, we view the hippocampus as including in its information processing capacities certain operations that are crucial for the maintenance and elaboration of anxiety. In particular, in the present edition, we see anxiety as resulting, in its most fundamental form, from interaction between the septo-hippocampal system and the amygdala. (Gray and McNaughton, 2000, p. viii; see also p. 282)

That is, in a substantial revision of the theory, the authors concluded that the amygdala serves as part of the BIS and is the structure responsible for the increased arousal (and increased autonomic activity) as a result of BIS activation (pp. 106–110, 281–282). However, there is no implication that arousal and autonomic activity are specific to anxiety—only that anxiety acts to increase the already existing levels of arousal and autonomic activity. The amygdala mediates both this anxiety-based increase in arousal and increases in arousal due to fear.

In the first edition of the book, the increased arousal output from the BIS (tentatively) was attributed to the noradrenergic innervation of the hypothalamus (Gray, 1982, p. 358; see also Gray & McNaughton, 2000, p. 108). In the intervening years, the well-known fear-potentiated startle paradigm provided conclusive evidence that the amygdala is responsible for this increased arousal in anxiety. In this paradigm, the amplitude of a startle response increases considerably if the startle stimulus (e.g., a loud noise) occurs shortly after the presentation of a CS associated with shock. This potentiation of startle reflects increased arousal, depends on the integrity of the amygdala but not the hippocampus, is blocked by a majority of anxiolytic drugs, and is affected by the drugs through a direct action in the amygdala (Gray & McNaughton, 2000, pp. 107–109)—evidence converging on the conclusion that the amygdala mediates increased arousal from BIS activation. Although this potentiation, as the name implies, is traditionally attributed to fear rather than anxiety, Gray and McNaughton saw the attenuation by anxiolytic drugs as indicating that anxiety rather than fear is involved. In that context, a discussion of goal conflicts in this paradigm and the importance of freezing during the CS for potentiation led the authors to conclude that "the paradigm is one of anxiety-potentiated startle, not fear-potentiated startle" (p. 109).

Further clarification of the role of the amygdala, as well as a better understanding of the fundamental importance of defensive direction, requires a consideration of the fear system. Integrating the work of (1) the Blanchards (e.g., Blanchard & Blanchard, 1990; Blanchard, Griebel, Henrie, & Blanchard, 1997) on a categorical distinction between anxiety and fear plus the concept of defensive distance, and (2) that of Graeff (1994) on hierarchical brain structures mapping onto hierarchical functions with their own work, Gray and McNaughton described a hierarchical defense system (pp. 6–8, 29–35, 94–114). One component of this system is concerned with *avoidance* of or moving away from danger (usually couched in terms of a predator), called the "defensive avoidance" or the "danger avoidance" hierarchy. The hierarchy has to do with the degree of crudeness or sophistication of the avoidance as a function of "defensive distance"—that is, how much time there is for defensive maneuvers (pp. 29–35). Beginning at the bottom, the dorsal periaqueductal grey controls "undirected escape"—the immediate responses of fight, flight, freezing, analgesia, and autonomic arousal (the fight–flight system). Panic attacks derive from activation of this system (pp. 8, 31, 99). It is also the structure through which higher-level systems effect an increase in arousal and autonomic activity. When time permits, the medial hypothalamus controls less impulsive, more sophisticated escape responses, called "directed escape." Still another step up, the amygdala implements simple "active avoidance." At the top of the hierarchy, the anterior cingulate cortex (p. 31) (or, more broadly, the anterior cingulate working in combination with the "ventral trend" of prefrontal cortex; pp. 122–139) is responsible for more complex or discriminated active avoidance.

The second component of the hierarchical defense system is concerned with "defensive or danger approach." At a level comparable in skill to that of the amygdala, the SHS controls passive avoidance or danger approach. At a level comparable to that of the anterior cingulate for defensive avoidance, the posterior cingulate controls discriminated avoidance in the context of defensive approach (pp. 29–35).

To return to the role of the amygdala in anxiety, as noted above, Gray and McNaughton (p. 281) proposed that anxiety requires the activation of both the SHS and the amygdala. It is activation of the amygdala that produces the increases in arousal and autonomic activity (p. 100), which are common to activation of the BIS and the fight–flight system. At the same time, the inhibitory output from the BIS acts to block the behavioral outputs that otherwise would arise from activation of the fight–flight system. The authors suggested that this activation of the fight–flight system is adaptive, in the sense that under conditions that generate anxiety, there is a real possibility of a need to engage in fight or flight. The switch from defensive approach to avoidance can be implemented quickly by releasing the BIS restraint of the behavioral output from the fight–flight system.

Although Gray and McNaughton concluded that the amygdala and its activation of the fight–flight system is part of the BIS, for several reasons they strongly rejected the idea that the amygdala itself can be identified as the central structure in an anxiety system. First, the amygdala is a crucial structure for fear (pp. 103–104, 106): It is the primary higher structure implementing responses to *actual* threat, where the danger is imminent rather than potential (p. 100). Second, the behavioral effects of lesions of the amygdala do not completely parallel the behavioral effects of anxiolytic drugs (pp. 103–104). Importantly, anxiolytic drugs and septal and hippocampal lesions affect behavior in delayed-matching-to-sample tasks (p. 76) and fixed-interval schedules, whereas lesions of the amygdala have no effect (p. 103). Third, lesions of the amygdala do not only decrease anxiety. The amygdala appears to endow sensory stimuli with emotional and motivational significance in general, not just aversive motivation (p. 100). Lesion-induced loss of this capacity alters dietary and sexual preferences, maternal behavior, and (in humans) a range of social and emotional behavior (p. 100). Of these arguments, the second point seems the most definitive, and it underscores the importance of the strategy of using the anxiolytic drugs to identify the processes associated with anxiety.

Even though this incorporation of the amygdala into the BIS resolves some conflicts in the literature, Gray and McNaughton acknowledged and regretted that it has come at a major cost: The effects of the anxiolytic drugs can no longer be attributed to a single site of action, and the BIS no longer can be mapped onto a neurally unified set of structures (pp. 109, 284). The contribution of the amygdala in effecting the arousal and autonomic outputs of the BIS is not affected by hippocampal lesions, and thus is substantially independent of the SHS (p. 283). In addition, of the two major effects of the anxiolytic drugs on hippocampal theta noted above, only the elimination of the 7.7-Hz theta-driving dip in connection with septal stimulation can be attributed to the attenuation of ascending monoaminergic (noradrenaline and serotonin) activity (p. 283). The effects on the reticular control of hippocampal theta frequency produced by injections of benzodiazepine into the supramammillary nucleus do not involve these monoamines, indicating an independent effect on anxiety that, even though operating on the SHS, cannot be subsumed under some unitary neural mechanism. To some extent, this was already a problem with Gray's (1982) invocation of both noradrenaline and serotonin as supporting anxiolytic action—but these could be unified via the common action of all anxiolytics on GABA$_A$ receptors. By 2000, however, the finding that the behavioral and electrophysiological (theta) effects of novel anxiolytics are effected through mechanisms other than increasing transmission at GABA$_A$ receptors precluded invoking this GABA-focused effect as a unitary mechanism for the anxiolytic drugs and the BIS (pp. 283–284).

These considerations caused Gray and McNaughton (2000) to propose that the BIS consists of parallel distributed systems, in which the impressively specific effects of anxiolytic drugs on the behavioral manifestations of anxiety can be attributed to a simultaneous effect on "quite separate nodes" within these systems (p. 92). The integration of the BIS may depend on coordinating links within the organism and via the environment. With respect to the latter point, they suggested (pp. 281–282) that pure fear or pure frustration (i.e., without goal conflict) activates the amygdala with its arousal and autonomic component, whereas goal conflict activates the SHS. Anxiety results only when the environment contains input for both fear-frustration and goal conflict. Although this shift from a unitary neural model to one of parallel distributed systems sacrifices elegant simplicity and is in some contrast to the work of others on the fear system, it should perhaps not be unexpected, given the complexity of the concept of anxiety. It is also consistent with modern network models for various processes, containing multiple, reciprocally connected structures that can be viewed as distributed systems (pp. 31–32).

Summary

The emergence of novel anxiolytics, with mechanisms of action qualitatively different from those of the classic anxiolytic drugs, has provided tests of the prior predictions of the theory with dramatically positive results. However, the conceptualization of the BIS has changed in subtle ways. The BIS controls behavior when achieving a goal requires moving toward danger. All inputs to the hippocampus represent goals, and the function of the BIS is to detect and resolve goal conflict. As a result, the stimuli to which the BIS responds include any stimulus that signals potential threat in a context of moving toward a source of danger (hence involving goal or motivational conflict). The list of stimulus inputs to the BIS include innate anxiety stimuli (as opposed to a set of less clearly defined innate fear stimuli in the past). The outputs of the BIS remain behavioral inhibition and increases in attention and arousal, but the output pathways have been delineated more fully. Behavioral inhibition and increased attention to the environment proceed by way of projections from the subiculum to the nucleus accumbens, while increased arousal and autonomic activity is achieved by way of projections to the amygdala.

Whereas in the earlier theory the SHS was believed to perform relatively complex functions, in the more recent theory these complex functions were seen as requiring the interaction of the SHS with other structures. The SHS serves an information-processing or computational function of detecting goal conflict and making decisions, and, through recursive networks, generates output that selectively increases the valence of affectively negative stimuli until the goal conflict is resolved. While the conflict continues, the SHS also generates output that facilitates obtaining new information from the environment relevant to the goal conflict.

Based on theoretical developments in the literature since earlier statements of the theory, Gray and McNaughton (2000) described a hierarchical defense system in which the direction of movement (toward or away from danger) and defensive distance are important parameters. The amygdala is the crucial structure for fear and is the primary higher-level structure in the component of the defense system concerned with moving away from danger. The SHS is a parallel structure concerned with moving toward danger. In a major theoretical development, the amygdala is added to the BIS, serving especially to increase arousal and autonomic activity. Its importance is underscored by the statement that anxiety results from the interaction of the SHS and the amygdala. The amygdala has not replaced the SHS as the primary contributor to anxiety, however, inasmuch as lesions to the amygdala produce behavioral effects different from those associated with the anxiolytic drugs. In addition, the amygdala has functions different from anxiety (e.g., fear conditioning, endowing a broad range of sensory stimuli with emotional and motivational significance).

As a result of these changes, the BIS can no longer be seen as mapping onto a neurally unified set of structures. Similarly, the effects of the anxiolytic drugs cannot be attributed to a single mode of action. Gray and McNaughton (2000) proposed that the BIS consists of parallel distributed systems in which the specific effects of anxiolytic drugs can be attributed to a simultaneous effect on quite separate components; the simultaneity depends to some extent on links within the organism and to some extent on multiple effects of the environment that gives rise to anxiety.

PERSONALITY AND PSYCHOPATHOLOGY

As would be expected, Gray's contributions to understanding personality/temperament and psychopathology consisted largely of trying to relate these phenotypic features to individual differences in the strength or reactivity of underlying neurobiological systems as he understood them. Of course, individual differences in the strength of the BIS were of greatest interest, but he also viewed two other systems as relevant. One of those is the fight–flight system already discussed. The third system has been implied throughout the discussion of anxiety above, but it requires more explicit description before Gray's contributions to personality are discussed.

The Behavioral Activation or Behavioral Approach System

Even in his early writings, Gray (1970; 1973, pp. 422–423; Gray & Smith, 1969) described three affective–motivational systems: approach, stop, and fight–flight. The BIS and fight–flight systems are discussed above, but the approach system is not, other than by implication. The approach or appetitive system, with its "reward mechanism," responds to appetitive CSs (Rew-CSs and nonPun-CSs) and is involved in approach learning, active avoidance, skilled escape, and predatory aggression (a form of approach). Its outputs are activation of approach behavior and, as in the BIS, an increase in (nonspecific) arousal. Behavior associated with activation of the approach system is the object of inhibition by the BIS; that is, the two systems act in opposition to each other in the various conflict paradigms, as described in a formal model by Gray and Smith (1969). In an early publication, I (Fowles, 1980) coined the term "behavioral activation system" (BAS), to parallel Gray's emphasis on inhibition of behavior in naming the BIS. Gray also referred to the system as the "behavioral activation system" (Pickering et al., 1997), but elsewhere he (Gray, 1991) preferred the term "behavioral approach system" (also abbreviated BAS), consistent with his having called it the "approach system" from the very beginning. Both usages are found in the literature.

Gray (e.g., 1973) cited the famous work of Olds and Olds (1965) on rewarding electrical self-stimulation, identifying this effect as focusing on the medial forebrain bundle and the lateral hypothalamus, along with projections of the medial forebrain bundle to the septal area. By 1983, Gray and colleagues (Gray, Owen, Davis, & Tsaltas, 1983), referring to the brain processes that mediate responses to stimuli associated with reward and nonpunishment, said that "the picture is now more ambiguous than ever before," that self-stimulation provides a poor guide to the functions of the region of stimulation, and that the authors were "unable to contribute much to the physiology of reward" (pp. 210–211). Four years later, however, Gray (1987, pp. 308–309, 330) identified the mesolimbic dopaminergic projections from the brainstem ventral tegmental area to the ventral striatum (including the nucleus accumbens) as playing a key role in "transmitting incentive motivation to motor systems" (p. 308) and as a major substrate for the rewarding effects of electrical self-stimulation of the brain. He also noted that this system "mediates some of the addictive effects" of heroin and amphetamine (pp. 282–283). Gray (1991), and Pickering and Gray (1999), described the BAS and its interconnections more fully and added cocaine, alcohol, and nicotine to the list of addictive drugs that promote release of dopamine into the nucleus accumbens. Gray, Kumari, Lawrence, and Young (1999) concluded that evidence for the mediation of the behavioral effects of rewards by the mesolimbic dopamine pathways is extremely strong (and added cannabis to the list of addictive drugs that activate this system). However, they also reviewed compelling evidence that all *salient* stimuli (including aversive stimuli unrelated to reward) activate the mesolimbic system, producing output that enhances sensory processing. Thus, in addition to the mesolimbic system's effect on motor behavior, it has an equally prominent role in sensory processing. Pickering and Gray (1999), although focusing on the involvement of the mesolimbic dopamine system's role in mediation of the BAS, similarly emphasized that it is not exclusively involved in positive incentive motivational effects, but rather responds to stimulus salience.

It should be mentioned that Depue's work (Depue & Collins, 1999; Depue, Collins, & Luciana, 1996; Depue & Iacono, 1989; Depue & Lenzenweger, 2001; Depue & Morrone-Strupinsky, 2005) has strongly supported this role of the mesolimbic (and perhaps mesocortical) dopamine system in the mediation of the incentive effects of CSs for reward. Depue uses the term "behavioral facilitation system" (BFS) to describe a system almost identical to the BAS, and he has written extensively on the relevance to personality and affective disorders. In addition, the contribution of the same dopaminergic pathways to the rewarding effects of all addictive drugs is so well documented that there is an increasing consensus that this system is critical to addiction (e.g., Leshner, 1997; Robinson & Berridge, 2003; Wise & Bozarth, 1987; Wise & Rompre, 1989). Thus the BAS (or BFS) is well supported as a third neurobiological affective–motivational system.

The Biological Basis of Personality

In an early paper, Gray (1973) proposed that (1) one should find explanations for temperament dimensions in terms of underlying psychological functions; (2) these functions are essentially similar in humans and other animals; (3) one can study the personality or temperament correlates of these functions in humans; and (4) one can identify the biological basis of these functions in terms of enduring structures in the neuroendocrine system (i.e., one can look for the biological basis of temperament). To transcend the gap between humans and (other) animals, it is necessary to match behavior patterns across species—an inherently theoretical enterprise, because of the difficulty of identifying similar behaviors in humans and animals. Furthermore, Gray proposed that there is more continuity across species if one examines the way species solve problems facing all of them: how to learn to approach rewards, and how to keep away from danger. The study of emotion is important, because emotions are modes of reactions to various classes of reinforcers. Emotions enjoy more phylogenetic longevity than more cortically based cognitive functions and are centered in the midbrain and limbic forebrain—structures that are found in a wide range of species. In keeping with this perspective, he argued that this phylogenetically old behavior (characterized by general laws of behavior that apply across species) is likely to be substantially under genetic control, consistent with findings for the temperament dimensions in humans.

Gray suggested that the study of emotional behavior in animals is the way to achieve this goal. Animal learning theory provided him with an excellent starting point, because that field really is about the learning of emotional responses and about behavioral regulation of the occurrence of emotion-provoking stimuli. He then went on to describe the approach, stop, and fight–flight systems discussed above.

Gray (1970, 1973) took Eysenck's personality dimensions as the point of departure for this effort. These (orthogonal) dimensions consisted of the famous "neuroticism" and "introversion–extraversion" factors, as well as the less well-established "psychoticism." For the two-factor space defined by neuroticism and introversion–extraversion, Gray proposed that the underlying causal dimensions lay on the approximately 45° diagonals and represented the BIS and the approach systems. That is, the BIS/anxiety dimension lay in the diagonal between neuroticism and introversion, whereas the approach system/impulsivity dimension lay in the diagonal between neuroticism and extraversion. For the BIS diagonal, Gray suggested that it corresponded roughly to the location (in two-factor space) of trait anxiety as defined by the Taylor Manifest Anxiety scale. Gray took for granted that impulsivity reflected heightened reactivity to cues for reward; in other words, he did not suggest that impulsivity might reflect a weak BIS with resultant poor inhibitory control. By this theoretical proposal, neuroticism was understood to reflect increased sensitivities to both reward (Rew-CSs + nonPun-CSs) and punishment (Pun-CSs + nonRew-CSs). Similarly, extraversion was seen as reflecting a greater sensitivity to reward than punishment, whereas introversion was seen as reflecting a greater sensitivity to punishment than reward. Thus the primary dimensions were anxiety (BIS) and impulsivity (approach), with Eysenck's factors understood as being derived from these primary dimensions.

In what he described as rash speculation, Gray (1973) suggested that the third factor, psychoticism, reflected the influence of the third system, fight–flight. He noted that the items on this scale that discriminate nonpsychotic subjects from psychotic subjects relate to aggressive, cruel actions and a general hostility toward other people. He also noted that subjects with aggressive psychopathy scored particularly high on this scale. However, again, he acknowledged that the attractiveness of symmetry (using the three behavioral systems to account for three temperament dimensions) influenced him to speculate.

In proposing and pursuing this approach to understanding temperament, Gray was following in the pioneering footsteps of Eysenck (e.g., 1957, 1967). Before Gray, Eysenck had conceptualized temperament in terms of individual differences in constructs derived from learning theory and biology. I myself still recall my excitement at first reading Eysenck's 1957 book, which at the time represented a groundbreaking and extremely appealing approach of attempting to integrate an understanding of individual differences with the basic science approach of the then-dominant Hullian learning theory—one of the early contributions to the emerging discipline of experimental personality and psychopathology (see also Pickering et al., 1997). To provide an analogy to illustrate the importance of this development, it was as if practitioners of medicine had first discovered that they could use the basic science understanding of physiology and biochemistry to understand pathology.

Gray's major contribution to this effort was at least twofold. First, Eysenck's learning theory and biology had become outdated over time and was badly in need of revision to make it consistent with current knowledge, which Gray provided. Second, and more important, Gray was much more heavily involved in—and had much greater expertise in—both learning theory and behavioral neuroscience. This expertise resulted in a reversal of Eysenck's approach. Eysenck started with temperament and, in top-down fashion, borrowed constructs from learning theory and biology. In contrast, Gray proceeded in a bottom-up approach by beginning with established behavioral mechanisms in animals and asking what temperament characteristics individual differences in these mechanisms would produce in humans. Whereas Eysenck was a temperament theorist who tried to assimilate basic science findings, Gray was a basic scientist who extended his research to understand temperament and psychopathology. As such, Gray served as the earliest and most influential model for this approach, and his writings were better informed and more influential by virtue of that expertise.

Gray's formulation of the contribution of the BIS and BAS to personality changed over time. Pickering and colleagues (1997) and Gray and

McNaughton (2000, pp. 335–342) continued to propose that individual differences in the strength or reactivity of the BIS and BAS produce dimensions of anxiety and impulsivity, respectively, and to relate the fight–flight system to the dimension of psychoticism. The application to personality was modified over time to acknowledge that neuroticism is correlated more strongly with trait anxiety than with impulsivity, resulting in a portrayal of anxiety at a 30° rotation from neuroticism. Impulsivity, still orthogonal to anxiety, falls at a 60° rotation from neuroticism (30° from extraversion) (Gray & McNaughton, 2000, p. 337). However, Pickering and colleagues and Pickering and Gray (1999) noted that psychoticism is more closely related to impulsivity than is extraversion. This point is consistent with the generally held view that psychoticism in Eysenck's scales is misnamed and reflects disinhibition more than psychosis (Clark & Watson, 1999). Pickering and Gray (1999) also noted the association of impulsivity with psychoticism, as well as (perhaps more weakly) with extraversion, in the Eysenck scales.

More than in any of Gray's other publications, Pickering and Gray (1999) focused on the contribution of individual differences in BAS reactivity to personality. They conceptualized BAS-based impulsivity as "impulsive sensation seeking" (ISS), referring to engaging in dangerous behavior and seeking danger, thrills, and arousal, as well as acting without thoughtful deliberation. Although these authors cited Depue and Collins (1999) as proposing that the BAS/BFS relates directly to extraversion, Pickering and Gray concluded after an extensive review of the literature that ISS is a better phenotype for individual differences in the BAS.

Pickering and colleagues (1997) reviewed the extensive experimental literature relating behavioral task performance and, to a lesser extent, physiological responsiveness to dimensions of personality as predicted by Gray's theory. As a result of the diversity of findings, the authors stated, "We clearly cannot reach any kind of optimistic conclusion about the degree to which the theory is supported by the available data" (p. 62). At the same time, the frequency of positive results was impressive enough to support the view of strong links between individual differences in sensitivity to reinforcement and personality traits; that is, the basic approach was deemed sound, but more research was felt to be needed. They strongly recommended that the field continue to develop theoretically sound experimental tasks until the relationships between sensitivity to reinforcement and temperament become clear.

The Pickering and colleagues (1997) conclusion seems a fair one. The enterprise of relating biological individual differences to personality phenotypes is an extraordinarily difficult and complicated one. It is not surprising that we, as a field, have not yet solved this problem. Gray's work and theoretical proposals have stimulated an enormous amount of research. It is highly likely that in the end, we will find that he has pointed us in the right direction, and that the neurobiological systems he has identified are indeed extremely important for personality.

Psychopathology as Related to Systems Underlying Personality: Anxiety Disorders

The obvious application of Gray's work to psychopathology is to anxiety disorders. As already discussed, Gray and McNaughton (2000) related the BIS to GAD and the fight–flight system to panic attacks and responses to phobic stimuli. This conceptualization plays a central role in Barlow's (e.g., 2000, 2002) comprehensive theory of the anxiety disorders, and Barlow cites Gray's work as a basis for some of his theorizing. In addition, Gray and McNaughton (pp. 34–35, 289–290) proposed that the well-established strong cognitive/attentional components (an excessively strong focus on potential threats) of GAD can be understood as manifestations of excessive activity in the BIS.

As noted above, Gray and McNaughton (2000) viewed the BIS as activated only when danger stimuli must be approached and when stimulus input produces conflict between incompatible goals. In their theoretical approach, *by definition*, only BIS activation constitutes "anxiety." In consequence, they suggested that neuroticism or trait anxiety may reflect "general sensitivity to threat" (p. 338), which would presumably include overall defense system sensitivity, and that only a subset of threat-related stimuli (i.e., conflict-producing stimuli) increase anxiety as they defined it. Consistent with this perspective, they used the terms "neuroticism" and "trait anxiety" to refer to "susceptibility to anxiety-related disorders" (p. 341). In spite of this conceptual distinction between trait anxiety and BIS reactivity, it appears that Gray and McNaughton viewed individual differences in BIS reactivity as major contributors to trait anxiety. Nevertheless, important processes such as classical aversive conditioning or exposure to uncontrollable aversive stimuli, which do not involve motivational conflict, may affect susceptibility to anxiety disorders apart from BIS functioning. More work is needed to resolve the question of the degree to which BIS reactivity underlies trait anxiety (N. McNaughton, personal communication, March 2005).

Psychopathology as Related to Systems Underlying Personality: Psychopathy

Although Gray did not extensively discuss psychopathy, he did suggest that those with this disorder seek rewards "with no fear of punishment," and that their persistent antisocial behavior reflects "a relative insensitivity to punishment" (Gray, 1970, p. 255)—implying a weak BIS combined with a normal (or possibly strong) BAS. Pickering and Gray (1999) suggested that individuals with psychopathy are at the extreme low end of the trait anxiety continuum. This hypothesis was attractive, because weak BIS activation in conflict situations predicts that persons with psychopathy would be less anxious than other individuals in such contexts and would be approach-dominant. Thus the weak-BIS hypothesis seemed to account for both the low anxiety and the behavioral disinhibition observed clinically in patients with psychopathy (Cleckley, 1982) and confirmed in laboratory investigations (Lykken, 1957, 1995). I (Fowles, 1980) used the weak-BIS hypothesis to account for discrepancies between heart rate and electrodermal responding (palmar skin conductance) in anticipation of shock in persons with psychopathy. In a major review of the psychopathy literature, Lykken (1995, Ch. 10) embraced the weak-BIS hypothesis; that is, he attbuted the fear deficit in psychopathy to a weak BIS. Thus Gray's suggestions concerning the application of the BIS to psychopathy have had a major influence.

There is, however, a major question about the extent of the relative contributions of low fear and low anxiety to psychopathy, raised especially by Patrick's (e.g., in press; Patrick, Bradley, & Lang, 1993; Patrick & Lang, 1999) research on psychopathy. In a review of this literature, we (Fowles & Dindo, 2006) found that the core features of psychopathy are associated with both low trait anxiety and high scores on questionnaire measures that reflect engaging in dangerous behaviors (e.g., low Harm Avoidance, high Thrill and Adventure Seeking). A case can be made that the latter personality scales reflect the effects of fear on behavior. The core features of psychopathy are also are associated with a diminished responsiveness to aversive pictures, as indexed by the fear–potentiated startle response. This startle potentiation appears to be more related to phobias (and thus the fight–flight system) than to anxiety. At present, therefore, it is not clear whether the core features of psychopathy are more strongly associated with Gray's BIS or with the fight–flight system.

GENERAL SUMMARY AND COMMENT

Jeffrey Gray's work focused on understanding anxiety at a behavioral, emotional, and neurobiological level. He brought to bear his extensive knowledge of animal learning theory and his expertise in behavioral neuroscience, with the two working synergistically in a manner that is rare. His brilliant insight that he could understand anxiety by defining it as the process affected by anxiolytic drugs productively guided his research throughout his career. This fundamental strategy provided a firm criterion for defining anxiety and facilitated the integration of behavioral and biological approaches.

It would be impossible to exaggerate Jeffrey Gray's impact on the fields of behavioral neuroscience, affective neuroscience, personality, and psychopathology. His direct contributions to these fields have been tremendous, as his obituary in one U.K. newspaper indicated (see Figure 2.1). Beyond that, however, he influenced the work of uncountable others by defining and demonstrating the general strategy for such research. Thus, even when his work is not directly cited, it is likely that Gray has fundamentally affected the way in which such work is, and will continue to be, conducted in many cases.

Jeffrey Gray

Experimental psychologist and accomplished linguist

Nick Rawlins

Thursday May 13, 2004

Guardian

Professor Jeffrey Gray, who has died aged 69, was one of the leading, and most highly cited, experimental psychologists in the UK. He had an extraordinarily wide range of professional interests—from the study of simple learning in the medicinal leech to theories of human consciousness, and from the translation of inaccessible Russian experimental work to the development of stem-cell transplantation for the treatment of brain damage.

He wholeheartedly pursued whatever information he needed, and was never embarrassed to ask straightforward questions when drawn into areas in which he was not yet expert. This intellectual courage was a great strength, enabling him to access and contribute to new ideas and technologies all his professional life. His research was very much concerned with big issues that were clinically relevant or conceptually challenging: anxiety (two books, each extending to a radically revised second edition); schizophrenia (one of the most highly cited papers ever written in the field); synaesthesia (something of a late arrival); and consciousness were all tackled, at levels that could range from the molecular to the philosophical. His work on neural transplants as a possible clinical treatment for brain damage led to the creation of a spin-out company, called ReNeuron.

Gray was born in the east end of London. His father was a tailor, but died when Jeffrey was only seven. He was brought up by his mother, who ran a haberdasher's shop. He took A-levels in Latin, Greek and history at Ilford County high school for boys, where he also won the school boxing championship. He undertook military service from 1952 until 1954, during which period he learned Russian, at the time a key interest for Army intelligence. He greatly admired the language teaching that he received, because he felt it taught him general principles which made it relatively easy for him to acquire other languages: in addition to Russian, he spoke French, Spanish, Italian and Persian, which was his wife's native language. He could as readily give a lecture in Russian; translate Mallarmé from French; negotiate a land sale with a Greek peasant; or conduct an interview in Persian on Iranian television.

The army taught him to type as well. It turned out that before a crucial typing test he had been told that those who did really well might be sent to Supreme Headquarters Allied Powers Europe (SHAPE) at Fontainebleau, whereas those who failed might be sent to Korea. He reported that his typing had quite suddenly dramatically improved.

Following military service, he took up a MacKinnon scholarship at Magdalen College, Oxford, with a place to read law. In the event he negotiated a switch to modern languages, obtaining a first in French and Spanish. He stayed on to take a second BA, this time in psychology and philosophy, which he completed in 1959. He managed to offset some of the financial costs by giving jive lessons, as well as by language teaching—he was approached by New College to become their French tutor when he was 23.

His postgraduate work both broadened and deepened his interests in psychology. In 1959–60 he undertook a course in clinical psychology at the institute of Psychiatry, in London, which led to the award of a Dip Psychol, with distinction, after which he stayed on at the institute to study for a PhD in the department of psychology, at that time

(continued)

FIGURE 2.1. Jeffrey Gray's obituary in a U.K. newspaper. Reprinted by permission of *The Guardian.*

headed by Professor Hans Eysenck. His PhD was awarded in 1964, and was a quite extraordinary work. Part was concerned with experimental studies of environmental, genetic and hormonal influences on emotional behaviour in animals, foreshadowing contemporary work in behavioural genetics; the other part presented translations of work from key Russian psychological laboratories, plus his own 300-page commentary on the Russian work. This component of the thesis was published as a book, Pavlov's Typology; the formidable Professor Stuart Sutherland regarded it as the best exegesis and clarification of Russian work to be produced by any western psychologist.

Later that year, Jeffrey was appointed to a university lectureship in experimental psychology at Oxford, and in 1965 was elected to an associated tutorial fellowship at University College. He remained at Oxford until he replaced Eysenck at the Institute of Psychiatry in 1983. He retired from the chair of psychology in 1999, but continued his experimental research as an emeritus professor, and spent a very happy and productive year at the Centre for Advanced Studies at Stanford University, California, where he essentially completed a new book on consciousness, due to appear very shortly.

From his earliest student days, he was immensely energetic, imaginative and productive. Where others might simply write some research articles and a review paper, he might well write a book, too. He received a president's award from the British Psychological Society in 1983, and became president of the Experimental Psychology Society in 1996 (and a lifetime honorary member in 1999).

His energy and enthusiasm were just as clear outside the laboratory. Throughout his life he loved drama—he directed The Winter's Tale in the Deer Park at Magdalen, casting the young Dudley Moore as Autolycus—as well as dance, opera, jazz and the cinema. He also developed passions for skiing and horse riding. He had enjoyed a wonderful ski trip shortly before the final stage of his illness began: he thought he had never skied better. He is survived by his wife, Venus, and his four children, Ramin, Babak, Leila and Afsaneh.

—Jeffrey Alan Gray, psychologist, born May 26 1934; died April 30 2004

FIGURE 2.1. *(continued)*

ACKNOWLEDGMENTS

I wish to thank Neil McNaughton for extensive, invaluable comments and suggestions that have substantially improved this chapter.

REFERENCES

Barlow, D. H. (2000). Unraveling the mysteries of anxiety and its disorders from the perspective of emotion theory. *American Psychologist, 55,* 1247–1263.

Barlow, D. H. (2002). *Anxiety and its disorders: The nature and treatment of anxiety and panic* (2nd ed.). New York: Guilford Press.

Blanchard, R. J., & Blanchard, D. C. (1990). An ethoexperimental analysis of defense, fear and anxiety. In N. McNaughton & G. Andrews (Eds.), *Anxiety* (pp. 124–133). Dunedin, New Zealand: Otago University Press.

Blanchard, R. J., Griebel, G., Henrie, J. A., & Blanchard, D. C. (1997). Differentiation of anxiolytic and panicolytic drugs by effects on rat and mouse defense test batteries. *Neuroscience and Biobehavioral Reviews, 21,* 783–789.

Bouton, M. E., Mineka, S., & Barlow, D. H. (2001). A modern learning theory perspective on the etiology of panic disorder. *Psychological Review, 108,* 4–32.

Clark, L. A., & Watson, D. (1999). Temperament: A new paradigm for trait psychology. In L. Pervin & O. P. John (Eds.), *Handbook of personality: Theory and research* (2nd ed., pp. 399–423). New York: Guilford Press.

Cleckley, H. (1982). *The mask of sanity* (6th ed.). St. Louis, MO: Mosby.

Coop, C. F., McNaughton, N., Warnock, K., & Laverty, R. (1990). Effects of ethanol and Ro 15-4513 in an electrophysiological model of anxiolytic action. *Neuroscience, 35,* 669–674.

Davis, M., Walker, D. L., & Lee, Y. (1999). Neurophysiology and neuropharmacology of startle and its affective modification. In M. E. Dawson, A.M. Schell, & A. H. Bohmelt (Eds.), *Startle modification: Implications for neuroscience, cognitive science, and clinical science* (pp. 95–113). New York: Cambridge University Press.

Depue, R. A., & Collins, P. F. (1999). Neurobiology of the structure of personality: Dopamine, facilitation of incentive motivation, and extraversion. *Behavioral and Brain Sciences, 22,* 491–517.

Depue, R. A., Collins, P. F., & Luciana, M. (1996). A model of neurobiology–environment interaction in developmental psychopathology. In M. F. Lenzenweger & J. J. Haugaard (Eds.), *Frontiers of developmental psychopathology* (pp. 44–77). New York: Oxford University Press.

Depue, R. A., & Iacono, W. G. (1989). Neurobehavioral aspects of affective disorders. *Annual Review of Psychology, 40,* 457–492.

Depue, R. A., & Lenzenweger, M. F. (2001). A neurobehavioral dimensional model. In W. J. Livesley (Ed.), *Handbook of personality disorders: Theory, research, and treatment* (pp. 136–176). New York: Guilford Press.

Depue, R. A., & Morrone-Strupinsky, J. V. (2005). A neurobehavioral model of affiliative bonding: Implications for conceptualizing a human trait of affiliation. *Behavioral and Brain Sciences, 28,* 313–395.

Eysenck, H. J. (1957). *The dynamics of anxiety and hysteria.* New York: Praeger.

Eysenck, H. J. (1967). *The biological basis of personality.* Springfield, IL: Thomas.

Fowles, D. C. (1980). The three arousal model: Implications of Gray's two-factor learning theory for heart rate, electrodermal activity, and psychopathy. *Psychophysiology, 17,* 87–104.

Fowles, D. C., & Dindo, L. (2006). A dual-deficit model of psychopathy. In C. J. Patrick (Ed.), *Handbook of psychopathy* (pp. 14–34). New York: Guilford Press.

Graeff, F. G. (1994). Neuroanatomy and neurotransmitter regulation of defensive behaviors and related emotions in mammals. *Brazilian Journal of Medical and Biological Research, 26,* 67–70.

Gray, J. A. (1970). The psychophysiological basis of introversion–extraversion. *Behaviour Research and Therapy, 8,* 249–266.

Gray, J. A. (1971). *The psychology of fear and stress.* London: Weidenfeld & Nicolson.

Gray, J. A. (1973). Causal theories of personality and how to test them. In J. R. Royce (Ed.), *Multivariate analysis and psychological theory* (pp. 409–463). New York: Academic Press.

Gray, J. A. (1975). *Elements of a two-process theory of learning.* New York: Academic Press.

Gray, J. A. (1976a). The behavioural inhibition system: A possible substrate for anxiety. In M. P. Feldman & A. Broadhurst (Eds.), *Theoretical and experimental bases of the behaviour therapies* (pp. 3–41). London: Wiley.

Gray, J. A. (1976b). The neuropsychology of anxiety. In I. G. Sarason & C. D. Spielberger (Eds.), *Stress and anxiety* (Vol. 3, pp. 3–26). Washington, DC: Hemisphere.

Gray, J. A. (1977). Drug effects on fear and frustration: Possible limbic site of action of minor tranquilizers. In L. L. Iversen, S. D. Iversen, & S. H. Snyder (Eds.), *Handbook of psychopharmacology: Vol. 8. Drugs, neurotransmitters, and behavior* (pp. 433–529). New York: Plenum Press.

Gray, J. A. (1978). The neuropsychology of anxiety. *British Journal of Psychology, 69*, 417–434.

Gray, J. A. (1979). A neuropsychological theory of anxiety. In C. E. Izard (Ed.), *Emotions in personality and psychopathology* (pp. 303–335). New York: Plenum Press.

Gray, J. A. (1982). *The neuropsychology of anxiety: An enquiry into the functions of the septo-hippocampal system.* Oxford: Oxford University Press.

Gray, J. A. (1987). *The psychology of fear and stress* (2nd ed.). Cambridge, UK: Cambridge University Press.

Gray, J. A. (1991). The neuropsychology of temperament. In J. Strelau & A. Angleitner (Eds.), *Explorations in temperament: International perspectives on theory and measurement* (pp. 105–128). London: Plenum Press.

Gray, J. A. (2004). *Consciousness: Creeping up on the hard problem.* Oxford: Oxford University Press.

Gray, J. A., Kumari, V., Lawrence, N., & Young, A. M. J. (1999). Functions of the dopaminergic innervation of the nucleus accumbens. *Psychobiology, 27*, 225–235.

Gray, J. A., & McNaughton, N. (2000). *The neuropsychology of anxiety: An enquiry into the functions of the septo-hippocampal system* (2nd ed.). Oxford: Oxford University Press.

Gray, J. A., Owen, S., Davis, N., & Tsaltas, E. (1983). Psychological and physiological relations between anxiety and impulsivity. In M. Zuckerman (Ed.), *The biological bases of sensation seeking, impulsivity and anxiety* (pp. 181–217). Hillsdale, NJ: Erlbaum.

Gray, J. A., & Smith, P. T. (1969). An arousal-decision model for partial reinforcement and discrimination learning. In R. Gilbert & N. S. Sutherland (Eds.), *Animal discrimination learning* (pp. 243–272). London: Academic Press.

Lang, P. J., Davis, M., & Öhman, A. (2000). Fear and anxiety: Animal modes and human cognitive psychophysiology. *Journal of Affective Disorders, 61*, 137–159.

LeDoux, J. E. (1996). *The emotional brain.* New York: Simon & Schuster.

LeDoux, J. E. (2000). Emotion circuits in the brain. *Annual Review of Neuroscience, 23*, 155–184.

LeDoux, J. E. (2002). *The synaptic self.* New York: Viking Penguin.

Leshner, A. I. (1997). Addiction is a brain disease, and it matters. *Science, 278*, 45–47.

Lykken, D. T. (1957). A study of anxiety in the sociopathic personality. *Journal of Abnormal and Social Psychology, 55*, 6–10.

Lykken, D. T. (1995). *The antisocial personalities.* Hillsdale, NJ: Erlbaum.

McNaughton, N., & Coop, C. F. (1991). Neurochemically dissimilar anxiolytic drugs have common effects on hippocampal rhythmic slow activity. *Neuropharmacology, 30*, 855–863.

McNaughton, N., & Corr, P. J. (2004). A two-dimensional neuropsychology of defense: fear/anxiety and defensive distance. *Neuroscience and Biobehavioral Reviews, 28,* 285–305.

McNaughton, N., & Mason, S. T. (1980). The neuropsychology and neuropharmacology of the dorsal ascending noradrenergic bundle: A review. *Progress in Neurobiology, 14,* 157–219.

McNaughton, N., Panickar, K. S., & Logan, B. (1996). The pituitary–adrenal axis and the different behavioral effects of buspirone and chlordiazepoxide. *Pharmacology, Biochemistry and Behavior, 54,* 51–56.

McNaughton, N., & Sedgwick, E. M. (1978). Reticular stimulation and hippocampal theta rhythm in rats: Effects of drugs. *Neuroscience, 3,* 629–632.

Olds, J., & Olds, M. (1965). Drives, rewards, and the brain. In F. Barron, W. C. Dement, W. Edwards, H. Lindmann, L. D. Phillips, J. Olds, & M. Olds (Eds.), *New directions in psychology* (Vol. 2, pp. 329–410). New York: Holt, Rinehart & Winston.

Patrick, C. J. (in press). Getting to the heart of psychopathy. In H. Herve & J. C. Yuille (Eds.), *Psychopathy: Theory, research, and social implications.* Mahwah, NJ: Erlbaum.

Patrick, C. J., Bradley, M. M., & Lang, P. J. (1993). Emotion in the criminal psychopath: Startle reflex modulation. *Journal of Abnormal Psychology, 102,* 82–92.

Patrick, C. J., & Lang, A. R. (1999). Psychopathic traits and intoxicated states: Affective concomitants and conceptual links. In M. E. Dawson, A. M. Schell, & A. H. Boehmelt (Eds.), *Startle modification: Implications for neuroscience, cognitive science, and clinical science* (pp. 209–230). New York: Cambridge University Press.

Pickering, A. D., Corr, P. J., Powell, J. H., Kumari, V., Thornton, J. C., & Gray, J. A. (1997). Individual differences in reactions to reinforcing stimuli are neither black nor white: To what extent are they Gray? In H. Nyborg (Ed.), *The scientific study of human nature: Tribute to Hans J. Eysenck at eighty* (pp. 36–67). London: Elsevier.

Pickering, A. D., & Gray, J. A. (1999). The neuroscience of personality. In L. A. Perrin & O. P. John (Eds.), *Handbook of personality theory and research* (2nd ed., pp. 277–299). New York: Guilford Press.

Robinson, T. E., & Berridge, K. C. (2003). Addiction. *Annual Review of Psychology, 54,* 25–53.

Wise, R. A., & Bozarth, M. A. (1987). A psychomotor stimulant theory of addiction. *Psychological Review, 94,* 469–492.

Wise, R. A., & Rompre, P.-P. (1989). Brain dopamine and reward. *Annual Review of Psychology, 40,* 191–225.

Zhu, X. O., & McNaughton, N. (1995). Similar effects of buspirone and chlordiazepoxide on a fixed interval schedule with long-term, low-dose administration. *Journal of Psychopharmacology, 9,* 326–330.

II

Studies of Extraversion and Related Traits

3

Biosocial Bases of Sensation Seeking

Marvin Zuckerman

The term "biosocial," as used in the title of this chapter, is often a mere nod to the idea of interaction, but is often just a cover for an exclusively biological or social approach. The genome, and the biological systems it controls, are in constant interaction with the environment; however, this fact is minimized by behavior genetic approaches that parcel deterministic influences into genetic, shared environment, and specific or nonshared environment. The third category is a wastebasket for what remains after genetic and shared environmental influences are partialed out. In most analyses of personality traits it accounts for at least half of the variance, but it also includes error of measurement (unreliability), which is not usually subtracted from the term. Shared environment is usually insignificant in these analyses.

Despite this evidence that minimizes the role of shared environment (possibly because it does not adequately deal with gene–environment interaction), I believe that both nature *and* nurture shape personality traits. Figure 3.1 shows two pathways from the distal to the proximal influences in personality. Evolution plays a distal role in both pathways, modifying the genome in the biological pathway and choosing among successful and unsuccessful cultures in group survival. Changes in the genome are slow, but those in cultures can be rapid and are influenced by technological changes (e.g., the advent of the computer). The genome expresses itself through the shaping of neurological systems and their biochemistry and physiology. Physiological activations and inhibitions are proximal to the moment-to-moment adaptations to environmental changes and instrumental and classical "conditioning." The social influences from the distal to the proximal range from culture, to society, to neighborhood and peer and family influences. They have their major effects in

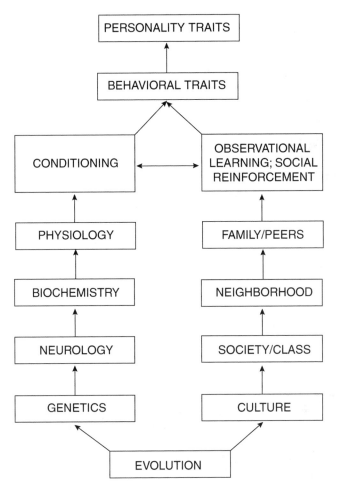

FIGURE 3.1. Two pathways to individual differences in personality: the biological and the social. From Zuckerman (2003, Fig. 4.1, p. 86). Copyright 2003 by John Wiley & Sons, Inc. Reprinted by permission.

observational learning reinforced by instrumental consequences and social reinforcements. Of course, what is learned depends in part upon intra-individual differences already shaped by previous biosocial interactions.

   McCrae (2004) argues that the basis for personality traits is entirely biological. Culture may influence "characteristic adaptations" and their behavioral expressions, but, according to this theory, personality traits (or temperament) influence the characteristic adaptations and are not influenced by them. However, the outcomes of "characteristic adaptations" may affect personality, particularly in its developmental stages. Most children are not entirely indifferent to the rewards and punishments of their parents. McCrae does note differences in measured personality traits in different parts of the world, and in some ethnic groups between indigenous and American-born populations, but he attributes these to test response biases or selective migration. I would suggest that there are differences in modal personality traits influenced by culture as expressed through family and peer influences. Two Asian populations, Japanese and Thai, were lower on the General Sensation Seeking Scale (SSS) than American norms (see Zuckerman, 1979). Comparisons of American, Canadian, Australian, and Spanish students show national differences, but primarily among the women (see Zuckerman, 1994).

GENETICS

Twin Studies

The first twin study of sensation seeking showed a high heritability (58%) for the SSS Total score, with the remainder of the variance due to specific or nonshared environmental influence and to error of measurement (Fulker, Eysenck, & Zuckerman, 1980). There was no influence of shared environment as indicated in the model used in the study (Jinks & Fulker, 1970). The heritability for the trait is at the upper limits of heritabilities found for personality traits, which average about .44 and usually fall between .40 and .50 (Bouchard, 1993; Loehlin, 1992).

If there is no effect of shared environment, then twins separated at birth and raised in different adopted families should show about the same heritability as those raised in the same families. D. T. Lykken (personal communication, 1992) reported correlations of .54 for separated monozygotic (MZ) twins and .32 for separated dizygotic (DZ) twins. The correlation between separated MZ twins was very close to the correlation of .58 in the Fulker and colleagues (1980) study and represents the heritability of the trait. The separated DZ twin correlation must be doubled to get the heritability and therefore would be .64. Averaging these two values gives a heritability of .59, nearly the same as found in the Fulker et al. study.

Eysenck (1983) analyzed the genetic variance in the four subscales of the SSS in the Fulker and colleagues (1980) study in men and women separately, and found high heritabilities (.42–.56) for the Experience Seeking, Disinhibition, and Thrill and Adventure Seeking subscales. A study of Dutch twins found even higher heritabilities (.56–.63) for these three subscales (Koopmans, Boomsma, Heath, & Lorenz, 1995). Hur and Bouchard (1997) analyzed the subscale data from the separated twins reported by Fulker and colleagues. Heritabilities for the three subscales were also high (.46–.55). Heritabilities across the studies were high for these three subscales (means = .50–.57) but lower for the fourth subscale, Boredom Susceptibility (.43), probably because of the lower reliability of this scale.

In nearly all of these biometric twin studies of sensation seeking, the analyses showed moderately strong effects of genetic factors and little or no effect of shared environment. However, in a Dutch study of nearly 2,000 pairs of twins, the investigators examined the effects of being raised in a religious home environment versus growing up in a nonreligious home (Boomsma, de Geus, van Baal, & Koopmans, 1999). The analysis was focused on the Disinhibition subscale of the SSS, because it showed the greatest difference between religious and nonreligious homes for fathers and mothers as well as sons and daughters. Not surprisingly, those in religious homes had lower scores on this subscale. It is important to note, however, that although twins raised in a religious environment had lower scores on Disinhibition than those from nonreligious homes, there were no differences in the variance of scores in these two groups. It is also important to note that genetic influences did not contribute to variation in religious practice of the grown children; nearly all of this variance was due to shared environment.

When the twins were subdivided on the basis of religious or nonreligious families, the genetic and shared environment effects depended on the family environment. For the twins raised in nonreligious families, the effects were like those in most studies of sensation seeking: a strong genetic effect (61% for females and 49% for males) and the absence of a significant shared environment effect (0% for females and 11% for males). Analyses of the twins raised in a religious environment showed no genetic effect for males and a weak one for females (37%), with a substantial shared environment effect for males (62%) and a lower although significant one for females (25%).

This shared environment effect would not be seen if the total population of twins had been used; it suggests that religious upbringing not only influences the absolute levels of disinhibition, but also its genetic architecture. In a family atmosphere in which genetic effects are free to express themselves, they play a prominent role, but in one where the environment imposes constraints, the genetic effects are attenuated and depend on some complex interactions with environments.

Family Studies

An early study of the relationship between parents and children on the SSS General scale found only a significant correlation between fathers and daughters (r =.39) and between the average of fathers' and mothers' scores and children's scores (midparent r = .28) (Kish & Donnenwerth, 1972). A more recent study of the correlations between SSS Form V scores of parents and their adolescent children was done in Croatia (Bratko & Butković, 2004). Only the fathers' score on the Total SSS correlated significantly with the daughters' scores (r = .36), as in the previous study. Fathers' Thrill and Adventure Seeking scores correlated with the sons' scores on this subscale.

Midparent scores correlated significantly (r = .31) with the Total scores of their offspring. If we assume only an additive genetic mechanism, the midparent offspring correlation represents the heritability. However, this heritability is only about half of that found in twin studies of sensation seeking. This is not an unusual finding for personality traits; it could be due to nonadditive sources of genetic variance, or to unequal environments for MZ and DZ twins (MZ twins tend to be treated more similarly).

Parenting: Affection and Control

In most analyses based on children's reports of parental behavior and attitudes, two or three main factors emerge: love or affection, punishment, and control. Correlations between children's personalities and parental behaviors and attitudes cannot establish any direction of causal effects, but they can show whether there are any such effects at all. We (Kraft & Zuckerman, 1999) correlated college students' scores on the Zuckerman–Kuhlman Personality Questionnaire (ZKPQ) with their reports of parental behavior and attitudes in intact families and broken families with a stepfather. The Impulsive Sensation Seeking (ImpSS) scores of males and females did not correlate with any of their perceptions of parental behavior and attitudes in intact families. In families with a stepfather, the daughters' ImpSS scores correlated positively with mother punishment and control scores and negatively with mother love scores, perhaps suggesting mothers' reactions to rebellious teenage daughters.

Bratko and Butković (2003) gave parental behavior scales directly to the parents of their adolescents and compared the parents' self-reported and partners' estimates of their parental behaviors and attitudes with their children's SSS scores. Only the fathers' Control scores correlated with the children's Total SSS and Disinhibition subscale scores. Fathers who were more permissive in regard to disinhibitory behavior in their children had children who were more disinhibited. Whether the fathers' relaxed control influenced the disinhibited pattern in their children or was a reaction to it cannot be determined from these correlational data. Another possibility is a shared genetic influence.

Assortative Mating

Bratko and Butković (2003) found a moderate correlation of .44 between husbands and wives on the Total SSS. Moderate to high spousal correlations on sensation seeking has been found in many previous studies (Zuckerman, 1994). Even in long-term premarital relationships, there is a moderate correlation between partners on the Total SSS (Thornquist & Zuckerman, 1995). These relationships suggest assortative mating. In effect, men and women are attracted to mates who are similar in their sensation-seeking levels. This is not true for most other personality traits, for which correlations between spouses are low or close to zero (Ahern, Johnson, Wilson, McClearn, & Vandenberg, 1982; Eysenck, 1990). Assortative mating could inflate additive-type heritability, although it does not appear to do so for sensation seeking. But the fact that sensation seeking is an important basis for mating attraction indicates its evolutionary biological significance.

Molecular Genetics

Advances in the field of molecular genetics have created the possibility of finding specific genes accounting for some part of the variance in personality traits. Ebstein and colleagues (1996) found that an allele (7 repeats) of the dopamine D4 receptor gene (*DRD4*) was associated with higher scores on Cloninger's Novelty Seeking (NS) scale, in contrast to lower scores with shorter alleles (commonly a 4-repeat sequence). NS is highly correlated (r = .68) with ImpSS (Zuckerman & Cloninger, 1996). Ebstein and colleagues used an Israeli sample.

This exciting finding was followed by many attempts at replication with different populations in different countries, some using other personality measures of novelty seeking. A meta-analysis of results from 21 groups in 14 studies found no overall effect when the 7-repeat sequence was contrasted with shorter-repeat alleles (Schinka, Letsch, & Crawford, 2002), but studies comparing all short and all long sequences yielded a small significant effect.

The long forms of the *DRD4* have been associated with heroin and alcohol abuse in several but not all studies (Ebstein & Kotler, 2002). The long-form alleles have also been related to pathological gambling and attention-deficit/hyperactivity disorder. In newborn infants, the long form is associated with indicators of approach behavior such as orientation to novel stimuli and less distress in reaction to such stimuli (Ebstein & Auerbach, 2002). In these studies there was an interaction between the *DRD4* and the serotonin (5-HT) transporter gene-linked promoter region (*5-HTTLPR*) alleles. The short form of the *5-HTTLPR* has been associated with anxiety in humans. The long form enhances the effect of the long form of the *DRD4* on orientation reactions, whereas the short form in combination with the short form of the *DRD4* reduces orientation and increases negative emotionality and distress to limitations. Ebstein and Auerbach (2002) summarize their results: "Our provisional findings are consistent with both human and animal studies that activation of dopaminergic pathways promotes exploratory and impulsive behavior, whereas serotonergic pathways are generally inhibitory and advance avoidance behavior" (p. 145).

PSYCHOPHYSIOLOGY

Optimal Levels of Stimulation and Arousal

The first theory of sensation seeking based the trait on the concept of individual differences in optimal levels of arousal (OLAs), with the hypothesis that individuals scoring high on the SSS ("high sensation seekers") were in a basal state of underarousal and therefore needed more stimulation to reach an OLA (Zuckerman, 1969, 1979). An alternative hypothesis was that people differ in their OLAs: For some, higher levels of arousal are more hedonically positive and facilitative, and they therefore require stronger stimulation to reach these levels. A third hypothesis involved arousability rather than arousal: Some persons react less to stimulation, and although they have the same basal level of arousal, they need more intense stimuli to reach an OLA. The first definition of sensation seeking involved the novelty, variety, and complexity of stimuli as qualities favored by high sensation seekers, but it did not mention the intensity of stimuli (Zuckerman, 1979). The optimal level theories are based on intensity of stimulation. In the later definition of sensation seeking (Zuckerman, 1994), intensity was included for reasons that are subsequently described.

Orienting and Defensive Reflexes

The first psychophysiological studies of sensation seeking used the orienting response (OR) to novel stimuli, as measured by the skin conductance response (SCR) to novel and repeated visual stimuli (Neary & Zuckerman, 1976). There was no difference between high and low sensation seekers in basal levels of electrodermal measured arousal. Studies by other investigators, using SCR, heart rate, blood pressure, and electroencephalogram, did not yield any consistent differences in basal arousal (Zuckerman, 1990, 1994).

High sensation seekers had a larger-amplitude SCR to novel stimuli, which quickly habituated to the level of the low sensation seekers' response on subsequent trials when the same stimulus was repeated (Neary & Zuckerman, 1976). Replication results were mixed. However, a series of studies by Smith and colleagues showed that the content of novel stimuli was important (Smith, Perstein, Davidson, & Michael, 1986). High sensation seekers did have larger SCRs than low sensation seekers to initial presentations of words with strong emotional associations (a combination of novelty and intensity), but did not differ in response to neutral words.

Changes in heart rate (HR) have also been used as measures of OR and the defensive reflex (DR). Deceleration of HR in the first few seconds after presentation of a stimulus is a measure of OR, whereas HR acceleration is a measure of either a DR or a startle response (SR). Orlebeke and Feij (1979) used a moderately high-intensity (80-dB) tone and found that subjects scoring high on the Disinhibition subscale of the SSS ("high disinhibiters") showed a deceleratory response (strong OR), whereas the low disinhibiters showed an acceleratory (DR or SR) pattern. The differences disappeared quickly on repetition of the stimulus. These results were more or less replicated in two subsequent studies (Ridgeway & Hare, 1981; Zuckerman, Simons, & Como, 1988).

The results for both SCR and HR indicate a stronger arousal by novelty in high disinhibiters, but a rapid habituation. The OR can be regarded as a measure of interest and attention, and its habituation a measure of uninterest and inattention. The stronger OR of high sensation seekers may be related to their preference for novelty in many forms of sensation and experience, and its rapid habituation to their boredom susceptibility in the absence of novelty or change.

Augmenting and Reducing of the Cortical Evoked Potential

The early components of the cortical evoked potential (EP) are sensitive to intensity of stimulation. Normally one would expect the amplitude of the EP to increase in direct relation to the intensity of the stimulus. The slope of the EP–stimulus intensity is one expression of the relationship. Buchsbaum (1971) found a range of individual differences in this relationship: Some individuals showed a marked positive slope ("augmenters"), and some showed a negligible slope and even a reduction in EP amplitudes in response to the highest intensities of stimuli ("reducers"). Another study (Zuckerman, Murtaugh, & Siegel, 1974) related EP augmenting and reducing (A-R) patterns in response to visual stimuli to the SSS and found a relationship with the Disinhibition scale, as shown in Figure 3.2. High disinhibiters commonly showed the augmenting pattern, whereas low disinhibiters demonstrated a reducing pattern with significant reduction of EP amplitude at the brightest intensity of flashing lights. Fair replication of results was achieved in 4 of 8 attempts at replication (described in Zuckerman, 1990, 1994). Efforts to replicate the relationship

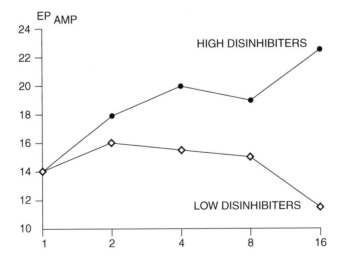

FIGURE 3.2. Visual evoked potentials (EPs) of high and low scorers on the Disinhibition subscale of the Sensation Seeking Scale as a function of stimulus intensity. From Zuckerman, Murtaugh, and Siegel (1974, p. 539). Copyright 1974 by the Society for Psychophysiological Research. Reprinted by permission of Blackwell Publishing, Ltd.

using auditory stimuli were even more successful, with replication in 8 of 10 studies. Further replications have been reported since the 1990 review (e.g., Brocke, Beauducel, John, Debener, & Heileman, 2000).

This kind of finding raises questions about the more molecular mechanisms underlying the psychophysiological phenomena. Such questions can be more easily addressed if the paradigm can be applied to other species of animals. Siegel and his colleagues applied the paradigm to cats and found that augmenter cats were more active, exploratory, and aggressive than reducer cats, and more likely to approach than to withdraw from novel stimuli (Lukas & Siegel, 1977; Saxton, Siegel, & Lukas, 1987).

Saxton and colleagues (1987) tested their cats in controlled learning experiments. One experiment involved responding on a fixed-interval (FI) bar-pressing task with food as a reward, and the other was differential reinforcement for a low rate of response (DRL). The FI task merely required an adjustment to the novel test chamber and the maintenance of a high rate of response. The DRL task, however, required inhibition or modulation of response rate. Cats that were augmenters did well on the FI task but poorly on the DRL, because they could not modulate their responding for food reward. Cats that were reducers had the opposite pattern: They did poorly on the FI task because they were too fearful in initial response to the novel environment, but they were more successful than augmenters in the task that demanded more restraint and inhibition. These studies demonstrated the validity of the A-R paradigm in cats with clear analogues of human sensation seeking. Our latest trait version of human sensation seeking combines impulsivity with sensation seeking, or "impulsive sensation seeking" (Zuckerman, 1996). Augmenting cats, like human impulsive sensation seekers, are unable to inhibit approach responses in the seeking of reward, even though unrestrained response may lead to loss of reward.

Siegel, Sisson, and Driscoll (1993) extended the A-R paradigm to another species, the rat, using two strains selectively bred from a parent strain (Wistar) for their ability to learn to avoid punishment. The Roman High Avoidance (RHA) rats are good at learning to avoid punishment by actively seeking an effective response. The Roman Low Avoidance (RLA) rats are slow to learn an active avoidance response and tend to freeze in response to shock. Nearly all of the RHA rats examined by Siegel and colleagues were augmenters, and almost all of the RLA rats were reducers (visual EPs were used to define A-R). The members of a selectively bred strain are genetically homogeneous, so we can look at other studies contrasting the two strains to elucidate behavioral and biological differences related to the A-R animal model for human sensation seeking. These results are summarized in Table 3.1.

In an open-field test, RHAs are more active and exploratory, whereas RLAs are more inhibited and fearful. RHAs are more aggressive in response to shock. RHAs are more ready to drink alcohol and have a high tolerance for barbiturates. Female RHAs are not good mothers, spending little time in their nests with their young pups. RLA females are more nurturing mothers.

TABLE 3.1. Differences between the RHA and RLA Rat Strains

Variable	Main difference
VEP augmenting–reducing	RHAs augmenters, RLAs reducers
Exploration (open-field test)	RHAs more active, less emotional
Shock-induced aggression	RHAs more aggressive
Alcohol drinking	RHAs drink alcohol (in solution), RLAs abstain
Barbiturates	RHAs high tolerance, RLAs low tolerance
Maternal behavior	RHA females less time in nest with pups
Hypothalamic self-stimulation: High and low intensities	RHAs less sensitive to low intensities, more responsive to high intensities; RLAs more sensitive to low intensities, more escape from high intensities

Stress effects: Monoamines and hormones	Main difference
Prefrontal cortex	RHAs increased dopamine, RLAs no change in dopamine
Hypothalamus	RLAs increased serotonin (5-HT), RHAs less change in 5-HT; RLAs increased corticotropin-releasing factor (CRF), RHAs less CRF
Pituitary	RLAs increased adrenocorticotropic hormone (ACTH), RHAs less change in ACTH

Note. VEP, visual evoked potential. From Zuckerman (2002). Copyright 2002 by Kluwer Academic Publishers. Reprinted by permission.

Brain electrical self-stimulation in rats is a model for biological reward seeking, as is drug use in humans. However, the intensity of the stimulus reward can affect the rate of response for reward. When lateral hypothalamic self-stimulation of low and high intensities was used, it was found that RHAs are less responsive to low intensities of stimulation but more responsive to high intensities than RLAs. RLAs respond more for the low intensities of stimulation reward, but show more escape reactions in response to high intensities. This paradigm has some resemblance to the A-R one, except that the stimulation is in a reward area of the brain rather than the cortex.

The two strains differ in neurotransmitter and hormonal responses to stress. The RHA rats show increases in dopamine in the prefrontal cortex, whereas the RLAs show no change. The RLAs react with increased serotonin (5-HT) in the hypothalamus; the RHAs show less change in 5-HT.

The hypothalamic–pituitary–adrenocortical (HYPAC) axis is a hormonal pathway for stress. The RLAs show increased corticotropin-releasing factor from the hypothalamus, which results in increased adrenocorticotropic hormone from the pituitary gland. The end result of this pathway would be increased release of cortisol from the adrenal cortex. The RHAs are less responsive in the HYPAC stress reactive pathway.

The increased dopaminergic response in the prefrontal cortex (PFC) is consistent with the hypotheses suggesting a more reactive dopaminergic system in human sensation seekers. But this hypothesis generally involves dopamine reactivity in the reward system of the medial forebrain bundle, including the nucleus accumbens (NA). Research suggests that dopamine release in the PFC actually blunts the responsiveness of the subcortical limbic dopamine system and the NA, suggesting an inverse relationship between the two (Grace, 2002).

Dellu, Piazza, Mayo, Le Moal, and Simon (1996) developed another rat model, based on exploratory reactivity to a novel environment (a circular maze). "High reactives" (HRs) are more exploratory and self-administer amphetamine at a higher rate than "low reactives" (LR). HRs are models for high sensation seeking and LRs for low sensation seeking. Interestingly, the HRs show a higher level of the dopamine metabolite 3,4-dihydroxyphenylacetic acid (DOPAC) in the NA. Dellu and colleagues found a positive correlation between DOPAC content in the NA and exploratory response to novelty. When the rats were stressed, dopamine in the NA increased more in the HR than in the LR rats. However, basal levels of dopamine activity in the PFC of LR rats were higher, based on a ratio of DOPAC to dopamine. If we extrapolate up to the human species, we would have to say that sensation seekers have a high level of dopamine reactivity in the NA reward center and are therefore more attracted to drugs and experiences that stimulate release in this area. The situation in the PFC is not clear. Are high sensation seekers characterized by low or high activity in the PFC? Although basal levels of activity may be low, stress may potentiate the activity, allowing for more active behavioral responses (active avoidance or aggression, depending on the stressors).

The heightened response of the HYPAC hormonal stress system in the LR rats suggests that they also have high levels of norepinephrine (NE), since NE (at low doses) and 5-HT stimulate corticotropin-releasing factor release. Therefore, we might expect to find low levels of NE and 5-HT in high sensation seekers, and high levels in low sensation seekers.

Human Correlational Studies

A large body of studies relates the enzyme monoamine oxidase (MAO) to sensation seeking and to forms of behavior and psychopathology that are related to sensation seeking. A review (Zuckerman, 1994) showed that levels of platelet MAO Type B (MAO-B) were inversely and significantly related to scores on the SSS General or Total scales in 9 out of 13 groups from 9 studies. The correlations were negative in 11 of the 13 studies. The median correlation was only –.24, a weak but relatively consistent effect. The strongest effect among the subscales was with Disinhibition.

Low MAO levels are also found in various forms of psychopathology, including attention-deficit/hyperactivity disorder, antisocial and borderline personality disorders, alcoholism and drug abuse, pathological gambling disorder, and paranoid schizophrenia (see Table 3.2). With the possible excep-

TABLE 3.2. Psychopathology and MAO

Low MAO is found in these conditions:	References
High sensation seeking (normal trait)	Zuckerman (1994)
Attention-deficit/hyperactivity disorder	Shekim et al. (1986)
Antisocial personality disorder	Lidberg et al. (1985)
Chronic criminality	Klinteberg (1996)
Borderline personality disorder	Reist et al. (1990)
Alcoholism	Major and Murphy (1978)
Relatives of alcoholics	Schuckit (1994), Sher (1993)
Drug abuse	Von Knorring et al. (1987)
Bipolar disorder	Murphy and Weiss (1972)
Relatives of bipolar disorder	Leckman et al. (1977)
Pathological gamblers	Blanco et al. (1996)
Schizophrenia with paranoid delusions and hallucinations (high MAO in schizophrenia with withdrawal and behavioral retardation)	Zureik and Meltzer (1988)

tion of paranoid schizophrenia (sensation seeking is actually low in more withdrawn individuals with schizophrenia), these are disorders characterized by impulsive and sensation-seeking behaviors in their active stages. Mania is a caricature of sensation seeking in its active stage, but even when patients with bipolar disorder are not having a manic episode, they score high on the SSS. Relatives of persons with alcoholism and sons of individuals with bipolar disorder also have low levels of MAO, even though they do not yet have the disorders; this suggests that MAO is a latent biological trait common to all of them.

MAO-B has a preferential affinity for dopamine (Murphy, Aulakh, Garrick, & Sunderland, 1987), and MAO-B inhibition is associated with enhanced activity of dopamine (Deutch & Roth, 1999). Low levels of MAO-B in high sensation seekers may therefore be related to higher levels of available dopamine, although this is not certain. It has also been suggested that platelet MAO activity is determined by the same set of genes that regulate levels of 5-HT turnover, implying a positive correlation between MAO and 5-HT. Sensation seekers therefore might be expected to have low levels of available 5-HT. In one study platelet MAO was negatively correlated with the dopamine metabolite homovanillic acid (HVA) in cerebrospinal fluid (CSF), but it was also correlated negatively with the 5-HT metabolite 5-hydroxyindoleacetic acid (5-HIAA) (Ballenger et al., 1983). The problem is that HVA and 5-HIAA are highly and positively correlated in CSF, for reasons that probably have little to do with their relationship in the brain.

Correlations between levels of HVA and 5-HIAA in CSF and sensation seeking are not significant (Ballenger et al., 1983; Limson et al., 1991). However, Ballenger and colleagues (1983) did find a significant negative correlation between NE in CSF and sensation seeking. This correlation suggests underarousal in high sensation seekers, but as far as I know, no one has attempted to replicate this finding.

Depue (1995) assessed prolactin response to a 5-HT stimulant and found negative correlations with the SSS Disinhibition and Boredom Susceptibility scales, as well as scales of impulsivity and control (see Table 3.3). The prolactin response, indicative of 5-HT reactivity, was also negatively related to measures of aggression and hostility. These tend to support the hypothesis of low 5-HT reactivity in high sensation seekers, particularly those of the impulsive kind. Dopamine reactivity, however, was not related to the SSS scales, but only to Eysenck's Venturesomeness and Risk Taking scales. Eysenck's Psychoticism scale, which tends to be positively correlated with sensation seeking, correlated negatively with both the 5-HT and dopamine reactions. The dopamine-induced prolactin was in response to an inhibitor, so that a negative correlation means a lack of inhibition of dopamine.

Netter, Hennig, and Roed (1996) also used drugs that stimulate or inhibit activity in the serotonergic and dopaminergic systems. Effects were measured in terms of hormonal, emotional state, and behavioral reactions. Their results were consistent with a blunted serotonergic response in high sensation seekers, but no association with the dopaminergic response to a stimulant. However, craving for nicotine was increased more by a dopamine stimulant in high sensation seekers. Other studies have shown more intense "highs" in response to these nicotine or amphetamine by high sensation seekers who had little or no experience with these drugs (no smoking history and no history of drug use). Perhaps the dopamine receptors of high sensation seekers are more sensitive, even if the absolute levels of dopamine do not differ in high and low sensation seekers.

TABLE 3.3. Correlations of Dopamine- and Serotonin-Induced Prolactin with Impulsivity and Sensation-Seeking Scales

Scales	5-HT-PRL	DA-PRL
MPQ Control	−.44*	−.13
EPQ Psychoticism	−.39*	−.39*
SSS Disinhibition	−.44*	−.12
SSS Boredom Susceptibility	−.44*	−.06
Barratt Impulsivity	−.51*	−.27
Eysenck Venturesomeness	−.13	.40*
Eysenck Risk Taking	−.10	.33*

Note. DA, dopamine; 5-HT, serotonin; PRL, prolactin; MPQ, Maudsley Personality Questionnaire; EPQ, Eysenck Personality Questionnaire; SSS, Sensation Seeking Scale. From Depue (1995). Copyright 1995 by John Wiley & Sons. Reprinted by permission.

Cloninger (1987) has proposed that "high novelty seekers" (individuals scoring high on his NS scale) are low in dopaminergic basal activity. This seems at odds with the observations that patients with Parkinson's disease are extremely low in sensation seeking, as expressed by a depressed lack of interest in their environment and reductions in spontaneous activity that are not entirely attributable to reduced striatal dopamine. Dopamine is also reduced in other pathways, including the mesolimbic, the postulated site of sensation-seeking motivation. Individuals with pathological gambling, in contrast, seem to have decreased dopamine with increased levels of the dopamine metabolites DOPAC and HVA, consistent with increased dopamine activity (Bergh, Eklund, & Soderstein, 1997). Such individuals have also been found to have low levels of MAO, consistent with dysregulated high levels of dopamine activity (Blanco, Orensnz-Munoz, Blanco-Jerez, & Saiz-Ruiz, 1996).

Dominance is a salient trait in primates and is regarded as an aspect of surgent-type extraversion in humans. Sensation seeking correlates with measures of the dominance trait in humans. Dominant monkeys in social groups were found to have higher concentrations of HVA in their CSF than subordinate monkeys (Kaplan, Manuck, Fontenot, & Mann, 2002). Serotonin-depleted rats are exploratory, aggressive, and socially dominant in their familiar environments (Ellison, 1977). Even though direct correlational evidence is lacking in humans, these kinds of comparative findings suggest that dopamine activity and certainly reactivity are high and serotonergic activity or reactivity is low in sensation seekers.

Biochemical Bases of A-R of the Cortical EP

I have discussed how the A-R of the EP is related to sensation seeking and analogous behavior in cats and rats. It is interesting, therefore, that visual EP augmenters tend to have low MAO levels and low levels of 5-HIAA (the 5-HT metabolite) in CSF (Von Knorring & Pervin, 1981). They also found lower levels of dopamine-beta-hydroxlase (DBH) in augmenters. DBH is the enzyme that converts dopamine to NE, and therefore low DBH is consistent with the lowered levels of NE found along with low levels of DBH in high sensation seekers (Ballenger et al., 1983).

Von Knorring and Johansson (1980) gave a drug selectively inhibiting 5-HT uptake to typical subjects and observed a reduction in the amplitude–intensity slope of the EP—experimental evidence of the serotonergic control of A-R. A genetic study found an interaction of the 5-HTTLPR allele associated with lower serotonergic activity, and the DRD4 allele associated with novelty seeking, in increased augmenting of the auditory EP (Strobel et al., 2003).

The genes, neurotransmitters, and enzymes associated with sensation seeking also influence the A-R phenomenon, increasing its claim to validity as a psychophysiological marker for the sensation-seeking trait and tying together the biological levels hypothesized to underlie this trait.

Hormones

Gonadal hormones were the first biochemicals studied in relationship to sensation seeking. The reasons for this selection were based on the gender differences (males higher than females) and age changes (a peak in late adolescence and a drop at subsequent ages) on the SSS. Testosterone has similar gender and age differences. Another finding suggestive of gonadal differences is that high sensation seekers tend to have more sexual experience with more partners than low sensation seekers (Zuckerman, Tushup, & Finner, 1976). Indeed, in males testosterone and estradiol were correlated with both SSS scores (particularly Disinhibition) and sexual experience (Daitzman & Zuckerman, 1980). Estradiol in males is produced by conversion of androgens to estradiol. The aromatization hypothesis suggests that androgens in males have their major motivational effects after conversion to estrogenic metabolites (Brain, 1983). SSS scores of hypogonadal men with low testosterone levels were compared to those of men with sexual dysfunctions but average testosterone levels (O'Carroll, 1984). The men with sexual dysfunctions who had average testosterone levels scored higher than the hypogonadal men on the General and Disinhibition scales of the SSS. Subsequent administration of testosterone to both groups did not change their personality scores, although it increased their sexual interest and functioning. The hormonal influence on personality probably occurs before puberty—even as early as the fetal period of life, where it affects the developing brain.

RLA rats (the models for low sensation seeking in humans, as discussed earlier) show increased hormonal stress response in the HYPAC system, as previously noted. Cortisol is the end product of the HYPAC system and is related to chronic stress in humans. Ballenger and colleagues (1983) found that cortisol in the CSF correlated negatively with the SSS Disinhibition scale, and other scales in a factor that also included the SSS General scale, the Eysenck Psychoticism scale, and the Minnesota Multiphasic Personality Inventory Hypomania scale (Zuckerman, Ballenger, & Post, 1984). Low levels of cortisol and NE in CSF formed the negative pole of this factor. Low levels of cortisol were related to novelty seeking in veterans with posttraumatic stress disorder (Wang, Mason, Charney, & Yehuda, 1997). Low cortisol and NE may indicate a lack of stress reactivity that is an advantage in some situations, but may also be associated with a lack of inhibition that leads to risky and sometimes antisocial forms of behavior.

SUMMARY

Putting together a biosocial-levels approach to personality is like assembling the pieces of a jigsaw puzzle or fitting words into a crossword puzzle. In the jigsaw puzzle, one has two pieces that seem to be related but require a third piece to fit them together. In the crossword puzzle, horizontal words (relation-ships between traits and behaviors) require vertical words (between traits and behaviors and underlying biological traits) to confirm them. The puzzle for sensation seeking is beginning to form some semblance of a theoretical model, although many pieces are missing and many words are disconnected. The comparative approach relies on connecting findings from human correlational studies, using normal and disordered populations, with animal experimental and correlational data.

At the bottom of the puzzle, we find alleles of specific genes related to the trait at the top level and to its behavioral expressions. Alleles of a dopamine receptor gene (*DRD4*) and a serotonin transporter gene (*5-HTTLPR*) in inter-action seem to be involved in (1) the trait of sensation seeking in adults; (2) behavioral expressions such as orientation, activity, and emotional reactivity in infants; (3) positive reactions to novelty in children; and (4) psycho-pathologies such as opiate use, attention-deficit/hyperactivity disorder, and pathological gambling. These genetic variations account for only a small part of the genetic variance, however, and other genes (pieces of the puzzle) remain to be discovered.

At the next levels, we find serotonin and dopamine neurotransmitter activity related to the sensation-seeking trait, probably also in interaction. Studies on other species and some human correlational research suggest that these neurotransmitters and their receptors in particular areas of the brain are involved in the personality trait. Dopamine reactivity is involved in approach behavior to novel stimuli and environments, whereas serotonergic reactivity is implicated in inhibition or passive avoidance of risky behavior in novel situa-tions. Enzymes like MAO, which regulate the neurotransmitters, show similar relationships with traits and behaviors. Gonadal hormones and hormones in the HYPAC stress response system are also involved, although their effects on the neurotransmitters are not clear. Norepinephrine and cortisol seem to be involved in producing inhibition at the opposite pole of the disinhibition dimension.

At the level of psychophysiology, we find that sensation seekers have strong orienting responses to novel stimuli, which habituate quickly on repetititon. Dopamine has not yet been connected with this behavior, al-though it is interesting that the dopamine–serotonergic gene interaction affects orientation in young infants (Ebstein & Auerbach, 2002). The first definition of sensation seeking included the need for novel stimuli and experiences. The current definition (Zuckerman, 1994) adds intensity to the qualities of stimuli that are attractive to high sensation seekers.

Intensity of stimuli is the major influence in the EP augmenting-reducing (A-R) paradigm. In three species (human, cat, rat), augmenting of the cortical EP in response to increasing stimulus intensity is related to disinhibited impul-sive behavior. Connections between the A-R paradigm and dopamine and serotonin also fit neatly into the model. Cortical augmenting in response to intense stimuli may represent "strength of the nervous system," to use the old Pavlovian term.

The capacity to function and feel well in response to intense stimuli has an obvious adaptive value and plays a role in the risk taking related to sensation seeking. It may be a function of strong dopaminergic and weak serotonergic reactivity. Reducing seems to serve a protective function in the nervous system of low sensation seekers. It may be mediated by strong serotonergic or gamma-aminobutyric acid (GABA) activity triggered by intense stimuli.

The theoretical model proposed here is pictured in Figure 3.3. Essentially, Impulsive Unsocialized Sensation Seeking (P-ImpUSS) is a function of the relative strengths and interactions of three behavioral mechanisms: approach, inhibition, and arousal. The biochemical mechanisms underlying these are also shown in the figure. Note that interactions occur at all of the biological levels. Simple isomorphisms, like those shown between the behavioral mechanisms and the neurotransmitters are unlikely. An accurate biosocial model would require arrows connecting everything with nearly everything else. It would also need more two-way arrows reflecting the interactions of behavior and biology in both directions, like the one between approach and inhibition. Although simple elegant models may be fine for physics, they are problematic for biobehavioral science, even at the most molecular levels such as the gene. We must simplify in order to converse in a coherent manner, recognizing that the subtext is more complex.

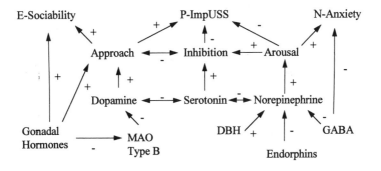

FIGURE 3.3. A psychopharmacological model for extraversion–sociability (E-Sociability), impulsive unsocialized sensation seeking (P-ImpUSS), and neuroticism–anxiety (N-Anxiety), showing the underlying behavioral mechanisms (approach, inhibition, and arousal) and neurotransmitters, enzymes, and hormones involved. Agonistic interactions between factors are indicated by a plus sign, and antagonistic interactions between factors are indicated by a minus sign. MAO, monoamine oxidase; DBH, dopamine-beta-hydroxylase; GABA, gamma-aminobutyric acid. From Zuckerman (1995, Fig. 1, p. 331). Copyright 1995 by Blackwell Publishing, Ltd. Reprinted by permission.

LOOKING FORWARD

There are two fronts on which biopersonality can make foreseeable advances: molecular genetics and brain imaging. The identification of specific genes with major effects related to personality, and the discovery of their roles in the intermediate biological mechanisms, will bring "consilience" between levels of biosocial phenomena. There have been some real problems in replicating the few gene–trait relationships found, but larger samples and better techniques may resolve these problems. Perhaps in the future we will even be able to identify genes of smaller effects. At present our best bet is to use "candidate" genes, identified as such through neurochemical theories or data on the physiological bases of the traits. Gene interactions are already being reported, and any study should investigate several genes putatively involved in order to investigate their interactions.

New methods of brain imaging can use experimental treatments, such as exposure to emotionally provoking stimuli, to examine differences in brain reactions in specific brain areas and assess the activations of specific neurotransmitter systems. These methods have so far been largely limited to studies of psychopathology and cognitive function. There is no reason why personality variables cannot be used in normal control groups in psychopathology studies and studies of cognitive functions in persons without psychopathology.

Of course, it would be preferable if personality brain imaging studies could be conducted on large, randomly selected samples. One could reduce the necessary sample size by selecting groups with extreme scores on a single personality variable. But given the present state of knowledge, it would be foolish to put all of our eggs in the one trait basket. There are likely to be interactions of traits related to genes, as well as interactions of genes involved in traits. The best strategy is to use personality tests that assess the major dimensions of personality—whether there are three, four, five, or more of these. There is now too much reliance on the "Big Five" trait model. This particular model was developed from a lexical analysis of human language rather than an analysis of temperament or biobehavioral traits. At least, representative scales from several methods should be used to assess basic traits. A number of psychometric analyses have identified factors common to several major tests. Group testing is not expensive and is a worthwhile addition to any biobehavioral study.

ACKNOWLEDGMENTS

I acknowledge an intellectual debt to colleagues and friends who were sources of theoretical insights and research on sensation seeking in humans or animal models of this trait or related ones. On the theoretical side, I owe much to the late Hans Eysenck and Jeffrey Gray. Hans got me started on the idea of biological explanations of personality using genetic and psychophysiological methods. Jeffrey introduced me to the more fundamental neuropsychology of personality from a "bottom-up" viewpoint.

My colleague and friend at the University of Delaware, Jerome Siegel, extended the EP A-R paradigm from humans to cats and then rats, providing an important comparative dimension to the trait of sensation seeking. His last study on rats indicated genetic origins of differences in behavior and psychopharmacology of rat models for high and low sensation seeking. Another colleague and friend at the university, Michael Kuhlman, was an essential collaborator in the development of the alternative five-factor model and the questionnaire embodying it (the ZKPQ).

The biosocial research on sensation seeking and related constructs has been done by colleagues from both Europe and America, including Alois Angleitner, Burkhard Brocke, Juergen Hennig, Petra Netter, Thomas Rammsayer, and Paul Schmitz (Germany); Britt af Klinteberg, Lars Von Knorring, Lars Oreland, and the late Daisy Schalling (Sweden); Sybil Eysenck, Adrian Furnham, and Alan Pickering (United Kingdom); Jan Strelau (Poland); Vilfredo De Pascalis (Italy); Andrew Johnson, Robert Stelmack, and P. Vernon (Canada); and Samuel Ball, Michael Bardo, Ernest Barratt, Lewis Donohew, Richard Haier, Jeffrey Joireman, Gerald Matthews, and Rick Zimmerman (United States).

Chapters written by all of these scientists, describing their work, may be found in the recent festschrift edited by Robert Stelmack (2004). Others who have contributed significant biobehavioral research include D. Boomsma, Jan Feij, and J. Orlebeke (The Netherlands), and F. Dellu, P. V. Piazza, W. Mayo, M. Le Moal, and H. Simon (France). The last-named group from France developed a new biobehavioral animal model for sensation seeking.

REFERENCES

Ahern, F. M., Johnson, R. C., Wilson, J. R., McClearn, G. E., & Vandenberg, S. G. (1982) Family resemblance in personality. *Behavior Genetics, 12,* 261–280.

Ballenger, J. C., Post, R. M., Jimerson, D. C., Lake, C. R., Murphy, D. L., Zuckerman, M., et al. (1983). Biochemical correlates of personality traits in normals: An exploratory study. *Personality and Individual Differences, 4,* 615–625.

Bergh, C., Eklund, T., & Soderstein, P. (1997). Altered dopamine function in pathological gambling. *Psychological Medicine, 27,* 473–475.

Blanco, C., Orensnz-Munoz, L., Blanco-Jerez, C., & Saiz-Ruiz, J. (1996). Pathological gambling and platelet MAO activity: A psychobiological study. *American Journal of Psychiatry, 153,* 119–121.

Boomsma, D. I., de Geus, E. J. C., van Baal, G. C. M., & Koopmans, J. R. (1999). A religious upbringing reduces the influence of genetic factors on disinhibition: Evidence for interaction between genotype and environment on personality. *Twin Research, 2,* 115–125.

Bouchard, T. J., Jr. (1993). Genetic and environmental influences on adult personality. In J. Hettema & I. J. Deary (Eds.), *Foundations of personality* (pp. 15–44). Dordrecht, The Netherlands: Kluwer.

Brain, P. F. (1983). Pituitary–gonadal influences on social aggression. In B. B. Svare (Ed.), *Hormones and aggressive behavior* (pp. 1–26). New York: Plenum Press.

Bratko, D., & Butković, A. (2003). Family study of sensation seeking. *Personality and Individual Differences, 35,* 1559–1570.

Brocke, B., Beauducel, A., John, R., Debener, S., & Heilemann, H. (2000). Sensation seeking and affective disorders: Characteristics in the intensity dependence of acoustic evoked potentials. *Neuropsychobiology, 41,* 24–30.

Buchsbaum, M. S. (1971). Neural events and the psychophysical law. *Science, 172,* 502.

Cloninger, C. R. (1987). A systematic method for clinical description and classification of personality variants. *Archives of General Psychiatry, 44,* 573–588.

Daitzman, R. J., & Zuckerman, M. (1980). Disinhibitory sensation seeking, personality, and gonadal hormones. *Personality and Individual Differences, 1,* 103–110.

Dellu, F., Piazza, P. V., Mayo, W., Le Moal, M., & Simon, H. (1996). Novelty-seeking in rats: Biobehavioral characteristics and possible relationship with the sensation-seeking trait in man. *Neuropsychobiology, 34,* 136–145.

Depue, R. A. (1995). Neurobiological factors in personality and depression. *European Journal of Personality, 9,* 413–439.

Deutch, A. Y., & Roth, R. H. (1999). Neurochemical systems in the central nervous system. In D. S. Charney, E. J. Nestler, & B. S. Bunney (Eds.), *Neurobiology of mental illness* (pp. 10–25). New York: Oxford University Press.

Ebstein, R. P., & Auerbach, J. G. (2002). Dopamine D4 receptor and serotonin transporter promoter polymorphisms and temperament in early childhood. In J. Benjamin, R. P. Ebstein, & R. H. Belmaker (Eds.), *Molecular genetics and the human personality* (pp. 137–149). Washington, DC: American Psychiatric Press.

Ebstein, R. P., & Kotler, M. (2002). Personality, substance abuse, and genes. In J. Benjamin, R. P. Ebstein, & R. H. Belmaker (Eds.), *Molecular genetics and the human personality* (pp. 151–163). Washington, DC: American Psychiatric Press.

Ebstein, R. P., Novick, O., Umansky, R., Priel, B., Osher, Y., Blaine, D., et al. (1996). Dopamine D4 receptor (D4DR) exon III polymorphism associated with the human personality trait of novelty seeking. *Nature Genetics, 12,* 78–80.

Ellison, G. D. (1977). Animal models of psychopathology: The low-norepinephrine and low-serotonin rat. *American Psychologist, 32,* 1036–1045.

Eysenck, H. J. (1983). A biometrical genetical analysis of impulsive and sensation seeking behavior. In M. Zuckerman (Ed.), *Biological bases of sensation seeking, impulsivity and anxiety* (pp. 1–27). Hillsdale, NJ: Erlbaum.

Eysenck, H. J. (1990). Genetic and environmental contributions to individual differences: Three major dimensions of personality. *Journal of Personality, 58,* 245–261.

Fulker, D. W., Eysenck, S. B. G., & Zuckerman, M. (1980). A genetic and environmental analysis of sensation seeking. *Journal of Research in Personality, 14,* 261–281.

Grace, A. A. (2002). Dopamine. In K. L. Davis, D. Charney, J. T. Coyle, & C. Nemeroff (Eds.), *Neuropsychopharmacology: The fifth generation of progress* (pp. 119–132). Philadelphia: Lippincott, Williams & Wilkins.

Hur, Y.-M., & Bouchard, T. J., Jr. (1997). The genetic correlation between impulsivity and sensation seeking traits. *Behavior Genetics, 27,* 455–463.

Jinks, J. L., & Fulker, D. W. (1970). Comparison of the biometrical genetical, MAVA, and the classical approaches to the analysis of human behavior. *Psychological Bulletin, 73,* 311–349.

Kaplan, J. R., Manuck, S. B., Fontenot, B., & Mann, J. J. (2002). Central nervous system monoamine correlates of social dominance in cynomolgus monkeys (*Macaca fascicularis*). *Neuropsychopharmacology, 26,* 431–443.

Kish, G. B., & Donnenwerth, G. V. (1972). Sex differences in the correlates of sensation seeking. *Journal of Consulting and Clinical Psychology, 38,* 42–49.

Klinteberg, B. (1996). Biology, norms, and personality: A developmental perspective. *Neuropsychobiology, 34,* 146–154.

Koopmans, J. R., Boomsma, D. I., Heath, A. C., & Lorenz, J. P. D. (1995). A multivariate genetic analysis of sensation seeking. *Behavior Genetics, 25,* 349–356.

Kraft, M. R., Jr., & Zuckerman, M. (1999). Parental behaviors and attitudes of their parents reported by young adults from intact and stepparent families and relationships between perceived parenting and personality. *Personality and Individual Differences, 27,* 453–476.

Leckman, J. F., Gershon, E. S., Nichols, A. S., & Murphy, D. L. (1977). Reduced MAO activity in first degree relatives of individuals with bipolar affective disorders. *Archives of General Psychiatry, 34,* 601–606.

Lidberg, L., Modlin, I., Oreland, L., Tuck, J. R., & Gillner, A. (1985). Platelet monoamine oxidase and psychopathy. *Psychiatry Research, 16,* 339–343.

Limson, R., Goldman, D., Roy, A., Lamparski, D., Ravitz, B., Adinoff, B., et al. (1991). Personality and cerebrospinal monoamine metabolites in alcoholics and normals. *Archives of General Psychiatry, 48,* 437–441.

Loehlin, J. C. (1992). *Genes and environment in personality development.* Newbury Park, CA: Sage.

Lukas, J. H., & Siegel, J. (1977). Cortical mechanisms that augment or reduce evoked potentials in cats. *Science, 196,* 73–75.

Major, L. F., & Murphy, D. L. (1978). Platelet and plasma amine oxidase activity in alcoholic individuals. *British Journal of Psychiatry, 132,* 548–554.

McCrae, R. R. (2004). Human nature and culture: A trait perspective. *Journal of Research in Personality, 38,* 3–14.

Murphy, D. L., Aulakh, C. S., Garrick, N. A., & Sunderland, T. (1987). Monoamine oxidase inhibitors as antidepressants: Implications for the mechanism of action of antidepressants and the psychology of affective disorders and some related disorders. In H. Y. Meltzer (Ed.), *Psychopharmacology: The third generation of progress* (pp. 545–552). New York: Raven Press.

Murphy, D. L., & Weiss, R. (1972). Reduced monoamine oxidase activity in blood platelets from bipolar depressed patients. *American Journal of Psychiatry, 128,* 1351–1357.

Neary, R. S., & Zuckerman, M. (1976). Sensation seeking trait and state anxiety, and the electrodermal orienting reflex. *Psychophysiology, 13,* 205–211.

Netter, P., Hennig, J., & Roed, I. S. (1996). Serotonin and dopamine as mediators of sensation seeking behavior. *Neuropsychobiology, 34,* 155–165.

O'Carroll, R. E. (1984). Androgen administration to hypogonadal and eugonadal men: Effects on measures of sensation seeking, personality and spatial ability. *Personality and Individual Differences, 5,* 595–598.

Orlebeke, J. F., & Feij, J. A. (1979). The orienting reflex as a personality correlate. In E. H. van Holst & J. F. Orlebeke (Eds.), *The orienting reflex in humans* (pp. 567–585). Hillsdale, NJ: Erlbaum.

Reist, C., Haier, R. J., De Met, E., & Cicz-De Met, A. (1990). Platelet MAO activity in personality disorders and normal controls. *Psychiatry Research, 30,* 221–227.

Ridgeway, D., & Hare, R. D. (1981). Sensation seeking and psychophysiological responses to auditory stimulation. *Psychophysiology, 18,* 613–618.

Saxton, P. M., Siegel, J., & Lukas, J. H. (1987). Visual evoked potential augmenting-reducing slopes in cats: 2. Correlations with behavior. *Personality and Individual Differences, 8,* 511–519.

Schinka, J. A., Letsch, E. A., & Crawford, F. C. (2002). DRD4 and novelty seeking: Results of meta-analyses. *American Journal of Medical Genetics, 114,* 643–648.

Schuckit, M. A. (1994). Familial alcoholism. In T. A. Widiger, A. J. Francis, H. A. Pincus, M. B. First, R. Ross, & W. Davis (Eds.), *DSM-IV sourcebook* (Vol. 1, pp. 159–167). Washington, DC: American Psychiatric Association.

Shekim, W. O., Bylund, D. B., Alexson, J., Glaser, R. D., Jones, S. B., Hodges, K., et al. (1986). Platelet MAO and measures of attention and impulsivity in boys with attention deficit and hyperactivity. *Psychiatry Research, 18,* 179–188.

Sher, K. J. (1993). Children of alcoholics and the intergenerational transmission of alcoholism: A biopsychosocial perspective. In J. S. Baer, A. Marlatt, & R. J. McMahon (Eds.), *Addictive behaviors across the life span* (pp. 3–33). Newbury Park, CA: Sage.

Siegel, J., Sisson, D. F., & Driscoll, P. (1993). Augmenting and reducing of visual evoked potentials in Roman High- and Low-Avoidance rats. *Physiology and Behavior, 54,* 707–711.

Smith, B. D., Perlstein, W. M., Davidson, R. A., & Michael, K. (1986). Sensation seeking: Differential effects of novel stimulation on electrodermal activity. *Personality and Individual Differences, 4,* 445–452.

Stelmack, R. M. (Ed.). (2004). *On the psychobiology of personality: Essays in honor of Marvin Zuckerman.* New York: Elsevier.

Strobel, A., Debener, S., Schmidt, D., Hünnerkopf, R., Lesch, K. P., & Brocke, B. (2003). Allelic variation in serotonin transporter function associated with the intensity dependence of the auditory evoked potential. *American Journal of Medical Genetics: Part B. Neuropsychiatric Genetics, 118B,* 41–47.

Thornquist, M. H., & Zuckerman, M. (1995). Psychopathy, passive-avoidance learning and basic dimensions of personality. *Personality and Individual Differences, 19,* 525–534.

Von Knorring, L., & Johansson, F. (1980). Changes in the augmenter–reducer tendency and in pain measures as a result of treatment with a serotonin reuptake inhibitor—zimelidine. *Neuropsychobiology, 6,* 313–478.

Von Knorring, L., Oreland, L., & Von Knorring, A. L. (1987). Personality traits and platelet MAO activity in alcohol and drug abusing teenage boys. *Acta Psychiatrica Scandinavica, 75,* 307–314.

Von Knorring, L., & Pervin, C. (1981). Biochemistry of the augmenting-reducing response in visual evoked potentials. *Neuropsychobiology, 7,* 1–8.

Wang, S., Mason, J., Charney, D., & Yehuda, R. (1997). Relationships between hormonal profile and novelty seeking in combat-related posttraumatic stress disorder. *Biological Psychiatry, 41,* 145–151.

Zuckerman, M. (1969). Theoretical formulations. In J. P. Zubek (Ed.), *Sensory deprivation: Fifteen years of research* (pp. 407–432). New York: Appleton-Century-Crofts.

Zuckerman, M. (1979). *Sensation seeking: Beyond the optimal level of arousal.* Hillsdale, NJ: Erlbaum.

Zuckerman, M. (1990). The psychophysiology of sensation seeking. *Journal of Personality, 58,* 313–345.

Zuckerman, M. (1994). *Behavioral expressions and biosocial bases of sensation seeking*. New York: Cambridge University Press.

Zuckerman, M. (1995). Good and bad humors: Biochemical bases of personality and its disorders. *Psychological Science, 6,* 325–332.

Zuckerman, M. (1996). The psychobiological model for impulsive unsocialized sensation seeking: A comparative approach. *Neuropsychobiology, 34,* 125–129.

Zuckerman, M. (2002). Personality and psychopathy: Shared behavioral and biological traits. In J. Glicksohn (Ed.), *Neurobiology of criminal behavior* (pp. 27–49). Boston: Kluwer Academic.

Zuckerman, M. (2003). Biological bases of personality. In I. B. Weiner (Series Ed.) and T. Millon & M. J. Lerner (Vol. Eds.), *Handbook of psychology: Vol. 5. Personality and social psychology* (pp. 85–116). New York: Wiley.

Zuckerman, M., Ballenger, J. C., & Post, R. M. (1984). The neurobiology of some dimensions of personality. In J. R. Smythies & R. J. Bradley (Eds.), *International review of neurobiology* (Vol. 25, pp. 391–434). New York: Academic Press.

Zuckerman, M., & Cloninger, C. R. (1996). Relationships between Cloninger's, Zuckerman's, and Eysenck's dimensions of personality. *Personality and Individual Differences, 21,* 283–285.

Zuckerman, M., Murtaugh, T. T., & Siegel, J. (1974). Sensation seeking and cortical augmenting–reducing. *Psychophysiology, 11,* 535–542.

Zuckerman, M., Simons, R. F., & Como, P. G. (1988). Sensation seeking and stimulus intensity as modulators of cortical, cardiovascular, and electrodermal response: A cross modality study. *Personality and Individual Differences, 9,* 361–372.

Zuckerman, M., Tushup, R., & Finner, S. (1976). Sexual attitudes and experience: Attitude and personality correlations and changes produced by a course in sexuality. *Journal of Consulting and Clinical Psychology, 44,* 7–19.

Zureik, J. L., & Meltzer, H. Y. (1988). Platelet MAO activity in hallucinating and paranoid schizophrenics. A review and meta-analysis. *Biological Psychiatry, 24,* 63–78.

4

Interpersonal Behavior and the Structure of Personality

NEUROBEHAVIORAL FOUNDATION OF AGENTIC EXTRAVERSION AND AFFILIATION

Richard A. Depue

The structure of temperament and personality consists of a relatively small number (four or five) of higher-order traits. As originally proposed by Gray (1973) and extended by others (Cloninger, 1986; Depue & Collins, 1999; Depue & Morrone-Strupinsky, 2005; Netter et al., 1996; White & Depue, 1999; Zuckerman, 1994), higher-order traits reflect emotional–motivational systems that evolved to increase adaptation to classes of stimuli associated with positive and negative reinforcement. Individual differences in personality traits thereby reflect variation in the sensitivity to such stimuli, and, overall, personality represents the relative strength of sensitivities to various stimulus classes. Within this framework, "sensitivity" ultimately means reactivity of neurobiological processes closely associated with a motivational system.

In view of the interdependence of personality traits, reinforcing stimuli, and motivational systems, it is not surprising that the higher-order structure of personality is substantially associated with the domain of interpersonal behavior. Other people are critical to the preservation of our species in mating, caring for offspring, and providing the social cooperation required in tasks critical to survival. Until relatively recently, the interpersonal domain of personality was embodied largely in one higher-order trait termed "extraversion," which, despite terminological variation, is identified in virtually every taxonomy of personality (Digman, 1997; Tellegen & Waller, in press).

60

More recent structural work in personality, including a five-factor structure of personality, has demonstrated that the interpersonal nature of extraversion is not unitary, but rather is composed of two independent higher-order traits (Digman, 1997; Tellegen & Waller, in press). One trait has been variably called "communion," "social closeness," and "agreeableness" (in the five-factor model), but my colleagues and I prefer the more generic term "affiliation" to maintain a conceptual bridge to animal neurobehavioral work (Carter, Lederhendler, & Kirkpatrick, 1997). Affiliation reflects enjoying and valuing close interpersonal bonds, and being warm and affectionate. The other trait associated with extraversion, "agency," reflects social dominance and the enjoyment of leadership roles, assertiveness, and a subjective sense of potency in accomplishing goals. These two traits are consistent with the two major independent traits identified in the theory of interpersonal behavior: "warm–agreeable" and "assured–dominant" (Wiggins, 1991). These latter two traits are poles of the two major orthogonal dimensions in Figure 4.1, and they are accompanied by two additional traits identified by Wiggins that further characterize interpersonal behavior: "gregarious–extraverted" (vs. "aloof") and "arrogant" (vs. "unassuming"). Within this multidimensional structure (referred to as a "circumplex"), much of interpersonal behavior can be represented as a combination of the two major traits.

Church and Burke (1994) supported a two-trait structure of extraversion by demonstrating that the lower-order traits of extraversion measured by the NEO Personality Inventory factored into agency (assertiveness, activity) and affiliation (warmth, positive emotions, agreeableness). Furthermore, when general affiliation and agency traits were derived in joint factor analyses of several multidimensional personality questionnaires (Church, 1994; Tellegen & Waller, in press), two general traits were identified in each case as affiliation and agency. This made it possible to plot the loadings of lower-order traits from several studies in relation to the general affiliation and agency traits (see Appendix A in Depue & Morrone-Strupinsky, 2005). When trait loadings are plotted from different studies, the interrelations among traits will only be approximations in a quantitative sense, but the pattern with respect to the general affiliation and agency traits is instructive. For purposes of comparison, the lower-order traits are plotted within the interpersonal trait structure of Wiggins (1991) in Figure 4.1. Lower-order traits of achievement, persistence, social dominance, and activity all load much more strongly on agency than on affiliation, whereas traits of sociability and agreeableness show a reverse pattern. Lower-order traits of well-being and positive emotions are associated with both agency and affiliation about equally, which is probably why affiliation and agency were combined in extraversion previously. But when positive emotion components are statistically removed, the associations among affiliative and agentic scales approach zero (range = .11– –.08; Watson & Clark, 1997). Similar independence of affiliative and agentic traits have been demon-

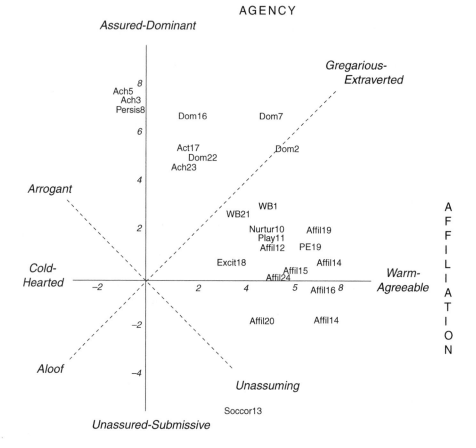

FIGURE 4.1. A structure of interpersonal behavior composed of four adjective-labeled dimensions, with the two predominant orthogonal dimensions labeled "Agency" and "Affiliation." The figure illustrates that the interpersonal engagement characteristic of extraversion is composed of two different dispositions of affiliation and agency. Within the structure, lower-order traits representing either agency or affiliation components of extraversion are plotted according to their loadings on the general agency and affiliation traits derived in several studies. See Appendix A in Depue and Morrone-Strupinsky (2005) for the identity of the abbreviations of trait measures (shown with numbers), the questionnaires to which the abbreviations correspond, and the studies providing the trait loadings.

strated by analysis of peer ratings after extensive social interaction experience (Hurley, 1998), and the human psychometric studies are supported by comparative studies in nonhuman personality, including the use of primates, where independent affiliative and agentic traits have been demonstrated. Indeed, Gosling (2001) has argued that the traits of sociability (affiliation) and confidence (agency) are fairly widespread in the animal kingdom.

ASSOCIATION OF AGENTIC EXTRAVERSION AND AFFILIATION WITH TWO NEUROBEHAVIORAL SYSTEMS

Behavioral systems may be understood as behavior patterns that evolved to adapt to stimuli critical for survival and species preservation (Gray, 1973; MacLean, 1986). As opposed to specific behavioral systems that guide interaction with very specific stimulus contexts, *general* behavioral systems are more flexible, and have less immediate objectives and more variable topographies. General systems are activated by broad classes of stimuli (Depue & Collins, 1999; Gray, 1973), and regulate general emotional–behavioral dispositions, such as desire–approach, fear–inhibition, or affiliative tendencies, that modulate goal-directed activity. The general systems are what directly influence the structure of mammalian behavior at higher-order levels of organization, because, like higher-order personality traits, their pervasive modulatory effects on behavior derive from frequent activation by broad stimulus classes. *Thus the higher-order traits of personality, which are general and few, most likely reflect the activity of the few general neurobehavioral systems.*

We have suggested that the two traits of agentic extraversion and affiliation reflect the activity of two neurobehavioral systems involved in guiding behavior to *rewarding* goals (Depue & Collins, 1999; Depue & Morrone-Strupinsky, 2005). Reward involves several dynamically interacting neurobehavioral processes occurring across two phases of goal acquisition: appetitive and consummatory. Although both phases are elicited by unconditioned incentive (reward-connoting) stimuli, their temporal onset, behavioral manifestations, and putative neural systems differ (Berridge, 1999; Depue & Collins, 1999; DiChiara & North, 1992; Wyvell & Berridge, 2000), and they are dissociated in factor-analytic studies based on behavioral characteristics of animals (Pfaus, Smith, & Coopersmith, 1999).

An appetitive, preparatory phase of goal acquisition represents the first step toward attaining biologically important goals (Hillard, Domjan, Nguyen, & Cusato, 1998). It is based on a mammalian behavioral system that is activated by, and serves to bring an animal into contact with, unconditioned and conditioned rewarding incentive stimuli. This system is consistently described in all animals across phylogeny, and we define this system as "behavioral approach based on incentive motivation" (Depue & Collins, 1999).

The nature of this behavioral system, as well as the system associated with a consummatory phase of reward (discussed next), can be most efficiently described by using an affiliative object (e.g., a potential mate) as the rewarding goal object. Thus an affiliative goal is used throughout this and the next sections. In the appetitive phase of affiliation (see Figure 4.2), specific, *distal* affiliative stimuli of potential bonding partners (e.g., facial features and smiles, friendly vocalizations and gestures, and bodily features; Porges, 2001) serve as unconditioned incentive stimuli based on their distinct patterns of sensory properties, such as smell, color, shape, and temperature (DiChiara & North, 1992; Hilliard et al., 1998). For instance, Breiter, Aharon, Kahneman, Dale, and Shizgal (2001) and Aharon and colleagues (2001) have shown that even passive viewing of attractive female faces unconditionally activates the anatomical areas that integrate reward, incentive motivation, and approach behavior in heterosexual males. These incentives are inherently evaluated as positive in valence, and activate incentive motivation, increased energy through sympathetic nervous system activity, and forward locomotion as a means of bringing individuals into close proximity (DiChiara & North, 1992). Moreover, the incentive state is inherently rewarding but in a highly activated manner, and animals will work intensively to obtain that reward without evidence of satiety (Depue & Collins, 1999).

In humans, the incentive state is associated with subjective feelings of desire, wanting, excitement, elation, enthusiasm, energy, potency, and self-efficacy; these are distinct from, but typically co-occur with, feelings of pleasure and liking (Berridge, 1999; Watson & Tellegen, 1985). This subjective experience is concordant with the nature of the lower-order traits of social dominance, achievement, endurance, persistence, efficacy, activity, and energy that all load strongly on the agency personality factor, and with the adjectives defining the subjective state of positive affect that is so closely associated with agentic extraversion ("activated," "peppy," "strong," "enthused," "energetic"; Watson & Tellegen, 1985). Therefore, we have proposed that agentic extraversion reflects the activity of a behavioral approach system based on *positive incentive motivation*.

When close proximity to a rewarding goal is achieved, the incentive-motivational approach gives way to a consummatory phase of goal acquisition (Herbert, 1993). In this phase, specific *interoceptive* and *proximal exteroceptive* stimuli related to critical primary biological aims elicit behavioral patterns that are relatively specific to those conditions (e.g., sexual, social, or food-related) (Hilliard et al., 1998; MacLean, 1986; Timberlake & Silva, 1995). Performance of these behavioral patterns is inherently rewarding (Berridge, 1999). In the case of potential mate acquisition, examples of affiliative behavioral patterns are courtship, gentle stroking and grooming, actual mating, and certain maternal patterns such as breastfeeding, all of which may include facial, caressive tactile, gestural, and certain vocal behaviors (Polan & Hofer, 1998). Tactile stimulation may be particularly effective in activating affiliative reward processes in animals and

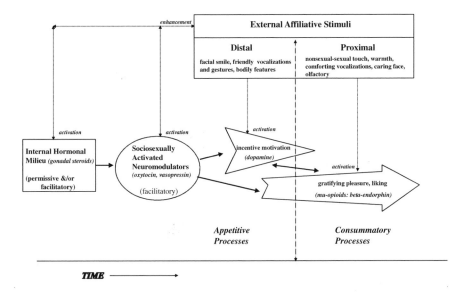

FIGURE 4.2. The development and maintenance of affiliative bonds across two phases of reward. Distal affiliative stimuli elicit an incentive-motivated approach to an affiliative goal, accompanied by strong emotional–motivational feelings of wanting, desire, and positive activation. The approach phase ensures not only sociosexual interaction with an affiliative object, but also acquisition of a memory ensemble or network of the context in which approach, reward, and goal acquisition occur. Next, proximal affiliative stimuli emanating from interaction with the affiliative object elicit strong feelings of consummatory reward, liking, and physiological quiescence, all of which become associated with these stimuli as well as with the context predictive of reward. As discussed in text, dopamine encodes the incentive salience of contextual stimuli predictive of reward during the approach phase and, in collaboration with μ-opiate-mediated consummatory reward, encodes the incentive salience of proximal stimuli directly linked to the affiliative object. The end result of this sequence of processes is an incentive-encoded affiliative memory network that continues to motivate approach toward and interaction with the affiliative object. Specialized processes ensure that affiliative stimuli are weighted as significant elements in the contextual ensembles representing affiliative memory networks. These specialized processes include the construction of a contextual ensemble via affiliative stimulus-induced opiate potentiation of dopamine processes, and the influence of permissive and/or facilitatory factors such as gonadal steroids, oxytocin, and vasopressin on (1) sensory, perceptual, and attentional processing of affiliative stimuli; and (2) formation of social memories. See Depue and Morrone-Strupinsky (2005) for details. From Depue and Lenzenweger (2005, p. 398). Copyright 2005 by The Guilford Press. Reprinted by permission.

humans (Fleming, Korsmit, & Dellard, 1994). Significantly, light, pleasant touch, such as that occurring in caress-like, skin-to-skin contact between individuals, is transmitted by different afferents than hard or unpleasant touch (Olausson et al., 2002). Light, pleasant touch is transmitted by slow-conducting unmyelinated afferents that project to the insular cortex but not to somatosensory areas S1 and S2, whereas hard, unpleasant touch is transmitted by fast-conducting myelinated afferents to anterior insular cortex. The insular cortex is a paralimbic region known to integrate several sensory modalities, including autonomic, gustatory, visual, auditory, and somatosensory, in order to characterize the emotional nature of sensory input (Damasio, 2003).

As opposed to an incentive-motivational state of activation, desire, and wanting, the expression of *consummatory* behavioral patterns elicits intense feelings of pleasure, gratification, and liking, plus physiological quiescence characterized by rest, sedation, anabolism, and parasympathetic nervous system activity, thereby reinforcing the production and repetition of those behaviors (Adolphs, 2003; Berridge, 1999; DiChiara & North, 1992; Porges, 2001). Thus, whereas appetitive approach processes bring an individual into contact with unconditioned incentive stimuli, consummatory processes bring behavior to a gratifying conclusion (Hilliard et al., 1998). Whether the pleasurable state generated in affiliative interactions shares a common neurobiology with the pleasure generated by other consummatory behaviors (e.g., feeding) is not certain, but it is assumed by some to be so (DiChiara & North, 1992; Panksepp, 1998).

The core content of affiliation scales seems to reflect the operation of neurobehavioral processes that (1) create a warm, affectionate, gratifying subjective emotional state elicited by others, which (2) motivate close interpersonal behavior. Our hypothesis is that the subjective experience of warmth and affection reflects the capacity to experience consummatory *reward* that is elicited by a broad array of affiliative stimuli (Depue & Morrone-Strupinsky, 2005). This capacity is viewed as providing the key element utilized in additional psychobiological processes that permit the development and maintenance of longer-term affective bonds—defined as the long-term selective social attachments that are observed most intensely between infants and parents and between adult mates, and that are characteristic of social organization in human and other primate societies (Gingrich, Liu, Cascio, Wang, & Insel, 2000). It is important to emphasize that a core capacity for affiliative reward and bonding is not viewed as a sufficient determinant of close social relationships—only as a necessary one, a sine qua non. Such affiliative reward is hypothesized to underlie all human social relationships having a positive affective component. Other interpersonal constructs of sociability, attachment, and separation anxiety are accordingly viewed as either broader than affiliation as defined here, and/or as based on different neurobehavioral systems (see Depue & Morrone-Strupinsky, 2005, for a full discussion).

NEUROBIOLOGY OF INCENTIVE MOTIVATION AND AFFILIATIVE REWARD

By drawing an association between traits and behavioral systems—agentic extraversion and incentive motivation, affiliation and affiliative reward—we are able to utilize the literature on behavioral neurobiology in animals to discern the neurobiology associated with these behavioral systems and, by analogy, with the personality traits of agentic extraversion and affiliation. As reviewed recently (Depue & Collins, 1999), animal research demonstrates that the positive incentive motivation and experience of reward that underlies a behavioral system of approach is dependent on the functional properties of the midbrain ventral tegmental area (VTA) dopamine (DA) projection system. DA agonists or antagonists in the VTA or nucleus accumbens (NA), which is a major terminal area of VTA DA projections, in rats and monkeys facilitate or markedly impair, respectively, a broad array of incentive-motivated behaviors. Furthermore, dose-dependent DA receptor activation in the VTA-NA pathway facilitates the acute rewarding effects of stimulants, and the NA is a particularly strong site for intracranial self-administration of DA agonists (Le Moal & Simon, 1991; Pich et al., 1997). DA agonists injected into the NA also modulate behavioral responses to *conditioned* incentive stimuli in a dose-dependent fashion (Cador, Taylor, & Robbins, 1991; Wolterink, Cador, Wolterink, Robbins, & Everitt, 1989). In single-unit recording studies, VTA DA neurons are activated preferentially by appetitive incentive stimuli (Schultz, Dayan, & Montague, 1997). DA cells, most numerously in the VTA, respond vigorously to and in proportion to the magnitude of both conditioned and unconditioned incentive stimuli and in anticipation of reward (Schultz et al., 1997).

Finally, incentive motivation is associated in humans with both positive *emotional* feelings such as elation and euphoria, and *motivational* feelings of desire, wanting, craving, potency, and self-efficacy. In humans, DA-activating psychostimulant drugs induce both sets of feelings (Drevets et al., 2001). Also, neuroimaging studies of subjects addicted to cocaine found that during acute administration, the intensity of a subject's subjective euphoria increased in a dose-dependent manner in proportion to cocaine binding to the DA uptake transporter (and hence to DA levels) in the striatum (Volkow et al., 1997). Moreover, cocaine-induced activity in the NA was linked equally strongly (if not more strongly) to motivational feelings of desire, wanting, and craving, as to the emotional experience of euphoric rush (Breiter et al., 1997). And the degree of amphetamine-induced DA release in healthy human ventral striatum assessed by positron emission tomography was correlated strongly with feelings of euphoria (Drevets et al., 2001). Hence, taken together, the animal and human evidence demonstrates that the VTA DA-NA pathway is a primary neural circuit for incentive motivation and its accompanying subjective state of reward.

With respect to consummatory reward and affiliative behavior, a broad range of evidence suggests a role for endogenous opiates. Endogenous opiate release or receptor binding is increased in rats, monkeys, and humans by lactation and nursing, sexual activity, vaginocervical stimulation, maternal social interaction, brief social isolation, and grooming and other nonsexual tactile stimulation (Depue & Morrone-Strupinsky, 2005; Keverne, 1996; Silk, Alberts, & Altmann, 2003). The opiate receptor (OR) antagonists naltrexone and naloxone in small doses apparently reduce the reward derived from social interactions, since they increase attempts to obtain such reward, manifested as increases in (1) the amount of maternal contact by young monkeys, and (2) solicitations for grooming and frequency of being groomed in mature female monkeys, which have been associated with increased cerebrospinal fluid levels of β-endorphin (Graves, Wallen, & Maestripieri, 2002; Martel, Nevison, Simpson, & Keverne, 1995). In addition, the endogenous opiate β-endorphin stimulates play behavior and grooming in juvenile rats, whereas naltrexone leads to reduced grooming of infants and other group members in monkeys and rats, and to maternal neglect in monkeys and sheep that is similar to the neglect shown by human mothers who abuse opiates (Keverne, 1996; Martel et al., 1995). Similarly, human females who were administered the opiate antagonist naltrexone showed an increased amount of time spent alone, a reduced amount of time spent with friends, and a reduced frequency and pleasantness of their social interactions relative to females receiving a placebo (Depue & Morrone-Strupinsky, 2005). Such findings suggest that opiates provide a critical part of the neural basis on which primate sociality has evolved (Nelson & Panksepp, 1998). Particularly important is the relation between μ-opiates and grooming, because the primary function of primate grooming may well be to establish and maintain social bonds (Matheson & Bernstein, 2000).

Perhaps most relevant to affiliative reward is the mu (μ) OR family, which is the main site for the effects of exogenously administered opiate drugs (e.g., morphine) and of endogenous endorphins (particularly β-endorphin) (LaBuda, Sora, Uhl, & Fuchs, 2000; Schlaepfer et al., 1998; Shippenberg & Elmer, 1998; Stefano et al., 2000; Wiedenmayer & Barr, 2000). μORs also appear to be the main site for the effects of endogenous β-endorphins and endogenous morphine on the subjective feelings in humans of increased interpersonal warmth, euphoria, well-being, and peaceful calmness, as well as of decreased elation, energy, and incentive motivation (Schlaepfer et al., 1998; Shippenberg & Elmer, 1998; Stefano et al., 2000).

The facilitatory effects of opiates on affiliative behavior are thought to be exerted by fibers that arise mainly from the hypothalamic arcuate nucleus and terminate in brain regions that typically express μORs. μORs may facilitate the rewarding effects associated with many motivated behaviors (Nelson & Panksepp, 1998; Niesink, Vanderschuen, & van Ree, 1996; Olive, Koenig, Nannini, & Hodge, 2001; Olson, Olson, & Kastin, 1997; Stefano et al., 2000). For instance, whereas DA antagonists block appetitive behaviors in pursuit of reward but not the acutal consumption of reward (e.g., sucrose;

Ikemoto & Panksepp, 1996), µOR antagonists block rewarding effects of sucrose and sexual behavior, and in neonatal rats persistently impair the response to the inherently rewarding properties of novel stimulation (Herz, 1998). Rewarding properties of µOR agonists are directly indicated by the fact that animals will work for the prototypical µOR agonists morphine and heroin, and that they are dose-dependently self-administered in animals and humans (Di Chiara, 1995; Nelson & Panksepp, 1998; Olson et al., 1997; Shippenberg & Elmer, 1998). There is a significant correlation between an agonist's affinity at the µOR and the dose that maintains maximal rates of drug self-administration behavior (Shippenberg & Elmer, 1998).

The rewarding effects of opiates may be especially mediated by µORs located in the NA and VTA, both of which support self-administration of µOR agonists that is attenuated by intracranially administered µOR antagonists (David & Cazola, 2000; Herz, 1998; Schlaepfer et al., 1998; Shippenberg & Elmer, 1998). When opiate and DA antagonists were given prior to cocaine or heroin self-administration, the opiate antagonist selectively altered opiate self-administration, while DA antagonists selectively altered the response to the DA agonist cocaine (Shippenberg & Elmer, 1998). Destruction of DA terminals in the NA also showed that opiate self-administration is independent of DA function, at least at the level of the NA (Dworkin, Guerin, Goeders, & Smith, 1988). Furthermore, NA DA functioning was specifically related to the incentive salience of reward cues, but was unrelated to the hedonic state generated by consuming the rewards (Wyvell & Berridge, 2000). *Thus DA and opiates appear to interact functionally in the NA, but they apparently provide independent contributions to rewarding effects.* This appears to be particularly the case for the *acute* rewarding effects of opiates, which are thought to occur through a DA-independent system that is mediated through brainstem reward circuits, including the tegmental pedunculo-pontine nucleus (Laviolette, Gallegos, Henriksen, & van der Kooy, 2004).

Rewarding effects of opiates are also directly indicated by the fact that a range of µOR agonists, when injected intracerebroventricularly or directly into the NA, serve as unconditioned rewarding stimuli in a dose-dependent manner in producing a conditioned place preference—a behavioral measure of reward (Narita, Aoki, & Suzuki, 2000; Nelson & Panksepp, 1998; Shippenberg & Elmer, 1998). VTA-localized µORs, particularly in the rostral zone of the VTA (Carlezon et al., 2000), mediate (1) rewarding effects such as self-administration behavior and conditioned place preference (Carlezon et al., 2000; Shippenberg & Elmer, 1998; Wise, 1998); (2) increased sexual activity and maternal behaviors (Callahan, Baumann, & Rabil, 1996; van Furth & van Ree, 1996); and (3) the persistently increased play behavior, social grooming, and social approach of rats subjected to morphine *in utero* (Hol, Niesink, van Ree, & Spruijt, 1996). Indeed, microinjections of morphine or a selective µOR agonist into the VTA produced marked place preferences, whereas selective antagonism of µORs prevented morphine-induced conditioned place preference. Indeed, transgenic mice lacking the μOR gene show neither morphine-induced place preferences nor physical dependence from morphine consumption, whereas morphine induces both of these behaviors in wild-type mice (Matthes et al., 1996; Simonin et al., 1998). And significantly, opiate but not oxytocin antagonists block the development of partner preference that is induced specifically by *repeated* exposure and *repeated* sexual activity in rodents (Carter et al., 1997).

An *interaction* of DA and μ-opiates in the experience of reward throughout appetitive and consummatory phases of affiliative engagement appears to involve two processes. During the anticipatory phase of goal acquisition, μOR activation in the VTA can increase DA release in the NA and hence the experience of reward (Marinelli & White, 2000). Subsequently, the firing rate of VTA neurons decreases following delivery and consumption of appetitive reinforcers (e.g., food, sex, liquid) (Schultz et al., 1997). At the same time, μOR activation in the NA (perhaps by opiate release from higher-threshold NA terminals that colocalize DA and opiates; Le Moal & Simon, 1991) decreases NA DA release, creating an opiate-mediated experience of reward associated with consummation that is independent of DA. Thus, in contrast to the incentive-motivational effects of DA during the anticipation of reward, opiates may subsequently induce calm pleasure and bring consummatory behavior to a gratifying conclusion. This may explain the fact that higher doses of μOR agonists administered into the NA can block the self-administration of certain psychostimulant drugs of abuse in animals and reduce appetitive behaviors (Johnson & Ait-Daoud, 2000; Kranzler, 2000).

In sum, as illustrated in Figure 4.2, distal affiliative cues (e.g., friendly smiles and gestures, sexual features) serve as incentive stimuli that activate DA-facilitated incentive/reward motivation, desire, wanting, and approach to affiliative objects. As these objects are reached, more proximal affiliative stimuli (e.g., pleasant touch) strongly activate μ-opiate release, which promotes an intense state of pleasant reward, warmth, affection, and physiological quiescence, and brings approach behavior to a gratifying conclusion.

INDIVIDUAL DIFFERENCES IN DA INCENTIVE AND μOR REWARD PROCESSES

Individual differences in agentic extraversion and affiliation are subject to strong genetic influence (Tellegen et al., 1988). Animal research demonstrates, as does much human work, that individual differences in DA functioning contribute significantly to variation in incentive-motivated behavior (Depue & Collins, 1999; Depue, Luciana, Arbisi, Collins, & Leon, 1994). Inbred mouse and rat strains with variation in the number of neurons in the VTA DA cell group or in several indicators of enhanced DA transmission show marked differences in behaviors dependent on DA transmission in the VTA-NA pathway, including levels of spontaneous exploratory activity and DA agonist-induced locomotor activity, and increased acquisition of self-administration of psychostimulants (Depue & Collins, 1999).

Similar findings for μ-opiates exist (Depue & Morrone-Strupinsky, 2005). Individual differences in humans and rodents have been demonstrated in levels of μOR expression and binding that are associated with a preference for μOR agonists such as morphine (Uhl, Sora, & Wang, 1999; Zubieta et al., 2001). In humans, individual differences in central nervous system (CNS) μOR densities show a range of up to 75% between the lower and upper thirds of the distribution (Uhl et al., 1999)—differences that appear to be related to variation in the rewarding effects of alcohol in humans and rodents (Berrettini, Hoehe, Ferraro, De Maria, & Gottheil, 1997; Olson et al., 1997).

Differences of this magnitude in the *expressive* properties of the μ-OR gene could contribute substantially to individual variation in μOR-induced *behavioral* expression via an effect on β-endorphin functional potency. For instance, one source of this individual variation is different single-nucleotide polymorphisms (SNPs) in the μOR gene, *OPRM1* (Berrettini et al., 1997; Bond et al., 1998; Gelernter, Kranzler, & Cubells, 1999). The most prevalent of these is A118G, which is characterized by a substitution of the amino acid Asn by Asp at codon 40, with an allelic frequency of 10% in a mixed sample of individuals who formerly abused heroin and controls without drug abuse (Bond et al., 1998). Although this SNP did not bind all opiate peptides more strongly than other SNPs or the normal nucleotide sequence, it did bind β-endorphin three times more tightly than the most common allelic form of the receptor (Bond et al., 1998). Furthermore, β-endorphin is three times more effective in agonist-induced activation of G-protein-coupled potassium channels at the A118G, variant receptor, compared to the most common allelic form (Bond et al., 1998).

Genetic variation in μOR properties is related to response to rewarding drugs, such as morphine, alcohol, and cocaine, and to opiate self-administration behavior in animals (Berrettini et al., 1997). For instance, when transgenic insertion was used to increase μOR density specifically in mesolimbic areas thought to mediate substance abuse via VTA DA neurons, transgenic mice showed increased self-administration of morphine compared to wild-type mice, even when the amount of behavior required to maintain drug intake increased 10-fold (Elmer, Pieper, Goldberg, & George, 1995). Thus the efficacy of morphine as a reinforcer was substantially enhanced in transgenic mice. Conversely, μOR knockout mice do not develop conditioned place preference and physical dependence on morphine, whereas morphine induces both of these behaviors in wild-type mice (Matthes et al., 1996).

Taken together, these studies suggest that genetic variation in DA and μOR properties in humans and rodents (1) is substantial; (2) is an essential element in the variation in the rewarding value of DA and opiate agonists; and (3) is critical in accounting for variation in the Pavlovian learning that underlies the association between contextual cues and reward, as occurs in partner and place preferences (Elmer et al., 1995; Matthes et al., 1996). This lack of response to reward in μOR knockout mice apparently interferes with the association of cues emanating from mother mice, since μOR knockout infant mice fail to bond to their mothers (Moles, Kieffer, & D'Amato, 2004). This latter finding provides direct support for our hypothesis that μOR activation serves as a critical factor in affiliative reward and bonding (Depue & Morrone-Strupinsky, 2005).

CONCEPTUALIZING INDIVIDUAL DIFFERENCES UNDERLYING EXTRAVERSION AND AFFILIATION

Elicitation of behavior can be modeled neurobiologically by use of a minimum threshold construct, which represents a CNS weighting of the external and internal factors that contribute to the probability of response expression (Depue & Collins, 1999; Depue & Morrone-Strupinsky, 2005). A response threshold is weighted most strongly by the joint function of two main variables: (1) magnitude of eliciting stimulation, and (2) level of postsynaptic receptor activation of the neurobiological variable thought to contribute most variance to the behavioral process in question (in our case, this would be DA to incentive motivation and μ-opiates to affiliative reward). The relation between these two variables is represented in Figure 4.3 as a tradeoff function (White, 1986), where pairs of values (of stimulus magnitude and receptor activation) specify a diagonal representing the minimum threshold value for elicitation of a behavioral process. Findings reviewed above show that agonist-induced *state* changes in DA and μOR activation influence the threshold of incentive-motivated behavior and affiliative reward, respectively. Because the two input variables (stimulus magnitude and receptor activation) are interactive, independent variation in either one not only modifies the probability of eliciting the behavioral process, but also simultaneously modifies the value of the other variable that is required to reach a minimum threshold of elicitation.

It is important to note that neurobiological variables that are not directly related to a trait's neurobiological foundation may nonetheless provide a marked influence on a trait's elicitation thresholds. In particular, functional levels of neuromodulators that provide a strong, relatively generalized *tonic inhibitory* influence on responding of many behaviors are good candidates as significant modulators of a response elicitation threshold. We and others (Coccaro & Siever, 1991; Depue & Spoont, 1986; Lesch, 1998; Panksepp, 1998; Spoont, 1992; Zald & Depue, 2001; Zuckerman, 1994) have suggested that serotonin (5-HT), acting at multiple receptor sites in most brain regions, is such a modulator (Azmitia & Whitaker-Azmitia, 1997; Tork, 1990). As reviewed many times in both the animal and human literatures, 5-HT modulates a diverse set of functions—including emotion, motivation, motor, affiliation, cognition, food intake, sleep, sexual activity, and sensory reactivity (Coccaro & Siever, 1991; Depue & Spoont, 1986; Lesch, 1998; Spoont, 1992; Zald & Depue, 2001). Thus 5-HT plays a substantial modulatory role in gen-

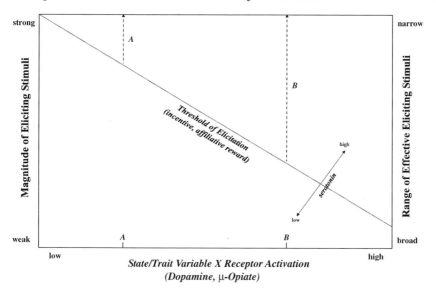

FIGURE 4.3. A minimum threshold for elicitation of a behavioral process (e.g., incentive motivation–positive affect or affiliative reward–affection) is illustrated as a tradeoff function between eliciting stimulus magnitude (left vertical axis) and variable X (e.g., dopamine, μ-opiate) postsynaptic receptor activation (horizontal axis). Range of effective (eliciting) stimuli is illustrated on the right vertical axis as a function of level of receptor activation. Two hypothetical individuals with low and high trait postsynaptic receptor activation (demarcated on the horizontal axis as A and B, respectively) are shown to have narrow (A) and broad (B) ranges of effective stimuli, respectively. Threshold effects due to serotonin modulation are illustrated as well. From Depue and Lenzenweger (2005, p. 424). Copyright 2005 by The Guilford Press. Adapted by permission.

eral neurobiological functioning that affects many forms of motivated behavior. This effect is illustrated in Figure 4.3, where variation in 5-HT functioning modulates (increases or decreases) the threshold of response elicitation.

A trait dimension of postsynaptic receptor activation of variable X (e.g., DA or μ-opiate) is represented on the horizontal axis of Figure 4.3, where two individuals with divergent trait levels are demarcated: *A* (low trait level) and *B* (high trait level). As Figure 4.3 indicates, for any given eliciting stimulus, the degree of variable *X*'s reactivity will, on average, be larger in individual *B* than in individual *A*.

Hence the subjective emotional and motivational experiences that are facilitated by variable *X* (e.g., incentive, affection) will also be more enhanced in *B* than in *A* (Depue & Collins, 1999; Depue & Morrone-Strupinsky, 2005). In addition, the difference between individuals *A* and *B* in magnitude of subjective experience may contribute to variation in the contemporaneous encoding of a stimulus's intensity or salience (a form of state-dependent learning), and hence in the stimulus's encoded salience in subsequent memory consolidation. Accordingly, individuals *A* and *B* may develop differences in the capacity of mental representations of (incentive, affiliative) contexts to activate the relevant motivational (incentive, affiliative) processes; these differences are significant because of the predominant motivation of behavior in humans by symbolic representations of goals.

If individual differences in encoding apply across the full range of stimulus magnitudes, trait differences in the reactivity of variable *X* may have marked effects on the *range* of effective (i.e., eliciting) stimuli. This is illustrated in Figure 4.3, where the right vertical axis represents the range of effective (eliciting) stimuli. Increasing trait levels of variable *X* (horizontal axis) are associated with an increasing efficacy of weaker stimuli (left vertical axis), and thus with an increasing range of effective stimuli (right vertical axis). In Figure 4.3, individuals *A* and *B* are shown to have a narrow and a broad range, respectively. Significantly, the broader range for individual *B* suggests that, on average, *B* will experience more frequent elicitation of subjective emotional experiences associated with variable *X*'s activity (incentive, affection). This means that the probability at any point in time of being in an *X*-facilitated state for individual *B* is higher than for *A*. Therefore, when subsequent relevant stimuli are encountered, their subjectively evaluated magnitude will show a stronger positive bias for *B* than for *A*. Thus trait differences in variable *X* may *proactively* influence the evaluation and encoding of relevant stimuli, and may not be restricted to *reactive* emotional processes.

DA AND μ-OPIATE FUNCTIONING IN HUMANS IN RELATION TO EXTRAVERSION AND AFFILIATION

The above-described neurobehavioral framework for agentic extraversion and affiliation is based overwhelmingly on the animal literature. There is now a significant need to extend this work to humans. Although this is being done in the area of genetics, especially assessing the relation of polymorphisms in neurotransmitter variables to personality (Munafo et al., 2003), there is a paucity of human research on the manner in which neuromodulators relate to the behavioral variation associated with personality traits. Therefore, we briefly present two recent findings from our laboratory that suggest a strong relation between DA and opiate functioning and interpersonal traits.

DA and Contextual Activation of Extraverted Behavior

Through Pavlovian associative learning, the experience of reward generated throughout appetitive and consummatory phases (Figure 4.2) is associated with previously affectively neutral stimulus contexts (objects, acts, events, places) in which pleasure occurred, thereby forming conditioned incentive stimuli that are predictive of reward, and that have gained the capacity to elicit anticipatory pleasure and incentive motivation (Berridge, 1999; Ostrowski, 1998; Timberlake & Silva, 1995). Because of the predominance of symbolic (conditioned) processes in guiding human behavior in the absence of unconditioned stimuli, conditioned incentives are likely to be particularly important elicitors of *enduring* reward processes. Thus the acquisition and maintenance of a mate relationship, for example, depends closely on Pavlovian associative learning that links the experience of reward with (1) the salient contextual cues that predict reward during the appetitive phase (e.g., features of a laboratory cage), and (2) a mate's individualistic cues associated directly with consummatory reward (e.g., individual characteristics of a sexually receptive female rat) (Domjan, Cusato, & Villareal, 2000). Taken together, the processes described above support acquisition of affiliative memories, where contextual ensembles are formed and weighted in association with the reward provided by interaction with the potential mate.

DA and μ-opiates play a critical role in facilitating long-term associations between contextual cues and reward (Depue & Morrone-Strupinsky, 2005). In the case of DA, when DA agonist drugs are used in a distinctive, neutral context, that context is attributed an incentive salience proportional to the magnitude of drug-induced reward (Kelley, 1999; Robinson & Berridge, 2000). Both the magnitude of incentive salience attributed to drug-paired contexts, and the subsequent contextual facilitation of conditioned responses, are dependent on the degree of stimulation of DA D1 receptors in the NA (Berke & Hyman, 2000; Kelley, 1999; Robinson & Berridge, 2000). This potentially explains why animals with constitutionally elevated activity in VTA DA neurons and/or increased DA release in the NA attribute a markedly enhanced incentive salience to drug-paired contexts (Cabib, 1993; Hooks, Jones, Neill, & Justice, 1992; Jodogne, Marinelli, Le Moal, & Piazza, 1994; Robinson & Berridge, 2000). Conversely, animals with very low DA activity in the NA attribute minimal incentive salience to drug-paired contexts, as shown by little or no contextual facilitation of responding (Cabib, 1993; Hooks et al., 1992; Jodogne et al., 1994; Piazza & Le Moal, 1996). Thus DA modulates the extent to which environmental cues become salient incentives, and hence the extent to which they can subsequently activate behavior.

The trait of extraversion, which indexes human variation in incentive-motivated behavior, is strongly associated with indicators of DA neurotransmission similar to those in animals, including locomotor activity, DA agonist-induced hormonal secretion, and DA receptor functioning (Depue & Collins, 1999; Depue et al., 1994). The importance of such variation is that once incentive salience is reliably associated with a distinctive context, DA release in the NA, the rewarding effects of drugs, and the activation of incentive-motivated behavior can be completely dependent on the facilitating effect of that context (Duvauchelle, Flemming, & Kornetsky, 2000; Koob & Le Moal, 1997). Therefore, humans with opposing extreme levels of extraversion may, as in animals, attribute different degrees of incentive salience to drug- or natural-reward-paired contexts, and hence may vary in the extent to which incentive contexts activate their behavior. Put simply, variation in extraverted behavior may result from differential context–reward conditioning and hence contextual activation of extraverted behavior.

To assess this possibility, we (Depue, Morrone-Strupinsky, & Dahkal, 2005) used a standard, double-blind design with three consecutive phases (Figure 4.4A):

1. *Association*: The potent DA agonist methylphenidate (MP) or placebo (lactose) was associated with a laboratory context for 3 days.
2. *Test*: Contextual facilitation of responding was assessed under MP conditions for all subjects. Because psychostimulants strongly amplify conditioned-cue activation of behavior via DA release in the NA shell (Everitt, Dickinson, & Robbins, 2001; Robinson & Berridge, 2000), all conditions received MP on the test day.
3. *Extinction*: 3 days of placebo. The first extinction day occurred in the absence of unconditioned drug effects, and so would provide direct evidence of a conditioned motivational effect of context (Everitt et al., 2001).

High- and low-extraversion subgroups ("high extraverts" and "low extraverts") were randomly selected from the top and bottom deciles, respectively, of Multidimensional Personality Questionnaire (MPQ) extraversion scores, and then were randomly assigned to the three experimental conditions. The final 55 subjects by subgroup sizes and condition were as follows: low extraverts—paired = 11, unpaired (UP) = 10, placebo (PB) = 4; high extraverts—paired = 16, UP = 10, PB = 4. Males (ages 19–21 years) were used, because DA efficacy varies markedly across the menstrual cycle. The three experimental conditions, each with subgroups of high and low extraverts, either paired MP with a laboratory context (paired) or did not (UP and PB). On each association day, all experimental conditions received MP or placebo in each of two contextually distinct labs (Labs A and B, Figure 4.4A), which equated paired and UP conditions on MP exposure but within different lab contexts (Parkinson, Olmstead, Burns, Robbins, & Everitt, 1999). Following previous research (Anagnostaras & Robinson, 1996), the context of Labs A and B differed in physical dimensions, flooring, wall colors and decorations, lighting, furniture, and research assistants. Participants completed the 2½-hour protocol between noon and 6:00 P.M. for 7 consecutive days.

In addition to general laboratory context, specific isolated drug cues also facilitate conditioned responses (Anagnostaras & Robinson, 1996; Everitt et al., 2001). Therefore, five 15-second audiovisual clips were developed. Three clips were initially incentive-neutral, but differed in their association with drug reward: (1) the front of Cornell's main library (Library), (2) the front of Lab A which subjects faced (LabFront), and (3) a large poster of a female portrait in the front of Lab A (Portrait). Facilitated responding on test day was a direct test was an acquired incentive salience for LabFront and Portrait com-

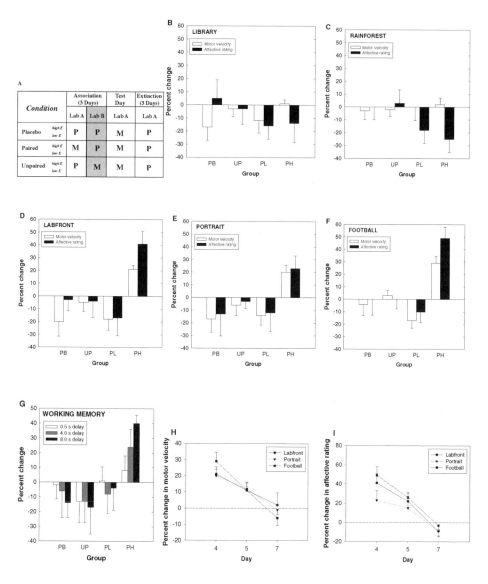

FIGURE 4.4. Contextual facilitation of motor velocity, affect, and visuospatial working memory during association and extinction phases for four groups. (A) Study design and experimental conditions. M, methylphenidate; P, placebo. (B–F) Degree of contextual facilitation (percentage of change in responding from association day 1 to test day) of motor and affective responding to five audiovisual clips. (G) Degree of contextual facilitation of visuospatial working memory accuracy. (H, I) Percentage of change in motor and affective responding on days 4, 5, and 7 compared to day 1. PB, placebo; UP, unpaired; PL, paired low extraverts; PH, paired high extraverts. Adapted with permission of the authors from Depue, Morrone-Strupinsky, and Dahkal (2005).

pared to Library (Everitt et al., 2001). Two additional previously validated (Morrone, Depue, Scherer, & White, 2000) clips had no association with drug reward or general laboratory context, but differed in incentive value: (4) rainforest scenes (Rainforest) and (5) a triumphant football game sequence (Football). Since unconditioned facilitatory effects of psychostimulants on responding depend on the incentive salience of eliciting stimuli (Robinson & Berridge, 2000; Schultz et al., 1997), MP-induced contextual facilitation on test day was expected to potentiate responding to Football but not to Rainforest.

Three variables, each dependent on VTA DA projections to the NA or prefrontal cortex, indexed incentive effects. Two of these variables were measured after each of the video clips. First, motor velocity (which was indexed by finger tapping on a laptop) is specifically related to incentive motivational processes facilitated by DA, predominantly in the NA shell (Depue & Collins, 1999); is activated by drug-associated cues (Berke & Hyman 2000); and correlates ($r = .68$, $p < .01$) with percentage of DA uptake binding in human NA (Volkow, Wang, Fischman, Foltin, & Fowler, 1998). The second variable rated was positive affective activation, which correlates with (1) percentage of DA uptake binding specifically in human NA (Volkow et al., 1997); (2) DA agonist challenge and responses to the video material used here ($r = .57$, $p < .01$) (Depue & Collins, 1999; Morrone et al., 2000); and (3) extraversion ($r = .34$, $p < .01$) (Morrone et al., 2000). The stimulus–response sequence in all conditions was as follows: (1) an audiovisual prompt on a TV monitor, preparing the subject for the video clip; (2) the video clip; (3) positive activation rating (~3 seconds); (4) 6 seconds of tapping, the timing of which started with the first tap and ended with an audio stop beep produced by a laptop; and (5) a 1-minute rest interval.

The third measure, reflecting incentive effects of general laboratory context, used a previously validated (Luciana, Collins, & Depue, 1998) visuospatial delayed-response task to assess working memory. The task is dependent in primates and humans on VTA DA projections to dorsolateral prefrontal cortex that are distinct from VTA DA projections to the NA (Oades & Halladay, 1987). The task involved the following trial sequence, with each subject in a chin–forehead rest with eyes 27 cm from a monochrome computer monitor: (1) a central fixation point for 3 seconds (black "+"); (2) a randomly, peripherally localized visual cue (black circle) within a 360° circumference for 200 milliseconds; (3) randomly presented delay intervals of either 0.5, 4, or 8 seconds (eight trials per delay, each within a different location, two per quadrant); (4) spatial location response with lightpen touching of a computer monitor; and (5) a 2-second intertrial interval. Spatial location error on each trial was calculated by computer, using the Pythagorean theorem.

Tasks and measures occurred only in Lab A over a 1-hour period, beginning 1 hour after drug ingestion. Tasks and measures occurred only on the first association day and on test day, to avoid excessive task repetition. During extinction, motor and affective responses to video clips were measured on the first and final days.

Within the PB and UP conditions, high- and low-extraversion subgroups were combined, since they did not differ statistically in percentage of change from association day 1 to test day on any variable. Statistical analyses of the video clips (Table 4.1) showed that the four groups (PB, UP, PL [paired low extraverts], and PH [paired high extraverts]) did not differ significantly in percentage of change in motor or affective responding for the Library and Rainforest scenes (Figures 4.4B, 4.4C). For the LabFront, Portrait, and Football scenes (Figures 4.4D, 4.4E, and 4.4F), PH showed both a significant increase from day 1 to test day in motor and affective responses to each scene, and also significantly exceeded percentage of change in responding of all other groups to each scene, none of which differed statistically from each other. The increased responding of PH was substantial, ranging from 20% to 52%. For PH, within-subject increases in motor and affective variables were correlated significantly for LabFront ($r = .43$, $p < .05$) and Football ($r = .45$, $p < .05$).

A similar pattern of responding was found for visuospatial working memory (Figure 4.4G, Table 4.2), where only PH showed significant increases in accuracy from day 1 to test day at both 4- and 8-second delays. All other groups decreased in accuracy and did not differ significantly from each other. The percentage of increased accuracy of PH became significantly more marked across the three increasing delay intervals: 8%, 24%, and 40% (Table 4.2). For PH, within-subject increases in 8-second delay accuracy correlated significantly with motor ($r = .41$, $p < .05$) and affective ($r = .46$, $p < .05$) increases to Football.

Because only PH demonstrated conditioning effects (all other groups showed a flat line across days 4–7), only this group's extinction data were analyzed (Figure 4.4H, 4.4I; Table 4.1). Whereas PH showed a significant decrease in responding on the first day of extinction (day 5) relative to test day (day 4) for LabFront, Portrait, and Football, responding on day 5 was significantly greater than on the first association day (day 1) and also than on the last extinction day (day 7) for all three scenes. This pattern indicates that contextual facilitation of conditioned responses occurred on day 5 even in the absence of unconditioned MP effects.

These findings suggest that extraversion is positively related to brain processes that attribute incentive salience to contexts associated with psychostimulant reward. The robustness of this conclusion is indicated by the acquired contextual facilitation across motor, affective, and cognitive processes, and by the magnitude of the enhanced responding by PH on test day, with increases ranging from of 20% to 52%. Several lines of evidence suggest that DA modulation of these brain processes contributes to the relation between extraversion and degree of attributed incentive salience. First, DA functioning in the NA is strongly correlated with the extent of incentive attributed to context in animals (Cabib, 1993; Hooks et al., 1992; Jodogne et al., 1994; Robinson & Berridge, 2000), and subsequently with the efficacy of drug cues to markedly enhance DA release and gene expression in the NA shell (Everitt et al., 2001). Second, MP is a potent DA agonist whose pairing

TABLE 4.1. Statistical Analyses of the Motor Velocity and Affective Ratings for Association and Extinction Phases

	Association phase					
	Motor velocity			Affective rating		
Stimulus	$F(df = 3,51)$	p	Post hoc comparisons	$F(df = 3,51)$	p	Post hoc comparisons
Library	1.919	.138		1.275	.273	
Rainforest	.455	.715		2.033	.121	
LabFront	22.228	.001	PH vs. PL = .001 PH vs. UP = .001 PH vs. PB = .001 None other sig.	14.346	.001	PH vs. PL = .003 PH vs. UP = .001 PH vs. PB = .001 None other sig.
Portrait	15.662	.001	PH vs. PL = .001 PH vs. UP = .001 PH vs. PB = .001 None other sig.	6.526	.001	PH vs. PL = .007 PH vs. UP = .048 PH vs. PB = .003 None other sig.
Football	36.857	.001	PH vs. PL = .001 PH vs. UP = .001 PH vs. PB = .001 None other sig.	16.761	.001	PH vs. PL = .001 PH vs. UP = .001 PH vs. PB = .001 None other sig.

	Extinction phase					
	Motor velocity			Affective rating		
Stimulus	$F(df = 3,45)$	p	Post hoc comparisons	$F(df = 3,45)$	p	Post hoc comparisons
LabFront	26.105	.001	4 vs. 5 = .001 5 vs. 1 = .001 5 vs. 7 = .001 1 vs. 7 = .669	38.333	.001	4 vs. 5 = .001 5 vs. 1 = .003 5 vs. 7 = .001 1 vs. 7 = .083
Portrait	53.596	.001	4 vs. 5 = .001 5 vs. 1 = .001 5 vs. 7 = .001 1 vs. 7 = .468	14.143	.001	4 vs. 5 = .001 5 vs. 1 = .056 5 vs. 7 = .003 1 vs. 7 = .188
Football	105.871	.001	4 vs. 5 = .001 5 vs. 1 = .001 5 vs. 7 = .001 1 vs. 7 = .262	48.498	.001	4 vs. 5 = .001 5 vs. 1 = .001 5 vs. 7 = .001 1 vs. 7 = .718

Note. In the association phase, one-way analyses of variance (ANOVAs) are based on percentage of change in responding (day 4 – day 1/range of day 1 scores obtained by the subject's respective group) to each stimulus scene for the four groups. Tukey post hoc analyses are shown for statistically significant ANOVAs, where significant *group* comparisons are displayed. In the extinction phase, only PH is analyzed. Primary analyses are one-way repeated-measures ANOVAs with Greenhouse–Geisser correction on raw data across days 1, 4, 5, and 7 for each of the stimulus scenes on which conditioning was observed (LabFront, Portrait, Football). Tukey post hoc analyses are shown for statistically significant ANOVAs, where the comparisons between *pairs of days* are displayed. PB, placebo; UP, unpaired; PL, paired low extraverts; PH, paired high extraverts. Adapted with permission of the authors from Depue, Morrone-Strupinsky, and Dahkal (2005).

TABLE 4.2. Data and Analyses for Visuospatial Working Memory in the Association Phase

Delay interval	PB		UP		PL		PH	
	M	SD	M	SD	M	SD	M	SD
0.0 sec	−4	49	−8	43	1	36	−2	40
0.5 sec	−2	19	−13	29	1	19	8	20
4.0 sec	−6	36	−13	29	−8	26	24	24
8.0 sec	−14	20	−17	36	−4	30	40	11

A. Comparison of % change between the four groups by delay interval:
   0.0 sec (accuracy): $F = 1.011$, $p = .342$.
   0.5 sec: $F = 2.44$, $p = .075$.
   4.0 sec: $F = 6.886$, $p < .0001$; PH vs. PL, $p = .016$; PH vs. PB, $p = .046$; PH vs. UP, $p < .0001$. No other comparisons were significant.
   8.0 sec: $F = 14.751$, $p = .001$; PH vs. PL, $p < .0001$; PH vs. PB, $p < .0001$; PH vs. UP, $p < .0001$. No other comparisons were significant.

B. Comparison of % change values across delay intervals for PH only:
   $F = 25.007$, $p < .0001$; 0.5 sec vs. 4.0 sec, $p = .017$; 4.0 sec vs. 8.0 sec, $p = .009$.

C. Comparison of reaction time (RT) and accuracy between the four groups by delay interval:
   4.0 sec, day 1: $F = 1.261$, $p = .320$ (RT); $F = 1.131$, $p = .314$ (accuracy).
   4.0 sec, day 4: $F = .587$, $p = .628$ (RT); $F = 1.329$, $p = .338$ (accuracy).
   8.0 sec, day 1: $F = 1.959$, $p = .141$ (RT); $F = 1.551$, $p = .211$ (accuracy).
   8.0 sec, day 4: $F = .349$, $p = .790$ (RT); $F = 1.324$; $p = .335$ (accuracy).

D. Comparison of biletter cancellation performance between the four groups by day:
   Day 1: $F = 1.355$, $p = .301$.
   Day 4: $F = 1.289$, $p = .311$.

Note. Means (M) and standard deviations (SD) of percentage (%) of change (day 4 – day 1/range of day 1 scores obtained by the subject's respective group) in working memory accuracy as a function of response delay interval are shown. One-way ANOVAs are used, with Tukey post hoc comparisons for significant F's to compare (A) the four groups on % change for each delay interval; (B) only PH on % change values across the three delay intervals (repeated measures), since PH was the only group to have demonstrated a significant facilitation effect across days as a function of delay interval; (C) reaction time and accuracy between the four groups at each delay interval and day as a test of drug effects on perceptual and/or sensorimotor functioning; and (D) biletter cancellation performance between the four groups on each day as a test of drug effects on nonspecific attentional, arousal, and motor, processes. Tasks C and D indicate group results and are not due to variation in reaction time of attention. PB, placebo; UP, unpaired; PL, paired low extraverts; PH, paired high extraverts. Adapted with permission of the authors from Depue, Morrone-Strupinsky, and Dahkal (2005).

with context in the current study was critical to demonstrating contextual facilitation in PH subjects, in that PB and UP subjects did not acquire such facilitation. Third, the presence of a conditioned response in PH subjects on the first day of extinction is also consistent with cue-induced DA activity in the NA (Ranaldi, Pocock, Zereik, & Wise, 1999). Fourth, the dependence of facilitation of motor velocity, positive affect, and visuospatial working memory processes on VTA DA projections to the NA and dorsolateral prefrontal cortex, respectively, is well established in both animals and humans (Depue & Collins, 1999; Luciana et al., 1998). The increasing efficacy of contextual facilitation of working memory with longer response delays found here, when demands on DA facilitation were increasing, is also consistent with a role for DA (Luciana et al., 1998). Fifth, the finding that only PH but not PL subjects acquired context–incentive associations may reflect the positive relation between DA functioning and extraversion found elsewhere (Depue & Collins, 1999).

The fact that both incentive motivational processes (as reflected by motor and affective variables) and cognitive processes (indexed by working memory) evidenced contextual facilitation suggests that afferents from cortico-limbic regions carrying contextual information to the VTA (Berke & Hyman, 2000; Carr & Sesack, 2000; Groenewegen, Wright, Beijer, & Voorn, 1999; Taber, Das, & Fibiger, 1995) have broad effects across VTA DA nuclear subgroups. Motor velocity and affect are influenced by laterally located VTA DA nuclei that project to the NA (Oades & Halliday, 1987). In contrast, working memory processes subserved by prefrontal cortex are modulated by medially located VTA DA nuclei (Luciana et al., 1998; Oades & Halliday, 1987). Contexts attributed incentive salience due to association with reward, then, apparently facilitate not only incentive motivational processes, but also cognitive processes that mediate behavioral strategies and outcome expectancies that guide goal-directed behavior (Berke & Hyman, 2000).

μ-Opiates and Affiliative Behavior

We have begun to study the association of opiate functioning to a human trait of affiliation. From a sample of 2981 college students who all took Tellegen's MPQ, including the Social Closeness (SC) scale, we (Depue & Dahkal, 2005) randomly selected high-SC (top-decile) and low-SC (bottom-decile) females (19–21 years of age). The general experimental approach involved assessing two dependent variables: (1) *state* affiliation ratings and (2) tolerance to heat, both measured after participants viewed either a film clip that specifically induced subjective experience of affection, warmth, and affiliation or a neutral film clip of a rainforest. The 15-minute affiliative film clip portrayed the development of a close mate relationship (without sex scenes), as the partners encountered struggles and joys while they were expecting their first child and after the birth of their child. The affiliative film was found to induce strong, significant changes in our rating scale for warmth and affection, which were specifically and significantly associated with MPQ SC but not with any other MPQ scale, including agentic Extraversion (Morrone et al., 2000; Morrone-Strupinsky & Depue, 2004). The neutral film was a 10-minute narrated segment of tropical rainforest scenes and had no significant effect on ratings of warmth and affection (Morrone et al., 2000).

Heat tolerance was chosen as a dependent variable because it is a well-established measure of μ-opiate activity in animals, is blocked by naltrexone (a potent μ-opiate antagonist), and is correlated with reward effects of opiates (Carlezon et al., 2000; Stefano et al., 2000; Uhl et al., 1999). Heat tolerance estimation involved placing the nondominant hand on a Plexiglas plate located over a high-intensity light source. Subjects reported verbally (1) first detection of "painful," and (2) "stop" with removal of the hand. The first report indicated the time to pain detection, and the second indicated the length of time pain was tolerated. Of course, it is not possible to separate purely physiological pain detection and tolerance from psychological factors, because they are essentially nonseparable aspects of pain in self-report under natural conditions (Zubieta et al., 2001). No significant group differences were found in any condition in pain detection level, or in time of reaching that detection level, on a scale rating heat feelings. Therefore, the results focused on tolerance.

Film-induced changes were measured under two drug conditions: placebo and an opiate antagonist, naltrexone (25 mg orally), which was used to demonstrate an opiate relation to the dependent variables. Naltrexone is a potent opiate antagonist that has high affinity for μORs and has no opiate agonist properties. Importantly, in humans naltrexone blocks the rewarding and tension-reducing effects of alcohol, morphine, and sexual orgasm, and the euphoric subjective effects of opioids, all of which are mediated largely by μORs (Uhl et al., 1999). It also blocks the development of vaginocervically induced mother–infant bonds in sheep, causes maternal neglect in monkeys (Keverne, 1996), blocks a preference for a novel odor or taste paired previously with morphine, and blocks the establishment of odor–mother and male–female recognition associations in rodents (Nelson & Panksepp, 1998; Panksepp, 1998).

Fifteen high-SC and 15 low-SC females were run in two randomized, crossover, double-blind drug conditions (separated by a 4-day interval) of placebo (lactose) and 25 mg oral naltrexone (identical gel capsules were used for the two conditions). Both conditions involved watching in counterbalanced order neutral and affiliative film segments (separated by a 10-minute interval) in both drug conditions. After each film segment, affect ratings (also measured before each film) and heat tolerance were assessed. The left half of Figure 4.5 shows the increase in affiliation ratings induced by the affiliative film relative to the neutral film in both drug conditions. A 2 groups × 2 films × 2 drugs analysis of variance (ANOVA) with repeated measures on the last two factors showed a significant three-way interaction ($F = 17.4$, $p < .01$). Post hoc Tukey testing of the placebo condition data showed that high-SC subjects significantly increased their affiliation ratings of the affiliative film relative to the

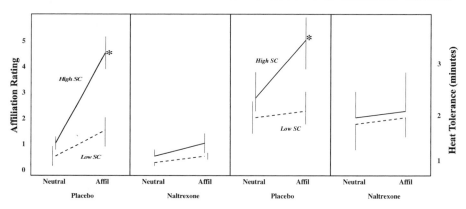

FIGURE 4.5. Data showing that (1) affiliative film material induced a stronger state of warmth and affection (left half of figure) and heat tolerance (right half of figure) in subjects who were high versus low in trait affiliation on Tellegen's Social Closeness (SC) scale under placebo conditions; and (2) elimination of these differences between groups under administration of the opiate antagonist naltrexone. See text for details. Neutral, neutral film condition; Affil, affiliative film condition. Adapted with permission of the authors from Depue and Dahkal (2005).

neutral film ($p < .01$), whereas low-SC subjects showed no significant increase in affiliation ratings ($p > .30$). Moreover, the affiliative ratings of the affiliative film were significantly higher in the high-SC than in the low-SC subjects ($p < .01$), whereas the groups did not differ significantly in ratings of the neutral film ($p > .20$). That opiates may have been involved in the film-induced increased affiliative state under placebo conditions in high-SC subjects is suggested by the lack of significant increase in ratings by the high-SC subjects of the affiliative film relative to the neutral film in the naltrexone condition ($p > .30$). Indeed, in the naltrexone condition, high- and low-SC groups were statistically indistinguishable in their ratings of either film.

The right half of Figure 4.5 shows the increase in heat tolerance (time to "stop") induced by the affiliative film relative to the neutral film in both drug conditions. The ANOVA showed a significant three-way interaction ($F = 12.7$, $p < .05$) mirroring the affiliation rating data: In the placebo condition, Tukey testing showed that (1) high-SC subjects showed significantly greater increases in heat tolerance after the affiliative film relative to the neutral film ($p < .01$), whereas the low-SC subjects showed no significant rating changes ($p > .30$); and (2) high-SC subjects had significantly higher heat tolerance scores after the affiliative film than low-SC subjects ($p < .01$), but the groups did not differ after the neutral film ($p > .30$). However, in the naltrexone condition, these various comparisons showed no significant differences between high- and low-SC subjects.

Thus naltrexone-induced blockade of opiate receptors eliminated the significant effects of affiliative film material on affiliative ratings and heat tolerance in high-SC subjects, such that the high- and low-SC groups became statistically indistinguishable in their responses to either film. This suggests that the differences in affiliative stimulus-induced feelings of affection and warmth and heat tolerance between high- and low-SC subjects are in part due to variation in opiate functioning. Although differences between the two groups did not appear to be related to social desirability and its correlates (self-esteem, diffidence), other unmeasured factors that might affect affiliative ratings to affiliative film material (e.g., attachment styles, rejection sensitivity, mate experiences) need to be controlled in future research.

LOOKING FORWARD

Although there is fairly high agreement on the structure of personality, there has been less robust research on the lines of causal influence underlying that structure. One reason for this is that the neurobehavioral foundation of higher-order traits has not been clearly delineated and empirically validated. This is the major reason why we have attempted to provide such a foundation for agentic extraversion (Depue & Collins, 1999) and affiliation (Depue & Morrone-Strupinsky, 2005), which is outlined herein. Genetic research on polymorphisms of neurotransmitter variables has begun to illuminate neurobiological associations with personality traits (Munafo et al., 2003), but there is a serious lack of *human* research on the manner in which neurobiology relates functionally to the behavior associated with these traits. We have discussed above two recent studies that suggest a strong relation between (1) DA and contextual activation of agentic extraverted behavior, and (2) μ-opiate functioning and a trait of affiliation. But clearly, this is just a beginning, and much more work is required on these and other traits if we are to understand the neurobehavioral foundation of personality. This area, then, represents a major research focus in the area of personality for years to come.

ACKNOWLEDGMENT

The writing of this chapter and the research reported herein were supported by National Institute of Mental Health Research Grant No. MH55347 awarded to Richard A. Depue.

REFERENCES

Adolphs, R. (2003). Cognitive neuroscience of human social behavior. *Nature Reviews Neuroscience, 4*, 165–178.

Aharon, I., Etcoff, N., Ariety, D., Chabris, C., O'Connor, E., & Breiter, H. (2001). Beautiful faces have variable reward value: fMRI and behavioral evidence. *Neuron, 32*, 537–551.

Anagnostaras, S. G., & Robinson, T. E. (1996). Sensitization to the psychomotor stim- ulant effects of amphetamine: Modulation by associative learning. *Behavioral Neuroscience, 110*, 1397–1414.

Azmitia, E., & Whitaker-Azmitia, P. (1997). Development and adult plasticity of sero- tonergic neurons and their target cells. In H. Baumgarten & M. Gothert (Eds.), *Serotoninergic neurons and 5HT receptors in the CNS* (pp. 1–39). New York: Springer.

Berke, J. D., & Hyman, S. E. (2000). Addiction, dopamine, and molecular mechanisms of memory. *Neuron, 25*, 515–532.

Berrettini, W. H., Hoehe, M., Ferraro, T. N., DeMaria, P., & Gottheil, E. (1997). Human mu opioid receptor gene polymorphisms and vulnerability to substance abuse. *Addiction and Biology, 2*, 303–308.

Berridge, K. C. (1999). Pleasure, pain, desire, and dread: Hidden Core processes of emotion. In D. Kahneman, E. Diener, & N. Schwarz (Eds.), *Well-being: The foundations of hedonic psychology* (pp. 525–557). New York: Russell Sage Foun- dation.

Bond, C., LaForge, K. S., Tian, M., Melia, D., Zhang, S., Borg, L., et al. (1998). Single- nucleotide polymorphism in the human mu opioid receptor gene alters β-endor- phin binding and activity: Possible implications for opiate addiction. *Proceedings of the National Academy of Sciences USA, 95*, 9608–9613.

Breiter, H. C., Aharon, I., Kahneman, D., Dale, A., & Shizgal, P. (2001). Functional imaging of neural responses to expectancy and experience of monetary gains and losses. *Neuron, 30*, 619–639.

Breiter, H. C., Gollub, R. L., Weisskoff, R. M., Kennedy, D. N., Makris, N., Berke, J. D., et al. (1997). Acute effects of cocaine on human brain activity and emotion. *Neuron, 19*, 591–611.

Cabib, S. (1993). Strain-dependent behavioural sensitization to amphetamine: role of environmental factors. *Behavioral Pharmacology, 4*, 367–374.

Cador, M., Taylor, J., & Robbins, T. (1991). Potentiation of the effects of reward- related stimuli by dopaminergic-dependent mechanisms in the nucleus accum- bens. *Psychopharmacology, 104*, 377–385.

Callahan, P., Baumann, M., & Rabil, J. (1996). Inhibition of tuberoinfundibular dopaminergic neural activity during suckling: Involvement of mu and kappa opi- ate receptor subtypes. *Journal of Neuroendocrinology, 8*, 771–776.

Carlezon, W., Haile, C., Coopersmith, R., Hayashi, Y., Malinow, R., Neve, R., et al. (2000). Distinct sites of opiate reward and aversion within the midbrain identified using a herpes simplex virus vector expressing GluR1. *Journal of Neuroscience, 20*(RC62), 1–5.

Carr, D., & Sesack, S. (2000). Projections from the rat prefrontal cortex to the ventral tegmental area: Target specificity in the synaptic associations with mesoac- cumbens and mesocortical neurons. *Journal of Neuroscience, 20*, 3864–3873.

Carter, C. S., Lederhendler, I., & Kirkpatrick, B. (1997). The integrative neurobiology of affiliation. *Annals of the New York Academy of Sciences, 807*, xiii–xviii.

Church, A. T. (1994). Relating the Tellegen and five-factor models of personality structure. *Journal of Personality and Social Psychology, 67*, 898–909.

Church, A. T., & Burke, P. (1994). Exploratory and confirmatory tests of the big five and Tellegen's three- and four-dimensional models. *Journal of Personality and Social Psychology, 66*, 93–114.

Coccaro, E., & Siever, L. (1991). *Serotonin and psychiatric disorders*. Washington, DC: American Psychiatric Press.

Damasio, A. R. (2003). *Looking for Spinoza*. Orlando, FL: Harcourt.

David, V., & Cazala, P. (2000). Anatomical and pharmacological specificity of the rewarding effect elicited by microinjections of morphine into the nucleus accumbens of mice. *Psychopharmacology, 150*, 24–34.

Depue, R. A., & Collins, P. F. (1999). Neurobiology of the structure of personality: Dopamine, facilitation of incentive motivation, and extraversion. *Behavioral and Brain Sciences, 22*, 491–569.

Depue, R. A., & Dahkal, S. (2005). *Opiate functioning and social bonding in human subjects*. Manuscript under review.

Depue, R. A., & Lenzenweger, M. F. (2005). A neurobehavioral dimensional model of personality disturbances. In M. F. Lenzenweger & J. F. Clarkin (Eds.), *Major theories of personality disorders* (2nd ed., pp. 391–453). New York: Guilford Press.

Depue, R. A., Luciana, M., Arbisi, P., Collins, P., & Leon, A. (1994). Dopamine and the structure of personality: Relation of agonist-induced dopamine activity to positive emotionality. *Journal of Personality and Social Psychology, 67*, 485–498.

Depue, R. A., & Morrone-Strupinsky, J. V. (2005). A neurobehavioral model of affiliative bonding: Implications for conceptualizing a human trait of affiliation. *Behavioral and Brain Sciences, 28*, 313–395.

Depue, R. A., Morrone-Strupinsky, J. V., & Dahkal, S. (2005). *On the nature of extraversion: Contextual activation of dopamine-facilitated behavior*. Manuscript under review.

Depue, R. A., & Spoont, M. (1986). Conceptualizing a serotonin trait: A behavioral dimension of constraint. *Annals of the New York Academy of Sciences, 487*, 47–62.

Di Chiara, G. (1995). The role of dopamine in drug abuse viewed from the perspective of its role in motivation. *Drug and Alcohol Dependence, 38*, 95–137.

Di Chiara, G., & North, R. A. (1992). Neurobiology of opiate abuse. *Trends in the Physiological Sciences, 13*, 185–193.

Digman, J. M. (1997). Higher-order factors of the Big Five. *Journal of Personality and Social Psychology, 73*, 1246–1256.

Domjan, M., Cusato, B., & Villarreal, R. (2000). Pavlovian feed-forward mechanisms in the control of social behavior. *Behavioral and Brain Sciences, 23*, 1–29.

Drevets, W. C., Gautier, C., Price, J. C., Kupfer, D. J., Kinahan, P. E., Grace, A. A., et al. (2001). Amphetamine-induced dopamine release in human ventral striatum correlates with euphoria. *Biological Psychiatry, 49*, 81–96.

Duvauchelle, C. L., Flemming, S., & Kornetsky, C. (2000). Effects of cocaine context on NAcc dopamine and behavioral activity after repeated intravenous cocaine administration. *Brain Research, 862*, 49–58.

Dworkin, S., Guerin, G., Goeders, N., & Smith, J. (1988). Kainic acid lesions of the nucleus accumbens selectively attenuate morphine self-administration. *Pharmacology, Biochemistry, and Behavior, 29*, 175–181.

Elmer, G. I., Pieper, J. O., Goldberg, S. R., & George, F. R. (1995). Opioid operant self-administration, analgesia, stimulation and respiratory depression in μ-deficient mice. *Psychopharmacology, 117*, 23–31.

Everitt, B. J., Dickinson, A., & Robbins, T. W. (2001). The neuropsychological basis of addictive behaviour. *Brain Research Reviews, 36*, 129–138.

Fleming, A. S., Korsmit, M., & Deller, M. (1994). Rat pups are potent reinforcers to the maternal animal: Effects of experience, parity, hormones, and dopamine function. *Psychobiology, 22*(1), 44–53.

Gelernter, J., Kranzler, H., & Cubells, J. (1999). Genetics of two m opioid receptor gene (OPRM1) exon I polymorphisms: Population studies, and allele frequencies in alcohol- and drug-dependent subjects. *Molecular Psychiatry, 4*, 476–483.

Gingrich, B., Liu, Y., Cascio, C., Wang, Z., & Insel, T. R. (2000). Dopamine D2 receptors in the nucleus accumbens are important for social attachment in female prairie voles (*Microtus ochrogaster*). *Behavioral Neuroscience, 114*(1), 173–183.

Gosling, S. (2001). From mice to men: What can we learn about personality from animal research? *Psychological Bulletin, 127*, 45–86.

Graves, F. C., Wallen, K., & Maestripieri, D. (2002). Opioids and attachment in rhesus macaque abusive mothers. *Behavioral Neuroscience, 116*, 489–493.

Gray, J. A. (1973). Causal theories of personality and how to test them. In J. R. Royce (Ed.), *Multivariate analysis and psychological theory* (pp. 409–463). New York: Academic Press.

Groenewegen, H., Wright, C., Beijer, A., & Voorn, P. (1999). Convergence and segregation of ventral striatal inputs and outputs. *Annals of the New York Academy of Sciences, 877*, 49–63.

Herbert, J. (1993). Peptides in the limbic system: Neurochemical codes for coordinated adaptive responses to behavioural and physiological demand. *Progress in Neurobiology, 41*, 723–791.

Herz, A. (1998). Opioid reward mechanisms: A key role in drug abuse? *Canadian Journal of Physiology and Pharmacology, 76*, 252–258.

Hilliard, S., Domjan, M., Nguyen, M., & Cusato, B. (1998). Dissociation of conditioned appetitive and consummatory sexual behavior: Satiation and extinction tests. *Animal Learning and Behavior, 26*(1), 20–33.

Hol, T., Niesink, M., van Ree, J., & Spruijt, B. (1996). Prenatal exposure to morphine affects juvenile play behavior and adult social behavior in rats. *Pharmacology, Biochemistry and Behavior, 55*, 615–618.

Hooks, M., Jones, G., Neill, D., & Justice, J. (1992). Individual differences in amphetamine sensitization: Dose-dependent effects. *Pharmacology, Biochemistry and Behavior, 41*, 203–210.

Hurley, J. R. (1998). Agency and communion as related to the "big five" self-representations and subsequent behavior in small groups. *Journal of Psychology, 132*, 337–356.

Ikemoto, S., & Panksepp, J. (1996). Dissociations between appetitive and consummatory responses by pharmacological manipulations of reward-relevant brain regions. *Behavioral Neuroscience, 110*, 331–345.

Insel, T. R. (1997). A neurobiological basis of social attachment. *American Journal of Psychiatry, 154*, 726–733.

Jodogne, C., Marinelli, C. M., Le Moal, M., & Piazza, P. V. (1994). Animals predisposed to develop amphetamine self-administration show higher susceptibility to develop contextual conditioning of both amphetamine-induced hyperlocomotion and sensitization. *Brain Research, 657*, 236–244.

Johnson, B., & Ait-Daoud, N. (2000). Neuropharmacological treatments for alcoholism: Scientific basis and clinical findings. *Psychopharmacology, 149*, 327–344.

Kelley, A. (1999). Neural integrative activities of nucleus accumbens subregions in relation to learning and motivation. *Psychobiology, 27*, 198–213.

Keverne, E. B. (1996). Psychopharmacology of maternal behaviour. *Journal of Psychopharmacology, 10*, 16–22.

Koob, G., & Le Moal, M. (1997). Drug abuse: Hedonic homeostatic dysregulation. *Science, 278*, 52–58.

Kranzler, H. R. (2000). Pharmacotherapy of alcoholism: Gaps in knowledge and opportunities for research. *Alcohol and Alcoholism, 35*, 537–547.

LaBuda, C. J., Sora, I., Uhl, G. R., & Fuchs, P. N. (2000). Stress-induced analgesia in mu-opioid receptor knockout mice reveals normal function of the delta-opioid receptor system. *Brain Research, 869*, 1–10.

Laviolette, S. R., Gallegos, R. A., Henriksen, S. J., & van der Kooy, D. (2004). Opiate state controls bi-directional reward signaling via GABA-A receptors in the ventral tegmental area. *Nature Neuroscience, 10*, 160–169.

Le Moal, M., & Simon, H. (1991). Mesocorticolimbic dopaminergic network: Functional and regulatory roles. *Physiological Reviews, 71*, 155–234.

Lesch, K.-P. (1998). Serotonin transporter and psychiatric disorders. *The Neuroscientist, 4*, 25–34.

Luciana, M., Collins, P. F., & Depue, R. A. (1998). Opposing roles for dopamine and serotonin in the modulation of human spatial working memory functions. *Cerebral Cortex, 8*, 218–226.

MacLean, P. (1986). Ictal symptoms relating to the nature of affects and their cerebral substrate. In E. Plutchik & H. Kellerman (Eds.), *Emotion: Theory, research, and experience. Vol 3. Biological foundations of emotion.* Orlando, FL: Academic Press.

Marinelli, M., & White, F. (2000). Enhanced vulnerability to cocaine self-administration is associated with elevated impulse activity of midbrain dopamine neurons. *Journal of Neuroscience, 20*, 8876–8885.

Martel, F., Nevison, C., Simpson, M., & Keverne, E. (1995). Effects of opioid receptor blockade on the social behavior of rhesus monkeys living in large family groups. *Developmental Psychobiology, 28*, 71–84.

Matheson, M. D., & Bernstein, I. S. (2000). Grooming, social bonding, and agonistic aiding in rhesus monkeys. *American Journal of Primatology, 51*, 177–186.

Matthes, H. W., Maldonado, R., Simonin, F., Valverde, O., Slowe, S., Kitchen, I., et al. (1996). Loss of morphine-induced analgesia, reward effect and withdrawal symptoms in mice lacking the μ-opioid-receptor gene. *Nature, 383*, 819–823.

Moles, A., Kieffer, B. L., & D'Amato, F. R. (2004). Deficit in attachment behavior in mice lacking the μ-opioid receptor gene. *Science, 304*, 1983–1986.

Morrone, J. V., Depue, R. D., Scherer, A. J., & White, T. L. (2000). Film-induced incentive motivation and positive activation in relation to agentic and affiliative components of extraversion. *Personality and Individual Differences, 29*, 199–216.

Morrone-Strupinsky, J. V., & Depue, R. A. (2004). Differential relation of two distinct, film-induced positive emotional states to affiliative and agentic extraversion. *Personality and Individual Differences, 36*, 1109–1126.

Munafo, M. R., Clark, T. G., Moore, L. R., Payne, E., Walton, R., & Flint, J. (2003). Genetic polymorphisms and personality: A systematic review and meta-analysis. *Molecular Psychiatry, 8*, 471–484.

Narita, M., Aoki, T., & Suzuki, T. (2000). Molecular evidence for the involvement of NR2B subunit containing *N*-methyl-D-aspartate receptors in the development of morphine-induced place preference. *Neuroscience, 101*, 601–606.

Nelson, E. E., & Panksepp, J. (1998). Brain substrates of infant–mother attachment: Contributions of opioids, oxytocin, and norepinephrine. *Neuroscience and Biobehavioral Reviews, 22*(3), 437–452.

Niesink, R. J. M., Vanderschuen, L. J. M. J., & van Ree, J. M. (1996). Social play in juvenile rats in utero exposure to morphine. *Neurotoxicology, 17*(3–4), 905–912.

Oades, R., & Halliday, G. (1987). Ventral tegmental (A10) system: Neurobiology. 1. Anatomy and connectivity. *Brain Research Reviews, 12*, 117–165.

Olausson, H., Lamarre, Y., Backlund, H., Morin, C., Wallin, B. G., Starck, G., et al. (2002). Unmyelinated tactile afferents signal touch and project to insular cortex. *Nature Neuroscience, 5*, 900–904.

Olive, M., Koenig, H., Nannini, M., & Hodge, C. (2001). Stimulation of endorphin neurotransmission in the nucleus accumbens by ethanol, cocaine, and amphetamine. *Journal of Neuroscience, 21*, RC184.

Olson, G., Olson, R., & Kastin, A. (1997). Endogenous opiates: 1996. *Peptides, 18*, 1651–1688.

Ostrowski, N. L. (1998). Oxytocin receptor mRNA expression in rat brain: Implications for behavioral integration and reproductive success. *Psychoneuroendocrinology, 23*(8), 989–1004.

Panksepp, J. (1998). *Affective neuroscience: The foundations of human and animal emotions*. New York: Oxford University Press.

Parkinson, J. A., Olmstead, M. C., Burns, L. H., Robbins, T. W., & Everitt, B. J. (1999). Dissociation in effects of lesions of the nucleus accumbens core and shell on appetitive Pavlovian approach behavior and the potentiation of conditioned reinforcement and locomotor activity by D-amphetamine. *Journal of Neuroscience, 19*, 2401–2421.

Pfaus, J. G., Smith, W. J., & Coopersmith, C. B. (1999). Appetitive and consummatory sexual behaviors of female rats in bilevel chambers: I. A correlational and factor analysis and the effects of ovarian hormones. *Hormones and Behavior, 35*, 224–240.

Piazza, P. V., & Le Moal, M. (1996). Pathophysiological basis of vulnerability to drug abuse: Role of an interaction between stress, glucocorticoids, and dopaminergic neruons. *Annual Review of Pharmacology and Toxicology, 36*, 359–378.

Pich, E., Pagliusi, S., Tessari, M., Talabot-Ayer, D., van Huijsduijnen, R., & Chiamulera, C. (1997). Common neural substrates for the addictive properties of nicotine and cocaine. *Science, 275*, 83–86.

Polan, H. J., & Hofer, M. A. (1998). Olfactory preference for mother over home nest shavings by newborn rats. *Developmental Psychobiology, 33*, 5–20.

Porges, S. (2001). The polyvagal theory: Phylogenetic substrates of a social nervous system. *International Journal of Psychophysiology, 42*, 123–146.

Ranaldi, R., Pocock, D., Zereik, R., & Wise, R. A. (1999). Dopamine fluctuations in the nucleus accumbens during maintenance, extinction, and reinstatement of intravenous D-amphetamine self-administration. *Journal of Neuroscience, 19*, 4102–4115.

Robinson, T. E., & Berridge, K. C. (2000). The psychology and neurobiology of addiction: An incentive–sensitization view. *Addiction, 95*(Suppl. 2), S91–S117.

Schlaepfer, T. E., Strain, E. C., Greenberg, B. D., Preston, K. L., Lancaster, E., Bigelow, G. E., et al. (1998). Site of opioid action in the human brain: Mu and kappa agonists' subjective and cerebral blood flow effects. *American Journal of Psychiatry, 155*(4), 470–473.

Schultz, W., Dayan, P., & Montague, P. (1997). A neural substrate of prediction and reward. *Science, 275,* 1593–1595.

Shippenberg, T. S., & Elmer, G. I. (1998). The neurobiology of opiate reinforcement. *Critical Reviews in Neurobiology, 12*(4), 267–303.

Silk, J. B., Alberts, S. C., & Altmann, J. (2003). Social bonds of female baboons enhance infant survival. *Science, 302,* 1231–1234.

Simonin, F., Valverde, O., Smadja, C., Slowe, S., Kitchen, I., Dierich, A., et al. (1998). Disruption of the kappa-opioid receptor gene in mice enhances sensitivity to chemical visceral pain, impairs pharmacological actions of the selective kappa-agonist U-50,488H and attenuates morphine withdrawal. *EMBO Journal, 17,* 886–897.

Spoont, M. (1992). Modulatory role of serotonin in neural information processing: Implications for human psychopathology. *Psychological Bulletin, 112,* 330–350.

Stefano, G., Goumon, Y., Casares, F., Cadet, P., Fricchione, G., Rialas, C., et al. (2000). Endogenous morphine. *Trends in Neurosciences, 23,* 436–442.

Taber, M., Das, S., & Fibiger, H. J. (1995). Cortical regulation of subcortical dopamine release: Mediation via the ventral tegmental area. *Neurochemistry, 65,* 1407–1410.

Tellegen, A., Lykken, D. T., Bouchard, T. J., Wilcox, K. J., Segal, N. L., & Rich, S. (1988). Personality similarity in twins reared apart and together. *Journal of Personality and Social Psychology, 54,* 1031–1039.

Tellegen, A., & Waller, N. G. (in press). Exploring personality through test construction: Development of the multidimensional personality questionnaire. In S. Briggs & J. Cheek (Eds.), *Personality measures: Development and evaluation* (Vol. 1). Amsterdam: JAI Press.

Timberlake, W., & Silva, K. (1995). Appetitive behavior in ethology, psychology, and behavior systems. In N. Thompson (Ed.), *Perspectives in ethology: Vol. 11. Behavioral design* (pp. 211–253). New York: Plenum Press.

Tork, I. (1990). Anatomy of the serotonergic system. *Annals of the New York Academy of Sciences, 600,* 9–32.

Uhl, G. R., Sora, I., & Wang, Z. (1999). The μ opiate receptor as a candidate gene for pain: Polymorphisms, variations in expression, nociception, and opiate responses. *Proceedings of the National Academy of Sciences USA, 96,* 7752–7755.

van Furth, W., & van Ree, J. (1996). Sexual motivation: Involvement of endogenous opioids in the ventral tegmental area. *Brain Research, 729,* 20–28.

Volkow, N. D., Wang, G., Fischman, M., Foltin, R., & Fowler, J. (1998). Association between decline in brain dopamine activity with age and cognitive and motor impairment in healthy individuals. *American Journal of Psychiatry, 155,* 344–349.

Volkow, N. D., Wang, G., Fischman, M., Foltin, R., Fowler, J., Abumrad, N., et al. (1997). Relationship between subjective effects of cocaine and dopamine transporter occupancy. *Nature, 386,* 827–829.

Watson, C., & Clark, L. (1997). Extraversion and its positive emotional core. In R. Hogan, J. Johnson, & S. Briggs (Eds.), *Handbook of personality psychology* (pp. 767–793). San Diego, CA: Academic Press.

Watson, D., & Tellegen, A. (1985). Towards a consensual structure of mood. *Psychological Bulletin, 98,* 219–235.

White, N. (1986). Control of sensorimotor function by dopaminergic nigrostriatal neurons: Influence on eating and drinking. *Neuroscience and Biobehavioral Reviews, 10,* 15–36.

White, T. L., & Depue, R. A. (1999). Differential association of traits of fear and anxiety with norepinephrine- and dark-induced pupil reactivity. *Journal of Personality and Social Psychology, 77*(4), 863–877.

Wiedenmayer, C. P., & Barr, G. A. (2000). Mu opiod receptors in the ventrolateral periaqueductal grey mediate stress-induced analgesia but not immobility in rat pups. *Behavioral Neuroscience, 114,* 125–138.

Wiggins, J. (1991). Agency and communion as conceptual coordinates for the understanding and measurement of interpersonal behavior. In D. Cicchetti & W. Grove (Eds.), *Thinking clearly about psychology: Essays in honor of Paul Everett Meehl* (pp. 89–113). Minneapolis: University of Minnesota Press.

Wise, R. (1998). Drug-activation of brain reward pathways. *Drug and Alcohol Dependence, 51,* 13–22.

Wolterink, G., Cador, M., Wolterink, I., Robbins, T., & Everitt, B. (1989). Involvement of D1 and D2 receptor mechanisms in the processing of reward-related stimuli in the ventral striatum. *Society for Neuroscience Abstracts, 15,* 490.

Wyvell, C. L., & Berridge, K. C. (2000). Intra-accumbens amphetamine increases the conditioned incentive salience of sucrose reward: Enhancement of reward "wanting" without enhanced "liking" or response reinforcement. *Journal of Neuroscience, 20,* 8122–8130.

Zald, D., & Depue, R. (2001). Serotonergic modulation of positive and negative affect in psychiatrically healthy males. *Personality and Individual Differences, 30,* 71–86.

Zubieta, J.-K., Smith, Y., Bueller, J., Xu, Y., Kilbourn, M., Jewett, D., et al. (2001). Regional mu opioid receptor regulation of sensory and affective dimensions of pain. *Science, 293,* 311–315.

Zuckerman, M. (1994). An alternative five-factor model for personality. In C. Halverson, G. Kohnstamm & R. Marten (Eds.), *The developing structure of temperament and personality from infancy to adulthood* (pp. 75–102). Hillsdale, NJ: Erlbaum.

5

Genomic Imaging of Extraversion

Turhan Canli

Some people are best known for their laughter. Wherever they are, that's where the party is. They draw others in, they value social contact, and they thoroughly enjoy good times shared with anybody. Drop them into a room of strangers, and they'll be best friends with everyone within the hour. These are the individuals who make the trait concept of extraversion come to life. What makes these people behave this way? Where do they get their energy? If I am not like that, but would like to be, could I? Can extraversion be acquired, or must one be born that way? Since all behavior must be represented in the brain, what are the neural differences between extraverts and introverts?

This focus on individual differences in complex behaviors is familiar to geneticists and personality psychologists, but less so to cognitive neuroscientists, who have traditionally regarded individual differences in their data sets as unwanted statistical noise (Plomin & Kosslyn, 2001). In neuroimaging of cognitive processes, individual differences may reduce statistical reliability. For example, if in a sample of 10 participants 5 showed activation in a certain brain region and 5 did not, what could we conclude? In the absence of any additional information, we would probably have to settle for stating that this region is not reliably activated. But how would the interpretation of the data change if additional information were available? For example, what if the 5 activators all happened to be female, and the 5 nonactivators all happened to be male? In this case, the inclusion of a specific dimension of individual differences (in this case, the sex of the participants) could reveal something about the brain's function ("Women activate, men don't") that otherwise would have been missed.

A focus on individual differences in neuroimaging is a relatively recent phenomenon. One of the earliest references comes from a neuroimaging study of language (Steinmetz & Seitz, 1991), in which the authors drew attention to individual differences in the localization of language. Since then, the publication record has steadily grown: A database search (MEDLINE) of the terms "individual difference" and either "PET" or "fMRI" returned 5 publications from 1990–1994, 11 from 1995–1999, and 57 from 2000–2004.

MAPPING EXTRAVERSION IN THE BRAIN: DECONSTRUCTION AND REDUCTION

How can an individual-difference approach be applied to the study of extraversion or related personality traits in the brain? Work to date has correlated responses on personality questionnaires with structural brain features (Knutson, Momenan, Rawlings, Fong, & Hommer, 2001; Onitsuka et al., 2005); neuroimaging of dopamine or serotonin function (Knutson et al., 1998; Laakso et al., 2003; Suhara et al., 2001); and brain activation at rest (Ebmeier et al., 1994; Johnson et al., 1999; Stenberg, Risberg, Warkentin, & Rosen, 1990; Suguira et al., 2000; Youn et al., 2002), during nonemotional cognitive processing (Fink, Schrausser, & Neubauer, 2002; Fischer, Wik, & Fredrikson, 1997; Gray & Braver, 2002; Gurrera, O'Donnell, Nestor, Gainski, & McCarley, 2001; Haier, Sokolski, Katz, & Buchsbaum, 1987; Kumari, Ffytche, Williams, & Gray, 2004; Stenberg, Wendt, & Risberg, 1993), or in response to emotional stimuli or mood states (Bartussek, Becker, Diedrich, Naumann, & Maier, 1996; Canli, 2004; Fischer, Tillfors, Furmark, & Fredrikson, 2001; Keightley et al., 2003).

My approach has been to use emotional stimuli to draw out individual differences in personality, and to look for brain regions where individual differences in emotional reactivity are associated with measures of personality (Canli, 2004). This approach takes advantage of the fact that extraversion is strongly linked with positive affect. For example, extraverts report more positive experiences than introverts (Costa & McCrae, 1980) and are more responsive to positive mood induction procedures (Larsen & Ketelaar, 1991). Indeed, extraversion is strongly correlated with dispositional positive affect across a large set of different subject samples (Watson, Wiese, Vaidya, & Tellegen, 1999), although the two are not interchangeable constructs (Gross, Sutton, & Ketelaar, 1998; Vaidya, Gray, Haig, & Watson, 2002).

To apply this approach to the biological study of traits, I deconstruct complex traits into simpler psychological domains of cognitive processing, and then pursue a reductionist agenda to move from behavioral levels of analysis to neural systems to molecular mechanisms (Figure 5.1).

For example, extraversion is a broad trait that encompasses interpersonal elements (see Depue, Chapter 4, this volume) as well as positive affect (Costa & McCrae, 1980; Watson & Clark, 1997). In an experimental setting, it is advantageous to study the association between extraversion and narrowly defined behaviors that may reflect individual differences in emotional experience, mem-

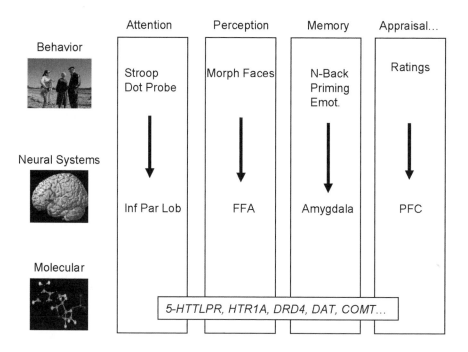

FIGURE 5.1. Figure depicting different levels of analysis in the deconstruction of personality into narrowly defined psychological domains. The illustration of the molecular level is courtesy of Juergen Suehnel at the Jena Image Library of Biological Macromolecules (jsuehnel@imb-jena.de); the molecular structure of adenosine monophosphate is depicted. Names in the row corresponding to the behavioral level of analysis correspond to various cognitive test paradigms such as perception of ambiguously morphed faces, the N-Back working memory tasks, or memory tasks using priming methods or emotional stimuli. Names in the row corresponding to the neural systems level of analysis correspond to the following brain structures: Inf Par Lob, inferior parietal lobule; FFA, fusiform face area; PFC, prefrontal cortex. Names in the row corresponding to the molecular level of analysis correspond to gene polymorphisms known to be associated with individual differences in emotion or personality.

ory, attention, or perception. For each of these domains of psychological processing, cognitive psychologists have developed tests that can capture and quantify behavior very precisely. For example, attention to emotional stimuli can be assessed by using the emotional variant of the classic Stroop task (Stroop, 1935). In the original version, words that denote colors are printed in colored fonts that are either congruent (e.g., the word "blue" printed in blue ink) or incongruent (e.g., the word "blue" printed in red ink) with the item's semantic content. Participants are asked to state, as quickly as possible, the color in which each word is printed. Reaction time (RT) to incongruent stimuli is slower than to congruent stimuli, suggesting that the semantic dimension of the word stimulus draws attentional resources away from the task itself.

In the emotional version of the Stroop task, participants view emotional or neutral word stimuli that are printed in colored fonts; they then indicate, as quickly and accurately as possible, the color in which each stimulus is printed. As in the classic version, the semantic content of the word is irrelevant to the task. Nonetheless, some individuals respond more slowly to negative than to neutral words, indicating that the words' meaning interferes with task performance. Indeed, emotional words are associated with slower reaction times than neutral words in trait-anxious individuals, presumably because attentional resources are diverted from compliance with task instructions (Richards, French, Johnson, Naparstek, & Williams, 1992).

A reductionist agenda would seek to identify the neural substrate associated with this task. As I discuss later in this chapter, neuroimaging studies have been conducted that implicate the anterior cingulate cortex (ACC) as a brain region associated with attentional processing, as measured by the Stroop task (Bush et al., 1998; Canli, Amin, Haas, Omura, & Constable, 2004; George et al., 1994; Whalen, Bush, et al., 1998).

Until recently, a further reduction toward the identification of cellular and molecular mechanisms required invasive methodologies that could only be applied in animal studies (see, e.g., Chiavegatto, Chapter 18, this volume). However, advances in the mapping of the human genome have revealed common variants within genes known as "polymorphisms," some of which are associated with personality traits. For example, a functional repeat length polymorphism in the transcriptional control or promoter region (5-HTTLPR) of the serotonin (5-HT) transporter gene (5-HTTLPR, SLC6A4) that results in a short and a long version has been described (Heils et al., 1996). The presence of the short variant of the repetitive sequence, which results in low 5-HT uptake function, is associated with anxiety-related traits and neuroticism (Lesch et al., 1996). Weinberger, Hariri, and colleagues were the first to show that the presence of the short allele is also associated with increased amygdala reactivity to negative emotional stimuli (Hariri et al., 2002), demonstrating that genetic variation can modulate brain function. Because the molecular and cellular processes of the 5-HTTLPR polymorphism have been identified (Lesch et al., 1996), one can begin constructing molecular models that explain how individuals differ in brain reactivity to emotional stimuli as a function of specific gene polymorphisms. In the following sections, I begin to outline how this agenda can be applied to the study of extraversion—the personality trait shared by those people who are most fun to be around.

NEUROIMAGING OF EXTRAVERSION

Given the association of extraversion with positive affect, one would expect that extraversion should correlate with brain reactivity to positive emotional stimuli. In earlier work, we had found evidence that brain activation patterns in response to emotional stimuli can vary dramatically as a function of individual differences in subjective emotional experience of the stimulus material (Canli, Desmond, Zhao, Glover, & Gabrieli, 1998), but it was unknown whether they would also vary as a function of extraversion. We therefore conducted a study using functional magnetic resonance imaging (fMRI), in which participants completed a personality questionnaire (Costa & McCrae, 1992) and then passively viewed alternating blocks of positive and negative stimuli (Canli et al., 2001).

The stimuli were complex visual scenes compiled by Lang, Bradley, and Cuthbert (2001) in the International Affective Picture System, and were normed for emotional valence and arousal. Positive images depicted happy babies, puppies and kittens, appetizing foods, and joyful people, whereas negative images depicted snarling dogs, spiders and sharks, disgusting objects (most notably a soiled toilet), tumors, or corpses. As a manipulation check, we asked participants to rate each image for valence and arousal after the scan was completed.

We found that activation to positive, relative to negative, images varied as a function of extraversion across many cortical and subcortical regions (Canli et al., 2001). For example, extraversion was correlated with activation of the ACC. This region is associated with emotional awareness (Lane, 2000; Lane, Fink, Chau, & Dolan, 1997; Lane et al., 1998) and with attention to emotional stimuli (Canli et al., 2004; George et al., 1994; Whalen, Bush, et al., 1998). The observation that a neural system associated with attention varies as a function of extraversion is consistent with a cognitive study's report of attentional bias for positive stimuli in extraverted individuals, who were found to be slow in shifting attention away from spatial locations associated with reward (Derryberry & Reed, 1994).

Activation of the ACC as a function of extraversion may indicate the involvement of an attention-related neural system, but our study could not make such a strong claim, because the task was not constrained to assess attention. Instead, participants' passive viewing of emotional stimuli may have activated a number of different cognitive processes within or between individuals. Some of the images shown may have triggered autobiographical recollections, free associations, visceral responses, internal verbal commentary, emotion regulation, or a host of other cognitive–affective processes.

In order to better isolate the presumed cognitive processes associated with brain regions that exhibit differential activation as a function of extraversion, subsequent studies used better-defined cognitive tasks. For example, we conducted an fMRI study of emotional attention, using the so-called "dot probe" task (Amin, Constable, & Canli, 2004). In this task, participants press a button as soon as they notice a probe stimulus (a simple dot) that is initially obscured by one of two images. Both images are displayed as a pair on a screen and then disappear simultaneously, with the probe stimulus emerging behind one or the other stimulus. RT is taken as an indirect measure of spatial attention: Faster RTs suggest that the participant attends to the picture behind which the probe is located, whereas slower RTs suggest that the participant attends to the other picture. When both images are of differing emotional content, biases in emotional attention can be revealed, as demonstrated by cognitive studies of anxious and depressed participants (Mogg, Bradley, & Williams, 1995).

We hypothesized that extraversion would be associated with individual differences in response to picture pairs that contained a positive image, and that brain regions associated with emotional or spatial attention should show activation differences as a function of extraversion. These a priori regions of interest included the amygdala (Davis & Whalen, 2001), the ACC (Whalen, Bush, et al., 1998), and the posterior fusiform region (Donner et al., 2000).

Behavioral data from this study found a significant effect of extraversion on participants' RTs. Interestingly, this effect was driven by negative stimuli, because participants showed faster RTs when the probe was obscured by a neutral picture of a neutral–negative pair, compared to a neutral–neutral pair. This suggests that highly extraverted individuals directed their attention *away from* negative stimuli, which might reflect an emotion regulation strategy (Gross, 1999).

If extraverts avoid negative pictures, then presentation of a probe behind the negative item of a negative–neutral pair should be associated with greater search effort and greater activation of brain regions associated with visual attention (compared to when the probe is behind the neutral item of the negative–neutral pair). This was indeed the case in the fusiform gyrus (Figure 5.2), one of our a priori regions of interest (when significance thresholds were relaxed from $p < .001$ to $p < .01$, the other a priori regions, the amygdala and the ACC, also emerged as significantly correlated with extraversion).

Another study focused on emotional facial expressions (Canli, Sivers, Whitfield, Gotlib, & Gabrieli, 2002). Functional neuroimaging studies using photographs of emotional facial expressions have consistently identified the amygdala as a brain region that is sensitive to expressions of fear (Breiter et al., 1996; Morris et al., 1996; Whalen, Rauch, et al., 1998). This is consistent with a large animal learning literature showing that the amygdala is involved in learned fear (Davis, Walker, & Myers, 2003; Fanselow & Poulos, 2005; LeDoux, 2003; Maren, 2005; Pare, Quirk, & LeDoux, 2004; Rodrigues, Schafe, & LeDoux, 2004; Rosen, 2004). On the other hand, there is less agreement as to whether the amygdala is also activated by positive, happy facial expressions. Some studies reported significant activation in the amygdala (Breiter et al., 1996; Killgore & Yurgelun-Todd, 2001; Yang et al., 2002), whereas others did not (Kesler-West et al., 2001; Morris et al., 1996; Phillips et al., 1998). We hypothesized that amygdala activation to happy facial expressions may reflect individual differences in extraversion (Pervin & John, 1999), given our earlier finding that amygdala activation to positive emotional scenes varied as a function of this trait (Canli et al., 2001). Indeed, this turned out to be the case (Figure 5.3). Additional analyses confirmed that

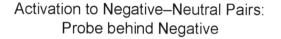

Activation to Negative–Neutral Pairs: Probe behind Negative

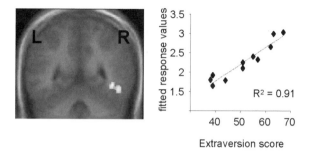

FIGURE 5.2. Correlation between fusiform activation and extraversion. Left panel shows coronal section through the region of interest. Right panel shows scatterplot of fusiform activation plotted against subjects' extraversion scores. From Amin, Constable, and Canli (2004). Copyright 2004 by Elsevier, Inc. Adapted by permission.

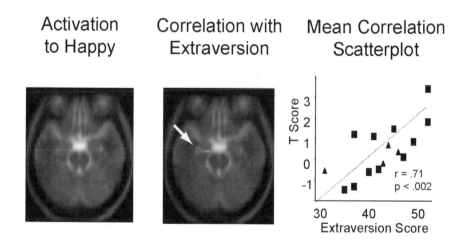

FIGURE 5.3. Amygdala activation to happy, relative to neutral, faces as a function of extraversion. Left panel shows result of group-level contrast analysis, showing no significant amygdala activation for the sample as a whole in response to happy, relative to neutral, faces. Middle panel shows a significant cluster in the amygdala, where degree of activation to happy faces correlated with degree of subject's extraversion. Right panel shows scatterplot from the same cluster. Squares represent females; triangles represent males. From Canli, Sivers, Whitfield, Gotlib, and Gabrieli (2002). Copyright 2002 by the American Association for the Advancement of Science. Adapted by permission.

the observed correlation was specific to extraversion and amygdala activation to happy facial expressions, since there were no significant correlations when other trait variables or emotional facial expressions were investigated.

DISSOCIATING TRAITS AND STATES

In the preceding section, I have illustrated the idea that personality traits can be studied by focusing on narrowly defined domains of psychological function, such as emotional experience, attention, or face processing. Given the strong association between extraversion and dispositional positive affect (Watson et al., 1999), is it possible that some of these associations are not due to stable traits, but rather due to mood states? Our next study addressed this question (Canli et al., 2004).

To dissociate personality trait and mood state variables, we administered the Revised NEO Personality Inventory (NEO PI-R; Costa & McCrae, 1992) and the Profile of Mood States (POMS; McNair, Lorr, & Droppleman, 1992) to 12 participants prior to scanning. We focused on the ACC as the a priori region of interest, because it responds to emotional stimuli (Devinsky, Morrell, & Vogt, 1995), is associated with emotional awareness (Canli, Desmond, Zhao, & Gabrieli, 2002; Lane et al., 1997, 1998), and varies in activation to positive stimuli as a function of individual differences in extraversion (Canli et al., 2001).

To activate the ACC, we selected the emotional Stroop task (see above), using word stimuli that were selected from a standardized stimulus library, the Affective Norms for English Words set (Bradley & Lang, 1999). Versions of the emotional Stroop have been used by other laboratories to activate the ACC (George et al., 1994; Whalen, Bush, et al., 1998). In our own work (see preceding section), we had reported that passive viewing of emotional positive pictures is associated with ACC activation as a function of extraversion (Canli et al., 2001), but in that study we had not controlled for mood state. It is therefore possible that the reported activation was not associated as much with a stable personality trait as with subjects' positive mood state. Our analysis strategy was to include measures of extraversion (the NEO PI-R Extraversion scale) and positive mood state (the POMS includes separate scales for positive and for negative mood) and to analyze ACC activation data for one while controlling for the other. Because men and women differed in their mood state responses, we also controlled for the effects of sex.

Figure 5.4 shows ACC activation as a function of personality trait (controlled for positive mood state and sex). We found that increased ACC activation to positive, relative to neutral, words was associated with extraversion, but not with positive mood. We also discovered a fascinating double dissociation when we investigated ACC reactivity to negative stimuli as a function of neuroticism and negative mood state: ACC activation to negative, relative to neutral, words varied across individuals as a function of negative mood, but not neuroticism. Thus, ACC processing of negative stimuli appears to vary as

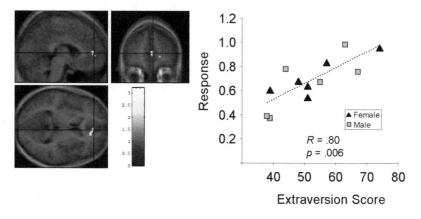

FIGURE 5.4. Activation of ACC in response to positive, relative to neutral, words as a function of extraversion (controlled for sex and positive mood). Left panel shows correlation cluster in the coronal, sagittal, and axial planes. Right panel shows scatterplot from this cluster. From Canli, Amin, Haas, Omura, and Constable (2004). Copyright 2004 by the American Psychological Association. Adapted by permission.

a function of mood state (and thus may vary within individuals), whereas ACC processing of positive stimuli appears to vary as a function of a stable personality trait (and may thus only vary across individuals). It should be noted, however, that the ACC was not the only brain region that exhibited activation differences to emotional stimuli as a function of mood state or personality trait. It is therefore expected that neural processing of trait and state variables involves larger networks of structures.

THE ENDOPHENOTYPE APPROACH: FROM TRAITS
TO COGNITIVE PROCESSES TO NEURAL SYSTEMS

In the two preceding sections, I have made the point that individual differences in brain activation to positive emotional stimuli can vary as a function of extraversion. But by what physiological mechanism does the degree of activation differ from one person to the next? One promising approach may be to include genomic information, which can account for some of the observed variance in terms of gene polymorphisms that have been associated with emotional reactivity or personality traits.

Several gene polymorphisms have been identified in which substitution of single nucleotides (single-nucleotide polymorphisms) or variation in the number of specific repeat sequences (variable number of tandem repeats) has been associated with individual differences in broad behavioral traits. For example, extraversion has been associated with variation in the dopamine D4 receptor

(*DRD4*) gene. The *DRD4* gene is located on chromosome 11p15.5 and contains a 48-base-pair repeat unit that varies between 2 and 11 times, producing gene variants of differing lengths. At the molecular level, the polymorphism has been shown to differentially affect receptor function (Asghari et al., 1995). At the behavioral level, Benjamin and colleagues (1996) and Ebstein and colleagues (1996), were the first to show that individuals who had at least one copy of the 7-repeat variant had significantly higher scores on self-report measures of extraversion (or novelty seeking) than those who had none.

These first reports prompted a significant number of replication studies. As reviewed by Reif and Lesch (2003), half of 34 replication studies reported evidence either in favor of or against an association between *DRD4* and personality traits related to extraversion. Reif and Lesch identified a number of factors that may have contributed to the reported null results, including small sample sizes, heterogeneous subject populations, unusual subject selection, and differing methods in personality assessment.

Another reason why gene–trait associations do not consistently replicate may be that self-reported personality traits are not sensitive enough a measure of behavior to capture the effect of genomic variation. This point was made by Hamer (2002), who regards the assumption of a linear relation between genes and behavior (as measured by personality questionnaires) as flawed, because it ignores the complex interactions between genes and the brain.

The endophenotype approach argues that genetic influences on behavior may be more sensitively captured by cognitive measures of behavior than by self-report (Castellanos & Tannock, 2002; de Geus, Wright, Martin, & Boomsma, 2001; Fossella et al., 2002; Goldberg & Weinberger, 2004; Gottesman & Gould, 2003; Hasler, Drevets, Manji, & Charney, 2004; Heiser et al., 2004; New & Siever, 2003; Siever, Torgersen, Gunderson, Livesley, & Kendler, 2002). Examples of cognitive endophenotypes may include attentional processes, executive functions, episodic memory, and language (for a review, see Goldberg & Weinberger, 2004). We have used this approach to investigate the effect of genetic variation within the 5-HT_{1A} receptor on cognitive measures of attention, using the emotional Stroop task (see Lesch & Canli, Chapter 13, this volume).

The endophenotype approach can be extended to the neural systems that mediate cognitive processes, as exemplified by the groundbreaking work of Weinberger and colleagues (Egan et al., 2001; Hariri et al., 2002, 2005; Hariri & Weinberger, 2003; Mattay et al., 2003). Some of this work is described in detail elsewhere in this volume (see Hariri, Chapter 14, this volume) and has focused on the amygdala, which was shown to vary in its response to negative emotional stimuli as a function of genetic variation within the *5-HTTLPR* (Hariri et al., 2002). This finding has since been replicated with a larger sample (Hariri et al., 2005) and by other groups (Furmark et al., 2004; Heinz et al., 2004).

The power of this genomic imaging approach is that the effect of genetic variation on brain activation is much more prominent than its effect on behavioral measures based on self-report. Indeed, Hamer (2002) has noted that while genes account for only a very modest amount of behavioral variance, they account for a considerably larger amount of variance when applied to specific brain regions. In support of this observation, he referred to Lesch and colleagues (1996), who reported that the *5-HTTLPR* polymorphism accounted for 3–4% of the total variance of their sample when self-report measures were used, and to the study by Hariri and colleagues (2002), in which genotype accounted for 20% of the variance when brain activation measures were used.

TOWARD GENOMIC IMAGING OF EXTRAVERSION

In this section, I illustrate how neuroimaging of extraversion can be integrated with a genomic imaging approach. As discussed above, it was previously shown that a number of brain regions respond to positive stimuli as a function of extraversion (Canli, 2004). Genetic variation within the dopamine D4 receptor gene (*DRD4*) is associated with extraversion. As noted earlier, this gene has a functional 48-base-pair repeat sequence in exon III that varies from 2 to 11 repeats (Cravchik & Goldman, 2000), and presence of the 7-repeat allele has been associated with extraversion or related personality traits (Benjamin et al., 1996, 2000; Ebstein et al., 1996; Strobel, Lesch, Jatzke, Paetzold, & Brocke, 2003). In collaboration with Klaus-Peter Lesch, we replicated this association in a sample of 100 Stony Brook students: participants who carried at least one copy of the 7-repeat allele ($n = 31$, NEO PI-R Extraversion mean = 55.0, *SEM* = 1.3) scored significantly higher in extraversion than participants who did not carry a 7-repeat allele ($n = 69$, NEO PI-R Extraversion mean = 49.0, *SEM* = 1.8), t (100) = 2.6, $p = .01$. If extraversion is associated with presence of the *DRD4* 7-repeat allele, then it may be possible that the *DRD4* genotype maps onto brain regions that respond to positive emotional stimuli as a function of extraversion.

To test this hypothesis, 30 healthy individuals with no history of psychopathology participated in a genomic imaging study, again in collaboration with Lesch. Each participant completed the NEO PI-R (Costa & McCrae, 1992) and was genotyped for the *DRD4* polymorphism.

While they were placed in the scanner, participants viewed 18-second blocks of neutral, happy, sad, and fearful face stimuli (four blocks per condition). Contrasts between activation to emotional versus neutral faces were calculated and correlated with subjects' extraversion scores. The regions identified by this procedure were then used as a mask for a subsequent one-sample t-test to determine whether there were any brain regions associated with extraversion, in which carriers of the *DRD4* 7-repeat allele ($n = 9$) showed significantly greater activation than noncarriers ($n = 21$). For this analysis, an activation threshold of $p < .05$ and cluster size threshold of 30 voxels was used, which reduces the probability of a false-positive error per pixel to an

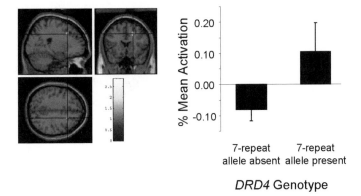

FIGURE 5.5. Brain activation associated with extraversion varies with *DRD4* genotype. Left panel shows activation within the middle frontal gyrus, where carriers of the *DRD4* 7-repeat allele exhibit significantly greater activation than noncarriers in the coronal, sagittal, and axial orientations. Right panel shows percentage of mean activation across the entire cluster as a function of genotype. From Canli (unpublished data).

estimated p = .003 (extrapolated from Forman et al., 1995). Two clusters were identified; one was located in the right middle frontal gyrus (37 voxels; Montreal Neurological Institute [MNI] coordinates: 22, 18, 38; p = .004) and the other in the left precuneus (40 voxels; MNI coordinates: −18, −46, 50; p = .01). Figure 5.5 shows data from the right middle frontal gyrus.

These results begin to suggest one mechanism by which brain activation to positive facial expressions differs between extraverted and introverted individuals. This mechanism may involve the twofold reduced inhibition in levels of cyclic adenosine monophosphate, a molecule that acts as an intracellular messenger, that is associated with the *DRD4* 7-repeat allele (Asghari et al., 1995). However, it is unknown what its effect on the functional activity of the dopamine receptor is. Thus future progress in the development of molecular models of personality is likely to require closer collaboration between investigators using genomic imaging approaches and investigators interested in molecular neurochemistry.

BEYOND SIMPLE GENE EFFECTS

The first studies have now been published that point to exciting discoveries about interactions between gene polymorphisms and other genes, environmental factors, and subjects' sex.

Gene–gene (epistatic) interactions relevant to personality have been reported by Ebstein and colleagues (1998), who reported a significant interaction between the *5-HTTLPR* and *DRD4* polymorphisms in neonatal orienting behavior (believed by the authors to be an antecedent to the adult novelty-seeking trait). They reported that the orientation score was lower in neonates homozygous for the *5-HTTLPR* short allele when they also lacked the long-allele form of the *DRD4* polymorphism (recall that the long, 7-repeat allele is associated with extraversion). A similar relation was reported in studies by Auerbach and colleagues (Auerbach et al., 1999; Auerbach, Benjamin, Faroy, Geller, & Ebstein, 2001), who found that infants homozygous for the *5-HTTLPR* short allele exhibited the highest scores in negative emotionality and distress when they were not carriers of the long *DRD4* allele. More complex gene–gene interactions have also been reported. Benjamin and colleagues (2000) found that novelty-seeking scores were related to the interplay of the *5-HTTLPR*, *DRD4*, and catechol-O-methyltransferase gene (*COMT*) polymorphisms. Specifically, they found that the association between subjects' novelty-seeking scores and the *DRD4* 7-repeat allele (previously associated with novelty seeking) was highest in subjects who did not carry the *5-HTTLPR* short allele (previously associated with neuroticism) and were homozygous for the *COMT* Val allele.

We recently found an interaction between dopaminergic and serotonergic gene polymorphisms in a study on impulsivity (Congdon, Lesch, & Canli, 2005). Forty-six Stony Brook University undergraduates were genotyped for the *5-HTTLPR*, 5-HT$_{1A}$ receptor gene (*HTR1A*), dopamine transporter gene (*DAT*), and *DRD4* polymorphisms. Participants then completed an impulsivity questionnaire, the Barratt Impulsiveness Scale–11 (BIS-11; Patton, Stanford, & Barratt, 1995), and were administered the Immediate Memory Task and Delayed Memory Task (IMT and DMT; Dougherty & Marsh, 2003). In the IMT, participants were instructed to respond only to target stimuli (a certain set of 5 digits) and not to respond to any other set of digits. Task instructions were identical for the DMT, except that participants needed to remember the sequence for the duration of a distracter stimulus.

An omnibus one-way multivariate analysis of variance, which included all four genotypes and three measures of impulsivity (BIS-11 score, IMT average commission errors, DMT average commission errors), revealed significant main effects for the *DRD4* and for the *DAT* genotypes, as well as significant interactions between the *5-HTTLPR* and *HTR1A* genotypes, and between the *5-HTTLPR* and *DRD4* genotypes. Univariate analyses showed that carriers of the *DRD4* 7-repeat allele committed more IMT commission errors than noncarriers. The interaction between the *DAT* and *DRD4* polymorphisms was evident in the DMT, in which more commission errors were associated with the presence of the *DRD4* 7-repeat allele and the *DAT* 10/10 genotype. This interaction is consistent with a study using ratings of hyperactivity–impulsivity, which also reported an interaction between the 7-repeat allele of the *DRD4* and the 10/10 genotype of the *DAT* (Roman et al., 2001). The interaction between *DRD4* and *5-HTTLPR* genotypes was evident in the IMT, in which the presence of the *DRD4* 7-repeat allele, in conjunction with the absence of the *5-HTTLPR* short allele, was associated with more commission errors than in any other group. This interaction is consistent with studies reporting that low levels of orienting behavior or high levels of distress in infants were associated with absence of the *DRD4* 7-repeat allele and presence of the *5-HTTLPR* short allele (Auerbach et al., 1999, 2001; Ebstein et al., 1998).

Gene–environment interactions have been reported in monkeys and in humans. For example, in rhesus macaques, *5-HTTLPR* genetic variation interacts with early rearing conditions to affect central 5-HT system homeostasis and emotionality in later life (Barr et al., 2004; Bennett et al., 2002; Lesch et al., 1997). In humans, Caspi and colleagues (2003) reported that the effect of life stress on depression and depression-related symptoms was moderated by the *5-HTTLPR* genotype. They followed a cohort of over 1000 participants over a period of 26 years to find that individuals who had experienced multiple life stress events and who carried at least one copy of the *5-HTTLPR* short allele had significantly higher rates of depressive symptoms, depression, and suicidality than individuals who were homozygous for the *5-HTTLPR* long allele. The neural systems that mediate this interaction are currently unknown.

Gene–sex interactions refer to observations suggesting that some gene polymorphisms exhibit sexually dimorphic associations. For example, one recent association study of the *DRD4* polymorphism with attention-deficit/hyperactivity disorder (ADHD) reported that ADHD was associated with long-repeat alleles in males and short-repeat alleles in females (Qian, Wang, Zhou, Yang, & Faraone, 2004). The same group also reported that the *COMT* polymorphism Met allele was preferentially transmitted to males with ADHD (Qian et al., 2003), but not to females with ADHD. Other reports also found greater association between the *COMT* Met allele and other forms of psychopathology in males, but not females (Karayiorgou et al., 1997, 1999; Nolan et al., 2000). The mechanisms by which these interactions operate in the brain are currently not understood.

LOOKING FORWARD

I think that personality psychology will undergo a dramatic makeover in the next decade or two, with the field shifting significantly toward molecular neuroscience. I am confident in this prediction for several reasons, which I outline below.

First, the trait approach has been criticized by some as being descriptive rather than explanatory (Mischel, 1999). Indeed, constructs such as the "Big Five" taxonomy of traits do not represent a specific theory (John & Srivastava, 1999). On the other hand, these traits have predictive validity and strong heritability (John & Srivastava, 1999), suggesting that they can explain behavior. Thus there should be strong motivation to utilize tools that can help develop explanatory theories of traits.

Second, there exists strong motivation outside the field of personality psychology to develop "real-world" predictive applications of genomic imaging. For example, the ability to predict aggressive behavior is relevant to law enforcement (Canli & Amin, 2002) and to homeland security (Canli, 2005). Strong economic or political motivation exists to improve the ability to predict an applicant's job performance, voter preferences, or consumer choices, using genomic imaging techniques (Canli, 2005). All of these behaviors, of course, also are of interest to personality psychologists

Third, recent developments in molecular biology, many driven by the Human Genome Project (Daiger, 2005), have found applications to the study of individual differences in humans. For example, the development of gene chips that can identify ten thousand, or even one hundred thousand, gene polymorphisms in humans today has revolutionized the ability to identify quantitative trait loci associated with complex traits (Butcher et al., 2004). The integration of such techniques with neuroimaging techniques can identify brain regions associated with individual differences and the genetic factors that contribute to these differences. The noninvasive nature of these techniques makes it possible to study the neuromolecular basis of personality in conscious, healthy human volunteers.

Fourth, some recently developed biological techniques make it possible to transition from associative to causal biological models of personality (Callaway, 2005). Specifically, methods have been developed to manipulate the genome and gene function (see Chiavegatto, Chapter 18, this volume). For example, animal "knockouts" have been developed in which specific genes have been removed from the genome, and conditional knockouts now make it possible to turn specific genes on or off at will. These techniques will make it possible to collect correlational data in humans, and then test causal predictions in genetically modified animals.

The preceding arguments in favor of a biological approach to personality are in no way intended to diminish the significance of environmental factors. Quite the opposite, in fact. The work of Caspi and colleagues has made it clear that life experience interacts with genetic variation in powerful ways (Caspi et al., 2002, 2003). A putative mechanism by which life experience can affect genetic function has been described in rats, where maternal behavior produced molecular changes within the glucocorticoid receptor gene in the hippocampus of rat pups (Weaver et al., 2004). Thus future neurogenetic models of personality must include explanations and predictions that articulate the interaction between genetic and environmental variables.

Personality psychology has traditionally been a discipline rooted within social psychology. A shift toward molecular neuroscience will undoubtedly alter the field's center of gravity, but biologically based models of personality will have to be able to integrate the insights of social psychologists. Thus biologically based models must ultimately explain and predict human behavior, even if they operate on the level of molecular events.

ACKNOWLEDGMENTS

The work described in this chapter was funded by Stony Brook University and by the National Science Foundation (Grant No. BCS-0224221). The conference was funded by a grant from the National Institute of Mental Health (No. 1R13MH06783501A1).

REFERENCES

Amin, Z., Constable, R. T., & Canli, T. (2004). Attentional bias for valenced stimuli as a function of personality in the dot-probe task. *Journal of Research in Personality, 38*, 15–23.

Asghari, V., Sanyal, S., Buchwaldt, S., Paterson, A., Jovanovic, V., & Van Tol, H. H. (1995). Modulation of intracellular cyclic AMP levels by different human dopamine D4 receptor variants. *Journal of Neurochemistry, 65*(3), 1157–1165.

Auerbach, J., Geller, V., Lezer, S., Shinwell, E., Belmaker, R. H., Levine, J., et al. (1999). Dopamine D4 receptor (D4DR) and serotonin transporter promoter (5-HTTLPR) polymorphisms in the determination of temperament in 2–month-old infants. *Molecular Psychiatry, 4*(4), 369–373.

Auerbach, J. G., Benjamin, J., Faroy, M., Geller, V., & Ebstein, R. (2001). *DRD4* related to infant attention and information processing: A developmental link to ADHD? *Psychiatric Genetics, 11*(1), 31–35.

Barr, C. S., Newman, T. K., Schwandt, M., Shannon, C., Dvoskin, R. L., Lindell, S. G., et al. (2004). Sexual dichotomy of an interaction between early adversity and the serotonin transporter gene promoter variant in rhesus macaques [Electronic version]. *Proceedings of the National Academy of Sciences USA, 101*(33), 12358–12363.

Bartussek, D., Becker, G., Diedrich, O., Naumann, E., & Maier, S. (1996). Extraversion, neuroticism, and event-related brain potentials in response to emotional stimuli. *Personality and Individual Differences, 20*(3), 301–312.

Benjamin, J., Li, L., Patterson, C., Greenberg, B. D., Murphy, D. L., & Hamer, D. H. (1996). Population and familial association between the D4 dopamine receptor gene and measures of novelty seeking. *Nature Genetics, 12*, 81–84.

Benjamin, J., Osher, Y., Kotler, M., Gritsenko, I., Nemanov, L., Belmaker, R. H., et al. (2000). Association between Tridimensional Personality Questionnaire (TPQ) traits and three functional polymorphisms: Dopamine receptor D4 (DRD4), serotonin transporter promoter region (5-HTTLPR) and catechol-O-methyltransferase (COMT). *Molecular Psychiatry, 5*(1), 96–100.

Bennett, A. J., Lesch, K. P., Heils, A., Long, J. C., Lorenz, J. G., Shoaf, S. E., et al. (2002). Early experience and serotonin transporter gene variation interact to influence primate CNS function. *Molecular Psychiatry, 7*(1), 118–122.

Bradley, M. M., & Lang, P. J. (1999). *Affective norms for English words (ANEW)*. Gainesville: NIMH Center for the Study of Emotion and Attention, University of Florida.

Breiter, H. C., Etcoff, N. L., Whalen, P. J., Kennedy, W. A., Rauch, S. L., Buckner, R. L., et al. (1996). Response and habituation of the human amygdala during visual processing of facial expression. *Neuron, 17*, 875–887.

Bush, G., Whalen, P. J., Rosen, B. R., Jenike, M. A., McInerney, S. C., & Rauch, S. L. (1998). The counting Stroop: An interference task specialized for functional neuroimaging—validation study with functional MRI. *Human Brain Mapping,* 6(4), 270–282.

Butcher, L. M., Meaburn, E., Liu, L., Fernandes, C., Hill, L., Al-Chalabi, A., et al. (2004). Genotyping pooled DNA on microarrays: A systematic genome screen of thousands of SNPs in large samples to detect QTLs for complex traits. *Behavior Genetics, 34*(5), 549–555.

Callaway, E. M. (2005). A molecular and genetic arsenal for systems neuroscience. *Trends in Neurosciences, 28*(4), 196–201.

Canli, T. (2004). Functional brain mapping of extraversion and neuroticism: Learning from individual differences in emotion processing. *Journal of Personality, 72*(6), 1105–1132.

Canli, T. (2005). When genes and brains unite: Ethical implications of genomic neuro-imaging. In J. Illes (Ed.), *Neuroethics in the 21st century* (pp. 169–184). New York: Oxford University Press.

Canli, T., & Amin, Z. (2002). Neuroimaging of emotion and personality: Scientific evidence and ethical considerations. *Brain and Cognition, 50,* 414–431.

Canli, T., Amin, Z., Haas, B., Omura, K., & Constable, R. T. (2004). A double disso-ciation between mood states and personality traits in the anterior cingulate. *Behavioral Neuroscience, 118*(5), 897–904.

Canli, T., Desmond, J. E., Zhao, Z., & Gabrieli, J. D. E. (2002). Sex differences in the neural basis of emotional memories. *Proceedings of the National Academy of Sci-ences USA, 99*(16), 10789–10794.

Canli, T., Desmond, J. E., Zhao, Z., Glover, G., & Gabrieli, J. D. E. (1998). Hemi-spheric asymmetry for emotional stimuli detected with fMRI. *NeuroReport, 9,* 3233–3239.

Canli, T., Sivers, H., Whitfield, S. L., Gotlib, I. H., & Gabrieli, J. D. (2002). Amygdala response to happy faces as a function of extraversion. *Science, 296,* 2191.

Canli, T., Zhao, Z., Desmond, J. E., Kang, E., Gross, J., & Gabrieli, J. D. E. (2001). An fMRI study of personality influences on brain reactivity to emotional stimuli. *Behavioral Neuroscience, 115*(1), 33–42.

Caspi, A., McClay, J., Moffitt, T. E., Mill, J., Martin, J., Craig, I. W., et al. (2002). Role of genotype in the cycle of violence in maltreated children. *Science, 297,* 851–854.

Caspi, A., Sugden, K., Moffitt, T. E., Taylor, A., Craig, I. W., Harrington, H., et al. (2003). Influence of life stress on depression: Moderation by a polymorphism in the 5-HTT gene. *Science, 301,* 386–389.

Castellanos, F. X., & Tannock, R. (2002). Neuroscience of attention-deficit/hyperac-tivity disorder: The search for endophenotypes. *Nature Reviews Neuroscience, 3*(8), 617–628.

Congdon, E., Lesch, K. P., & Canli, T. (2005). *The endophenotype of impulsivity in a non-clinical sample.* Manuscript submitted for publication.

Costa, P. T., Jr., & McCrae, R. R. (1980). Influence of extraversion and neuroticism on subjective well-being: Happy and unhappy people. *Journal of Personality and Social Psychology, 38,* 668–678.

Costa, P. T., Jr., & McCrae, R. R. (1992). *Professional manual of the Revised NEO Personality Inventory and NEO Five-Factor Inventory.* Odessa, FL: Psychologi-cal Assessment Resources.

Cravchik, A., & Goldman, D. (2000). Neurochemical individuality: Genetic diversity among human dopamine and serotonin receptors and transporters. *Archives of General Psychiatry, 57*(12), 1105–1114.

Daiger, S. P. (2005). Was the Human Genome Project worth the effort? *Science, 308,* 362–364.

Davis, M., Walker, D. L., & Myers, K. M. (2003). Role of the amygdala in fear extinction measured with potentiated startle. *Annals of the New York Academy of Sciences, 985,* 218–232.

Davis, M., & Whalen, P. J. (2001). The amygdala: Vigilance and emotion. *Molecular Psychiatry, 6*(1), 13–34.

de Geus, E. J., Wright, M. J., Martin, N. G., & Boomsma, D. I. (2001). Genetics of brain function and cognition. *Behavior Genetics, 31*(6), 489–495.

Derryberry, D., & Reed, M. A. (1994). Temperament and attention: Orienting towards and away from positive and negative signals. *Journal of Personality and Social Psychology, 66,* 1128–1139.

Devinsky, O., Morrell, M. J., & Vogt, B. A. (1995). Contributions of anterior cingulate cortex to behaviour. *Brain, 118*(Pt. 1), 279–306.

Donner, T., Kettermann, A., Diesch, E., Ostendorf, F., Villringer, A., & Brandt, S. A. (2000). Involvement of the human frontal eye field and multiple parietal areas in covert visual selection during conjunctive search. *European Journal of Neuroscience, 12,* 3407–3414.

Dougherty, D. M., & Marsh, D. M. (2003). *Immediate and Delayed Memory Tasks (IMT/DMT 2.0): A research tool for studying attention, memory, and impulsive behavior.* Houston: Neurobehavioral Research Laboratory and Clinic, University of Texas Health Science Center at Houston.

Ebmeier, K. P., Deary, I. J., O'Carroll, R. E., Prentice, N., Moffoot, A. P. R., & Goodwin, G. M. (1994). Personality associations with the uptake of the cerebral blood flow marker Tc-exametazime estimated with single photon emission tomography. *Personality and Individual Differences, 5,* 587–595.

Ebstein, R. P., Levine, J., Geller, V., Auerbach, J., Gritsenko, I., & Belmaker, R. H. (1998). Dopamine D4 receptor and serotonin transporter promoter in the determination of neonatal temperament. *Molecular Psychiatry, 3*(3), 238–246.

Ebstein, R. P., Novick, O., Umansky, R., Priel, B., Osher, Y., Blaine, D., et al. (1996). Dopamine D4 receptor (D4DR) exon III polymorphism associated with the human personality trait of novelty seeking. *Nature Genetics, 12,* 78–80.

Egan, M. F., Goldberg, T. E., Kolachana, B. S., Callicott, J. H., Mazzanti, C. M., Straub, R. E., et al. (2001). Effect of COMT Val108/158 Met genotype on frontal lobe function and risk for schizophrenia. *Proceedings of the National Academy of Sciences USA, 98*(12), 6917–6922.

Fanselow, M. S., & Poulos, A. M. (2005). The neuroscience of mammalian associative learning. *Annual Review of Psychology, 56*(1), 207–234.

Fink, A., Schrausser, D. G., & Neubauer, A. C. (2002). The moderating influence of extraversion on the relationship between IQ and cortical activation. *Personality and Individual Differences, 33,* 311–326.

Fischer, H., Tillfors, M., Furmark, T., & Fredrikson, M. (2001). Dispositional pessimism and amygdala activity: A PET study in healthy volunteers. *NeuroReport, 12,* 1635–1638.

Fischer, H., Wik, G., & Fredrikson, M. (1997). Extraversion, neuroticism and brain function: A PET study of personality. *Personality and Individual Differences, 23*(2), 345–352.

Forman, S. D., Cohen, J. D., Fitzgerald, M., Eddy, W. F., Mintun, M. A., & Noll, D. C. (1995). Improved assessment of significant activation in functional magnetic resonance imaging (fMRI): Use of a cluster-size threshold. *Magnetic Resonance in Medicine, 33*, 636–647.

Fossella, J., Sommer, T., Fan, J., Wu, Y., Swanson, J. M., Pfaff, D. W., et al. (2002). Assessing the molecular genetics of attention networks. *BMC Neuroscience, 3*(1), 14.

Furmark, T., Tillfors, M., Garpenstrand, H., Marteinsdottir, I., Langstrom, B., Oreland, L., et al. (2004). Serotonin transporter polymorphism related to amygdala excitability and symptom severity in patients with social phobia. *Neuroscience Letters, 362*(3), 189–192.

George, M. S., Ketter, T. A., Parekh, P. I., Rosinsky, N., Ring, H. A., Casey, B. J., et al. (1994). Regional brain activity when selecting a response despite interference: An H2-15O PET study of the Stroop and an emotional Stroop. *Human Brain Mapping, 1*, 194–209.

Goldberg, T. E., & Weinberger, D. R. (2004). Genes and the parsing of cognitive processes. *Trends in Cognitive Sciences, 8*(7), 325–335.

Gottesman, I. I., & Gould, T. D. (2003). The endophenotype concept in psychiatry: Etymology and strategic intentions. *American Journal of Psychiatry, 160*(4), 636–645.

Gray, J. R., & Braver, T. S. (2002). Personality predicts working-memory-related activation in the caudal anterior cingulate cortex. *Cognitive, Affective and Behavioral Neuroscience, 2*(1), 64–75.

Gross, J. J. (1999). Emotion and emotion regulation. In L. A. Pervin & O. P. John (Eds.), *Handbook of personality: Theory and research* (2nd ed., pp. 525–552). New York: Guilford Press.

Gross, J. J., Sutton, S. K., & Ketelaar, T. V. (1998). Relations between affect and personality: Support for the affect-level and affective-reactivity views. *Personality and Social Psychology Bulletin, 24*, 279–288.

Gurrera, R. J., O'Donnell, B. F., Nestor, P. G., Gainski, J., & McCarley, R. W. (2001). The P3 auditory event-related brain potential indexes major personality traits. *Biological Psychiatry, 49*(11), 922–929.

Haier, R. J., Sokolski, K., Katz, M., & Buchsbaum, M. S. (1987). The study of personality with positron emission tomography. In J. Strelau & H. J. Eysenck (Eds.), *Personality dimensions and arousal* (pp. 251–267). New York: Plenum Press.

Hamer, D. (2002). Genetics: Rethinking behavior genetics. *Science, 298*, 71–72.

Hariri, A. R., Drabant, E. M., Munoz, K. E., Kolachana, B. S., Mattay, V. S., Egan, M. F., et al. (2005). A susceptibility gene for affective disorders and the response of the human amygdala. *Archives of General Psychiatry, 62*(2), 146–152.

Hariri, A. R., Mattay, V. S., Tessitore, A., Kolachana, B., Fera, F., Goldman, D., et al. (2002). Serotonin transporter genetic variation and the response of the human amygdala. *Science, 297*, 400–403.

Hariri, A. R., & Weinberger, D. R. (2003). Imaging genomics. *British Medical Bulletin, 65*, 259–270.

Hasler, G., Drevets, W. C., Manji, H. K., & Charney, D. S. (2004). Discovering endophenotypes for major depression. *Neuropsychopharmacology, 29*(10), 1765–1781.

Heils, A., Teufel, A., Petri, S., Stober, G., Riederer, P., Bengel, D., et al. (1996). Allelic variation of human serotonin gene expression. *Journal of Neurochemistry, 66*(6), 2621–2624.

Heinz, A., Braus, D. F., Smolka, M. N., Wrase, J., Puls, I., Hermann, D., et al. (2004). Amygdala–prefrontal coupling depends on a genetic variation of the serotonin transporter. *Nature Neuroscience, 7*(12).

Heiser, P., Friedel, S., Dempfle, A., Konrad, K., Smidt, J., Grabarkiewicz, J., et al. (2004). Molecular genetic aspects of attention-deficit/hyperactivity disorder. *Neuroscience and Biobehavioral Reviews, 28*(6), 625–641.

John, O. P., & Srivastava, S. (1999). The Big Five trait taxonomy: History, measurement, and theoretical perspectives. In L. A. Pervin & O. P. John (Eds.), *Handbook of personality: Theory and research* (2nd ed., pp. 102–138). New York: Guilford Press.

Johnson, D. L., Wiebe, J. S., Gold, S. M., Andreasen, N. C., Hichwa, R. D., Watkins, G. L., et al. (1999). Cerebral blood flow and personality: A positron emission tomography study. *American Journal of Psychiatry, 156*, 252–257.

Karayiorgou, M., Altemus, M., Galke, B. L., Goldman, D., Murphy, D. L., Ott, J., et al. (1997). Genotype determining low catechol-O-methyltransferase activity as a risk factor for obsessive–compulsive disorder. *Proceedings of the National Academy of Sciences USA, 94*(9), 4572–4575.

Karayiorgou, M., Sobin, C., Blundell, M. L., Galke, B. L., Malinova, L., Goldberg, P., et al. (1999). Family-based association studies support a sexually dimorphic effect of COMT and MAOA on genetic susceptibility to obsessive–compulsive disorder. *Biological Psychiatry, 45*(9), 1178–1189.

Keightley, M. L., Seminowicz, D. A., Bagby, R. M., Costa, P. T., Fossati, P., & Mayberg, H. S. (2003). Personality influences limbic–cortical interactions during sad mood induction. *NeuroImage, 20*(4), 2031–2039.

Kesler-West, M. L., Andersen, A. H., Smith, C. D., Avison, M. J., Davis, C. E., Kryscio, R. J., et al. (2001). Neural substrates of facial emotion processing using fMRI. *Cognitive Brain Research, 11*(2), 213–226.

Killgore, W. D., & Yurgelun-Todd, D. A. (2001). Sex differences in amygdala activation during the perception of facial affect. *NeuroReport, 12*(11), 2543–2547.

Knutson, B., Momenan, R., Rawlings, R. R., Fong, G. W., & Hommer, D. (2001). Negative association of neuroticism with brain volume ratio in healthy humans. *Biological Psychiatry, 50*(9), 685–690.

Knutson, B., Wolkowitz, O. M., Cole, S. W., Chan, T., Moore, E. A., Johnson, R. C., et al. (1998). Selective alteration of personality and social behavior by serotonergic intervention. *American Journal of Psychiatry, 155*(3), 373–379.

Kumari, V., Ffytche, D. H., Williams, S. C., & Gray, J. A. (2004). Personality predicts brain responses to cognitive demands. *Journal of Neuroscience, 24*, 10636–10641.

Laakso, A., Wallius, E., Kajander, J., Bergman, J., Eskola, O., Solin, O., et al. (2003). Personality traits and striatal dopamine synthesis capacity in healthy subjects. *American Journal of Psychiatry, 160*(5), 904–910.

Lane, R. D. (2000). Neural correlates of conscious emotional experience. In R. D. Lane & L. Nadel (Ed.), *Cognitive neuroscience of emotion* (pp. 345–370). New York: Oxford University Press.

Lane, R. D., Fink, G. R., Chau, P. M., & Dolan, R. J. (1997). Neural activation during selective attention to subjective emotional responses. *NeuroReport, 8*, 3969–3972.

Lane, R. D., Reiman, E. M., Axelrod, B., Yun, L. S., Holmes, A., & Schwartz, G. E. (1998). Neural correlates of levels of emotional awareness: Evidence of an interaction between emotion and attention in the anterior cingulate cortex. *Journal of Cognitive Neuroscience, 10*(4), 525–535.

Lang, P. J., Bradley, M. M., & Cuthbert, B. N. (2001). *International Affective Picture System (IAPS): Instruction manual and affective ratings* (Technical Report No. A-5). Gainesville: Center for Research in Psychophysiology, University of Florida.

Larsen, R. J., & Ketelaar, T. (1991). Personality and susceptibility to positive and negative emotional states. *Journal of Personality and Social Psychology, 61,* 132–140.

LeDoux, J. (2003). The emotional brain, fear, and the amygdala. *Cellular and Molecular Neurobiology, 23*(4–5), 727–738.

Lesch, K. P., Bengel, D., Heils, A., Sabol, S. Z., Greenberg, B. D., Petri, S., et al. (1996). Association of anxiety-related traits with a polymorphism in the serotonin transporter gene regulatory region. *Science, 274,* 1527–1531.

Lesch, K. P., Meyer, J., Glatz, K., Flugge, G., Hinney, A., Hebebrand, J., et al. (1997). The 5-HT transporter gene-linked polymorphic region (5-HTTLPR) in evolutionary perspective: Alternative biallelic variation in rhesus monkeys. Rapid communication. *Journal of Neural Transmission, 104*(11–12), 1259–1266.

Maren, S. (2005). Building and burying fear memories in the brain. *Neuroscientist, 11*(1), 89–99.

Mattay, V. S., Goldberg, T. E., Fera, F., Hariri, A. R., Tessitore, A., Egan, M. F., et al. (2003). Catechol-O-methyltransferase Val158-Met genotype and individual variation in the brain response to amphetamine. *Proceedings of the National Academy of Sciences USA, 100*(10), 6186–6191.

McNair, M. L., Lorr, M., & Droppleman, L. F. (1992). *Profile of Mood States (POMS) manual.* San Diego, CA: Edits.

Mischel, W. (1999). Personality coherence and dispositions in a cognitive–affective processing system (CAPS) approach. In D. Cervone & Y. Shoda (Eds.), *The coherence of personality: Social-cognitive bases of consistency, variability, and organization* (pp. 37–60). New York: Guilford Press.

Mogg, K., Bradley, B. P., & Williams, R. (1995). Attentional bias in anxiety and depression: The role of awareness. *British Journal of Clinical Psychology, 34,* 17–36.

Morris, J. S., Frith, C. D., Perrett, D. I., Rowland, D., Young, A. W., Calder, A. J., et al. (1996). A differential neural response in the human amygdala to fearful and happy facial expressions. *Nature, 383,* 812–815.

New, A. S., & Siever, L. J. (2003). Biochemical endophenotypes in personality disorders. *Methods in Molecular Medicine, 77,* 199–213.

Nolan, K. A., Volavka, J., Czobor, P., Cseh, A., Lachman, H., Saito, T., et al. (2000). Suicidal behavior in patients with schizophrenia is related to COMT polymorphism. *Psychiatric Genetics, 10*(3), 117–124.

Onitsuka, T., Nestor, P. G., Gurrera, R. J., Shenton, M. E., Kasai, K., Frumin, M., et al. (2005). Association between reduced extraversion and right posterior fusiform gyrus gray matter reduction in chronic schizophrenia. *American Journal of Psychiatry, 162*(3), 599–601.

Pare, D., Quirk, G. J., & LeDoux, J. E. (2004). New vistas on amygdala networks in conditioned fear. *Journal of Neurophysiology, 92*(1), 1–9.

Patton, J. H., Stanford, M. S., & Barratt, E. S. (1995). Factor structure of the Barratt Impulsiveness Scale. *Journal of Clinical Psychology, 51*(6), 768–774.

Pervin, L. A., & John, O. P. (Eds.). (1999). *Handbook of personality: Theory and research* (2nd ed.). New York: Guilford Press.

Phillips, M. L., Bullmore, E. T., Howard, R., Woodruff, P. W., Wright, I. C., Williams, S. C., et al. (1998). Investigation of facial recognition memory and happy and sad facial expression perception: An fMRI study. *Psychiatry Research, 83*(3), 127–138.

Plomin, R., & Kosslyn, S. M. (2001). Genes, brain and cognition. *Nature Neuroscience, 4*, 1153–1154.

Qian, Q., Wang, Y., Zhou, R., Li, J., Wang, B., Glatt, S., et al. (2003). Family-based and case–control association studies of catechol-O-methyltransferase in attention deficit hyperactivity disorder suggest genetic sexual dimorphism. *American Journal of Medical Genetics, 118B*(1), 103–109.

Qian, Q., Wang, Y., Zhou, R., Yang, L., & Faraone, S. V. (2004). Family-based and case–control association studies of *DRD4* and DAT1 polymorphisms in Chinese attention deficit hyperactivity disorder patients suggest long repeats contribute to genetic risk for the disorder. *American Journal of Medical Genetics, 128B*(1), 84–89.

Reif, A., & Lesch, K. P. (2003). Toward a molecular architecture of personality. *Behavioral Brain Research, 139*(1–2), 1–20.

Richards, A., French, C. C., Johnson, W., Naparstek, J., & Williams, J. (1992). Effects of mood manipulation and anxiety on performance of an emotional Stroop task. *British Journal of Psychology, 83*, 479–491.

Rodrigues, S. M., Schafe, G. E., & LeDoux, J. E. (2004). Molecular mechanisms underlying emotional learning and memory in the lateral amygdala. *Neuron, 44*(1), 75–91.

Roman, T., Schmitz, M., Polanczyk, G., Eizirik, M., Rohde, L. A., & Hutz, M. H. (2001). Attention-deficit hyperactivity disorder: A study of association with both the dopamine transporter gene and the dopamine D4 receptor gene. *American Journal of Medical Genetics, 105*(5), 471–478.

Rosen, J. B. (2004). The neurobiology of conditioned and unconditioned fear: A neurobehavioral system analysis of the amygdala. *Behavioral and Cognitive Neuroscience Reviews, 3*(1), 23–41.

Siever, L. J., Torgersen, S., Gunderson, J. G., Livesley, W. J., & Kendler, K. S. (2002). The borderline diagnosis: III. Identifying endophenotypes for genetic studies. *Biological Psychiatry, 51*, 964–968.

Steinmetz, H., & Seitz, R. J. (1991). Functional anatomy of language processing: Neuroimaging and the problem of individual variability. *Neuropsychologia, 29*, 1149–1161.

Stenberg, G., Risberg, J., Warkentin, S., & Rosen, I. (1990). Regional patterns of cortical blood flow distinguish extraverts from introverts. *Personality and Individual Differences, 11*, 663–673.

Stenberg, G., Wendt, P. E., & Risberg, J. (1993). Regional cerebral blood flow and extraversion. *Personality and Individual Differences, 15*, 547–554.

Strobel, A., Lesch, K. P., Jatzke, S., Paetzold, F., & Brocke, B. (2003). Further evidence for a modulation of novelty seeking by *DRD4* exon III, 5-HTTLPR, and COMT Val/Met variants. *Molecular Psychiatry, 8*(4), 371–372.

Stroop, J. R. (1935). Studies of interference in serial verbal reactions. *Journal of Experimental Psychology, 18*, 643–662.

Suguira, M., Kawashima, R., Nakagawa, M., Okada, K., Sato, T., Goto, R., et al. (2000). Correlation between human personality and neural activity in the cerebral cortex. *NeuroImage, 11*, 541–546.

Suhara, T., Yasuno, F., Sudo, Y., Yamamoto, M., Inoue, M., Okubo, Y., et al. (2001). Dopamine D2 receptors in the insular cortex and the personality trait of novelty seeking. *NeuroImage, 13*(5), 891–895.

Vaidya, J. G., Gray, E. K., Haig, J., & Watson, D. (2002). On the temporal stability of personality: Evidence for differential stability and the role of life experiences. *Journal of Personality and Social Psychology, 83*(6), 1469–1484.

Watson, C., & Clark, L. A. (1997). Extraversion and its positive emotional core. In R. Hogan, J. Johnson, & W. J. S. Briggs (Eds.), *Handbook of personality psychology* (pp. 767–793). San Diego, CA: Academic Press.

Watson, D., Wiese, D., Vaidya, J., & Tellegen, A. (1999). The two general activation systems of affect: Structural findings, evolutionary considerations, and psychobiological evidence. *Journal of Personality and Social Psychology, 76*, 820–838.

Weaver, I. C., Cervoni, N., Champagne, F. A., D'Alessio, A. C., Sharma, S., Seckl, J. R., et al. (2004). Epigenetic programming by maternal behavior [Electronic version]. *Nature Neuroscience, 7*(8), 847–854.

Whalen, P. J., Bush, G., McNally, R. J., Wilhelm, S., McInerney, S. C., Jenike, M. A., et al. (1998). The emotional counting Stroop paradigm: A functional magnetic resonance imaging probe of the anterior cingulate affective division. *Biological Psychiatry, 44*(12), 1219–1228.

Whalen, P. J., Rauch, S. L., Etcoff, N. L., McInerney, S. C., Lee, M. B., & Jenike, M. A. (1998). Masked presentations of emotional facial expressions modulate amygdala activity without explicit knowledge. *Journal of Neuroscience, 18*, 411–418.

Yang, T. T., Menon, V., Eliez, S., Blasey, C., White, C. D., Reid, A. J., et al. (2002). Amygdalar activation associated with positive and negative facial expressions. *NeuroReport, 13*, 1737–1741.

Youn, T., Lyoo, I. K., Kim, J. K., Park, H. J., Ha, K. S., Lee, D. S., et al. (2002). Relationship between personality trait and regional cerebral glucose metabolism assessed with positron emission tomography. *Biological Psychology, 60*(2–3), 109–120.

6

Neural Substrates
for Emotional Traits?

THE CASE OF EXTRAVERSION

Brian Knutson and Jamil Bhanji

LOOKING BACK

The problem was common enough in academia, but unprecedented in this particular laboratory: How was a professor to deal with a stubborn student? The problem pupil had completed an experiment showing that after having tasted a black acid solution, dogs salivated profusely when simply shown a jug of sloshing black water. And the sight of the dark fluid did not summon just any type of spittle; it specifically evoked a watery type of saliva that dogs exude when aversive substances are placed in the mouth. The thin, watery saliva was probably useful for washing away noxious compounds, and could be contrasted with a thicker, mucus-like saliva elicited by tasty treats (e.g., a squirt of meat powder), which might facilitate sticking to the tongue. Although his advisor advocated a physiological hypothesis, the student was not satisfied, and insisted instead on a psychological explanation of the dogs' anticipatory salivation, referring to "emotions" and "desires"! How could the advisor resolve the dispute? In the short run, he retained his physiological view, writing that "after a considerable mental conflict, I decided finally in regard to so-called psychical stimulation to remain in the role of a pure physiologist" (quoted in Boakes, 1984, p. 121). In the long run, after winning the Nobel Prize, advisor Ivan Pavlov was enshrined in the canons of science, while student Anton Snarsky—who had conducted the first experimental demonstration of classical conditioning—faded into obscurity.

But the question of emotion's role in conditioning remained unresolved. Because Pavlov collected individual rather than group data on his dogs, he could not help noticing the temperamental variability that different dogs showed to identical conditioned stimuli. These differences became particularly apparent when Pavlov exposed dogs to difficult-to-discriminate cues signaling an upcoming shock: The cues put some to sleep and reduced others to whimpering wrecks. Later in his career, Pavlov documented these individual differences, drawing on the humoral theories of the ancient Greeks, and also his own speculations about interactions between subcortical excitation and cortical inhibition in the brain (Pavlov, 1927).

What: Identifying and Measuring Emotional Traits

Pavlov's speculations were later adopted and further developed by psychologist Hans Eysenck, who postulated that a human trait dubbed "extroversion" by Carl Jung reflects insufficient cortical arousal, resulting in stimulation seeking. (Eysenck's own spelling of this term, "extraversion," has remained in common use in the field.) According to Eysenck, cortical arousal is generated by a midbrain structure called the "ascending reticular activating system" (Eysenck, 1990), which (as researchers subsequently discovered) houses several distinct types of aminergic neurons, including dopamine. Although research failed to provide conclusive evidence for Eysenck's cortical hypoarousal hypothesis of extraversion, the behavioral traits of the extraverted phenotype remained robust. Eysenck later added a second and independent temperamental trait called "neuroticism," which he attributed to subcortical hyperarousal, resulting in emotional instability (Eysenck, 1967). Perhaps most importantly, Eysenck also developed a psychometrically reliable and valid instrument for measuring these traits, the Eysenck Personality Inventory (EPI; Eysenck, 1990).

Eysenck's successor, Jeffrey Gray, subsequently attempted to translate these traits to a behavioral framework in order to study the effects of psychotropic drugs on rats, and did so by rotating the extraversion/neuroticism axis 45° to form dimensions of "behavioral activation" and "behavioral inhibition" (Gray, 1987; see also Fowles, Chapter 2, this volume). Although Gray's maneuver had the intended effect of moving the focus of investigation away from measurable psychological experience to behavior, it also conceptually obfuscated aspects of Eysenck's constructs. For instance, a still rat might be described as showing behavioral inhibition, but could either be asleep or frozen in fear (i.e., at opposite ends of the arousal spectrum). In addition, because Gray's constructs were primarily inferred from rat behavior, Gray never developed a psychometric measure of his dimensions in humans (but see Carver & White, 1994).

More recently, the psychometric literature has built upon and expanded Eysenck's EPI to incorporate five rather than three factors. A commonly used inventory, called the Revised NEO Personality Inventory (NEO PI-R), assesses both Extraversion and Neuroticism, as well as three additional factors called Agreeableness, Conscientiousness, and Openness (Costa & McCrae, 1992). Both Extraversion and Neuroticism have retained core emotional characteristics, but not exactly in the manner conceptualized by Eysenck. Instead of a single dimension of arousal, a central feature of Extraversion involves the frequency of experiencing positive aroused affective states, while a central feature of Neuroticism involves the frequency of experiencing negative aroused affective states. These core affective sensitivities are evident not only in the content of NEO PI-R items, but also in self-report during experience sampling (Spain, Eaton, & Funder, 2000) and laboratory affect challenge studies (Gross, Sutton, & Ketelaar, 1998; Larsen & Ketelaar, 1989). Thus current research suggests that extraverts are more likely to experience positive arousal (e.g., excitement, energy), whereas neurotics are more likely to experience negative arousal (e.g., fear, tension; see Figure 6.1). Physiologically, these findings raise the possibility that common mechanisms underlie emotional states and traits.

To summarize, emotional traits appear to show robust and heritable individual differences in humans, as well as dogs, rats, and possibly other mammalian species (Gosling & John, 1999; see Mehta & Gosling, Chapter 20, this volume). Two of these traits have been clearly linked to the propensity to experience affective states. Specifically, extraversion is associated with an

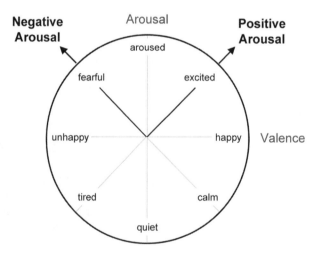

FIGURE 6.1. The affective circumplex. From Watson, Wiese, Vaidya, and Tellegen (1999). Copyright 1999 by the American Psychological Association. Adapted by permission.

increased likelihood of experiencing positive arousal, while neuroticism is associated with an increased likelihood of experiencing negative arousal. If the neural mechanisms responsible for positive and negative arousal were identified, one could then investigate whether the functioning of these mechanisms is also related to emotional traits (Depue, Luciana, Arbisi, Collins, & Leon, 1994; Knutson et al., 1998). Unfortunately, today as in Pavlov's time, the neural basis of affective experience is far from clear. Fortunately, we now have access to methods that could begin to provide answers. Even so, we must first know where in the brain to look for such an association, as well as when in time.

Where: Localizing Relevant Neural Circuitry

The emerging discipline of affective neuroscience aims at a mechanistic understanding of the physiological mechanisms that underlie affective experience. Two primary approaches have brought light to bear on this question. The first begins with studies of animal physiology and typically focuses on subcortical circuits (Panksepp, 1991); the second begins with studies of human physiology and typically focuses on cortical circuits (Davidson & Sutton, 1995). Although both have produced useful insights, we focus on the first (or comparative) approach, which primarily arose not only from the ancient observation of stock breeders that emotional traits are heritable (Bouchard, 1994), but also from brain stimulation research (Olds & Fobes, 1981).

Although earlier examples exist, such as the "sham rage" that Nobel laureate Walter Hess evoked by stimulating subcortical parts of the brain (Hess, 1959), the most relevant example to the present work is that of James Olds and Peter Milner. In 1954, they discovered that rats would work furiously and to the exclusion of other incentives (e.g., food, drink, sex, and sleep) to electrically stimulate their brains in certain subcortical locations (Olds & Milner, 1954). Histochemical visualization methods later clarified that many of these "self-stimulation" regions lay along the ascending path of the mesolimbic dopamine system (Hillarp, Fuxe, & Dahlstrom, 1966). Innervated by ventral tegmental area (VTA) dopamine neurons of the midbrain, these regions included not only the subcortical nucleus accumbens (NA), other ventral striatal regions, and the medial amygdala, but also parts of the orbital and the mesial prefrontal cortex (MPFC) (Nieuwenhuys, 1985). Regions that potently evoke electrical self-stimulation colocalize with an ascending "mesolimbic" dopamine pathway that runs from the VTA to the lateral hypothalamus, the ventral striatum (including the NA), and finally parts of the MPFC.

When: Temporally Deconstructing Incentive Processing

More recently, electrophysiological studies of monkeys demonstrated that VTA dopamine neurons fire not only when a monkey receives unexpected rewards (e.g., a juice squirt), but also when a cue is presented that predicts a reward (Schultz, Dayan, & Montague, 1997). These findings thus suggest a candidate neural mechanism for Pavlov's appetitive conditioning. However, although the VTA provides a "beacon of incentive motivation" in the brain, it is not clear where that beacon shines. Deconstructing Pavlov's paradigms in time, we can derive a matrix illustrating two valences (positive and negative) and phases (anticipation and outcome) of incentive processing (see Figure 6.2).

Presently, controversy swirls around the specificity of dopamine's role in incentive processing. Does dopamine fire in response only to positive incentives, or also to negative incentives? And after learning has taken place, does dopamine primarily fire during anticipation of incentives, or also in response to incentive outcomes? Answers to these questions depend critically upon methodological advances. Specifically, researchers must be able to visualize ongoing activity in mesolimbic regions with detailed enough spatial resolution to resolve small subcortical structures, and at a fine enough temporal resolution to distinguish anticipatory from consummatory activity.

Developments in methods for investigating brain function in rats and humans may help resolve the controversy. In rats, microdialysis probes provide good chemical resolution of dopamine release, but not good temporal resolution (i.e., on the order of 2 minutes) (Westerink, 1995). Thus, although microdialysis studies have clearly implicated NA and MPFC dopamine release in incentive processing, the temporal specificity of this involvement is not clear. However, a new method called "*in vivo* cyclic voltammetry," which provides better temporal resolution of dopamine release (i.e., on the order of 200 milliseconds), clearly indicates that dopamine release in the NA can precede reward outcomes, and thus can occur during anticipation (Wightman & Robinson, 2002).

Simultaneously, a parallel set of methodological advances has occurred in human brain imaging. Although variants of positron emission tomography (PET) provide chemically specific information about the release of dopamine

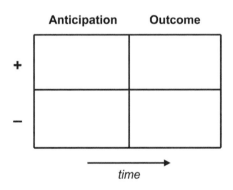

FIGURE 6.2. Simplified scheme for studying incentive processing.

in the brain, the temporal resolutions of these methods are limited to 2–3 minutes (Laruelle, 2000). As with microdialysis in comparative research, PET has implicated NA and MPFC dopamine release in incentive processing, but has not elucidated the time course of release (Koepp et al., 1998). On the other hand, event-related functional magnetic resonance imaging (fMRI) indexes oxygen utilization instead of dopamine release, but can do so at an enhanced temporal resolution (i.e., on the order of 1–2 seconds). Thus event-related fMRI studies have attempted to capture the time course of mesolimbic activity during all phases and types of incentive processing.

Integrating Where and When

Developing an incentive-processing task suitable for use with event-related fMRI raises a number of challenges, including what type of incentive to use. Our laboratory has developed a task that utilizes monetary incentives, descriptively dubbed the "monetary incentive delay" (MID) task. Although not a "primary" or unlearned incentive, money has three important advantages: It is compelling (i.e., most people will work for it), reversible (i.e., it can be given and taken away), and scalable (i.e., it can be parameterized). In addition to including incentives involving potential monetary gain or loss, the MID task incorporates both anticipatory and outcome phases of incentive processing. Specifically, on each trial of the MID task, participants see a cue indicating whether they can gain or avoid losing money and how much is at stake. Then, after a short delay (2–3 seconds), they must respond to a rapidly presented target with a button press. Depending on their success at pressing the button before the target disappears, they can either make or avoid losing money. Subsequent feedback indicates the outcome of that trial and the subject's cumulative total (Knutson, Westdorp, Kaiser, & Hommer, 2000). Thus brain activity during incentive anticipation and outcome phases can be separately visualized (see Figure 6.3).

Using event-related fMRI in combination with the MID task, our laboratory has focused in several studies on identifying neural markers for each type and phase of incentive processing. Monkey electrophysiological research indicated that one or more mesolimbic regions should "activate" during anticipation of positive outcomes. Indeed, as subjects anticipated increasing potential gains (i.e., +$0.00, +$0.20, +$1.00, +$5.00), activity in three subcortical regions increased. These regions included the thalamus, medial caudate, and NA. However, activity in the thalamus and medial caudate also increased when subjects anticipated increasing losses. But activation in the NA did not, suggesting that NA activation was proportionally associated with gain anticipation, but not with loss anticipation (Knutson, Adams, Fong, & Hommer, 2001). In addition, NA activation returned to baseline by the time subjects learned that they had succeeded in gaining money. Thus NA activation was more closely associated with gain anticipation than with gain outcomes (Knutson, Fong, Adams, Varner, & Hommer, 2001). On the other hand,

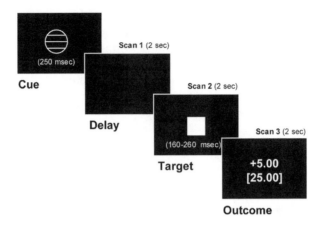

FIGURE 6.3. Trial structure of the monetary incentive delay (MID) task. From Knutson, Fong, Bennett, Adams, and Hommer (2003). Copyright 2003 by Academic Press. Adapted by permission.

when anticipation was controlled for, gain outcomes activated a part of the MPFC instead of the NA. Relative to anticipating and making no money, when people anticipated making a large amount (+$5.00) and succeeded, activation in the MPFC increased, but when they failed, activation decreased (Knutson, Fong, Bennett, Adams, & Hommer, 2003). Together, these results implicated the NA in processing of gain anticipation, but the MPFC in processing of gain outcomes.

BRAIN ACTIVITY AND POSITIVE AROUSAL

Armed with neural probes of reward processing, we could begin to examine the relationship between NA activation and positive arousal across individuals. PET research from a number of laboratories suggested not only that injections of amphetamine could powerfully induce positive arousal (e.g., euphoria) in some subjects, but also that individual differences in the degree to which subjects experienced positive arousal depended upon the amount of dopamine release in ventral striatal regions such as the NA (Drevets et al., 2001; Mawlawi et al., 2001; Volkow et al., 1999). If the NA activation we observed during gain anticipation was related to dopamine release and resultant postsynaptic modulation, and these physiological events were related to positive arousal, we might predict that NA activation during gain anticipation should predict cue-elicited positive arousal.

To test this hypothesis, we examined whether NA activation during gain anticipation predicted cue-elicited positive arousal in a number of studies.

After exiting the scanner, subjects rated their affective reactions to each of the cues they saw while participating in the MID task (i.e., varying in terms of both valence and arousal). Affective ratings were then mean-deviated across cue type, within subject and item. The resulting mean-deviated ratings could be conceptualized as capturing a subject's affective discrimination among different cues. Based on the finding that NA activation was highest when subjects anticipated large gains, we predicted that large gain cues would most potently increase positive arousal, whereas large loss cues would increase negative arousal. In addition, across individuals, we predicted that subjects who showed the most NA activation during anticipation of large gains would also report experiencing the most positive arousal in response to those cues.

In an initial study ($n = 8$), subjects participated in an MID task in which they saw cues indicating potential gain or loss of different amounts of money ($0.00, $0.20, $1.00, and $5.00) with equal probability (66%) while undergoing fMRI (Knutson, Adams, et al., 2001). This was the first study in which we observed NA activation proportional to the amount of anticipated gain, but not anticipated loss, across subjects. In addition, across subjects, large gain cues (+$1.00 and +$5.00) elicited significantly more happiness than nongain cues (+$0.00), whereas all loss cues (–$0.20, –$1.00, –$5.00) elicited more unhappiness than nonloss cues (–$0.00)—a pattern replicated in subsequent studies (Bjork et al., 2004; Knutson et al., 2003, 2004; Knutson, Taylor, Kaufman, Peterson, & Glover, 2005). Importantly, individual differences in NA activation during anticipation of large gains (+$5.00) predicted cue-elicited happiness ($r = .75$, $p < .05$), but not unhappiness. Thus individuals who had greater NA activation during anticipation of large gains subsequently reported experiencing greater cue-elicited happiness ("excitement" and "fear" were not measured in this study).

A second study of identical design involved a larger sample ($n = 24$), consisting of both adolescents (ages 12–17, $n = 12$) and young adults (ages 22–28, $n = 12$) (Bjork et al., 2004). Although the two groups showed similar patterns of brain activation, adolescents showed slightly less NA activation as a group while anticipating large gains (+$5.00), and age and NA activation were positively correlated. After exiting the scanner, subjects rated their reactions to cues on adjectives indexing aroused as well as valenced aspects of affect (i.e., "excited," "happy," "fearful," "unhappy"). As in the prior study, ratings were mean-deviated across cues, within item and subject. When age was controlled for, individual differences in NA activation to the large gain cue (+$5.00) did not predict cue-elicited unhappiness or fear. NA activation to the large gain cue also did not significantly predict cue-elicited happiness (although there was a nonsignificant trend toward such an association). However, NA activation to the large gain cue did predict cue-elicited excitement for both right (beta = .45, $p < .05$) and left (beta = .50, $p < .05$) NA volumes of interest. These findings indicated that during anticipation of large gains, individual differences in NA activation correlated with self-reported excitement independently of age, suggesting that NA activation was related to both positive and aroused aspects of affect.

A third study (n = 14) included an additional factor, such that cues indicated not only different amounts of potential gain and loss ($0.00, $1.00, or $5.00), but also different probabilities of successfully obtaining gains or avoiding losses (20%, 50%, or 80%) (Knutson et al., 2005). Group analyses replicated prior findings, revealing that anticipation of large gains activated both the VTA and the NA, regardless of probability. However, anticipated gain probability instead activated the MPFC. In this study, reactions to each cue were assessed with valence (good to bad) and arousal (high to low) rating scales. Mean-deviated ratings were then rotated 45° through a two-dimensional space to derive measures of positive arousal and negative arousal. Regardless of cued probability, individual differences in both right (r = .53, p < .05) and left (r = .48, p < .05) NA activation predicted positive arousal, but not negative arousal, elicited by large gain cues. Thus findings from this study confirmed not only that anticipated gain magnitude drives NA activation across a group of subjects, but also that individual differences in NA activation predict how much positive arousal individuals report experiencing to anticipated gains of the same amount.

The brain data from these studies also generated a novel behavioral prediction. Specifically, positive arousal should increase more robustly when people anticipate gain than when they receive gain outcomes. Thus, in further research, we probed subjects' valence and arousal online in response to gain anticipation and outcomes while they participated in the MID task in a behavioral laboratory. Consistent with the brain imaging prediction, subjects reported the most positive arousal (i.e., increases in both valence and arousal) while anticipating monetary gains, whereas gain outcomes primarily altered valence (positive for hits and negative for misses), but not arousal (Knutson, Nielsen, Larkin, & Carstensen, 2005). Since NA activation predicts individual differences in positive arousal, and research suggests that extraverts are more likely to experience positive arousal, we turned to examine whether extraversion is associated with NA activation.

BRAIN ACTIVITY AND EXTRAVERSION

Currently, a handful of studies have used fMRI to investigate neural activation correlates of extraversion and neuroticism, but none at the temporal resolution described above. In an initial study presented at a conference, prior to modeling anticipation and outcome phases separately, we simply modeled each trial of the MID task as a whole (Knutson, Kaiser, Westdorp, & Hommer, 1999). This less temporally specific method revealed activation in striatal, thalamic, and mesial prefrontal regions for incentive versus nonincentive trials at the group level, but not in NA or MPFC, as did later studies (Knutson et al., 2000). Within this group (n = 12), individual differences in extraversion were positively correlated with dorsal caudate ($r = .49$, $p < .05$) and thalamic ($r = .50$, $p < .05$) activation for incentive versus nonincentive trials, whereas individual differences in neuroticism were negatively correlated with thalamic ($r = -.43$, $p < .05$) activation for incentive versus nonincentive trials ($n = 12$).

Elements of these findings were consistent with the first work on this topic to be published in a peer-reviewed journal (Canli et al., 2001; see Canli, Chapter 5, this volume). Specifically, Canli and colleagues found that extraversion (but not neuroticism) was correlated with increased neural activation to positive versus negative pictures in a number of cortical regions, including lateral regions and the anterior cingulate, as well as subcortical regions, including the striatum and amygdala ($n = 14$, all female). Although that study did not feature a neutral control condition (later studies did) or temporal specificity, due to its block design, the findings suggested that individual differences in extraversion might predict enhanced neural activation to positive versus negative emotional stimuli in a number of cortical and subcortical regions.

The MID task complements existing work by both including a neutral control condition and offering temporal specificity. These methodological features potentially enable investigators to address questions about extraversion that have been extant since the time of Eysenck. For instance, do extraverts show increased neural responsiveness to anticipation of gain or gain outcomes? And do extraverts show increased neural responsiveness only to anticipation of gain, or also to anticipation of loss? Pooling across two fMRI studies that utilized a parametric variant of the MID task (Knutson, Adams, et al., 2001; Knutson et al., 2003), we have recently completed an investigation of the neural correlates of extraversion ($n = 26$; 13 female) (Knutson, Fong, Danube, Bhanji, & Hommer, 2005). Based on the comparative literature and our prior findings on positive arousal, we hypothesized that extraverts would show specific neural sensitivity to gain anticipation. In other words, we predicted that extraverts would show increased NA activation during anticipation of gain but not loss, and, furthermore, that extraverts would not show increased MPFC activation to gain outcomes. Finally, we included other demographic variables (e.g., sex, age) and measures of other personality constructs (e.g., neuroticism), with the hypothesis that they would not correlate as robustly with NA activation during gain anticipation.

Preliminary analyses of regions of interest along the ascending mesolimbic pathway revealed that for gain versus nongain anticipation, individual differences in extraversion were significantly correlated with activation foci in the NA, medial caudate, and MPFC. However, for loss versus nonloss anticipation, extraversion was only correlated with an activation focus in the caudate. In contrast, for nonloss versus loss outcomes, individual differences in neuroticism were correlated with activation foci in the NA, caudate, and MPFC (see Table 6.1).

Because our hypotheses focused on the NA, we structurally defined volumes of interest (VOIs) on the bilateral NA, using standard anatomical land-

TABLE 6.1. Maximum Foci Correlated with Emotional Traits
in Mesolimbic Regions

Extraversion	Gain vs. non (ant)	Loss vs. non (ant)	Gain vs. non (out)	Non vs. loss (out)
Extraversion				
NA	3.42* (4, 11, 0)			
Caudate	5.01* (−3, 4, 12)	3.63* (4, 11, 5)		
MPFC	4.10* (0, 41, −22)			
Neuroticism				
NA				3.42* (−11, 11, 0)
Caudate				3.49* (−4, 0, 4)
MPFC				5.31* (0, 49, 5)

Note. $n = 26$, t-scores, uncorrected; ant, anticipation; out, outcome.
*$p < .001$.

marks (Breiter et al., 1997). Contrast coefficients were then averaged and dumped from these VOIs and were correlated with individual-difference measures, including the NEO PI-R factors (Costa & McCrae, 1992), Behavioral Activation Scale (BAS) factors (Carver & White, 1994), Positive and Negative Affect Schedule (PANAS) Trait factors (Watson, Clark, & Tellegen, 1988), and the Barratt Impulsiveness Scale (Patton, Stanford, & Barratt, 1995), as well as the demographic variables of age and sex (see Table 6.2). As predicted,

TABLE 6.2. Association of Trait Measures with Contrast
Coefficients in the Left NA VOI

	Contrast coefficient	
	Gain vs. non (ant)	Loss vs. non (ant)
Age	−1.19	−1.11
Sex (female > male)	1.50	1.89
NEO PI-R Neuroticism	−0.44	−0.35
NEO PI-R Extraversion	2.26*	0.41
NEO PI-R Openness	−0.33	−0.20
NEO PI-R Agreeableness	−1.24	−0.65
NEO PI-R Conscientiousness	−1.97*	−0.70
BAS Drive	0.03	−1.83
BAS Fun Seeking	1.35	−0.68
BAS Reward Resp.	−0.03	−0.94
PANAS Trait Positive Affect	−0.60	−0.14
PANAS Trait Negative Affect	−0.06	0.09
Barratt Impulsiveness	0.92	0.86

Note. $n = 26$, z-scores, uncorrected; ant, anticipation.
*$p < .05$.

individual differences in extraversion were correlated with NA activation related to gain versus nongain anticipation, but not to loss versus nonloss anticipation. No other demographic or trait variable was correlated with NA activation during gain versus nongain anticipation, except for an unexpected negative correlation with NEO PI-R Conscientiousness. Surprisingly, this specificity even applied to theoretically related constructs such as BAS subscales, PANAS Trait Positive Arousal, and the Barratt Impulsiveness Scale.

Overall, voxel-wise analyses supported the predicted association between individual differences in extraversion and NA activation during gain versus nongain anticipation. Individual differences in extraversion were not associated with NA activation during loss anticipation, gain outcomes, and avoidance of loss outcomes. Thus NA sensitivity to gain anticipation may constitute a core feature of extraversion. However, individual differences in extraversion were also correlated with caudate activation to loss anticipation. Since caudate activation has been associated with motor preparation, this additional finding could lend some credence to an incentive salience hypothesis of extraversion, or the notion that extraverts have heightened sensitivity to anticipation of all incentives (Depue & Collins, 1999). Surprisingly, individual differences in neuroticism were associated with increased mesolimbic activation to loss avoidance, suggesting perhaps that neurotic subjects view loss avoidance in a manner analogous to gain outcomes. Though not predicted, this finding holds some face validity and deserves further exploration.

NA VOI analyses shed more light on the specificity of the association between extraversion and NA activation during gain anticipation. Of several demographic and trait constructs, extraversion alone correlated positively with NA activation during gain versus nongain anticipation. Even related constructs did not significantly correlate with NA activity—perhaps due to the superior psychometric properties (i.e., reliability and internal consistency) of the NEO PI-R. As suggested by the voxel-wise analyses, extraversion was not correlated with NA activation during loss versus nonloss anticipation, supporting the hypothesis of neural sensitivity to gain anticipation.

LOOKING FORWARD

In summary, event-related fMRI studies suggest not only that gain anticipation activates the NA while gain outcomes activate the MPFC, but also that individual differences in NA activation predict individual differences in positive arousal during gain anticipation. Another study suggests that individual differences in extraversion correlate with NA activation during gain anticipation. Together, these findings imply that a common neural substrate may contribute both to the state of positive arousal and to trait extraversion, which could help explain their natural covariance.

However, the story is far from complete. Replication is in order—and, ideally, verification that individual differences in positive arousal mediate the link between NA activation and extraversion. In addition, more work could be done on whether facets of extraversion most closely related to positive arousal correlate most robustly with NA activation during gain anticipation. Presently, although fMRI evidence for a neural signature for processing gain anticipation and outcomes looks promising, no similarly crisp index exists for processing of loss anticipation and outcomes. Identification of such a marker is essential for investigating neural correlates of the state of negative arousal and of trait neuroticism.

In addition to psychological questions, the findings also raise physiological questions. The development of localized markers of reward processing raises the question of how dopamine release and postsynaptic activity is related to activation visualized with fMRI. In addition, the fact that different mesolimbic substrates participate in different stages of reward processing suggests that these components must interact dynamically, and thus raises the possibility that these interactions could be computationally modeled. If activations are indeed due in part to the dynamics of neurotransmitter function, then pathways that create, transport, release, and degrade those neurotransmitters can be manipulated—through either genetic polymorphisms, drugs, or environmental manipulations (Knutson et al., 2004).

Findings that connect physiology to psychology thus open new avenues for scientific exploration. On the one hand, scientists studying phenotypic variables can benefit from understanding the physiological underpinnings of the systems they study. On the other, scientists studying genetic mechanisms need solid functional phenotypes to establish relevance. Thus researchers are now in a unique position to practice not only reductionism (understanding how physiology generates psychology), but also "expansionism" (understanding how psychology influences physiology). Here, rather than taking a broad approach that attempts to explain all of personality, we have taken a "deep" approach that seeks to link physiological and psychological levels of analysis for one prominent trait (see Figure 6.4). Translating across levels necessarily requires interdisciplinary thought and collaboration, but our hope is that bridges that span levels, once built, will last.

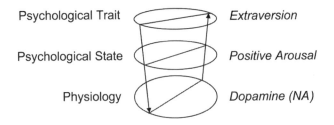

FIGURE 6.4. Linking levels of analysis bidirectionally.

The emergence of these findings critically depended upon the enhanced spatiotemporal resolution conferred by event-related fMRI. The explosive advance of fMRI over the past decade suggests that spatial and temporal resolution of physiological measurement will continue to improve at a rapid pace. Indeed, the history of personality psychology has been a history of technical innovation, beginning with the development of psychometrics (Galton, 1879). Psychometrics remain as relevant (and perhaps underestimated) today as over a century ago; trait phenotypes with superior reliability and validity will necessarily show stronger correlations with physiological signals. Further improvements in measuring both physiological and psychological signals will doubtless drive the field forward.

Linking physiology to psychology has not only obvious implications for advancing scientific theory, but also applications for clinical practice. In the case of extraversion, there is some evidence that extraversion can buffer against stress vulnerability, speeding remission from depression (Kasch, Rottenberg, Arnow, & Gotlib, 2002), and even conferring resistance to illnesses such as influenza (Cohen, Doyle, Turner, Alper, & Skoner, 2003) and viral infection (Cole, Kemeny, Fahey, Zack, & Naliboff, 2003). Because neuroticism is one of the strongest longitudinal predictors of subsequent anxiety and mood disorders (Hettema, Prescott, & Kendler, 2004; Krueger, Caspi, Moffitt, McGee, & Silva, 1996), understanding neuroticism has obvious clinical implications as well.

By placing physiological constraints on psychological theory, multilevel analyses can lead us beyond "black box" thinking to incremental progress. At some point, the mentor Pavlov turned away from the possibility of linking mechanism to mind. His stubborn student Snarsky would not. Whose view will ultimately prevail? Only time and data will tell.

ACKNOWLEDGMENTS

We thank Turhan Canli and Jeanne L. Tsai for feedback on prior drafts of this chapter. During the preparation of this chapter, Brian Knutson was supported by National Institute of Mental Health Grant No. MH066923 and a National Alliance for Research on Schizophrenia and Depression Young Investigator Award.

REFERENCES

Bjork, J. M., Knutson, B., Fong, G. W., Caggiano, D. M., Bennett, S. M., & Hommer, D. W. (2004). Incentive-elicited brain activation in adolescents: Similarities and differences from young adults. *Journal of Neuroscience, 24*, 1793–1802.

Boakes, R. (1984). *From Darwin to behaviourism.* Cambridge, UK: Cambridge University Press.

Bouchard, T. J. (1994). Genes, environment, and personality. *Science, 264,* 1700–1701.

Breiter, H. C., Gollub, R. L., Weisskoff, R. M., Kennedy, D. N., Makris, N., Berke, J. D., et al. (1997). Acute effects of cocaine on human brain activity and emotion. *Neuron, 19*, 591–611.

Canli, T., Zhao, Z., Desmond, J. E., Kang, E., Gross, J. J., & Gabrieli, J. D. E. (2001). An fMRI study of personality influences on brain reactivity to emotional stimuli. *Behavioral Neuroscience, 115*, 33–42.

Carver, C. S., & White, T. L. (1994). Behavioral inhibition, behavioral activation, and affective responses to impending reward and punishment. *Journal of Personality and Social Psychology, 67*, 319–333.

Cohen, S., Doyle, W. J., Turner, R., Alper, C. M., & Skoner, D. P. (2003). Sociability and susceptibility to the common cold. *Psychological Science, 14*, 389–395.

Cole, S. W., Kemeny, M. E., Fahey, J. L., Zack, J. A., & Naliboff, B. D. (2003). Psychological risk factors for HIV pathogenesis: Mediation by the autonomic nervous system. *Biological Psychiatry, 54*, 1444–1456.

Costa, P. T., Jr., & McCrae, R. R. (1992). *Professional manual of the Revised NEO Personality Inventory (NEO PI-R) and NEO Five-Factor Inventory (NEO FFI)*. Odessa, FL: Psychological Assessment Resources.

Davidson, R., & Sutton, S. (1995). Affective neuroscience: The emergence of a discipline. *Current Opinions in Neurobiology, 5*, 217–224.

Depue, R. A., & Collins, P. F. (1999). Neurobiology of the structure of personality: Dopamine, facilitation of incentive motivation, and extraversion. *Behavioral and Brain Sciences, 22*, 491–517.

Depue, R. A., Luciana, M., Arbisi, P., Collins, P., & Leon, A. (1994). Dopamine and the structure of personality: Relation of agonist-induced dopamine activity to positive emotionality. *Journal of Personality and Social Psychology, 67*, 485–498.

Drevets, W. C., Gautier, C., Price, J. C., Kupfer, D. J., Kinahan, P. E., Grace, A. A., et al. (2001). Amphetamine-induced dopamine release in human ventral striatum correlates with euphoria. *Biological Psychiatry, 49*, 81–96.

Eysenck, H. J. (1967). *The biological basis of personality*. Springfield, IL: Thomas.

Eysenck, H. J. (1990). Biological dimensions of personality. In L. A. Pervin (Ed.), *Handbook of personality: Theory and research* (pp. 244–276). New York: Guilford Press.

Galton, F . (1879). Psychometric experiments. *Brain: A Journal of Neurology, 2*, 149–162.

Gosling, S. D., & John, O. P. (1999). Personality dimensions in nonhuman animals: A cross-species review. *Current Directions in Psychological Science, 8*, 69–75.

Gray, J. A. (1987). *The psychology of fear and stress* (2nd ed.). Cambridge, UK: Cambridge University Press.

Gross, J. J., Sutton, S. K., & Ketelaar, T. (1998). Relations between affect and personality: Support for the affect-level and affective-reactivity views. *Personality and Social Psychology Bulletin, 24*, 279–288.

Hess, W. R. (1959). *The functional organization of the diencephalon*. New York: Grune & Stratton.

Hettema, J. M., Prescott, C. A., & Kendler, K. S. (2004). Genetic and environmental sources of covariation between generalized anxiety disorder and neuroticism. *American Journal of Psychiatry, 161*, 1581–1587.

Hillarp, N. A., Fuxe, K., & Dahlstrom, A. (1966). Demonstration and mapping of central neurons containing dopamine, noradrenaline, and 5–hydroxytryptamine and their reactions to psychopharmaca. *Pharmacological Review, 18*, 727–741.

Kasch, K. L., Rottenberg, J., Arnow, B. A., & Gotlib, I. H. (2002). Behavioral activation and inhibition systems and the severity and course of depression. *Journal of Abnormal Psychology, 111,* 589–597.

Knutson, B,. Adams, C. M., Fong, G. W., & Hommer, D. (2001). Anticipation of increasing monetary reward selectively recruits nucleus accumbens. *Journal of Neuroscience, 21,* RC159.

Knutson, B., Bjork, J. M., Fong, G. W., Hommer, D. W., Mattay, V. S., & Weinberger, D. R. (2004). Amphetamine modulates human incentive processing. *Neuron, 43,* 261–269.

Knutson, B., Fong, G. W., Adams, C. M., Varner, J. L., & Hommer, D. (2001). Dissociation of reward anticipation and outcome with event-related fMRI. *NeuroReport, 12,* 3683–3687.

Knutson, B., Fong, G. W., Bennett, S. M., Adams, C. M., & Hommer, D. (2003). A region of mesial prefrontal cortex tracks monetarily rewarding outcomes: Characterization with rapid event-related fMRI. *NeuroImage, 18,* 263–272.

Knutson, B., Fong, G. W., Danube, C., Bhanji, J., & Hommer, D. W. (2005). *Neural substrates for emotional traits.* Manuscript submitted for publication.

Knutson, B., Kaiser, E., Westdorp, A., & Hommer, D. (1999). Personality predicts brain activation to incentives. *NeuroImage, 8,* S360.

Knutson, B., Nielsen, L., Larkin, G., & Carstensen, L. L. (2005). *Affect dynamics: Tracking trajectories through affect space.* Manuscript submitted for publication.

Knutson, B., Taylor, J., Kaufman, M. T., Peterson, R., & Glover, G. (2005). Distributed neural representation of expected value. *Journal of Neuroscience, 25,* 4806–4812.

Knutson, B., Westdorp, A., Kaiser, E., & Hommer, D. (2000). fMRI visualization of brain activity during a monetary incentive delay task. *NeuroImage, 12,* 20–27.

Knutson, B., Wolkowitz, O. M., Cole, S. W., Chan, T., Moore, E. A., Johnson, R. C., et al. (1998). Selective alteration of personality and social behavior by serotonergic intervention. *American Journal of Psychiatry, 155,* 373–379.

Koepp, M. J., Gunn, R. N., Lawrence, A. D., Cunningham, V. J., Dagher, A., Jones, T., et al. (1998). Evidence for striatal dopamine release during a video game. *Nature, 393,* 266–268.

Krueger, R. F., Caspi, A., Moffitt, T. E., Silva, P. A., & McGee, R. (1996). Personality traits are differentially linked to mental disorders: A multitrait-multidiagnosis study of an adolescent birth cohort. *Journal of Abnormal Psychology, 105,* 299–312.

Larsen, R. J., & Ketelaar, T. (1989). Extraversion, neuroticism and susceptibility to positive and negative mood induction procedures. *Personality and Individual Differences, 10,* 1221–1228.

Laruelle, M. (2000). Imaging synaptic neurotransmission with in vivo binding competition techniques: A critical review. *Journal of Cerebral Blood Flow and Metabolism, 20,* 423–451.

Mawlawi, O., Martinez, D., Slifstein, M., Broft, A., Chatterjee, R., Hwang, D., et al. (2001). Imaging human mesolimbic dopamine transmission with positron emission tomography: I. Accuracy and precision of D2 receptor parameter measurements in ventral striatum. *Journal of Cerebral Blood Flow and Metabolism, 21,* 1034–1057.

Nieuwenhuys, R. (1985). *Chemoarchitecture of the brain.* New York: Springer-Verlag.

Olds, J., & Milner, P. (1954). Positive reinforcement produced by electrical stimulation of septal area and other regions of rat brain. *Journal of Comparative and Physiological Psychology, 47,* 419–427.

Olds, M. E., & Fobes, J. L. (1981). The central basis of motivation: Intracranial self-stimulation studies. *Annual Review of Psychology, 32,* 523–574.

Panksepp, J. (1991). Affective neuroscience: A conceptual framework for the study of emotions. In K. Strongman (Ed.), *International reviews of studies in emotions* (pp. 59–99). Chichester, UK: Wiley.

Patton, J. H., Stanford, M. S., & Barratt, E. S. (1995). Factor structure of the Barratt Impulsiveness Scale. *Journal of Clinical Psychology, 51,* 768–774.

Pavlov, I. P. (1927). *Conditioned reflexes: An investigation of the physiological activity of the cerebral cortex.* Oxford: Oxford University Press.

Schultz, W., Dayan, P., & Montague, P. R. (1997). A neural substrate of prediction and reward. *Science, 275,* 1593–1599.

Spain, J. S., Eaton, L. G., & Funder, D. C. (2000). Perspectives on personality: The relative accuracy of self versus others for the prediction of emotion and behavior. *Journal of Personality, 68,* 837–867.

Volkow, N. D., Wang, G., Fowler, J. S., Logan, J., Gatley, S. J., Wong, C., et al. (1999). Reinforcing effects of psychostimulants in humans are associated with increases in brain dopamine and occupancy of D2 receptors. *Journal of Pharmacology and Experimental Therapeutics, 291,* 409–415.

Watson, D., Clark, L. A., & Tellegen, A. (1988). Development and validation of brief measures of positive and negative affect: The PANAS scales. *Journal of Personality and Social Psychology, 54,* 1063–1070.

Watson, D., Wiese, D., Vaidya, J., & Tellegen, A. (1999). The two general activation systems of affect: Structural findings, evolutionary considerations, and psychobiological evidence. *Journal of Personality and Social Psychology, 76,* 820–838.

Westerink, B. H. C. (1995). Brain microdialysis and its application for the study of animal behaviour. *Behavioral Brain Research, 70,* 103–124.

Wightman, R. M., & Robinson, D. L. (2002). Transient changes in mesolimbic dopamine and their association with "reward. " *Journal of Neurochemistry, 82,* 721–735.

7

Mapping the Neural Correlates of Dimensions of Personality, Emotion, and Motivation

John D. Herrington, Nancy S. Koven, Gregory A. Miller, and Wendy Heller

It is well established that depression and anxiety are associated with abnormal patterns of asymmetrical brain activity, particularly in frontal regions (e.g., Heller, Nitschke, & Miller, 1998). Data in support of this finding have highlighted the relative roles of left and right frontal regions in positive and negative emotions, respectively (e.g., Davidson & Irwin, 1999). In recent years, it has become increasingly clear that asymmetrical brain function can be understood not only in terms of theories of emotion, but also in terms of specific personality constructs. Despite decades of electroencephalographic (EEG) research identifying frontal asymmetries in emotion and personality, these findings have been largely unreplicated by hemodynamic studies (e.g., functional magnetic resonance imaging [fMRI] and positron emission tomography [PET]). This chapter briefly reviews evidence regarding the contribution of frontal brain asymmetries to understanding components of emotion, motivation, and personality. The review is followed by a more detailed consideration of how frontal brain asymmetries can and should be quantified via hemodynamic imaging measures—methodologies that are currently highly underutilized in neuroimaging research. An example of a recent study in our laboratory that illustrates some of the methodology discussed is also presented (Herrington et al., 2005).

EMOTION, PERSONALITY,
AND FRONTAL BRAIN ASYMMETRIES

Evidence in favor of frontal brain asymmetries for emotion, personality, and psychopathology comes from numerous methodologies. Clinical case studies have shown that damage to the right hemisphere is associated with euphoric mood states, whereas damage to the left hemisphere results in dysphoric mood states (Borod, 1992; Gainotti, 1972). These findings parallel those for patients undergoing the Wada test, where one hemisphere of the brain is temporarily deactivated with sodium amytal (Alema, Rosadini, & Rossi, 1961; Lee, Loring, Meador, & Flanagan, 1987). Studies of eye movements, electro-convulsive therapy, and epilepsy have shown a similar pattern (Bear & Fedio, 1977; Decina, Sackeim, Prohovnik, Portnoy, & Malitz, 1985; Flor-Henry, 1979; Myslobodsky & Horesh, 1978). Finally, over the past two decades, numerous EEG studies have documented both state and trait changes in affect related to lateralized activity in frontal regions (Coan & Allen, 2004; Davidson, Pizzigalli, Nitschke, & Putnam, 2002).

Findings regarding the role of frontal cortex in emotion and personality have been crucially informed by specific models of the structure of emotion. Factor-analytic and multidimensional scaling approaches have shown that basic emotions (e.g., happiness, fear, etc.) can be represented by a two-dimensional structure with axes representing valence (pleasant vs. unpleasant) and arousal (e.g., Russell, 1980). This structure is the basis for the circumplex model of emotion, which has been applied to the interpretation of brain activity (e.g., Heller, Nitschke, Etienne, & Miller, 1997; Heller et al., 1998; Nitschke, Heller, Palmieri, & Miller, 1999). We and others have suggested that the pleasant–unpleasant axis (valence) can be used to describe patterns of relative activity in frontal cortex among nonclinical samples, and that abnormalities in these patterns are related to personality (e.g., Schmitke & Heller, 2004) and psychopathology, particularly depression and anxiety disorders (for reviews, see Coan & Allen, 2004; Heller et al., 1998).

The study of frontal lateralization of function has critically advanced the understanding of various forms of psychopathology, particularly mood and anxiety disorders. For example, Heller and colleagues (Heller, Etienne, & Miller, 1995; Heller et al., 1997; Keller et al., 2000; Nitschke et al., 1999) have argued that it is important to interpret frontal asymmetries for emotion and psychopathology in the context of the common co-occurrence of depression and anxiety. Their work is informed by an influential model positing that mood and anxiety disorders share a general distress factor referred to as "negative affect" (Clark & Watson, 1991). "Positive affect" and "negative affect" are terms for the axes formed after implementing a rotation of the circumplex model that subsumes arousal (Watson & Tellegen, 1985). Because elevated negative affect is related to frontal asymmetry in favor of the right hemisphere, depression and anxiety would both be expected to show right-lateralized patterns of frontal activity (Davidson, 2004). This common pattern would appear to suggest that measures of frontal lateralization cannot be used to distinguish depression and anxiety. However, some research suggests that frontal lateralization may be related to other dimensions of emotion along which depression and anxiety do differ. In particular, several studies have shown that a specific dimension of anxiety called "anxious apprehension" (e.g., worry) is related to increased left-hemisphere activity, possibly resulting in a pattern of frontal asymmetry distinct from depression (Heller et al., 1997, 1998; Nitschke et al., 1999). The robustness and reliability of this finding remain unclear, as comorbidity is seldom controlled for in studies of depression and anxiety. An additional possibility is that both the negative affect and anxious apprehension dimensions capture unique variance in frontal lateralization. Depression and anxiety may therefore share brain asymmetries in some regions of frontal cortex but not others. Appropriate electromagnetic or hemodynamic imaging studies of well-characterized clinical samples will be essential to answering these questions.

In recent years, it has become increasingly apparent that frontal brain asymmetries can also be understood in terms of specific personality dimensions. Numerous studies have posited that frontal lateralization associated with emotion reflects approach and avoidance motivation, with left activity more associated with approach motivation and right activity reflecting avoidance motivation (Davidson, 1992a, 1998). Because most positive emotions are associated with approach motivation and negative emotions with avoidance motivation, the valence and motivation perspectives are highly overlapping. Anger, however, is often cast as involving both unpleasant valence and approach motivation. A series of studies have suggested that the valence dimension may not account for the frontal asymmetry data as well as the motivational dimensions dichotomized as "approach–withdrawal" (Harmon-Jones, 2004). Recent work by Wacker, Heldmann, and Stemmler (2003), however, has emphasized that affective states can be characterized by both valence and motivational direction (e.g., anger is unpleasant, but it may be accompanied by approach motivation or withdrawal motivation, depending on the circumstances). In an experimental paradigm that examined both valence and motivation, neither model was sufficient to account fully for anterior EEG data (Wacker et al., 2003). Wacker et al. argued that a better account is provided by a combination of three systems based on Gray's (1994) theory, including the behavioral activation system (BAS, mediating approach behavior); the fight–flight–freezing system (FFFS, mediating avoidance); and the behavioral inhibition system (BIS, which serves to interrupt and/or inhibit ongoing goal-directed behavior). Furthermore, it is by no means obvious that anger should invariably be seen as a wholly negative emotion. In some circumstances, it may show clear hallmarks of pleasant valence. Some evidence (Harmon-Jones & Allen, 1998), however, suggests that frontal asymmetries in anger are better accounted for by approach motivation than by pleasant valence when both are present. Regardless, evidence that valence may be an important source of variance in the degree to which different brain regions are involved in cognition (e.g., Herrington et al., 2005; Perlstein, Elbert, & Stenger, 2002) indicates that it remains an important variable in investigations of emotion–cognition interactions.

A central goal of personality psychology has been to identify the basic structures of personality, and the valence and motivation models are just two of several approaches that have been used to classify personality dimensions. These also include trait adjective systems (e.g., yielding descriptors such as "extraversion" and "introversion"). Although debate continues regarding the nature of proposed dimensions (e.g., nomenclature, number, and orthogonality), these systems share the same core tenet that personality, at a basic level, consists of stable, heritable, biologically instantiated sensitivities to positive and negative stimuli (Elliot & Thrash, 2002). How one responds emotionally to positive and negative stimuli; how one regulates this response; and how the regulated response is characterized across experiential, language, behavioral, physiological, and interpersonal domains are all questions that extend from this premise. Scholars have identified conceptual overlap between neuroticism–extraversion and negative temperament–positive temperament (e.g., Carver, Sutton, & Scheier, 2000), behavioral inhibition–behavioral activation and negative temperament–positive temperament (e.g., Watson, 2000), and neuroticism–extraversion and behavioral inhibition–behavioral activation (e.g., Carver et al., 2000). Further empirical work, through factor-analytic and correlational studies, has identified relationships between extraversion and positive temperament, as well as neuroticism and negative temperament (e.g., Clark & Watson, 1999); between negative temperament and behavioral inhibition, as well as positive temperament and behavioral activation (e.g., Carver & White, 1994); between extraversion and behavioral activation (e.g., Gomez, Cooper, & Gomez, 2000); and between neuroticism and behavioral inhibition (e.g., Diaz & Pickering, 1993).

Elliot and Thrash (2002) have proposed that the variance shared among these constructs be interpreted as "approach temperament" and "avoidance temperaments." "Approach temperament" subsumes the personality qualities associated with extraversion, the affective style associated with positive temperament, and behavior patterns associated with the BAS, whereas "avoidance temperament" subsumes the personality qualities associated with neuroticism, the affective style associated with negative temperament, and behavior patterns associated with the BIS (Elliot & Thrash, 2002). This theoretical heuristic has been supported empirically through factor-analytic studies showing that measures of extraversion, neuroticism, positive temperament, negative temperament, BAS, and BIS yield a two-factor structure (approach temperament and avoidance temperament) that is unaffected by response bias (Elliot & Thrash, 2002).

Recent support for the intersection of personality, psychopathology, and emotional dimensions comes from work in our lab examining the relationship of the approach and avoidance temperaments, as defined by Elliot and Thrash (2002), to performance on neuropsychological tests sensitive to lateralized brain activity (Koven, 2003). In this study, relationships between approach and avoidance temperaments, patterns of anterior brain asymmetry, situational strategies to regulate negative emotion (suppression and reappraisal), and the outcomes of these strategies on emotion processes were examined. Emotional responses to a situational stressor were measured via self-report, facial affect coding, and salivary cortisol. Individuals characterized by approach temperament used reappraisal more advantageously than they did suppression. Reappraisal instructions were effective in reducing the degree of emotional responding in the self-report, behavioral, and physiological domains. Individuals characterized by avoidance temperament, in contrast, were more adept at using suppression to achieve the same results. A comparison of estimated marginal means revealed that the suppression technique facilitated approximately the same magnitude of emotion regulation for avoidance-biased individuals as the reappraisal technique did for approach-biased individuals. This finding is illustrated for changes in self-reported negative affect in Figure 7.1, and for frequency of facial displays of negative emotion in Figure 7.2. However, suppression was slightly less effective for participants with avoidance temperament than reappraisal was for partici-

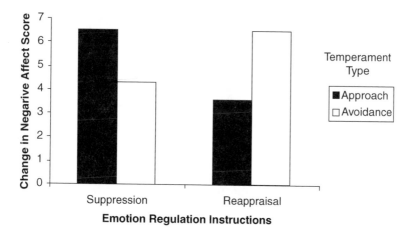

FIGURE 7.1. Relationship of temperament and task instruction to change in negative affect score. The *x*-axis represents groups of individuals classified as having either an approach (black bars) or an avoidance (white bars) temperament, according to a two-factor solution from a principal-components analysis using subscales of the NEO Five Factor Inventory (Costa & McCrae, 1992), the General Temperament Survey (Watson & Clark, 1993), and the Behavioral Inhibition and Behavioral Activation Scales (Carver & White, 1994). The *x*-axis also represents groups of individuals who completed the suppression and reappraisal conditions of Koven's (2003) experiment. The *y*-axis represents changes in negative affect after the experimental manipulation, as measures by the Positive and Negative Affect Schedule—Expanded Form (Watson & Clark, 1991). Adapted from Koven (2003), by permission of Nancy S. Koven.

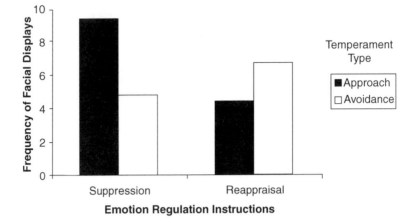

FIGURE 7.2. Relationship of temperament and instruction to facial reactivity score. The x-axis represents groups of individuals classified as having either an approach (black bars) or an avoidance (white bars) temperament, according to a two-factor solution from a principal-components analysis using subscales of the NEO Five Factor Inventory (Costa & McCrae, 1992), the General Temperament Survey (Watson & Clark, 1993), and the Behavioral Inhibition and Behavioral Activation Scales (Carver & White, 1994). The x-axis also represents groups of individuals who completed the suppression and reappraisal conditions of Koven's (2003) experiment. The y-axis represents the frequency of participants' emotional facial expressions after the experimental manipulation, as measured by the Facial Affect Coding System (Ekman, Friesen, & Hager, 2002). Adapted from Koven (2003), by permission of Nancy S. Koven.

pants with approach temperament in down-regulating cortisol reactivity (see Figure 7.3).

Of greatest relevance to this chapter, approach-biased participants outperformed avoidance-biased individuals on neuropsychological tests that required specialized cognitive functions of the left prefrontal lobe, whereas avoidance-biased participants excelled on neuropsychological tests involving specialized cognitive functions of the right prefrontal lobe (see Figure 7.4). These data complement findings from other studies that have used neuropsychological techniques in nonclinical samples to map relationships among patterns of anterior brain asymmetry and personality-, mood-, and coping-related variables, such as euphoric–dysphoric affect (Bartolic, Basso, Schefft, Glauser, & Titanic-Schefft, 1999; Gray, 2001; Greene & Noice, 1988; Isen & Daubman, 1984; Isen, Daubman, & Nowicki, 1987), hostility (Williamson & Harrison, 2003), anxiety (Everhart & Harrison, 2002), verbal–nonverbal cognitive style (Elfgren & Risberg, 1998; Gevins & Smith, 2000), extraversion–introversion (Henderson, 1992), self-control (O'Connell, Tucker, & Scott, 1987), flexibility–rigidity (Regard, 1983), engagement–disengagement (Fogel, 2000), and self-enhancement coping style (Tomarken & Davidson, 1994).

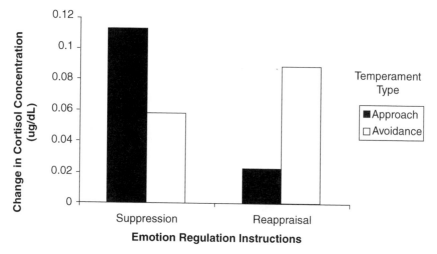

FIGURE 7.3. Relationship of temperament and instruction to change in cortisol concentration. The x-axis represents groups of individuals classified as having either an approach (black bars) or an avoidance (white bars) temperament, according to a two-factor solution from a principal-components analysis using subscales of the NEO Five Factor Inventory (Costa & McCrae, 1992), the General Temperament Survey (Watson & Clark, 1993), and the Behavioral Inhibition and Behavioral Activation Scales (Carver & White, 1994). The x-axis also represents groups of individuals who completed the suppression and reappraisal conditions of Koven's (2003) experiment. The y-axis represents changes in cortisol concentration after the experimental manipulation. Adapted from Koven (2003), by permission of Nancy S. Koven.

These studies provide strong evidence for hemisphericity of temperament variables. Specifically, they indicate that approach temperament, reflecting behavioral approach, extraversion, and positive temperament, is associated with greater left trait anterior brain activity, and that avoidance temperament, encompassing behavioral inhibition, introversion, and negative temperament, is associated with greater right trait anterior brain activity. Moreover, these neuropsychological findings provide additional support for earlier studies suggesting that the two-dimensional models of extraversion–neuroticism, positive–negative temperament, and behavioral inhibition–activation are different conceptualizations of the same psychobiological substrates that contribute to personality, affective, and motivation traits.

The considerable conceptual overlap between extraversion and neuroticism, approach and avoidance motivation, pleasant and unpleasant emotion, and positive and negative affect suggests that extraversion and neuroticism should be associated with lateralized brain function (Koven, 2003). Although results in the literature have been mixed in this regard, Schmidtke and Heller (2004) recently reported that increased neuroticism was associated with decreased alpha activity (indicating elevated brain activity) recorded over the

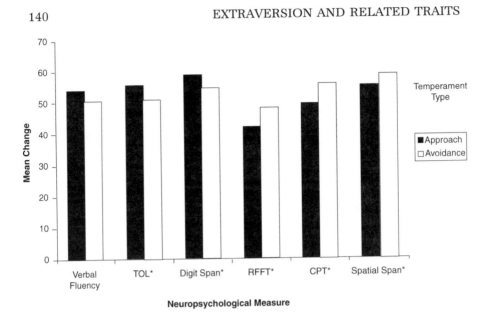

FIGURE 7.4. Mean change in neuropsychological test performance for approach- and avoidance-biased participants. The *x*-axis represents groups of individuals classified as having either an approach (black bars) or an avoidance (white bars) temperament, according to a two-factor solution from a principal-components analysis using subscales of the NEO Five Factor Inventory (Costa & McCrae, 1992), the General Temperament Survey (Watson & Clark, 1993), and the Behavioral Inhibition and Behavioral Activation Scales (Carver & White, 1994). The *x*-axis also represents neuropsychological tests related to left (Verbal Fluency Test [Gladsjo, Miller, & Heaton, 1999]; Tower of London [TOL; Culbertson & Zillmer, 2001]; Digit Span subtest of the Wechsler Memory Scale—Third Edition [Wechsler, 1997]) and right (Ruff Figural Fluency Test [RFFT; Ruff, 1996]; Conners Continuous Performance Test II [CPT; Conners, 2000]; Spatial Span subtest of the Wechsler Memory Scale—Third Edition [Wechsler, 1997]) frontal hemisphere functions. The *y*-axis shows mean scores in *t*-score units. *indicates that the mean difference between temperament types for the specified neuropsychological test is significant at *p* < .05. Adapted from Koven (2003), by permission of Nancy S. Koven.

right hemisphere. However, this lateralization was localized to posterior and not anterior regions. Although the lack of frontal findings failed to provide evidence for anterior asymmetries, the posterior findings were consistent with the hypothesis that neuroticism would be positively correlated with arousal, as indexed by activity in the right posterior cortex. Other studies have provided support for asymmetries in the predicted direction in anterior regions (e.g., Canli, Desmond, Zhao, Glover, & Gabrieli, 1998).

In summary, a substantial amount of evidence indicates that lateralized activity in frontal cortex is associated with specific dimensions of emotion and motivation, particularly positive emotion/approach motivation in favor of left frontal cortex and negative emotion/avoidance motivation in favor of right frontal cortex. Data in support of this pattern comes from numerous methodologies, including brain injury studies, Wada testing, EEG studies, and others (Borod, 1992; Davidson, 2004; Heller et al., 1997, 1998; Lee et al., 1987; Nitschke et al., 1999). This lateralization appears to have both state and trait components, responding to experimentally induced changes in mood and characterizing the emotional experience of individuals with depression and anxiety (Coan & Allen, 2003). Studies examining frontal lateralization have traversed a variety of theoretical perspectives in psychology, including emotion, psychopathology, and personality. The prominence of frontal brain lateralization research in human neuroscience attests to its potential importance for parsing complex, overlapping constructs such as depression and anxiety, or motivation and personality.

FRONTAL ASYMMETRY, ELECTROPHYSIOLOGY, AND HEMODYNAMICS

Although numerous EEG studies have found lateralized frontal activity in emotion and personality, studies using hemodynamic imaging generally have not (Coan & Allen, 2004; Wager, Phan, Liberzon, & Taylor, 2003). We submit that this replication failure may stem from the widespread use of data-analytic strategies that are inappropriate for identifying asymmetrical brain activity. This section reviews psychophysiological techniques for examining lateralized brain activity, with particular emphasis on techniques used in hemodynamic imaging studies.

EEG and the Study of Frontal Asymmetries

Coan and Allen (2004) estimated that over 70 published EEG studies have examined frontal asymmetries in emotion. As EEG methods have advanced, so has knowledge of the dynamics of these asymmetries. For example, analyses of spectral activity across frontal electrode sites have shown that important differences in left and right frontal activity in depression and anxiety are relative rather than absolute (Bell, Schwartz, Hardin, Baldwin, & Kline, 1998; Bruder et al., 1997; Gotlib, Ranganath, & Rosenfeld, 1998). Although data from EEG studies using few electrodes have generally supported the finding that individuals with depression and anxiety show relatively less left frontal activity, the limited spatial resolution of this methodology constrains the ability to localize this activity within frontal cortex. Recent years have seen dramatic improvements in the spatial resolution of EEG, due primarily to increased electrode densities, more common availability of structural MRIs, and improved source localization techniques. However, many previous studies of brain asymmetry have not capitalized on these advances. Very few of these EEG studies have reliably identified electrical signals from deep frontal regions (e.g., orbital and medial frontal cortex), as the observed scalp distribution of signals from these regions is often difficult to disambiguate from signals closer to the scalp (Davidson, 2004). The incorporation of structural MRI and fMRI information can greatly improve our ability to localize EEG signal in deep structures, but to date few studies of depression and anxiety have capitalized on this combined approach.

PET and fMRI have been used extensively in recent years to localize specific regions related to emotion, depression, and anxiety (for reviews, see Murphy, Nimmo-Smith, & Lawrence, 2003; Wager et al., 2003). Studies using these techniques can provide somewhat better localization information than EEG, particularly for deep structures. It is thus striking that virtually no PET or fMRI studies have robustly replicated the EEG asymmetry findings (Wager et al., 2003). As has been pointed out in recent articles, this represents a significant problem, calling into question either the asymmetry itself or the methods used to measure it (Canli, 1999; Davidson, 1998, 2002; Davidson & Irwin, 1999; Herrington et al., 2005).

In their recent meta-analysis, Wager and colleagues (2003) concluded that there was only "limited support for valence-specific lateralization of emotional activity in frontal cortex" (p. 513) in the hemodynamic literature. When analyzing studies designed to assess brain activity during approach–withdrawal and positive–negative affective states, they found only a trend toward increased activity in left versus right frontal cortex for approach versus withdrawal, and no effect of hemisphere for positive compared to negative stimuli or states. However, an examination of their methods calls this null finding into question. Of critical importance is that most of the studies used in their meta-analysis did not actually directly test laterality effects. In an effort to compensate for this critical shortcoming, Wager and colleagues used a form of conjunction analysis[1] in order to infer laterality effects in the studies they examined. As explained below, conjunction analyses are frequently insensitive to laterality effects in PET and fMRI; thus reliance on this approach limits the conclusions that can be drawn. This criticism also applies to a meta-analysis by Murphy and colleagues (2003), who also examined PET and fMRI studies to test the anterior asymmetry hypothesis in nonclinical populations. They concluded that theories of anterior asymmetries "may be too coarse, in terms of both their neural underpinnings and the aspect of emotion under consideration" (p. 227). However, in the absence of hemodynamic imaging studies using robust asymmetry analyses, the conclusions of these meta-analyses cannot be accepted with confidence.

Because of the failure of hemodynamic methods to replicate the EEG results, it remains to be seen which specific areas of prefrontal cortex are driving the EEG laterality effects. Some researchers have argued that dorsolateral prefrontal cortex (DLPFC) is the key region relating frontal EEG lateralization to emotional valence and motivation (Davidson, 2004; Herrington et al., 2005). However, it is quite possible that, due to the relative ease with which EEG can detect signals from regions near the scalp surface, electrical activity from DLPFC may overshadow important lateralized activity in deeper structures. For example, in addition to DLPFC, ventromedial prefrontal cortex (VMPFC) and regions of anterior cingulate cortex play important roles in emotion (Davidson & Irwin, 1999). It is possible that these regions also show lateralized activity patterns that explain important variance in emotion and motivation.

Because of the relative consistency of EEG techniques and findings in this area over the past two decades, it can be argued that limitations in hemodynamic imaging paradigms, techniques, and analyses are central to the failure of hemodynamic imaging to replicate EEG findings regarding frontal lateralization. The following sections examine theoretical and methodological areas where hemodynamic imaging studies may be falling short.

Hemodynamic Imaging and the Manipulation of Emotion

Findings regarding frontal asymmetries in emotion turn crucially on what component of the emotion construct is under investigation. The distinction between recognition and experience of different emotions is particularly important, as self-reported emotional experience is more frequently related to patterns of frontal lateralization than is recognition performance (Canli, 1999; Davidson, 1992; Ekman, Davidson, & Friesen, 1990). Studies examining self-reported emotional experience typically rely either on experimental mood manipulations or on comparisons between groups of individuals exhibiting abnormal, stable patterns of emotional function (e.g., depression or anxiety). Canli (1999) noted that many hemodynamic imaging studies of emotion have focused only on the perception of affective stimuli, rather than on other aspects of emotion processing, such as emotional experience per se. It is unclear whether hemodynamic studies have employed paradigms that examine changes in emotional experience to a lesser extent than have EEG studies. If so, robust laterality findings would be expected to occur less frequently in hemodynamic imaging studies.

Another critical issue is the extent to which specific psychophysiological measures alter moods. Although few if any data exist comparing individuals' emotional reactions to hemodynamic versus electrophysiological procedures, there is reason to suspect that the former may in fact be significantly more anxiety-inducing, in ways that could artifactually foster different results for the two types of measures. Both PET and MRI involve placement in tightly enclosed spaces; PET involves an intravenous injection, and MRI involves very loud noise. It is unclear what effect these procedural factors have on experiments concerning the neurobiology of emotion and personality. It is possible that a procedurally induced baseline increase in negative affect may attenuate the relative effect of an experimental mood manipulation or group comparison. Ultimately, this attenuation may play some part in the failure of hemodynamic imaging studies of emotion to replicate the EEG frontal asymmetry findings.

Hemodynamic Measures of Brain Asymmetry

PET and fMRI techniques for measuring brain asymmetry generally employ a few basic approaches, such as size/mass difference analyses, conjunction analyses, factorial designs, and connectivity analyses (Friston, 2003). Almost no studies directly compare relative strengths and weaknesses of these four approaches. The following discussion briefly examines the utility of these approaches in revealing lateralized brain activity. An examination of 52 hemodynamic imaging studies of frontal asymmetries in emotion carried out for the present chapter indicates that only a very small number of them used analyses that were sufficiently sensitive to hemispheric asymmetries.

Size/Mass Difference Analyses

Some studies (e.g., Canli et al., 1998) have examined laterality by counting the number of voxels within an active cluster and comparing that to the number of voxels in an active cluster in the same region of the contralateral hemisphere. It would be important in a study using this method to specify the criteria used to select a contralateral cluster (e.g., what sort of search field is allowed for a contralateral cluster to be considered truly homologous). This issue is both difficult and nontrivial, given that in many respects the brain is not truly symmetrical either structurally or functionally. For example, the volume that is contralateral according to three-dimensional coordinates may fall in a neighboring gyrus, a different portion of a somatotopic map, or the like. As a consequence, it is difficult to assess the validity or generalizability of this approach in testing asymmetries. Furthermore, this technique is vulnerable to a more significant problem: It may take only cluster size into account and not cluster intensity. Some studies attempt to overcome this limitation by deriving some type of index that reflects both the size and intensity of a cluster (such as "cluster mass"), or by simultaneously using size and intensity thresholds (e.g., Maddock, Buonocore, Kile, & Garrett, 2003). A third limitation of this strategy is that it ignores voxels that are just below the specified significance threshold. As a result, it is possible that a putative cluster in one hemisphere has a substantial amount of subthreshold activity, yet an observed voxel significance count of zero. Lastly, hemispheric asymmetries may be present in areas where activity in neither hemisphere reaches the a priori statistical threshold for inclusion in a cluster. A size/mass difference analysis would overlook such regions; even if a region failed to meet a statistical threshold in each hemisphere, the hemispheres might still differ from one another were the test done. Overall, this technique can lead to unacceptably high false-positive or false-negative laterality findings.

Conjunction Analyses

A so-called "conjunction analysis" involves a binary comparison of significant activity in two regions, conditions, or groups (Friston, 2003). If a particular region is considered active, based on a specific significance threshold, activity in that region can be considered asymmetrical if the analogous region in the contralateral hemisphere does not exceed that same threshold. As discussed by Davidson and Irwin (1999) and Friston (2003), this approach is problematic, as it does not directly test the *size* of the difference between a given region and its contralateral homologue. Failure to conduct a direct comparison violates basic tenets of conventional analysis of variance (ANOVA). This approach also drastically increases the vulnerability to both false positives and false negatives.

Factorial Designs

A direct comparison of asymmetrical activity can be obtained using a factorial design, where hemisphere is included as one of the factors (Davidson & Irwin, 1999; Friston, 2003). Very few hemodynamic studies examining the contribution of frontal regions to emotion have implemented this analytic strategy. Indeed, it is remarkably rare in hemodynamic studies in the cognitive neuroscience literature more generally. Although Friston (2003) outlined how it can be implemented in the program Statistical Parametric Mapping (one of the most widely used neuroimaging statistical packages; www.fil.ion.ucl.ac.uk/spm), it is not directly integrated into the analysis component of this program or into most other commonly used programs. This is surprising, because the inclusion of hemisphere as a factor in an ANOVA design is consistent with basic statistical approaches across numerous disciplines and is analytically trivial relative to the computations carried out by most hemodynamic imaging analysis packages.

Connectivity Analyses

"Connectivity analysis" is another approach to examining hemispheric asymmetries (Friston, 2003). This approach examines coactivation patterns in two or more brain regions. It can be implemented in many ways, most simply with correlational designs using voxels or clusters of voxels as inputs over time, conditions, or subjects. For example, Irwin and colleagues (2004) examined fronto-limbic correlations in depressed and nondepressed samples. A groupwise comparison of correlations between frontal and amygdalar regions, using Fisher's r-to-z test, showed a significant group difference.

Structural equation modeling, independent-components analysis, and dynamic causal modeling are techniques for testing specific relationships among brain regions (Friston et al., 1997). These techniques are presently rare in hemodynamic imaging studies, as they are computationally intensive and unfamiliar to most researchers, but they are receiving increasing attention.

Connectivity analyses can be used to address questions regarding brain asymmetries by examining the relationship between homologous (or non-homologous) regions in contralateral hemispheres. For example, a significant correlation between a frontal region in both hemispheres during an emotional task can indicate coordinated, bilateral activity. Correlations between paired regions can be calculated separately by subject group and then statistically compared to examine group differences in lateralized activity. Dynamic causal modeling and structural equation modeling can further the understanding of this sort of bilateral activity by testing whether activity in a subregion of one hemisphere is mediated or moderated by activity in a contralateral region (Friston, 2003). These and other techniques warrant considerably wider use in the systematic evaluation of brain asymmetries.

Methodological Complexities in Asymmetry Analyses

Although some of the statistical techniques discussed above are relatively triv-ial to implement, additional methodological complexities exist that may be responsible for their underutilization. There is a great deal of confusion in fMRI research regarding exactly what brain data, where, and how many should be submitted to statistical analyses. fMRI studies collect voxels of data that generally range in size from 1 to 10 mm per dimension, and then align and scale them to a standard anatomical template, so that ideally each voxel for each participant will be coregistered. Commonly, statistics are then carried out independently for each voxel. However, variations in participants' brain anatomy and imperfections in standardization procedures essentially preclude each recorded voxel aligning with an identical part of the brain across an entire sample or vis-à-vis a standard brain template. This problem is particu-larly relevant to analyses carried out between homologous voxels in different hemispheres, as the two hemispheres often differ morphologically in ways that are not readily accounted for when typical fMRI alignment procedures are used.

A number of strategies can be employed to address this problem. Most fMRI studies do not draw conclusions based on the findings of individual voxels. Low-pass spatial filters are typically applied, blurring the signal from individual voxels across their neighbors. This has the effect of decreasing spa-tial resolution (millimeter scale) while expanding signal across larger areas that can be more reliably identified (many millimeters or centimeters).

However, because many areas of the brain lack obvious morphological landmarks that are discernable from fMRI images, even these larger areas may be difficult to define stereotactically. This problem is generally handled by cre-ating some other type of boundary criterion to define signal from a number of voxels grouped together—either a predefined shape (e.g., a sphere encompassing all voxels within a specified radius) or a set of contiguous voxels that individually meet some statistical threshold. It is often unclear which of these approaches will most effectively minimize localization error on a given data set. Few studies have systematically compared them, and none has done so within the context of measuring brain asymmetries.

AN EXAMPLE OF LATERALIZED ACTIVITY MEASURED BY fMRI

We (Herrington et al., 2005) used FMRI to examine brain asymmetries associated with emotion using fMRI in an unselected sample of participants. The experimental paradigm was a variant on the color–word Stroop task, using pleasant, neutral, and unpleasant words as stimuli. In this emotional Stroop task, participants name the ink color in which a series of emotional and neutral words are written, while ignoring the meaning of each word. Changes in response time for emotionally valenced words are regarded as evidence of an effect of emotional information on cognition. This experiment set out to examine prefrontal cortical asymmetries for positive emotion, using a factorial design.

Analyses explored a variety of techniques for isolating bilateral regions in DFLPC. The most effective technique combined low-pass spatial filtering with the selection of a set of contiguous voxels in left DLPFC that was statistically significant on a per-voxel basis when data from the pleasant- and unpleasant-word conditions were compared. Data from this cluster as well as the homologous region in the right hemisphere were extracted and included as levels of an ANOVA factor. Functional image processing and analyses were implemented with FEAT (the Oxford Centre for Functional Magnetic Resonance Imaging of the Brain's [FMRIB's] Expert Analysis Tool, available from FMRIB's Software Library; www.fmrib.ox.ac.uk/analysis/research/feat) and the Statistical Package for the Social Sciences (SPSS). Each fMRI time series was motion-corrected, high-pass-filtered (to remove drift in signal intensity), intensity-normalized, and spatially smoothed by using a three-dimensional gaussian kernel (full width at half maximum 7 mm) prior to analysis.

Statistical maps were generated for each participant's time series data by applying a regression analysis to each intracerebral voxel (Woolrich, Ripley, Brady, & Smith, 2001). The fitted model was designed to predict observed brain activity from explanatory variables representing pleasant- and unpleasant-word trial blocks separately, convolved with a gamma variate function to model the hemodynamic response (Aguirre, Zarahn, & D'Esposito, 1998; Miezin, Maccotta, Ollinger, Petersen, & Buckner, 2000). Each explanatory variable in these analyses yielded a voxel-by-voxel map of parameter estimates (β) representing the correlation between the explanatory variable (e.g., pleasant- and unpleasant-word conditions) and the observed data. These maps were then converted to *t*-statistic maps by dividing each β by its standard error. Finally, each voxel in the *t*-statistic maps was converted into a *z*-statistic by comparing each *t*-value to a gaussianized *t*-distribution that follows a *z*-distribution.

For analyses across participants, *z*-maps representing the difference between pleasant- and unpleasant-word conditions for each participant were registered into a common stereotactic space (Talairach & Tornoux, 1988) with automated linear registration software (FMRIB's Linear Image Registration Tool, available from FMRIB's Software Library; see the website above). Statistical analyses were carried out with MEDx (version 3.4) via paired *t*-tests comparing each participant's *z*-map to zero (zero indicating no valence effect for that voxel). For ease of interpretation, the resulting *t*-values for each voxel were then converted into *z*-statistics following a gaussianized *t*-distribution (as above for individual participants' *z*-maps). This analysis was intended to identify specific regions of interest (ROIs) for subsequent ROI analyses. The probability of obtaining false positives was minimized by assigning a relatively liberal statistical threshold concurrently with requiring a large cluster size. Thus voxels were considered to show a significant valence effect if the *z*-score was greater than 2.3 or less than –2.3 ($p < .01$, two-tailed, uncorrected) and comprised at least 20 contiguous voxels (Compton et al., 2003; Forman et al., 1995).

This analysis revealed a significant cluster of greater activity for pleasant words in left DLPFC (see Figure 7.5). The center of mass for this cluster was located at $x = -32$, $y = 24$, and $z = 42$ in Talairach and Tournoux's (1988) coordinate space. The cluster was located in inferior and medial frontal gyri, with small intrusions into superior frontal and precentral gyri (between *z*-coordinates of 20 and 62). In order to test the hypothesis regarding the conjoint effects of emotion, laterality, and executive function, an ANOVA was implemented to examine activity within this DLPFC cluster and its homologue in the right hemisphere (see Figure 7.5). Average *z*-scores were calculated for this cluster within each participant's *z*-maps representing significant activity during pleasant and unpleasant conditions. A repeated-measures ANOVA was carried out on these ROI scores to examine main effects and interactions for word valence (pleasant or unpleasant) and hemisphere. In line with the voxel-wise *t*-tests in the left hemisphere, the ANOVA revealed a main effect for valence, $F(1, 19) = 5.216$, $p = .034$, with more bilateral DLPFC activity for pleasant than for unpleasant words. Importantly, the valence effect varied by hemisphere, $F(1, 19) = 6.712$, $p = .018$, indicating more left than right DLPFC activity for pleasant than for unpleasant words. There was no main effect of hemisphere $F(1, 19) = 0.017$, n.s.

As predicted, therefore, the results revealed an asymmetrical activation in favor of the left hemisphere's DLPFC for pleasant relative to unpleasant stimuli. This study is thus among the first to effectively use fMRI to complement EEG findings of asymmetrical brain activity for emotion, and to localize these findings within a specific frontal region.

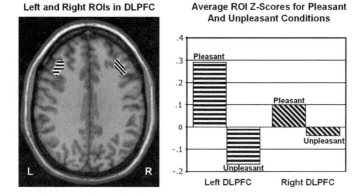

FIGURE 7.5. Differences in brain activity during presentation of pleasant versus unpleasant words. Left panel: Regions of interest (ROIs) used to quantify activity in left and right DLPFC on an axial image in radiological orientation (right hemisphere displayed on left) at a z-coordinate of 34 mm. Right panel: Mean z-scores for pleasant- and unpleasant-word conditions in right and left DLPFC; z-scores representing the relationship between brain activity and pleasant- or unpleasant-word conditions were averaged for all voxels inside the DLPFC ROIs. From Herrington et al. (2005). Copyright 2005 by the American Psychological Association. Reprinted by permission.

This study is also among the first to directly examine frontal asymmetry with fMRI by including hemisphere as a factor in statistical analyses. Notably, although an ANOVA design with two within-subject factors is modest relative to what SPSS can handle, it is beyond the capability of some common MRI analysis packages. An SPSS solution is viable for ROI analyses but not for the thousands of dependent variables in per-voxel, whole-brain analyses, and we have written Matlab software to accomplish this.

Another important component of the study concerned the use of multiple techniques for isolating homologous regions. Although the paper focused on an area of DLPFC shown to be statistically significant on a per-voxel basis, other techniques were initially used as well, including extracting spherically shaped regions of data centered around the area of highest statistical significance within left DLPFC. These techniques yielded comparable results, converging on a significant interaction between pleasant- versus unpleasant-word conditions and left versus right DLPFC.

In addition to directly testing asymmetrical brain activity, this study addressed another limitation pointed out by Canli (1999) as affecting the ability of hemodynamic imaging methods to replicate findings from EEG. There is some evidence that asymmetry findings emerge most robustly when pleasant emotions are compared directly to unpleasant emotions (Canli, 1999; Davidson, 1995; Herrington et al., 2005). Much more commonly, the comparison is of unpleasant to neutral or nonemotional stimuli. The direct comparison of pleasant and unpleasant conditions improved the likelihood that lateralized findings could be obtained.

In summary, our results (Herrington et al., 2005) suggest that the consistency between EEG and fMRI studies of emotion and laterality will improve to the extent that analysis methods in the two domains are similar. Including hemisphere as a factor in one's ANOVA is de rigeur in the EEG literature, but is remarkably rare in the fMRI literature. This problem is readily addressed with an ANOVA design that reflects hypotheses about hemispheric differences.

CONCLUSION

The past 20 years have witnessed a revolution in the technologies available to examine brain activity. These technologies allow us not only to relate specific brain regions and time courses more accurately to psychological processes, but also to refine psychological and biological theories describing these processes. As our technologies advance, so must our approaches to analyzing the complex data they produce. If hemodynamic imaging studies are going to advance our knowledge of brain asymmetries beyond what has already been achieved with low-density EEG, careful attention must be paid to the choice of analytic strategy. Foremost among these is the examination of voxel-wise statistical maps that typically fail to incorporate hemisphere as a formal factor. Furthermore, the methodologies of existing hemodynamic studies must be closely examined if inferences regarding lateralized brain function are to be made.

LOOKING FORWARD

Recent research examining frontal brain function has demonstrated the benefit of integrating multiple theoretical perspectives from personality psychology with decades-old theories regarding the frontal lateralization of emotion (e.g., Elliot & Thrash, 2002; Schmidtke & Heller, 2004; Wacker et al., 2003). As pointed out by Wacker and colleagues (2003), the valence perspective on frontal asymmetry has persisted for about 20 years, with very little direct examination of whether related constructs such as motivation or behavioral activation–inhibition may in fact capture the lateralization as well or better. Considerably more research is needed before findings regarding frontal asymmetry converge on one or more dimensions or resolve disagreements in favor of one dichotomy over another. For example, Wacker and colleagues and Elliot and Thrash (2002) reached somewhat different conclusions regarding whether one or many dimensions may be related to frontal lateralization. Whereas Elliot and Thrash found motivation (approach–avoidance temperament) to subsume numerous other constructions (extraversion and neuroticism, emotional valence, and behavioral activation and inhibition), Wacker and colleagues argued that the behavioral activation–inhibition model best accounted for frontal lateralization, and that valence and motivation models did not.

Which psychological construct ends up best explaining frontal lateralization may ultimately turn on which area of frontal cortex is being examined. Few researchers have tried to reconcile models of specific frontal regions related to emotion with patterns of EEG frontal lateralization. Perspectives on the roles of frontal subregions in emotion generally focus on DLPFC, VMPFC, and regions of anterior cingulate cortex (Davidson & Irwin, 1999). Although it has been suggested that the DLPFC in particular accounts for patterns of frontal EEG asymmetry (Davidson, 2004; Herrington et al., 2005), VMPFC and anterior cingulate may also show lateralized activity patterns. For example, lateralized activity in VMPFC may be more related to approach–avoidance motivation or the BIS and BAS than to valence, as VMPFC has been shown to play a role in the anticipation of rewards and punishments (Bechara, Damasio, Damasio, & Anderson, 1994). Hemodynamic imaging could be an invaluable tool for addressing this and many other questions, if appropriate data-analytic techniques are used.

ACKNOWLEDGMENTS

This research was supported by grants from the National Institute on Drug Abuse (No. R21 DA14111), the National Institute of Mental Health (NIMH Nos. R01 MH61358 and T32 MH19554), Carle Clinic, and the Beckman Institute. The research was conducted while John D. Herrington and Nancy S. Koven were predoctoral trainees in the Quantitative Methods program of the Department of Psychology, University of Illinois at Urbana–Champaign (NIMH Grant No. T32 MH14257). We thank Aprajita Mohanty, Joscelyn Fisher, Jennifer Stewart, Marie Banich, Andrew Webb, Joseph Barkmeier, and Tracey Wszalek for their contributions to this research.

NOTE

1. This description of Wager and colleagues' (2003) analysis holds if one defines "conjunction analysis" as including the binary examination of multiple regions within the same group or condition. Wager and colleagues conducted their meta-analysis by tallying the presence or absence of bilateral activity findings across emotion studies and statistically testing for the likelihood of obtaining these tallies. They went beyond typical conjunction analyses by directly testing the probabilities of finding multiple studies that had lateralized findings in a particular direction. But the underlying principle they used was conjunction—examining the co-occurrence, or lack thereof, of homologous activity across hemispheres.

REFERENCES

Aguirre, G. K., Zarahn, E., & D'Esposito, M. (1998). The variability of human BOLD hemodynamic response. *NeuroImage, 8*, 360–369.

Alema, G., Rosadini, G., & Rossi, G. F. (1961). Psychic reactions associated with intracarotid amytal injections and relation to brain damage. *Excerpta Medica, 37*, 154–155.

Bartolic, E. I., Basso, M. R., Schefft, B. K., Glauser, T., & Titanic-Schefft, M. (1999). Effects of experimentally-induced emotional states on frontal lobe cognitive task performance. *Neuropsychologia, 37*, 677–683.

Bear, D. M., & Fedio, P. (1977). Quantitative analysis of interictal behavior in temporal lobe epilepsy. *Archives of Neurology, 34*, 454–467.

Bechara, A., Damasio, A. R., Damasio, H., & Anderson, S. W. (1994). Insensitivity to future consequences following damage to human prefrontal cortex. *Cognition, 50*, 7–15.

Bell, I. R., Schwartz, G. E., Hardin, E. E., Baldwin, C. M., & Kline, J. P. (1998). Differential resting quantitative electroencephalographic alpha patterns in women with environmental chemical intolerance, depressives, and normals. *Biological Psychiatry, 43*, 376–388.

Borod, J. C. (1992). Interhemispheric and intrahemispheric control of emotion: A focus on unilateral brain damage. *Journal of Consulting and Clinical Psychology, 60*(3), 339–348.

Bruder, G. E., Stewart, J. W., Mercier, M. A., Agosti, V., Leite, P., Donovan, S., et al. (1997). Outcome of cognitive-behavioral therapy for depression: Relation to hemispheric dominance for verbal processing. *Journal of Abnormal Psychology, 106*, 138–144.

Canli, T. (1999). Hemispheric asymmetry in the experience of emotion: A perspective from functional imaging. *Neuroscientist, 5*(4), 201–207.

Canli, T., Desmond, J. E., Zhao, Z., Glover, G., & Gabrieli, J. D. E. (1998). Hemispheric asymmetry for emotional stimuli detected with fMRI. *NeuroReport, 9*(14), 3233–3239.

Carver, C. S., Sutton, S., & Scheier, M. F. (2000). Action, emotion, and personality: Emerging conceptual integration. *Personality and Social Psychology Bulletin, 26*, 741–751.

Carver, C. S., & White, T. (1994). Behavioral inhibition, behavioral activation, and affective responses to impending reward and punishment: The BIS/BAS scales. *Journal of Personality and Social Psychology, 67*, 319–333.

Clark, L. A., & Watson, D. (1991). Tripartite model of anxiety and depression: Psychometric evidence and taxonomic implications. *Journal of Abnormal Psychology, 100*, 316–336.

Clark, L. A., & Watson, D. (1999). Temperament: A new paradigm for trait psychology. In L. Pervin & O. John (Eds.), *Handbook of personality: Theory and research* (2nd ed., pp. 399–423). New York: Guilford Press.

Coan, J. A., & Allen, J. J. B. (2003). The state and trait nature of frontal EEG asymmetry in emotion. In K. Hugdahl & R. J. Davidson (Eds.), *The asymmetrical brain* (pp. 565–615). Cambridge, MA: MIT Press.

Coan, J. A., & Allen, J. J. (2004). Frontal EEG asymmetry as a moderator and mediator of emotion. *Biological Psychology, 67*, 7–50.

Compton, R. J., Banich, M. T., Mohanty, A., Milham, M. P., Herrington, J. D., Miller,

G. A., et al. (2003). Paying attention to emotion: An fMRI investigation of cognitive and emotional Stroop tasks. *Cognitive, Affective and Behavioral Neuroscience, 3*(2), 81–98.

Conners, C. K. (2000). *Conners Continuous Performance Test II: Computer technical guide and software manual* [Computer software]. North Tonawanda, NY: Multi-Health Systems.

Costa, P. T., & McCrae, R. (1992). *Revised NEO Personality Inventory (NEO PI-R) and Five Factor Inventory (NEO FFI) professional manual*. Odessa, FL: Psychological Assessment Resources.

Culbertson, W. C., & Zillmer, E. A. (2001). *Tower of London—Drexel University (TOL^{DX})*. North Tonawanda, NY: Multi-Health Systems.

Davidson, R. J. (1992a). Emotion and affective style: Hemispheric substrates. *Psychological Science, 3*, 39–43.

Davidson, R. J. (1992b). Prolegomenon to the structure of emotion: Gleanings from neuropsychology. *Cognition and Emotion, 6*, 245–268.

Davidson, R. J. (1995). Cerebral asymmetry, emotion, and affective style. In R. J. Davidson & K. Hugdahl (Eds.), *Brain asymmetry* (pp. 361–387). Cambridge, MA: MIT Press.

Davidson, R. J. (1998). Anterior electrophysiological asymmetries, emotion, and depression: Conceptual and methodological conundrums. *Psychophysiology, 35*, 607–614.

Davidson, R. J. (2002). Anxiety and affective style: Role of prefrontal cortex and amygdala. *Biological Psychiatry, 51*, 68–80.

Davidson, R. J. (2004). What does the prefrontal cortex "do" in affect: Perspectives on frontal EEG asymmetry research. *Biological Psychology, 67*, 219–233.

Davidson, R. J., & Irwin, W. (1999). The functional neuroanatomy of emotion and affective style. *Trends in Cognitive Sciences, 3*, 11–21.

Davidson, R. J., Pizzagalli, D., Nitschke, J. B., & Putnam, K. (2002). Depression: Perspectives from affective neuroscience. *Annual Review of Psychology, 53*(1), 545–574.

Decina, P., Sackeim, H. A., Prohovnik, I., Portnoy, S., & Malitz, S. (1985). Case report of lateralized affective states immediately after ECT. *American Journal of Psychiatry, 142*, 129–131.

Diaz, A., & Pickering, A. (1993). The relationship between Gray's and Eysenck's personality spaces. *Personality and Individual Differences, 15*, 297–305.

Ekman, P., Davidson, R. J., & Friesen, W. V. (1990). Duchenne's smile: Emotional expression and brain physiology, II. *Journal of Personality and Social Psychology, 58*, 342–353.

Ekman, P., Friesen, W. V., & Hager, J. C. (2002). *Facial Action Coding System*. Salt Lake City, UT: Network Information Research Corporation.

Elfgren, C. I., & Risberg, J. (1998). Lateralized frontal blood flow increases during fluency tasks: Influences of cognitive strategy. *Neuropsychologia, 36*, 505–512.

Elliot, A. J., & Thrash, T. M. (2002). Approach–avoidance motivation in personality: Approach and avoidance temperaments and goals. *Journal of Personality and Social Psychology, 82*, 804–818.

Everhart, D. E., & Harrison, D. W. (2002). Heart rate and fluency performance among high- and low-anxious men following autonomic stress. *International Journal of Neuroscience, 112*, 1149–1171.

Flor-Henry, P. (1979). On certain aspects of the localization of the cerebral systems regulating and determining emotion. *Biological Psychiatry, 14,* 677–698.

Fogel, T. G. (2000). Patterns of perceptual asymmetries in the perception of chimeric faces: Influences of depression, anxiety, and approach and withdrawal styles of coping. *Dissertation Abstracts International, 60,* 5223B.

Forman, S. D., Cohen, J. D., Fitzgerald, M., Eddy, W. F., Mintun, M. A., & Noll, D. C. (1995). Improved assessment of significant activation in functional magnetic resonance imaging. *Magnetic Resonance in Medicine, 33*(5), 636–647.

Friston, K. J. (2003). Characterizing functional asymmetries with brain mapping. In K. Hugdahl & R. J. Davidson (Eds.), *The asymmetrical brain* (pp. 162–196). Cambridge, MA: MIT Press.

Friston, K. J., Buechel, C., Fink, G. R., Morris, J., Rolls, E., & Dolan, R. J. (1997). Psychophysiological and modulatory interactions in neuroimaging. *NeuroImage, 6,* 218–229.

Gainotti, G. (1972). Emotional behavior and hemispheric side of the lesion. *Cortex, 8,* 41–55.

Gevins, A., & Smith, M. E. (2000). Neuropsychological measures of working memory and individual differences in cognitive ability and cognitive style. *Cerebral Cortex, 10,* 829–839.

Gladsjo, J. A., Miller, S. W., & Heaton, R. K. (1999). *Norms for letter and category fluency: Demographic corrections for age, education, and ethnicity.* Odessa, FL: Psychological Assessment Resources.

Gomez, R., Cooper, A., & Gomez, A. (2000). Susceptibility to positive and negative mood states: Test of Eysenck's, Gray's, and Newman's theories. *Personality and Individual Differences, 29,* 351–365.

Gotlib, I., Ranganath, C., & Rosenfeld, P. (1998). Frontal EEG alpha asymmetry, depression, and cognitive functioning. *Cognition and Emotion, 12,* 449–478.

Gray, J. A. (1994). Three fundamental emotion systems. In P. Ekman & R. J. Davidson (Eds.), *The nature of emotion: Fundamental questions* (pp. 243–247). New York: Oxford University Press.

Gray, J. R. (2001). Emotional modulation of cognitive control: Approach–withdrawal states double-dissociate spatial from verbal two-back task performance. *Journal of Experimental Psychology: General, 130,* 436–452.

Greene, T. R., & Noice, H. (1988). Influence of positive affect upon creative thinking and problem solving in children. *Psychological Reports, 63,* 895–898.

Harmon-Jones, E. (2004). Contributions from research on anger and cognitive dissonance to understanding the motivational functions of asymmetrical frontal brain activity. *Biological Psychology, 67,* 51–76.

Harmon-Jones, E., & Allen, J. J. (1998). Anger and frontal brain activity: EEG asymmetry consistent with approach motivation despite negative affective valence. *Journal of Personality and Social Psychology, 74*(5), 1310–1316.

Heller, W., Etienne, M. A., & Miller, G. A. (1995). Patterns of perceptual asymmetry in depression and anxiety: Implications for neuropsychological models of emotion and psychopathology. *Journal of Abnormal Psychology, 104,* 327–333.

Heller, W., & Nitschke, J. B. (1998). The puzzle of regional brain activity in depression and anxiety: The importance of subtypes and comorbidity. *Cognition and Emotion, 12*(3), 421–447.

Heller, W., Nitschke, J. B., Etienne, M. A., & Miller, G. A. (1997). Patterns of regional brain activity differentiate types of anxiety. *Journal of Abnormal Psychology, 106,* 376–385.

Heller, W., Nitschke, J. B., & Miller, G. A. (1998). Lateralization in emotion and emotional disorders. *Current Directions in Psychological Science, 7,* 26–32.

Henderson, J. R. (1992). Introverts' and extroverts' performance on the Wechsler Memory Scale—Revised. *Dissertation Abstracts International, 53,* 1064B.

Herrington, J. D., Mohanty, A., Koven, N. S., Fisher, J. E., Stewart, J. L., Banich, M. T., et al. (2005). Emotion-modulated performance and activity in left dorsolateral refrontal cortex. *Emotion, 5,* 200–207.

Irwin, W., Anderle, M. J., Abercrombie, H. C., Schaefer, S. M., Kalin, N. H., & Davidson, R. J. (2004). Amygdalar interhemispheric functional connectivity differs between the non-depressed and depressed human brain. *NeuroImage, 21,* 674–686.

Isen, A. M., & Daubman, K. A. (1984). The influence of affect on categorization. *Journal of Personality and Social Psychology, 46,* 1206–1217.

Isen, A. M., Daubman, K. A., & Nowicki, G. P. (1987). Positive affect facilitates creative problem solving. *Journal of Personality and Social Psychology, 52,* 1122–1131.

Keller, J., Nitschke, J. B., Bhargava, T., Deldin, P. J., Gergen, J. A., Miller, G. A., et al. (2000). Neuropsychological differentiation of depression and anxiety. *Journal of Abnormal Psychology, 109*(1), 3–10.

Koven, N. S. (2003). *An individual differences approach to emotion regulation using a neuropsychological model of approach and avoidance temperament.* Unpublished doctoral dissertation, University of Illinois at Urbana–Champaign.

Lee, G. P., Loring, D. W., Meador, K. J., & Flanagan, H. F. (1987). Emotional reactions and behavioral complications following intracarotid sodium amytal injection. *Journal of Clinical and Experimental Neuropsychology, 37,* 565–610.

Maddock, R. J., Buonocore, M. H., Kile, S. J., & Garrett, A. S. (2003). Brain regions showing increased activation by threat-related words in panic disorder. *NeuroReport, 14*(3), 325–328.

Miezin, F. M., Maccotta, L., Ollinger, J. M., Petersen, S. E., & Buckner, R. L. (2000). Characterizing the hemodynamic response: Effects of presentation rate, sampling procedure, and the possibility of ordering brain activity based on relative thinking. *NeuroImage, 11,* 735–739.

Meyer, G. J., & Shack, J. R. (1989). Structural convergence of mood and personality: Evidence for old and new directions. *Journal of Personality and Social Psychology, 57,* 691–706.

Murphy, F. C., Nimmo-Smith, I., & Lawrence, A. D. (2003). Functional neuroanatomy of emotions: A meta-analysis. *Cognitive, Affective and Behavioral Neuroscience, 3*(3), 207–233.

Myslobodsky, M. S., & Horesh, N. (1978). Bilateral electrodermal activity in depressive patients. *Biological Psychology, 6*(2), 111–120.

Nitschke, J. B., Heller, W., Palmieri, P. A., & Miller, G. A. (1999). Contrasting patterns of brain activity in anxious apprehension and anxious arousal. *Psychophysiology, 36,* 628–637.

O'Connell, T. R., Tucker, D. M., & Scott, T. B. (1987). Self-report of neuropsychological dimensions of self-control. In A. Glass (Ed.), *Individual differences in hemispheric specialization* (NATO ASI Series A: Life Sciences, No. 130, pp. 267–282). New York: Plenum Press.

Perlstein, W. M., Elbert, T., & Stenger, V. A. (2002). Dissociation in human prefrontal cortex of affective influences on working memory-related activity. *Proceedings of the National Academy of Sciences USA, 99*(3), 1736–1741.

Regard, M. (1983). Cognitive rigidity and flexibility: A neuropsychological study. *Dissertation Abstracts International, 43*, 2714B.

Ruff, R. M. (1996). *Ruff Figural Fluency Test.* Odessa, FL: Psychological Assessment Resources.

Russell, J. A. (1980). A circumplex model of affect. *Journal of Personality and Social Psychology, 39*, 1161–1178.

Schmidtke, J. I., & Heller, W. (2004). Personality, affect and EEG: Predicting patterns of regional brain activity related to extraversion and neuroticism. *Personality and Individual Differences, 36*, 717–732.

Talairach, J., & Tornoux, P. (1988). *Co-planar stereotactic atlas of the human brain.* Stuttgart: Thieme.

Tomarken, A. J., & Davidson, R. J. (1994). Frontal brain activation in repressors and nonrepressors. *Journal of Abnormal Psychology, 103*, 339–349.

Wacker, J., Heldmann, M., & Stemmler, G. (2003). Separating emotion and motivational direction in fear and anger: Effects on frontal asymmetry. *Emotion, 3*(2), 167–193.

Wager, T. D., Phan, K. L., Liberzon, I., & Taylor, S. F. (2003). Valence, gender, and lateralization of functional brain anatomy in emotion: A meta-analysis of findings from neuroimaging. *NeuroImage, 19*(3), 513–531.

Watson, D. (2000). *Mood and temperament.* New York: Guilford Press.

Watson, D., & Clark, L. (1991). *The PANAS-X: Manual for the Positive and Negative Affect Schedule—Expanded Form.* Iowa City: University of Iowa.

Watson, D., & Clark, L. A. (1993). Behavioral disinhibition versus constraint: A dispositional perspective. In D. Wegener & J. Pennebaker (Eds.), *Handbook of mental control* (pp. 506–527). Englewood Cliffs, NJ: Prentice-Hall.

Watson, D., & Tellegen, A. (1985). Toward a consensual structure of mood. *Psychological Bulletin, 98*(2), 219–235.

Wechsler, D. (1997). *Wechsler Memory Scale—Third Edition: Administration and scoring manual.* San Antonio, TX: Psychological Corporation.

Williamson, J. B., & Harrison, D. W. (2003). Functional cerebral asymmetry in hostility: A dual task approach with fluency and cardiovascular regulation. *Brain and Cognition, 52*, 167–174.

Woolrich, M. W., Ripley, B. D., Brady, M., & Smith, S. M. (2001). Temporal autocorrelation in univariate linear modeling of fMRI data. *NeuroImage, 14*, 1370–1386.

III

Age and Sex as Determinants of Individual Differences

8

The Affective Neuroscience of Aging and Its Implications for Cognition

Marisa Knight and Mara Mather

COGNITIVE AGING

Aging is accompanied by an overall reduction in brain volume (Morrison & Hof, 1997; Raz, 2000; Resnick, Pham, Kraut, Zonderman, & Davatzikos, 2003). However, there is considerable diversity in rates of decline for specific subregions. Likewise, there are variable rates of decline across different cognitive domains, with some functions remaining relatively intact, and others showing unambiguous impairment (Hedden & Gabrieli, 2004; Mather, 2004; Park et al., 2002; Prull, Gabrieli, & Bunge, 2000).

According to the "frontal aging hypothesis," age-related cognitive decline is driven by deterioration of the frontal brain areas, notably the prefrontal cortex (PFC) (for reviews, see Greenwood, 2000; West, 1996). Indeed, neural declines in volume are found to be greatest in the frontal lobes and smallest in the sensory cortices (for reviews, see Hedden & Gabrieli, 2004; Raz, 2000; Tisserand & Jolles, 2003). Functions involving the type of cognitive control mediated by PFC regions are particularly likely to decline with age. For example, impairments are seen in selective activation of goal-relevant information, episodic memory, prospective memory, and working memory (Hasher, Zacks, & May, 1999; Hedden & Gabrieli, 2004; Prull et al., 2000; Raz, 2000; West, 1996). Conversely, autobiographical and automatic memory processes, performance on theory-of-mind tasks, and vocabulary and semantic knowledge are all relatively stable across the adult life span, at least until the seventh or eighth decade (see Hedden & Gabrieli, 2004, for a review).

More general age-related changes in the brain also include reductions in synapse density, grey and white matter, and cerebral blood flow (Jernigan et al., 2001; Raz, 2000; Resnick et al., 2003). In healthy older adults, white matter lesions are associated with reductions in information-processing speed (De Carli et al., 1995; De Groot et al., 2000). Along with rapid declines observed in PFC volume and function, moderate declines have also been found to develop gradually across the adult life span in the striatum, a region that is responsible for dopamine production (Gunning-Dixon, Head, McQuain, Acker, & Raz, 1998; Raz, 2000). These changes are accompanied by declines in dopamine concentration and in dopamine and serotonin receptor availability in the frontal cortex (Volkow et al., 1998; Wang et al., 1995). Together, these age-related declines in PFC volume and in neurotransmitter systems are associated with declines in cognitive performance among aging adults (Volkow et al., 1998).

Several behavioral and neuroimaging studies have provided evidence to suggest that executive processes, such as those involving behavioral self-regulation, planning, working memory, inhibition, and strategic memory processes, are mediated by the ventrolateral and dorsolateral PFC (Bunge, Ochsner, Desmond, Glover, & Gabrieli, 2001; Kane & Engle, 2002; Rypma, Berger, & D'Esposito, 2002; Wagner, Maril, Bjork, & Schacter, 2001). There is evidence to suggest that the lateral regions of PFC show the largest age-related declines of all the subregions of the PFC (Tisserand et al., 2002).

Processes governing cognition and emotion appear to have different trajectories as people age (Carstensen, Isaacowitz, & Charles, 1999; Mather, 2004). Older adults show impairments on strategic memory tasks tapping frontal lobe function (see Prull et al., 2000, for a review), whereas their regulation of emotion and social behavior, also associated with the frontal lobes, is not compromised (see Mather, 2004, for a review). Researchers have recently attempted to account for the opposing trajectories in cognitive and emotional functioning by conceptualizing the frontal cortex as a collection of subregions, each with specialized functions, as opposed to a homogeneous unit (MacPherson, Phillips, & Della Salla, 2002; Mather, 2004; Tisserand & Jolles, 2003).

EMOTION RESEARCH

The neural circuits mediating emotion and cognition share many connections; thus emotion and cognition are likely to interact in complex ways. The pervasive nature of emotion is evidenced in its involvement in attention, decision making, learning, memory, and perception (see Lane, Nadel, Allen, & Kasniak, 2000, for a review). Emotions consist of behavioral, physiological, subjective/experiential, and expressive components that serve to index the significance of events (Bradley & Lang, 2000; Damasio, 1994; Dolan, 2002; LeDoux, 2000; Öhman, Flykt, & Lundqvist, 2000).

According to Damasio (2000), emotions can be defined as "specific and consistent collections of physiological responses triggered by certain brain systems when the organism represents certain objects or situations" (p. 15). These organized responses are assumed to have a genetic basis. The chain of physiological events that belong to an emotional response operate at a general level by changing the state of the body and at a more specific level by preparing the organism to respond appropriately to the emotion-inducing stimulus (Damasio, 2000). Although the collection of responses specific to each emotion is regarded as being highly routinized, there are individual differences in the strength and duration of the subprocesses belonging to each one. Sources of variability in the way emotions unfold and are experienced include learning, culture, and (as we will argue) age-related changes in neurophysiology and motivation.

In contrast with cognitive processes such as memory that decline with age, emotional processes show little decline. In fact, as people get older, subjective emotional experience improves (for reviews, see Carstensen et al., 1999; Mather, 2004; Mroczek, 2001). For example, when asked at random intervals during a week about their current emotions, older adults report less negative affect than younger adults (Carstensen, Pasupathi, Mayr, & Nesslroade, 2000); and in a longitudinal study including almost 3000 participants from four different generations, negative affect decreased across the life span (Charles, Reynolds, & Gatz, 2001). Socioemotional selectivity theory explains this relative stability and improvement in emotional functioning across the adult life span by proposing a shift in goals and motivation that is associated with the perceived amount of time left in life (Carstensen, 1995; Carstensen, Fung, & Charles, 2003). During young adulthood, the time left in life is perceived as being expansive and goals are future-oriented. With age this perception shifts from a future that is wide open to an end that is soon approaching. Along with this change in perception comes a shift in goals. Future-oriented goals that involve expanding horizons and acquiring information are given less priority and goals that focus on emotional well-being and emotionally meaningful aspects of life gain in importance.

The degree to which emotions are negative or positive is only one dimension of emotional experience. Emotional responses are defined in terms of two dimensions: "valence," which determines the direction of a behavioral response (approach or avoidance); and "arousal," which determines the magnitude of the response, or the degree of excitement–relaxation associated with it. Although the importance of each dimension in its contribution to emotion is still a matter of debate, valence and arousal are both fundamental components of emotion (see Bradley & Lang, 2000, for a review). Many studies on emotion have included stimuli from the International Affective Picture System (Lang, Bradley, & Cuthbert, 1995), a large collection of emotional and neutral images that have been standardized in terms of subjective ratings of valence and arousal. Images depicting threat, mutilation, and erotica are associated with the largest values in subjective reports of emotional arousal, as well as in physiological measures of skin conductance and startle reflex modulation (Bradley, Codispoti, Cuthbert, & Lang, 2001).

Older adults and younger adults show similar skin conductance responses to emotional pictures (Denberg, Buchanan, Tranel, & Adolphs, 2003). Older adults, however, demonstrate smaller changes in cardiovascular responses during such emotional events as recalling relived emotions, discussions about marital conflict, and viewing film clips (Levenson, Carstensen, & Gottman, 1994; Levenson, Friesen, Ekman, & Carstensen, 1991; Tsai, Levenson, & Carstensen, 2001). Across the various studies, this dampening of cardiovascular responses among older adults is not associated with any decrease in the degree of subjective emotion or behavioral responses to emotional events, compared with those of younger adults. Older adults report as much intensity in their everyday emotions as younger adults do (Carstensen et al., 2000). Apparently, changes in cardiovascular responsiveness to emotional events do not cause older adults to experience emotional events differently. Thus, on the whole, there seem to be few differences in emotional arousal, especially at the level of subjective experience.

AFFECTIVE NEUROSCIENCE

The amygdala consists of small bundles of nuclei located in the anterior temporal lobes (LeDoux, 2000). It shares connections with several brain regions, including the hippocampus (Cahill & McGaugh, 1996); the thalamus (LeDoux, 2003); and the frontal, occipital, and temporal cortices (Amaral, Price, Pitkanen, & Carmichael, 1992). The amygdala is involved in early processing of incoming sensory and cognitive information that has affective significance (see LeDoux, 2003, for a review). It plays a role in the perception of threatening information, the processing and appraisal of social signals that convey threat or danger, the acquisition of fear conditioned responses, and the enhancement of memory for emotionally arousing stimuli (Adolphs, 2003; Adolphs, Tranel, & Damasio, 1998; Cahill & McGaugh, 1998; LeDoux, 2000). Amygdala lesions are associated with deficits in the ability to accurately judge emotionally relevant social signals, such as eye gaze direction and basic emotions from facial expressions, especially fear (see Adolphs, 2003, for a review; see also Young, Hellawell, Van De Wal, & Johnson, 1996). In contrast to the atrophy observed in the PFC in late adulthood, amygdala volume shows less age-related decline (see Mather, 2004, for a review).

Thus the amygdala appears to be crucial in the rapid acquisition, stability, and persistence of learned emotional responses, especially those involving fear (Cahill, Babinsky, Markowitsch, & McGaugh, 1995; LeDoux, 2003). The persistence of such learning makes good evolutionary sense, as aversive reactions are often elicited by stimuli that have the potential to inflict harm. However, the disadvantage of such responses is that they may at times be out of proportion to the eliciting event or even incorrect. Survival requires flexibility in the ways we think about and respond to events. When our initial reactions are not well matched to our circumstances, how is it that we are able to change our minds?

Processing supported by the PFC may be one answer to the preceding question. In addition to its involvement in high-level cognitive control and executive processes, the PFC (especially the medial and orbito-frontal regions) has been shown to play a crucial role in emotion processing (Davidson & Irwin, 1999; Phan, Wager, Taylor, & Liberzon, 2002). Several studies have provided evidence linking the orbito-frontal PFC to processes governing emotion, social regulation, and self-regulation (Bechara, Damasio, & Damasio, 2000; Beer, Heerey, Keltner, Scabini, & Knight, 2003; Rolls, Hornack, Wade, & McGrath, 1994).

The orbito-frontal cortex plays a crucial role in the modification of reinforced behavior and the encoding of predicted reward value of stimuli on the basis of relevant sensory cues (Deco & Rolls, 2005; Gottfried, O'Doherty, & Dolan, 2003; Kringelbach & Rolls, 2004). In both humans and monkeys, the orbito-frontal cortex shows rapid activity changes when reward contingencies are reversed (Rolls, Critchley, Mason, & Wakeman, 1996). However, the amygdala continues to respond to the initially trained reward contingency (Sanghera, Rolls, & Roper-Hall, 1979). A recent neuroimaging study with humans showed both the orbito-frontal cortex and the medial amygdala to be involved in rapid, experience-dependent emotional learning. In contrast, ventral amygdala activity was associated with a persistent and relatively irreversible learned response to biologically relevant stimuli (Morris & Dolan, 2004). These findings suggest that amygdala-related modifications of emotional learning are resistant to change, whereas the orbito-frontal cortex allows for flexible updating of emotional learning as a function of rapid external changes (Morris & Dolan, 2004; Rolls, 1999). Additional evidence implicating the orbito-frontal cortex in affective situations that involve flexible executive control processes can be found in studies showing decision-making impairments and impulsive, socially inappropriate behavior in patients with orbito-frontal damage (Bechara et al., 2000; Beer et al., 2003).

The ventromedial PFC and anterior cingulate cortex (ACC) share many connections with limbic structures and, along with the dorsolateral PFC, are thought to play a crucial role in motivation and attention, the processing and regulation of emotion, and the guidance and control of behavior (Bush et al., 1998; Bush, Luu, & Posner, 2000; Dolan, 1999). In a recent meta-analysis including 55 positron emission tomography and functional magnetic resonance imaging (fMRI) studies investigating the neural correlates of emotion, the medial PFC was commonly activated across various emotion types and emotion induction methods (Phan et al., 2002). The same meta-analysis found the ACC to be significantly more responsive to emotion tasks coupled with cognitive demand compared to tasks involving emotion alone (Phan et al., 2002). The ACC, located on the medial surface of the frontal lobes, is thought to be an important interface between cognition and affect (Bush et al., 2000).

The dorsal ACC has been shown to play a role in error processing and the inhibition of prepotent response tendencies, and the ventral ACC is implicated in the processing of affective information (Bush et al., 2000). This structure shares connections with the PFC, thalamus, and brainstem. Recent evidence suggests that the ACC and PFC work together in the implementation and maintenance of cognitive control (Gehring & Knight, 2000).

There is little research examining the impact of age on the separate subregions of the PFC. Some evidence suggests that the orbito-frontal cortex and other areas associated with the regulation of emotion and social behavior may exhibit less age-related decline than other areas of the PFC do (Salat, Kaye, & Janowsky, 2001). In addition, in a recent study examining age differences on tests sensitive to dorsolateral PFC dysfunction (executive function and working memory) and ventromedial PFC dysfunction (emotion and social decision making), age-related performance differences occurred on all of the tasks dependent on the dorsolateral PFC, but did not occur on the majority of tasks dependent on the ventromedial PFC (MacPherson et al., 2002; but see Lamar & Resnick, 2004). Thus research examining the effects of aging on affective brain systems is consistent with behavioral findings showing emotional functioning to be an area of resiliency and even improvement over time (for reviews, see Carstensen et al., 2003; Mather, 2004).

EMOTION REGULATION

Emotion regulation is a crucial aspect of adaptive functioning. Emotional disequilibrium serves as one of many diagnostic criteria for many mental disorders (American Psychiatric Association, 2000). Fortunately, there is considerable evidence that we can, through various strategies, exert a considerable degree of control over our emotions in the service of our goals (Gross, 1998, 2001). In particular, the appraisals we make can determine the particular emotion that results (Gross, 2002; Lazarus, 1991; Roseman, 2004).

Of course, circumstances do not always allow us to anticipate emotional responses. Unexpected events sometimes leave us no choice but to deal with emotions after they are already well underway. Successful adaptation may depend on the capacity to up-regulate and down-regulate (enhance and diminish) emotion flexibly, to match the demands imposed by the situation. The link between flexibility in emotional control and successful adaptation was explored in a recent study in which New York City undergraduates, less than 1 month after beginning college, viewed positive and negative images (Bonanno, Papa, Lalande, Westphal, & Coifman, 2004). The participants were sometimes instructed to enhance their emotional expression, sometimes to suppress their emotional expression, or sometimes to respond to the images naturally.

By chance, this study was conducted just prior to the terrorist attacks of September 11, 2001, allowing the researchers to examine suppression and enhancement as a predictor of distress among participants immediately after the attacks and 1½ years later. The results indicated that ability to up-regulate and down-regulate emotion expression independently predicted the magnitude of the stress reduction at the 1½ year postattack measurement (Bonnano et al., 2004). These findings are consistent with previous research linking both the ability to diminish and enhance emotional responses to subjective well-being and stress adaptation (Diener, 1984; Nolen-Hoeksema & Morrow, 1991).

Research using various measures suggests that emotion regulation becomes more effective with age. Older adults report focusing more on controlling their emotions (Lawton, Kleban, Rajagopal, & Dean, 1992) and being better able to control their emotions (Gross et al., 1997). Compared with younger adults, older adults experience negative affect less often and for shorter durations (Carstensen et al., 2000; Charles et al., 2001). Furthermore, episodes of positive affect last longer for older adults than for younger adults (Carstensen et al., 2000).

Research with younger adults shows that different strategies have very different implications for affect, well-being, and social relationships (Gross & John, 2003). Reappraisal, an emotion regulation strategy that attempts to intervene early in the emotion-generative process, involves the use of cognitive control to reinterpret an emotion-eliciting event. Reappraisal may serve to flexibly modify an initial appraisal of an emotionally arousing stimulus in the service of self-regulatory goals (Ochsner & Gross, 2004). For example, if one were viewing an image of a car accident victim in a hospital bed, one might focus on imagining the individual fully recovering and resuming usual activities. This strategy is associated with greater experienced and expressed positive emotion and well-being than is chronic suppression, a strategy that attempts to mask physical expression of an emotion once it has been triggered (Gross & John, 2003). In contrast with reappraisal, the tendency to engage in suppression is associated with greater experienced and expressed negative emotion, increased sympathetic activity, memory impairment, and poor interpersonal functioning (Gross & John, 2003). Some researchers have suggested that older adults' success at emotion regulation is due to antecedent-focused strategies such as reappraisal, whereas younger adults are more likely to engage in the suppression of emotions after they have already begun to unfold (Carstensen, Gross, & Fung, 1998). However, there is little empirical evidence available to indicate how regulation processes may differ among younger and older adults.

Researchers using neuroimaging to investigate the roles played by the cognitive and emotional systems involved in reappraisal have observed activity in PFC regions and modulation of activity in brain areas associated with emotion, such as the amygdala and the ACC (Beauregard, Levesque, & Bourgouin, 2001; Levesque et al., 2003; Ochsner, Bunge, Gross, & Gabrieli, 2002). Nearly all of the neuroimaging studies that have examined the neural correlates of emotion regulation have looked at the intentional down-regulation of an emotional response.

In the first imaging study to examine both the enhancement and attenuation of an emotional response (Ochsner et al., 2004), participants who were previously trained in both kinds of strategies viewed a series of negative images. Prior to each image, they were instructed to enhance or diminish their emotional response, or just to look at the image. In comparison to "just look" trials, both up-regulation and down-regulation trials showed increased activation in left lateral PFC regions involved in working memory and response selection, along with increased activation in the dorsomedial PFC. Increased activation of the ACC also was observed. Interestingly, activation in the amygdala was modulated, such that enhancing emotional responses resulted in increased activation and diminishing emotional responses resulted in decreased activation in this structure.

Overall, these results suggest a crucial role for the PFC in emotion regulation in younger adults. Through its modulatory role on amygdala activation, the PFC seems to be involved in both the enhancement and attenuation of negative emotion. More research is needed to determine whether older adults engage the same neural circuitry to regulate emotion via reappraisal strategies, and whether the same brain regions are involved in the enhancement and attenuation of positive emotion.

Given the relative sparing of the neural mechanisms of emotion and the reprioritization of emotional goals across the adult life span, these findings suggest that older adults' success at emotion regulation involves both the complex collection of organized responses involved in emotion and the ability to implement cognitive control. In addition to the integrity of the neural circuitry involved in emotion processing, the ability to effectively engage the neural circuitry involved in goal-directed cognitive processing may also be predictive of successful emotion regulation. In the next section, we discuss research that highlights the interaction between emotion and cognitive systems involved in older adults' emotional memory.

MEMORY AND EMOTION

Events that carry emotional significance are often experienced as being very compelling and vivid. Emotionally arousing stimuli capture our attention and signal that a situation has a high degree of personal relevance (Öhman et al., 2000). Correspondingly, it comes as no surprise that a memory advantage for emotionally arousing over neutral information is a well-established finding (Buchanan & Adolphs, 2003; Dolan, 2002; Hamann, Ely, Grafton, & Kilts, 1999). Given the emphasis and high priority we assign to emotion, researchers have attempted to determine whether there are distinct neural mechanisms involved in the encoding, consolidation, and retrieval of emotional versus nonemotional events. Although the memory advantage for emotional stimuli probably derives in part from effortful, self-initiated cognitive control processes, a growing body of work suggests that memory for emotional events also involves specialized neural mechanisms (Buchanan & Adolphs, 2003; Hamann, 2001).

In several neuroimaging studies, amygdala activation during encoding has been found to correlate with later memory for emotional but not neutral stimuli (Canli, Zhao, Brewer, Gabrieli, & Cahill, 2000; Hamann et al., 1999; Kilpatrick & Cahill, 2003). The amygdala modulates memory formation via stress hormones that exert an influence on surrounding structures responsible for memory consolidation and storage, such as the hippocampus and PFC (Kilpatrick & Cahill, 2003; McGaugh, 2000; Roozendaal, 2002; Zola-Morgan, Squire, Alvarez-Royo, & Clower, 1991).

Evidence for the role of the amygdala in the modulation of memory comes from patients with bilateral amygdala damage, who have intact memory for nonemotional stimuli, but show specific impairments in memory for both visual and verbal emotional material in comparison to controls without brain damage (Cahill et al., 1995; Markowitsch et al., 1994). Impairments in memory for emotional material have also been observed in patients with unilateral amygdala damage (Adolphs, Tranel, & Denberg, 2000). In patients diagnosed with Alzheimer's disease, which is known to result in a dramatic reduction in amygdala volume (Callen, Black, Gao, Caldwell, & Szalai, 2001), there is evidence that the memory enhancement for emotional material typically found in healthy adults is absent for both verbal and pictorial information (Abrisqueta-Gomez, Bueno, Oliviera, & Bertolucci, 2002; Kensinger, Anderson, Growdon, & Corkin, 2004; Kensinger, Brierly, Medford, Growdon, & Corkin, 2002).

The medial temporal lobe, a collection of structures involved in explicit memory, includes the hippocampus and the immediately surrounding parahippocampal and perirhinal cortices (Prull et al., 2000). The medial temporal lobe helps bind together information from widely distributed neural systems into a coherent memory trace (Eichenbaum & Bunsey, 1995; Giovanello, Schnyer, & Verfaellie, 2004; Henke, Weber, Kneifel, Wieser, & Buck, 1999; Mitchell, Johnson, Raye, Mather, & D'Esposito, 2000). Bilateral medial temporal lobe damage has been associated with the inability to learn new episodic and semantic information and with impairments in spatial/contextual memory (Nadel, 1991; Squire & Zola-Morgan, 1991). In neuroimaging studies, hippocampal activity correlates with memory for neutral information (Alkire, Haier, Fallon, & Cahill, 1998).

Recent neuroimaging studies have begun to elucidate the amygdala's role in enhancing hippocampal activity during emotional memory encoding. In a recent study, a memory advantage for both negative arousing and nonarousing words over neutral words was observed when the words were encoded under full attention (Kensinger & Corkin, 2003). However, when a secondary task was added during the encoding phase, only the negative arousing words retained their memory advantage over neutral words and negative nonarousing words, which were remembered equally well. Results from the fMRI portion of this study showed amygdala and hippocampal activation to be correlated for successfully encoded arousing words, suggesting that hippocampal activity may be modulated by the amygdala (Kensinger & Corkin,

2003; see also Richardson, Strange, & Dolan, 2004). Patients with damage to hippocampal and diencephalic brain regions, in spite of their general impairment in overall memory performance, still show an intact recognition memory advantage for emotional material (Hamann, Cahill, & Squire, 1997), suggesting that the amygdala may also modulate nonhippocampal memory encoding processes as well.

Kensinger and Corkin's (2003) study provides support for a distinction between the cognitive and neural processes governing valence-related memory enhancement and those involved in arousal-related memory enhancement (see also Anderson et al., 2003; Cunningham, Raye, & Johnson, 2004). In comparison to neutral words, encoding of negative nonarousing words was associated with increased activation in the PFC, an area involved in effortful encoding. The behavioral results support this distinction by showing that taxing the PFC, and therefore interfering with self-initiated encoding strategies, eliminated the memory advantage for negative nonarousing words, while leaving the memory advantage for negative arousing words intact.

It appears that memory formation for highly arousing negative stimuli involves a relatively passive and automatic route, whereas negative stimuli ranking relatively low on the arousal scale require more effortful PFC-mediated processing. Although this study examined memory for negative stimuli only, the results have very interesting implications for how emotional well-being and functioning across the life span may be related to cognitive control.

In the cognitive domain of memory, the overall pattern of findings indicates both spared and impaired abilities in late adulthood. Those forms of memory that rely on automatic processes (i.e., priming, implicit, semantic, and recognition memory) have been shown to remain relatively intact, compared with forms of memory relying on self-initiated cognitive control processes (i.e., recall, source, and prospective memory) (Hedden & Gabrieli, 2004; West, 1996). A number of studies have examined the impact of age on the neural systems underlying memory processes (for reviews, see Moscovitch & Winocur, 1995; Prull et al., 2000; Tisserand & Jolles, 2003). Although hippocampal and parahippocampal volume reductions have been found in pathological aging, evidence for volume reductions in nonpathological aging is mixed, with some studies reporting volume reductions in these structures (Jack et al., 1998; Pruessner, Collins, Pruessner, & Evans, 2001; Raz, 2000) and others reporting either no evidence for volume reductions or relatively small reductions in comparison with other brain regions across the life span (Raz, 2000; Sullivan, Marsh, Mathalon, Lim, & Pfefferbaum, 1995). Likewise, the amygdala has been shown to exhibit very little volume loss across the adult life span (Good et al., 2001).

Behavioral research showing a preserved memory advantage for emotional over neutral material in older adults (see Mather, 2004, for a review) is in accord with preliminary evidence that the neural mechanisms of emotion decline little across the life span (e.g., amygdala–hippocampus complex—Good et al., 2001; Ohnishi, Matsuda, Tabira, Asada, & Uno, 2001; orbito-frontal cortex—Salat et al., 2001). In one study, older and younger adults were asked to participate in or merely to imagine participating in various scripted activities (Hashtroudi, Johnson, & Chrosniak, 1990). Their memories for the imagined and experienced events were assessed both immediately and after a 1-day delay. After a 1-day delay, older adults experienced thoughts and feelings as being more memorable, and reported more thoughts, feelings, and evaluative statements during recall, than younger adults did. Younger adults, in contrast, recalled more perceptual and contextual information. There were no age differences in responses immediately after experiencing the events, suggesting that emotional and evaluative information increased in importance over time for older adults. A similar pattern of results emerged from a study examining memory for a narrative containing emotional and neutral phrases in four age groups spanning the second decade (20s) through the eighth decade (80s). For each successive age group, the proportion of recall memory consisting of emotional information increased linearly (Carstensen & Turk-Charles, 1994).

This pattern of findings was extended to visual stimuli in a study examining age differences in memory for emotional images that were accompanied by one sentence narrative descriptions. Twenty-four hours after viewing the pictures and listening to the descriptions, adults ranging in age from 35 to 85 years took a surprise memory test. As expected, older adults had poorer memory overall for the images. However, recall memory was enhanced to a comparable extent across age groups for the emotionally arousing stimuli, which showed enhanced memory for gist and impaired memory for detail (Denberg et al., 2003). Comparable memory enhancement for emotional pictorial and verbal stimuli has been observed in healthy older and younger adults, but not in patients with Alzheimer's disease, in two separate studies (Kensinger et al., 2002, 2004).

Some studies reveal an age-related shift favoring positive over negative information in recognition, recall, and autobiographical memory (see Mather, 2004, for a review). In a study examining memory for choices, older adults were more likely to correctly recognize positive features from the choice options than negative features (Mather, Knight, & McCaffrey, 2005). In addition, another study found that older adults were more likely to misremember the features associated with a chosen option in a way that made their decisions look better than they actually were (Mather & Johnson, 2000). A similar pattern has been demonstrated in autobiographical memory, with older adults remembering their past health, daily habits, and emotional state as being better than they actually were (Kennedy, Mather, & Carstensen, 2004).

In a study examining memory for emotional pictures, younger (18–29 years), middle-aged (41–53 years), and older (65–80 years) adults viewed a series of positive, negative, and neutral pictures (Charles, Mather, & Carstensen, 2003). The presentation of the images was followed by recall and recognition memory tests 15 minutes later. The results showed a decrease across the adult life span in the proportion of negative images remembered, along with an increase in the proportion of positive pictures remembered (see Figure 8.1). The significant age × valence interaction was not influenced by gender, socioeconomic status, or ethnicity.

What cognitive processes or neural mechanisms might be driving this positivity effect observed in older adults' memory? Age-related cognitive impairments can be explained by the deterioration of brain regions highly susceptible to the aging process. However, the improvement in emotion regulation and experience in late adulthood may be driven in part by goal-directed processes. Whereas older adults seem to have chronic emotional goals that lead to positivity effects, younger adults only show positivity effects when primed to think about their emotions (Kennedy et al., 2004; Mather & Johnson, 2000).

Recent work in our lab has linked older adults' positivity effect in memory to their ability to recruit executive processes (Mather & Knight, 2005). Our work has examined the impact of repeated retrieval, cognitive control, and divided attention on age differences in emotional memory. Over a series of studies, older and younger adults viewed equal numbers of positive, negative, and neutral slides. We varied the number of retrieval attempts they engaged in, as well as the attentional resources they could dedicate to encod-

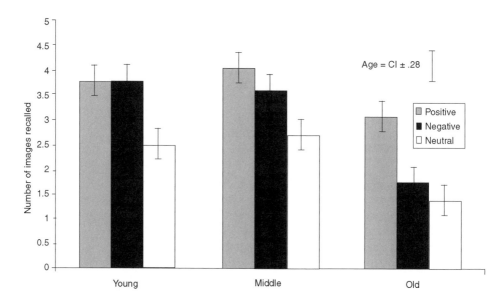

FIGURE 8.1. The average number of positive, negative, and neutral images recalled, with the confidence intervals (CIs) for the age × valence interaction (represented by the vertical lines) as well as the between-subjects factor (age). From Charles, Mather, and Cartensen (2003). Copyright 2003 by the American Psychological Association. Reprinted by permission.

ing. In addition to replicating the results of Charles and colleagues (2003), our findings showed that older adults given repeated retrieval opportunities showed an increased positivity effect, relative to older adults given a single retrieval opportunity. This finding suggests that older adults may have been recruiting executive processes that allowed for deeper encoding and successful retrieval of positive images than of negative images.

We found further evidence for the role of executive processes in the positivity effect with measures of executive ability. Older adults with high scores on these measures showed larger positivity effects than older adults with low scores. When we directly manipulated older adults' ability to engage executive processes by distracting them during encoding, they no longer showed positivity effects. These results indicate that older adults rely on executive processes in order to implement their emotional goals successfully. The increased focus on emotion that tends to accompany the aging process is necessary but not sufficient to guarantee success in emotion regulation and functioning. To regulate their emotions successfully, older adults must engage cognitive control processes.

In the next section, we discuss research on age differences in perception and attention that also implicates goal-directed processing in successful emotional functioning.

EMOTION, PERCEPTION, AND ATTENTION

Neuroimaging studies suggest that many of the brain areas involved in emotion evolved much earlier than the neural circuitry allowing for awareness of, and influence over, processes involved in the emotion-generative process (Damasio, 2000). Consistent with this view is research that shows the rapid mobilization of attentional resources by emotionally arousing stimuli (Canli et al., 2000; Koster, Crombez, Van Damme, Verschuere, & De Houwer, 2004; Lang et al., 1998). From an evolutionary perspective, the quick engagement of the systems underlying approach and avoidance tendencies would enhance survival chances for an organism, via efficient recruitment of adaptive behavioral responses (see Öhman et al., 2000, for a review).

Studies with younger adult participants suggest that attention is preferentially and automatically oriented toward threatening, evolutionarily relevant stimuli (Mogg & Bradley, 1999; Öhman, 2002; Öhman, Lundqvist, & Esteves, 2001). A study in our lab using a visual search paradigm showed age equivalence in the preferential orientation of attention to threatening stimuli (Mather & Knight, in press). In a visual search task (Öhman et al., 2001), older and younger adults viewed a grid containing nine schematic faces and indicated whether all of the faces were identical (all of their features matched) or whether there was a discrepant face present. On half of the trials, all of the faces had an identical neutral expression. The remaining trials contained a discrepant face with either a threatening or a happy expression.

A comparison of the reaction times for older and younger adults revealed that both groups were significantly faster to respond when the discrepant face was threatening compared to when the discrepant face was happy, and compared to trials on which all of the faces were identical. The absence of an age × valence interaction suggests that older adults derived the same threat detection advantage as younger adults in their perception of faces. Apparently, the neural mechanisms that enhance detection of threatening stimuli are intact in older adults.

In addition to evidence that the threat relevance of stimuli can influence attention, there is some evidence to indicate that attention may serve a self-regulatory function by reducing the emotional impact of negative events (Ellenbogen, Schwartzman, Stewart, & Walker, 2002). Previous research with healthy participants who reported being worried about future heart problems demonstrated an attentional bias against words related to such problems during a search task (Mogg, Bradley, & Hallowell, 1994). In addition, studies have shown successful control of attention in children to be predictive of later adaptive functioning (Derryberry & Rothbart, 1997; Kubzansky, Martin, & Buka, 2004).

As already reviewed, older adults favor positive over negative information in their memories. Several studies suggest that selective attention may contribute to these memory biases. In 1 study, older and younger adults viewed a pair of faces presented simultaneously on either side of a centrally located fixation cross (Mather & Carstensen, 2003). After 1 second, the face pairs disappeared, and one of them was replaced by a small dot. The dot would appear randomly behind either face. On each trial, a face with a neutral expression was paired with a face that had either a negative or a positive expression. Older and younger adults responded to the dot with a key press indicating which side of the screen the dot appeared on.

The results showed that older adults took significantly longer to respond when the dot appeared behind a negative face than when it appeared behind a neutral face. Younger adults were equally fast for all types of faces (see Figure 8.2). In unpublished data by the authors, when the duration of presentation of the face pairs was varied, and the presentation was decreased to 200 milliseconds, the attentional bias seen in older adults at the 1-second duration disappeared. If the negative bias demonstrated in older adults' response patterns were automatic, one would expect to see the same bias operating in both the 200-millisecond condition and the 1-second condition. The fact that the negative bias required an extended time course suggests that it might have been motivated by a strategic process.

The results from the visual search task suggest that the underlying attentional mechanisms responsible for detecting threatening stimuli are intact in older adults. The dot probe task suggests that older adults with sufficient time will direct attention away from negative stimuli. Negative information shows the same detection advantage in both age groups, but older adults may subsequently focus cognitive resources on denying it access to working memory.

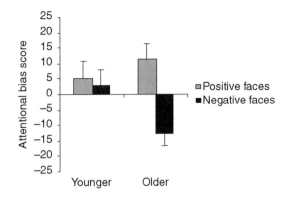

FIGURE 8.2. Attentional bias scores for positive and negative faces in Experiment 1. Results are shown separately for older and younger adults. Error bars display the standard error of the mean. From Mather and Cartensen (2003). Copyright 2003 by Blackwell. Reprinted by permission.

Also suggestive of goal-directed processing during encounters with emotional stimuli is neuroimaging research examining age differences in the processing of emotional facial expressions and emotionally arousing pictures. In one neuroimaging study, brain activity in the limbic and cortical regions of older and younger adults was compared while they engaged in emotion and age discrimination tasks (Gunning-Dixon et al., 2003). Participants viewed emotional facial expressions consisting of mostly negative expressions (anger, disgust, fear, happiness, and sadness) and neutral faces, and indicated whether a face displayed a positive or negative expression or whether the face belonged to an older or younger individual. For both tasks, younger adults activated bilateral PFC and visual cortex while processing emotional faces. In the emotion discrimination task, younger adults also recruited the right amygdala and other right-hemisphere temporo-limbic regions. In contrast, older adults did not show activity in the right amygdala and surrounding regions. For both tasks, older adults recruited the ACC, but they recruited bilateral PFC and parietal regions in the emotion discrimination task only (Gunning-Dixon et al., 2003).

In another neuroimaging study (Iidaka et al., 2002), older adults showed reduced amygdala activity compared with younger adults while evaluating the gender of negative faces. Consistent with the study previously discussed, older adults also showed reduced activity in several medial temporal lobe structures. The reduction of amygdala and surrounding temporo-limbic region activation in older adults may be interpreted as revealing neural circuitry that has been compromised by the aging process. However, older adults' greater recruitment of the PFC and ACC in response to negative stimuli may reflect attempts to down-regulate emotional responses to negative stimuli, leading to less amygdala activation.

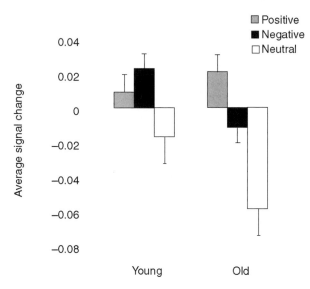

FIGURE 8.3. Mean arousal ratings for younger and older adults while seeing each type of picture (positive, negative, and neutral). Error bars indicate the standard error. From Mather et al. (2004). Copyright 2004 by Blackwell. Reprinted by permission.

This pattern of reduced amygdala reactivity to negative faces in older adults was recently replicated and extended to negative pictures (Mather et al., 2004). Brain activity in older and younger adults was measured while they viewed positive, negative, and neutral pictures. The results showed greater amygdala activity in older adults while viewing positive pictures relative to negative pictures. In young adults, activation in the amygdala was equivalent for both positive and negative pictures (see Figure 8.3).

Younger adults who most closely matched older adults in terms of arousal ratings showed a profile of amygdala activation similar to that of the older adults. Those younger adults whose arousal ratings were dissimilar from those of older adults also had different patterns of amygdala activity from those of the older adults. This pattern of results is consistent with a goal-directed process operating in older adults by which amygdala activity may be selectively diminished in order to reduce the impact of negative information (Mather et al., 2004).

CONCLUDING REMARKS

In comparison to the well-documented course of cognitive functioning across the adult life span, age-related changes in the neural mechanisms of emotion and their behavioral consequences are not as well understood. Although many cognitive processes seem to follow a downward trajectory, a growing body of behavioral evidence suggests relative stability and even improvement in emotion regulation and experience with age (for reviews, see Carstensen et al., 2003; Mather, 2004). These findings are predicted by socioemotional selectivity theory, which posits an increased emphasis on emotional goals motivated by the perception of the diminishing time left in life (Carstensen, 1995; Carstensen et al., 2003). Complementing behavioral evidence suggesting stability and improvement in emotion functioning are recent findings showing the relative sparing of the neural mechanisms of emotion across the life span (Mather, 2004). Consistent with the sparing of the neural mechanisms of emotion with age is research demonstrating a preserved memory advantage for emotional over neutral information among older adults (Carstensen & Turk-Charles, 1994; Denberg et al., 2003; Hashtroudi et al., 1990; Kensinger et al., 2003). Furthermore, older adults use executive processes to selectively enhance positive information and diminish negative information in attention and memory (Mather, 2004; Mather & Knight, 2005). Older adults' positive memory bias, increased focus on emotionally meaningful aspects of life, and enhanced emotion regulation skills fine-tuned by experience may mutually reinforce one another and help maintain positive affective states.

Initial findings suggest that the neural mechanisms that help people notice threatening stimuli quickly remain intact in older adults (Mather & Knight, 2003). But after detecting negative stimuli, older adults avoid attending to them (Mather & Carstensen, 2003; Mather & Knight, 2003). Given sufficient time and ability to implement their emotional goals, older adults can influence attention and memory in the service of these goals.

LOOKING FORWARD

Investigations into the affective neuroscience of aging are relatively new. The evidence reviewed thus far suggests several avenues for future investigation. Although many cognitive processes show evidence of age-related decline, emotion regulation and functioning show stability and even improvement. Although neuroimaging studies have begun to investigate the neural circuitry involved in emotion regulation strategies in younger adults, the specific emotion-regulating strategies invoked by older adults remain unexplored. How do older adults achieve success in carrying out their emotional goals? Does the neural circuitry involved in successful emotion regulation show evidence of stability or change across the life span? If there is a change, is it one that is quantitative, qualitative, or both? Research investigating older adults' positivity bias in memory suggests that this bias relies upon the recruitment of executive processes (Mather & Knight, 2005). Although older adults tend to show impairments in executive performance relative to their younger counterparts, they may still achieve their emotional goals by allocating more cognitive resources to the enhancement of positive emotional experiences. Future work is needed to establish which executive processes in particular are crucial to the achievement of emotional goals (selective attention, self-initiated encoding and retrieval, etc.). In addition, future work is needed to clarify the role of various subregions of the PFC in emotion regulation and functioning. Executive processes are closely associated with the dorsolateral PFC. However, this region shares many connections with ventromedial and orbito-frontal areas of PFC involved in emotion. What might be the ventromedial and orbito-frontal contributions to goal-directed behavior? How might these interactions change throughout the life span?

ACKNOWLEDGMENT

This chapter was supported by a grant from the National Institute on Aging (No. AG025340).

REFERENCES

Abrisqueta-Gomez, J., Bueno, O. F., Oliveira, M. G., & Bertolucci, P. H. (2002). Recognition memory for emotional pictures in Alzheimer's disease. *Acta Neurologica Scandinavica, 105,* 51–54.

Adolphs, R. (2003). Is the human amygdala specialized for processing social information? *Annals of the New York Academy of Sciences, 985,* 326–340.

Adolphs, R., Tranel, D., & Damasio, A. R. (1998). The human amygdala in social judgment. *Nature, 393,* 470–474.

Adolphs, R., Tranel, D., & Denberg, N. (2000). Impaired emotional declarative memory following unilateral amygdala damage. *Learning and Memory, 7,* 180–186.

Alkire, M. T., Haier, R. J., Fallon, J. H., & Cahill, L. (1998). Hippocampal, but not amygdala activity at encoding correlates with long-term, free recall of nonemotional information. *Proceedings of the National Academy of Sciences USA, 95,* 14506–14510.

Amaral, D. G., Price, J. L., Pitkanen, A., & Carmichael, S. T. (1992). Anatomical organization of the primate amygdaloid complex. In J. P. Aggleton (Ed.), *The amygdala: Neurobiological aspects of emotion, memory, and mental dysfunction* (pp. 1–66). New York: Wiley–Liss.

American Psychiatric Association. (2000). *Diagnostic and statistical manual of mental disorders* (4th ed., text rev.). Washington, DC: Author.

Anderson, A. K., Christoff, K., Stappen, I., Panitz, D., Ghahremani, D. G., Glover, G., et al. (2003). Neural correlates of the automatic processing of threat facial signals. *Journal of Neuroscience, 23,* 5627–5633.

Beauregard, M., Levesque, J., & Bourgouin, P. (2001). Neural correlates of conscious self-regulation of emotion. *Journal of Neuroscience, 21,* RC165.

Bechara, A., Damasio, H., & Damasio, A. R. (2000). Emotion, decision making, and the orbitofrontal cortex. *Cerebral Cortex, 10,* 295–307.

Beer, J. S., Heerey, E. A., Keltner, D., Scabini, D., & Knight, R. T. (2003). The regulatory function of self-conscious emotion: Insights from patients with orbitofrontal damage. *Journal of Personality and Social Psychology, 85,* 594–604.

Bonanno, G. A., Papa, A., Lalande, K., Westphal, M., & Coifman, K. (2004). The importance of being flexible: The ability to both enhance and suppress emotional expression predicts long-term adjustment. *Psychological Science, 15,* 482–487.

Bradley, M. M., Codispoti, M., Cuthbert, B. N., & Lang, P. J. (2001). Emotion and motivation: I. Defensive and appetitive reactions in picture processing. *Emotions, 1,* 276–298.

Bradley, M. M., & Lang, P. J. (2000). Measuring emotion: Behavior, feeling and physiology. In R. D. Lane & L. Nadel (Eds.), *Cognitive neuroscience of emotion* (pp. 242–276). New York: Oxford University Press.

Buchanan, T. W., & Adolphs, R. (2003). The neuroanatomy of emotional memory in humans. In D. Reisberg & P. Hertel (Eds.), *Memory and emotion* (pp. 42–75). Oxford: Oxford University Press.

Bunge, S. A., Ochsner, K. N., Desmond, J. E., Glover, G. H., & Gabrieli, J. D. (2001). Prefrontal regions involved in keeping information in and out of mind. *Brain, 124,* 2074–2086.

Bush, G., Luu, P., & Posner, M. (2000). Cognitive and emotional influences in anterior cingulate cortex. *Trends in Cognitive Sciences, 4,* 215–222.

Bush, G., Whalen, P. J., Rosen, B. R., Jenike, M. A., McInerney, S. C., & Rauch, S. L. (1998). The counting Stroop: An interference task specialized for functional neuroimaging—validation study with functional MRI. *Human Brain Mapping, 6,* 270–282.

Cahill, L., Babinsky, R., Markowitsch, H. J., & McGaugh, J. L. (1995). The amygdala and emotional memory. *Nature, 377,* 295–296.

Cahill, L., & McGaugh, J. L. (1998). Mechanisms of emotional arousal and lasting declarative memory. *Trends in Neurosciences, 21,* 294–299.

Callen, D. J. A., Black, S. E., Gao, F., Caldwell, C. B., & Szalai, J. P. (2001). Beyond the hippocampus: MRI volumetry confirms widespread limbic atrophy in AD. *Neurology, 57,* 1669–1674.

Canli, T., Zhao, Z., Brewer, J., Gabrieli, J. D. E., & Cahill, L. (2000). Event-related activation in the human amygdala associates with later memory for individual emotional experience. *Journal of Neuroscience, 20,* 1–5.

Carstensen, L. L. (1995). Evidence for a life-span theory of socioemotional selectivity. *Current Directions in Psychological Science, 4,* 151–156.

Carstensen, L. L., Fung, H. H., & Charles, S. T. (2003). Socioemotional selectivity theory and the regulation of emotion in the second half of life. *Motivation and Emotion, 27,* 103–123.

Carstensen, L. L., Gross, J. J., & Fung, H. H. (1998). The social context of emotional experience. *Annual Review of Gerontology and Geriatrics, 17,* 325–352.

Carstensen, L. L., Isaacowitz, D. M., & Charles, S. T. (1999). Taking time seriously: A theory of socioemotional selectivity. *American Psychologist, 54,* 165–181.

Carstensen, L. L., Pasupathi, M., Mayr, U., & Nesslroade, J. R. (2000). Emotional experience in everyday life across the adult life span. *Journal of Personality and Social Psychology, 79,* 644–655.

Carstensen, L. L., & Turk-Charles, S. (1994). The salience of emotion across the adult life course. *Psychology and Aging, 9,* 259–264.

Charles, S. T., Mather, M., & Carstensen, L. L. (2003). Aging and emotional memory: The forgettable nature of negative images for older adults. *Journal of Experimental Psychology: General, 132,* 310–324.

Charles, S. T., Reynolds, C. A., & Gatz, M. (2001). Age-related differences and change in positive and negative affect over 23 years. *Journal of Personality and Social Psychology, 80,* 136–151.

Cunningham, W. A., Raye, C. A., & Johnson, M. K. (2004). Implicit and explicit evaluation: fMRI correlates of valence, emotional intensity, and control in the processing of attitudes. *Journal of Cognitive Neuroscience, 16,* 1717–1729.

Damasio, A. R. (1994). *Descartes' error: Emotion, reason, and the human brain.* New York: Putnam.

Damasio, A. R. (2000). A second chance for emotion. In R. D. Lane & L. Nadel (Eds.), *Cognitive neuroscience of emotion* (pp. 12–23). New York: Oxford University Press.

Davidson, R. J., & Irwin, W. (1999). The functional neuroanatomy of emotion and affective style. *Trends in Cognitive Sciences, 3,* 11–21.

De Carli, C., Murphy, D. G., Tranh, M., Grady, C. L., Haxby, J. V., Gillette, J. A., et al. (1995). The effect of white matter hyperintensity volume on brain structure, cognitive performance, and cerebral metabolism of glucose in 51 healthy adults. *Neurology, 45,* 2077–2084.

Deco, G., & Rolls, E. T. (2005). Synaptic and spiking dynamics underlying reward reversal in the orbitofrontal cortex. *Cerebral Cortex, 15,* 15–30.

De Groot, J. C., De Leeuw, F. E., Oudkerk, M., van Gun, J., Hofman, A., Jolles, J., et al. (2000). Cerebral white matter lesions and cognitive function: The Rotterdam scan study. *Annals of Neurology, 47,* 145–151.

Denberg, N. L., Buchanan, T. W., Tranel, T., & Adolphs, R. (2003). Evidence for preserved emotional memory in normal older persons. *Emotion, 3,* 239–253.

Derryberry, D., & Rothbart, M. K. (1997). Reactive and effortful processes in the organization of temperament. *Development and Psychopathology, 9,* 633–652.

Diener, E. (1984). Subjective well-being. *Psychological Bulletin, 95,* 542–575,

Dolan, R. J. (1999). On the neurology of morals. *Nature Neuroscience, 2,* 927–929.

Dolan, R. J. (2002). Emotion, cognition, and behavior. *Science, 298,* 1191–1194.

Eichenbaum, H., & Bunsey, M. (1995). On the binding of associations in memory: Clues from studies on the role of the hippocampal region in paired-associate learning. *Current Directions in Psychological Science, 4,* 19–23.

Ellenbogen, M. A., Schwartzman, A. E., Stewart, J., & Walker, C. (2002). Stress and selective attention: The interplay of mood, cortisol levels, and emotional information processing. *Psychophysiology, 39,* 723–732.

Gehring, W., & Knight, R. (2000). Prefrontal cingulate interactions in action monitoring. *Nature Neuroscience, 3,* 516–520.

Giovanello, K. S., Schnyer, D. M., & Verfaellie, M. (2004). A critical role for the anterior hippocampus in relational memory: Evidence from an fMRI study comparing associative and item recognition. *Hippocampus, 14,* 5–8.

Good, C. D., Johnsrude, I. S., Ashburner, J., Henson, R. N. A., Friston, K. J., & Frackowiak, R. S. J. (2001). A voxel-based morphometric study of aging in 465 normal adult human brains. *NeuroImage, 14,* 21–36.

Gottfried, J. A., O'Doherty, J., & Dolan, R. J. (2003). Encoding predictive reward value in human amygdala and orbitofrontal cortex. *Science, 301,* 1104–1107.

Greenwood, P. M. (2000). The frontal aging hypothesis evaluated. *Journal of the International Neuropsychological Society, 6,* 705–726.

Gross, J. J. (1998). The emerging field of emotion regulation: An integrative review. *Review of General Psychology, 2,* 271–299.

Gross, J. J. (2001). Emotion regulation in adulthood: Timing is everything. *Current Directions in Psychological Science, 10*, 214–219.

Gross, J. J. (2002). Emotion regulation: Affective, cognitive, and social consequences. *Psychophysiology, 39*, 281–291.

Gross, J. J., Carstensen, L. L., Pasupathi, M., Tsai, J., Skorpen, C. G., & Hsu, A. Y. C. (1997). Emotion and aging: Experience, expression, and control. *Psychology and Aging, 12*, 590–599.

Gross, J. J., & John, O. P. (2003). Individual differences in two emotion regulation processes: Implications for affect, relationships, and well-being. *Journal of Personality and Social Psychology, 85*, 348–362.

Gunning-Dixon, F. M., Gur, R. C., Perkins, A. C., Schroeder, L., Turner, T., Turetsky, B. I., et al. (2003). Age-related differences in brain activation during emotional face processing. *Neurobiology of Aging, 24*, 285–295.

Gunning-Dixon, F. M., Head, D., McQuain, J., Acker, J. D., & Raz, N. (1998). Differential aging of the human striatum: A prospective MR imaging study. *American Journal of Neuroradiology, 19*, 1501–1507.

Hamann, S. B. (2001). Cognitive and neural mechanisms of emotional memory. *Trends in Cognitive Sciences, 5*, 394–400.

Hamann, S. B., Cahill, L., & Squire, L. R. (1997). Emotional perception and memory in amnesia. *Neuropsychology, 11*, 104–113.

Hamann, S. B., Ely, T. D., Grafton, S. T., & Kilts, C. D. (1999). Amygdala activity related to enhanced memory for pleasant and aversive stimuli. *Nature Neuroscience, 2*, 289–293.

Hasher, L., Zacks, R. T., & May, C. P. (1999). Inhibitory control, circadian arousal, and age. In D. Gopher & A. Koriat (Eds.), *Attention and performance XVII: Cognitive regulation of performance: Interaction of theory and application* (pp. 653–675). Cambridge, MA: MIT Press.

Hashtroudi, S., Johnson, M. K., & Chrosniak, L. D. (1990). Aging and qualitative characteristics of memories for perceived and imagined complex events. *Psychology and Aging, 5*, 119–126.

Hedden, T., & Gabrieli, J. D. E. (2004). Insights into the ageing mind: A view from cognitive neuroscience. *Neuroscience, 5*, 87–96.

Henke, K., Weber, B., Kneifel, S., Wieser, H. G., & Buck, A. (1999). Human hippocampus associates information in memory. *Proceedings of the National Academy of Sciences USA, 96*, 5884–5889.

Iidaka, T., Okada, T., Murata, T., Omori, M., Kosaka, H., Sadato, N., et al. (2002). Age-related differences in the medial temporal lobe responses to emotional faces as revealed by fMRI. *Hippocampus, 12*, 352–362.

Jack, C. R., Jr., Petersen, R. C., Xu, Y., O'Brien, P. C., Smith, G. E., Ivnik, R. J., et al. (1998). Rate of medial temporal lobe atrophy in typical aging and Alzheimer's disease. *Neurology, 51*, 993–999.

Jernigan, T. L., Archibald, S. L., Fennema-Notestine, C., Gamst, A. C., Stout, J. C., Bonner, J., et al. (2001). Effects of age on tissues and regions of the cerebrum and cerebellum. *Neurobiology of Aging, 22*, 581–594.

Kane, M. J., & Engle, R. W. (2002). The role of prefrontal cortex in working-memory capacity, executive attention, and general fluid intelligence: An individual-differences perspective. *Psychonomic Bulletin and Review, 9*, 637–671.

Kennedy, Q., Mather, M., & Carstensen, L. L. (2004). The role of motivation in the age-related positivity effect in autobiographical memory. *Psychological Science, 15*, 208–214.

Kensinger, E. A., Anderson, A. A., Growdon, J. H., & Corkin, S. (2004). Effects of Alzheimer disease on memory for verbal emotional information. *Neuropsychologia, 42*, 791–800.

Kensinger, E. A., Brierley, B., Medford, N., Growdon, J. H., & Corkin, S. (2002). Effects of normal aging and Alzheimer's disease on emotional memory. *Emotion, 2*, 118–134.

Kensinger, E. A., & Corkin, S. (2004). Two routes to emotional memory: Distinct neural processes for valence and arousal. *Proceedings of the National Academy of Sciences USA, 101*, 3310–3315.

Kilpatrick, L., & Cahill, L. (2003). Amygdala modulation of parahippocampal and frontal regions during emotionally influenced memory storage. *NeuroImage, 20*, 2091–2099.

Koster, E. H., Crombez, G., Van Damme, S., Verschuere, B., & De Houwer, J. (2004). Does imminent threat capture and hold attention? *Emotion, 4*, 312–317.

Kringelbach, M. L., & Rolls, E. T. (2004). The functional neuroanatomy of the human orbitofrontal cortex: Evidence from neuroimaging and neuropsychology. *Progress in Neurobiology, 72*, 341–372.

Kubzansky, L. D., Martin, L. T., & Buka, S. L. (2004). Early manifestations of personality and adult emotional functioning. *Emotion, 4*, 364–377.

Lamar, M., & Resnick, S. M. (2004). Aging and prefrontal functions: Dissociating orbitofrontal and dorsolateral abilities. *Neurobiology of Aging, 25*, 553–558.

Lane, R. D., Nadel, L., Allen, J. J. B., & Kasniak, A. W. (2000). The study of emotion from the perspective of cognitive neuroscience. In R. D. Lane & L. Nadel (Eds.), *Cognitive neuroscience of emotion* (pp. 3–11). New York: Oxford University Press.

Lang, P. J., Bradley, M. M., & Cuthbert, B. N. (1995). *International Affective Picture System (IAPS): Technical manual and affective ratings.* Gainesville: University of Florida, Center for Research in Psychophysiology.

Lang, P. J., Bradley, M. M., Fitzsimmons, J. R., Cuthbert, B. N., Scott, J. D., Moulder, B., et al. (1998). Emotional arousal and activation of the visual cortex: An fMRI analysis. *Psychophysiology, 35*, 199–210.

Lawton, M. P., Kleban, M. H., Rajagopal, D., & Dean, J. (1992). Dimensions of affective experience in three age groups. *Psychology and Aging, 7*, 171–184.

Lazarus, R. S. (1991). Progress on a cognitive–motivational–relational theory of emotion. *American Psychologist, 46*, 819–834.

LeDoux, J. E. (2000). Emotion circuits in the brain. *Annual Review of Neuroscience, 23*, 155–184.

LeDoux, J. E. (2003). The emotional brain, fear, and the amygdala. *Cellular and Molecular Neurobiology, 23*, 727–738.

Levenson, R. W., Carstensen, L. L., & Gottman, J. M. (1994). The influence of age and gender on affect, physiology, and their interrelations: A study of long-term marriages. *Journal of Personality and Social Psychology, 67*, 56–68.

Levenson, R. W., Friesen, W. V., Ekman, P., & Carstensen, L. L. (1991). Emotion, physiology and expression in old age. *Psychology and Aging, 6*, 28–35.

Levesque, J., Eugene, F., Joanette, Y., Paquette, V., Mensour, B., Beaudoin, G., et al. (2003). Neural circuitry underlying voluntary suppression of sadness. *Biological Psychiatry, 53*, 502–510.

MacPherson, S. E., Phillips, L. H., & Della Sala, S. (2002). Age, executive function, and social decision making: A dorsolateral prefrontal theory of cognitive aging. *Psychology and Aging, 17,* 598–609.

Markowitsch, H. J., Calabrese, P., Wurker, M., Durwen, H. F., Kessler, J., Babinsky, R., et al. (1994). The amygdala's contribution to memory: A study on two patients with Urbach–Wiethe disease. *NeuroReport, 5,* 1349–1352.

Mather, M. (2004). Aging and emotional memory. In D. Reisberg & P. Hertel (Eds.), *Memory and emotion* (pp. 272–307). Oxford: Oxford University Press.

Mather, M., Canli, T., English, T., Whitfield, S., Wais, P., Ochsner, K., et al. (2004). Amygdala responses to emotionally valenced stimuli in older and younger adults. *Psychological Science, 15,* 259–263.

Mather, M., & Carstensen, L. L. (2003). Aging and attentional biases for emotional faces. *Psychological Science, 14,* 409–415.

Mather, M., & Johnson, M. K. (2000). Choice-supportive source monitoring: Do our decisions seem better to us as we age? *Psychology and Aging, 15,* 596–606.

Mather, M., & Knight, M. (2005). *Goal-directed memory: The role of executive processes in older adults' emotional memory.* Manuscript submitted for publication.

Mather, M., & Knight, M. (in press). Angry faces get noticed quickly: Threat detection is not impaired among older adults. *Journal of Gerontology: Psychological Sciences.*

Mather, M., Knight, M., & McCaffrey, M. (2005). The allure of the alignable: Younger and older adults' false memories of choice features. *Journal of Experimental Psychology: General, 134*(1), 38–51.

McGaugh, J. L. (2000). Memory: A century of consolidation. *Science, 287,* 248–251.

Mitchell, K. J., Johnson, M. K., Raye, C. L., Mather, M., & D'Esposito, M. (2000). Aging and reflective processes of working memory: Binding and test load deficits. *Psychology and Aging, 15,* 527–541.

Mogg, K., & Bradley, B. P. (1999). Orienting of attention to threatening facial expressions presented under conditions of restricted awareness. *Cognition and Emotion, 13,* 713–740.

Mogg, K., Bradley, B. P., & Hallowell, N. (1994). Attentional bias to threat: Roles of trait anxiety, stressful events, and awareness. *Quarterly Journal of Experimental Psychology, 47,* 841–864.

Morris, J. S., & Dolan, R. J. (2004). Dissociable amygdala and orbitofrontal responses during reversal fear conditioning. *NeuroImage, 22,* 372–380.

Morrison, J. H., & Hof, P. R. (1997). Life and death of neurons in the aging brain. *Science, 278,* 412–419.

Moscovitch, M., & Winocur, G. (1995). Frontal lobes, memory, and aging. *Annals of the New York Academy of Sciences, 769,* 119–150.

Mroczek, D. K. (2001). Age and emotion in adulthood. *Current Directions in Psychological Science, 10,* 87–90.

Nadel, L. (1991). The hippocampus and space revisited. *Hippocampus, 1,* 221–229.

Nolen-Hoeksema, S., & Morrow, J. (1991). A prospective study of depression and distress following a natural disaster: The 1989 Loma Prieta earthquake. *Journal of Personality and Social Psychology, 61,* 105–121.

Ochsner, K. N., Bunge, S. A., Gross, J. J., & Gabrieli, J. D. E. (2002). Rethinking feelings: An fMRI study of the cognitive regulation of emotion. *Journal of Cognitive Neuroscience, 14,* 1215–1229.

Ochsner, K. N., & Gross, J. J. (2004). Thinking makes it so: A social cognitive neuroscience approach to emotion regulation. In R. F. Baumeister & K. D. Vohs (Eds.), *Handbook of self-regulation* (pp. 229–255). New York: Guilford Press.

Ochsner, K. N., Ray, R., Cooper, J., Robertson, E., Chopra, S., Gabrieli, J. D. E., et al. (2004). For better or for worse: Neural systems supporting the cognitive down- and up-regulation of negative emotion, *NeuroImage, 23,* 483–499.

Öhman, A. (2002). Automaticity and the amygdala: Nonconscious responses to emotional faces. *Current Directions in Psychological Science, 11,* 62–66.

Öhman, A., Flykt, A., & Lundqvist, D. (2000). Unconscious emotion: Evolutionary perspectives, psychophysiological data and neuropsychological mechanisms. In R. D. Lane & L. Nadel (Eds.), *Cognitive neuroscience of emotion* (pp. 296–327). New York: Oxford University Press.

Öhman, A., Lundqvist, D., & Esteves, F. (2001). The face in the crowd revisited: A threat advantage with schematic stimuli. *Journal of Personality and Social Psychology, 80,* 381–396.

Ohnishi, T., Matsuda, H., Tabira, T., Asada, T., & Uno, M. (2001). Changes in brain morphology in Alzheimer disease and normal aging: Is Alzheimer disease an exaggerated aging process? *American Journal of Neuroradiology, 22,* 1680–1685.

Park, D. C., Lautenschlager, G., Hedden, T., Davidson, N. S., Smith, A. D., & Smith, P. K. (2002). Models of visuospatial and verbal memory across the adult life span. *Psychology and Aging, 17,* 299–320.

Phan, K. L., Wager, T., Taylor, S. F., & Liberzon, I. (2002). Functional neuroanatomy of emotion: A meta-analysis of emotion activation studies in PET and fMRI. *NeuroImage, 16,* 331–348.

Pruessner, J. C., Collins, D. L., Pruessner, M., & Evans, A. C. (2001). Age and gender predict volume decline in the anterior and posterior hippocampus in early adulthood. *Journal of Neuroscience, 21,* 194–200.

Prull, M. W., Gabrieli, J. D. E., & Bunge, S. A. (2000). Age-related changes in memory: A cognitive neuroscience perspective. In F. I. M. Craik & T. A. Salthouse (Eds.), *The handbook of aging and cognition* (2nd ed., pp. 91–153). Mahwah, NJ: Erlbaum.

Raz, N. (2000). Aging of the brain and its impact on cognitive performance: Integration of structural and functional findings. In F. I. M. Craik & T. A. Salthouse (Eds.), *The handbook of aging and cognition* (2nd ed., pp. 1–90). Mahwah, NJ: Erlbaum.

Resnick, S. M., Pham, D. L., Kraut, M. A., Zonderman, A. B., & Davatzikos, C. (2003). Longitudinal magnetic resonance imaging studies of older adults: A shrinking brain. *Journal of Neuroscience, 23,* 3295–3301.

Richardson, M. P., Strange, B. A., & Dolan, R. J. (2004). Encoding of emotional memories depends on amygdala and hippocampus and their interactions. *Nature Neuroscience, 7,* 278–285.

Rolls, E. T. (1999). The functions of the orbitofrontal cortex. *NeuroCase, 5,* 301–312.

Rolls, E. T., Critchley, H. D., Mason, R., & Wakeman, E. A. (1996). Orbitofrontal cortex neurons: Role in olfactory and visual association learning. *Journal of Neurophysiology, 75,* 1970–1981.

Rolls, E. T., Hornack, J. Wade, D., & McGrath, J. (1994). Emotion-related learning in patients with social and emotional changes associated with frontal lobe damage. *Journal of Neurology, Neurosurgery and Psychiatry, 57,* 1518–1524.

Roozendaal, B. (2002). Stress and memory: Opposing effects of glucocorticoids on memory consolidation and memory retrieval. *Neurobiology of Learning and Memory, 78,* 578–595.

Roseman, I. J. (2004). Appraisals, rather than unpleasantness or muscle movements, are the primary determinants of specific emotions. *Emotion, 4,* 145–150.

Rypma, B., Berger, J. S., & D'Esposito, M. (2002). The influence of working-memory demand and subject performance on prefrontal cortical activity. *Journal of Cognitive Neuroscience, 14,* 721–731.

Salat, D. H., Kaye, J. A., & Janowsky, J. S. (2001). Selective preservation and degeneration within the prefrontal cortex in aging and Alzheimer's disease. *Archives of Neurology, 58,* 1403–1408.

Sanghera, M. K., Rolls, E. T., & Roper-Hall, A. (1979). Visual responses of neurons in the dorsolateral amygdala of the alert monkey. *Psychological Review, 103,* 403–428.

Squire, L. R., & Zola-Morgan, S. (1991). The medial temporal lobe memory system. *Science, 253,* 1380–1386.

Sullivan, E. V., Marsh, L., Mathalon, D. H., Lim, K. O., & Pfefferbaum, A. (1995). Age-related decline in MRI volumes of temporal lobe gray matter but not hippocampus. *Neurobiology of Aging, 16,* 591–606.

Tisserand, D. J., & Jolles, J. (2003). On the involvement of prefrontal networks in cognitive ageing. *Cortex, 39,* 1107–1128.

Tisserand, D. J., Pruessner, J. C., Arigita, E. J. S., van Boxtel, M. P. J., Evans, A. C., Jolles, J., et al. (2002). Regional frontal cortical volumes decrease differentially in aging: An MRI study to compare volumetric approaches and voxel-based morphometry. *NeuroImage, 17,* 657–669.

Tsai, J. L., Levenson, R. W., & Carstensen, L. L. (2000). Autonomic, subjective and expressive responses to emotional films in older and younger Chinese Americans and European Americans. *Psychology and Aging, 15,* 684–693.

Volkow, N. D., Gur, R. C., Wang, G. J., Fowler, J. S. Moberg, P. J., Ding, Y. S., et al. (1998). Association between decline in brain dopamine activity with age and cognitive and motor impairment in healthy individuals. *American Journal of Psychiatry, 155,* 344–349.

Wagner, A. D., Maril, A., Bjork, R. A., & Schacter, D. L. (2001). Prefrontal contributions to executive control: fMRI evidence for functional distinctions within lateral prefrontal cortex. *NeuroImage, 14,* 1337–1374.

Wang, G. J., Volkow, N. D., Logon, J., Fowler, J. S., Schlyer, D., MacGregor, R. R., et al. (1995). Evaluation of age-related changes in serotonin 5–HT2 and dopamine D2 receptor availability in healthy human subjects. *Life Sciences, 56,* 249–253.

West, R. L. (1996). An application of prefrontal cortex function theory to cognitive aging. *Psychological Bulletin, 120,* 272–292.

Young, A. W., Hellawell, D. J., Van De Wal, C., & Johnson, M. (1996). Facial expression processing after amygdalotomy. *Neuropsychologia, 34,* 31–39.

Zola-Morgan, S., Squire, L. R., Alvarez-Royo, P., & Clower, R. P. (1991). Independence of memory functions and emotional behavior: Separate contributions of the hippocampal formation and the amygdala. *Hippocampus, 1,* 207–220.

9

Sex Differences in Neural Responses to Sexual Stimuli in Humans

Stephan Hamann

Of all the kinds of human individual differences, the differences between men and women are the ones that seem to hold a particular fascination. Psychologists have investigated and documented a growing catalog of such sex differences, ranging from subtle to substantial, in domains such as memory and language (Gur et al., 2000); emotion (Hamann & Canli, 2004); emotional memory (Cahill, Uncapher, Kilpatrick, Alkire, & Turner, 2004; Canli, Desmond, Zhao, & Gabrieli, 2002); spatial reasoning and navigation; rates of aggression and mood disorders; and responses to pain (Naliboff et al., 2003). Some of the most striking behavioral differences between men and women occur in the domain of sexual behavior. To take a prominent example, men differ markedly from women in the role that visual stimuli play in the process of sexual arousal and motivation. Numerous studies have corroborated the popular stereotype that men are more psychologically and physiologically responsive to visual sexually arousing stimuli, and that they display a greater motivation to seek out and interact with such stimuli (Herz & Cahill, 1997; Kinsey, Pomeroy, & Martin, 1948; Laumann, Gagnon, Michael, & Michaels, 1994; Symons, 1979).

The origin of such behavioral sex differences in reproductive behavior—whether they arise from differential experiences and socialization, from genetic differences, or through some interactions of these influences—remains a hotly debated issue (Buss & Schmidt, 1993; Symons, 1979). Regardless of their origin, because these sex differences are ultimately mediated by the brain, their functional basis can be explored through modern, noninvasive brain imaging methods. A better understanding of how sex differences play out on the neural level may help inform the debate over their nature and origin, and perhaps may also illuminate mechanisms underlying sex differences in other cognitive domains.

This chapter examines the findings of recent studies that have explored the neural correlates of sex differences in responses to sexual stimuli in humans. The primary focus is on functional neuroimaging studies, including those using positron emission tomography (PET) and functional magnetic resonance imaging (fMRI). Where relevant, studies of the structural correlates of sex differences between men and women, and findings from studies with non-human animals, are covered as well. I also briefly consider theories of the possible origins of these neural sex differences, including evolutionary, neural, and cultural factors. I conclude by considering future directions for study and the possible implications of evidence from different levels of analysis that converge on the limbic regions as critical areas mediating behavioral differences in sexual response between men and women.

SEX DIFFERENCES IN SEXUAL BEHAVIOR

A casual perusal of the contemporary mass media quickly reveals that human males appear much more preoccupied with visual representations of sexual content than are human females. Sexually arousing publications, websites, videos, and advertisements directed at male consumers far outnumber those directed at females. Surveys and experimental studies of sexual behavior corroborate this impression (Herz & Cahill, 1997; Kinsey et al., 1948; Laumann et al., 1994). Stereotypes aside, by a variety of metrics, male sexual arousal is more centered around visual stimuli than is female sexual arousal: In general, men are more psychologically and physiologically responsive to visual sexually arousing stimuli, and they display a greater motivation to seek out and interact with such stimuli (Bradley, Codispoti, Sabatinelli, & Lang, 2001; Herz & Cahill, 1997; Laumann et al., 1994).

Why do men and women differ in this way? Two main theoretical views have been proposed: an evolutionary/sociobiological account and a social influences account. The evolutionary account traces its lineage back to Darwin, who proposed the notion of sexual selection, whereby the sex that has the lower degree of parental investment in reproduction is more likely to engage in competition for the opposite sex. More recently, this account has been revised and elaborated by several sociobiological theorists (Buss & Schmidt, 1993; Symons, 1979; Trivers, 1972). According to this view, men, who require a lesser investment of time and resources to reproduce, should aggressively compete with other males for access to females and should have a greater ability to become quickly sexually aroused and motivated to engage in sexual activity. Visual sexual cues should be more salient to males, because they allow for rapid identification and appraisal of mating opportunities with females in the visual field, and thus facilitate their mating with a maximal number of females. Conversely, because women have a much greater parental investment in time and resources in reproduction, it would be disadvantageous for their reproductive behavior to be driven primarily by visual stimuli, and for them to be as quickly and broadly responsive to mating opportunities as men are. Instead, women are predicted to place a greater emphasis on social status, genetic fitness, and the ability of a potential mate to provide long-term commitment and protection.

Rather than focusing on adaptive behaviors and reproductive strategies, the social influences account emphasizes the role of the socialization process in shaping the way men and women respond sexually, and point to the social construction of sexuality as the primary factor underlying sex differences in sexual behavior (Byrne, 1977; Gagnon, 1977; Gagnon & Simon, 1973). For example, Byrne (1977) has proposed that appraisals of sexual stimuli derive from an individual's life history of learning associations between positive and negative feelings and sexual stimuli. Thus, according to this account, differences in men's and women's responses to sexual stimuli arise from different degrees of positive and negative reinforcement that males and females have experienced during the process of socialization. A strong version of this view would predict that men and women would respond equivalently to sexual stimuli if they were exposed to the same history of positive and negative reinforcement associated with sexuality. Although social attitudes toward male and female sexuality have changed markedly in recent decades in many countries (particularly in Western societies), substantial differences in the socialization of males and females with respect to sexuality persist today (Gagnon, 1977; Gagnon & Simon, 1973); according to social influences theorists, these disparities continue to give rise to sex differences in sexual responses.

Although these two views are often portrayed as mutually exclusive, particularly in media reports dealing with human sex differences, it is clearly possible that both sets of processes could contribute to sex differences in sexual behavior. As noted above, the hope is that a better understanding of the brain mechanisms underlying these behavioral differences may help to clarify the origins of these differences and help inform this debate. Modern neuroimaging techniques offer the ability to identify sex differences in brain structure and function, and to relate them to differences in sexual behavior.

NEUROIMAGING STUDIES OF SEXUAL RESPONSE

Many neuroimaging studies have examined the neural correlates of fear, disgust, and other emotional states, but until recently little was known specifically about how the human brain responds to stimuli of a specifically sexual nature. Moreover, most of what is known about brain responses to sexual stimuli is limited to males, in part because it is generally easier to study male responses than female responses. These studies have primarily examined responses to erotic films or photographs, and have reported activations across a wide range of cortical and subcortical areas involved in perception, attention, emotion and motivation, and physiological responses (Beauregard, Levesque, & Bourgouin, 2001; Holstege et al., 2003; Redoute et al., 2000; Stoleru et al., 1999; for a comprehensive review of neuroimaging studies focusing on male sexual responses, see Sumich, Kumari, & Sharma, 2003). More recently, attention has turned to investigating women's responses to sexual stimuli and to characterizing sex differences.

To date, only two published neuroimaging studies have directly compared neural responses to visual sexual stimuli across the sexes (Hamann, Herman, Nolan, & Wallen, 2004; Karama et al., 2002). The rationale behind both of these studies was to examine sex differences in an effort to determine the neural correlates underlying the greater male response to visual sexual stimuli. Another similarity between these studies is that their choices of brain regions to focus on in their analyses were strongly influenced both by prior neuroimaging studies of emotion and responses to sexual stimuli in human males, and by studies using nonhuman animals. (See Figure 9.1 for a summary of key brain regions linked to sex differences in responses to visual sexual stimuli in human neuroimaging studies.)

Studies of nonhuman animals have identified several sex differences in brain regions that mediate reproductive behavior, which may provide clues to brain regions underlying sex differences in human sexual response. For example, the amygdala has long been known to play a role in primate sexual behavior, from landmark studies such as those of Klüver and Bucy (1939). Bilateral damage to the amygdala and surrounding cortical areas results in the so-called "Klüver–Bucy syndrome" in monkeys and, more rarely, in humans (Terzian & Dalle Ore, 1955); this is characterized by atypical and indiscriminate sexual behavior. Clinical evidence has also linked temporal lobe seizures located near the amygdala to abnormal sexual behavior such as sexual automatisms (Leutmezer et al., 1999). In work with rodents, Everitt (1990) demonstrated that lesions to the medial amygdala interfered with the ability of male rats to respond to olfactory and visual sexual cues from a receptive female, implicating this structure in male appetitive sexual motivation. In this study, male rats were trained to gain access to receptive female rats that were sequestered above them in a Plexiglas enclosure, by repeatedly pushing a lever that would open a trap door. Lesions to the medial amygdala markedly reduced bar-pressing behavior to obtain females, but did not interfere with sexual behavior such as intromissions when the females were placed next to the males. Because lesions to the medial amygdala do not affect female sexual receptivity, this demonstrates that in rats this structure is critical for male but not female responses to distal sexually salient stimuli. Another prominent sex difference has been identified in the hypothalamus. Male and female rats' sexual behaviors are controlled by different hypothalamic regions, with lesions to the

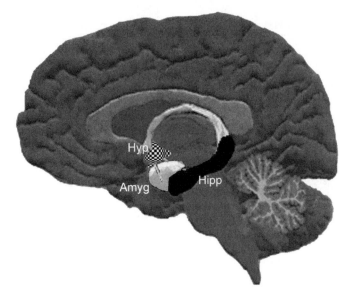

FIGURE 9.1. Some key regions implicated in sex differences in human responses to sexually arousing stimuli. The amygdala is a small almond-shaped structure located deep in the anterior temporal lobe; it plays a critical role in a variety of emotional processes, including adaptive responses to emotional stimuli, motivation, and emotional memory. The hypothalamus has direct connections with the amygdala and mediates a host of physiological and hormonal responses, including responses to sexual stimuli. Recent work suggests that differences between men and women in responses to visual sexually arousing stimuli are mediated by these two highly interconnected regions. In addition to the amygdala and hypothalamus, other structures, including those involved in memory (hippocampus) and other functions, have also been linked with these sex differences. Hyp, hypothalamus; Amyg, amygdala; Hipp, hippocampus.

medial preoptic area affecting male but not female sexual behavior, and lesions to the ventromedial hypothalamic nucleus having the converse effect (Everitt, 1990).

   These findings from animal studies have guided neuroimaging researchers in their search for brain regions that may underlie the greater male response to visual sexually arousing stimuli. As noted above, men are more psychologically and physiologically responsive to such stimuli, and they display a greater motivation to seek out and interact with them. This specific sex difference is predicted by evolutionary and sociobiological theories that it is adaptive for males to react rapidly to visual information signaling an opportunity to mate with a fertile female, because this tends to increase their probability of passing on their genes. Because of the greater maternal investment in time and resources for childrearing, a similar rapid arousal response to visual stimuli is not adaptive for females, and thus differences in neural responses between men and women should be observed.

The first study to examine this sex difference by directly comparing men and women on neural responses to visual sexual stimuli (Karama et al., 2002) examined brain activity with fMRI in 20 men and 20 women while they viewed erotic film clips (sexual interactions between a man and a woman) and neutral film clips (social interactions with no sexual content). All subjects were heterosexual young adult university students. Subjects were asked to refrain from sexual activity leading to orgasm for at least 24 hours before scanning, and the women were tested on days outside of their ovulatory period, to help minimize potential effects of cyclic hormonal fluctuations. Subjects viewed the erotic and neutral film segments through video goggles for 3 minutes each (film order was counterbalanced across subjects), with a short rest break between the two segments, during which a blank screen was presented. Following scanning, subjects were asked to rate their level of perceived sexual arousal experienced during the erotic film segment, on a scale ranging from 0 (lowest) to 8 (highest).

Consistent with prior studies showing that men respond more strongly to visual sexual stimuli, men rated the erotic films as significantly more sexually arousing than did women, although both groups rated the erotic films as being at least moderately sexually arousing. Interestingly, the majority of the activations elicited by the sexual stimuli were similar in magnitude for men and women, indicating considerable commonality between the neural responses of men and women to visual sexual stimuli. These regions of common activation included the anterior cingulate, medial prefrontal, orbito-frontal, insular, and occipito-temporal cortices, as well as subcortical areas involved in emotion, motivation, and reward, including the amygdala and ventral striatum.

When men and women were compared on their neural responses to the erotic films versus the neutral control films, the primary sex difference revealed was a greater activation in the hypothalamus for men than for women (Figure 9.2)—a finding that accords well with the predicted involvement of this structure in sex differences in sexual response, on the basis of converging evidence from prior neuroimaging studies and studies with nonhuman animals. Weaker evidence for a sex difference in thalamic activity was also found: Men showed greater activation in this structure than women did; however, the direct comparison between men and women on activity in the thalamus failed to find a significant group difference. Hypothalamic activity in males (but not in females) was also significantly correlated with higher self-ratings of sexual arousal experienced during the erotic films. This finding supports a link between hypothalamic activity and physiological correlates of sexual arousal in males, consistent with a previous neuroimaging study in men (Redoute et al., 2000) that reported a positive correlation between hypothalamic activity and a measure of genital tumescence.

This initial study of sex differences in brain responses to visual sexual stimuli provided considerable new information regarding both the overall commonality in patterns of neural responses in men and women, and a spe-

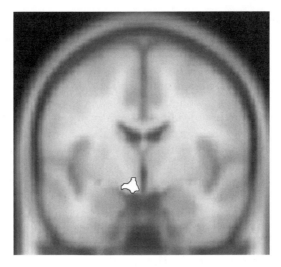

FIGURE 9.2. Greater hypothalamic activation for males versus females elicited by viewing erotic films (vs. emotionally neutral films) from an fMRI study, displayed on a coronal brain section at a statistical significance threshold of $p < .001$ ($z = 3.09$). Data from Karama et al. (2002).

cific sex difference in the response of the hypothalamus to sexual stimuli. However, one limitation of this study noted by its authors was its unusual experimental design. Most fMRI paradigms alternate frequently between two or more experimental conditions to avoid certain artifacts peculiar to this methodology, such as interference from low-frequency noise effects that can reduce sensitivity to experimental effects and introduce spurious activations. Because this study used only one alternation between the two 3-minute film conditions (the erotic and neutral films), its design was particularly vulnerable to interference from low-frequency noise effects and was relatively insensitive to rapid changes in amygdala activity, which may be critical for reliably detecting sex differences in the responses of this structure (Hamann et al., 2004). Thus some sex differences in brain response may have gone undetected because of limited sensitivity. Another important consideration is that the men in this study rated the sexual stimuli as substantially more sexually arousing than did the women, raising the possibility that the observed sex differences might reflect differences in arousal rather than a sex difference per se. Consistent with this possibility, when the authors conducted a regression analysis that factored in the effects of rated sexual arousal, the sex difference in hypothalamic activation was no longer statistically significant.

The results of an fMRI study my colleagues and I conducted (Hamann et al., 2004) both fit nicely with and extend those of Karama and colleagues (2002), and they also clarify a number of issues. As in the previous study, our objective was to investigate the neural basis underlying the greater male interest in and response to visual sexually arousing stimuli. We were particularly interested in possible sex differences in activity in the amygdala and hypothalamus, based both on prior converging evidence from animal studies and on the key role of the amygdala in mediating emotional and physiological responses to biologically salient stimuli (particularly visual stimuli). We specifically set out to test two alternative hypotheses concerning how sex differences in activations to sexual stimuli might arise. As mentioned in relation to the Karama and colleagues study above, if men exhibit greater brain activations than women in response to visual sexual stimuli, this neural difference may arise simply because the men typically respond with greater psychological and physiological arousal, rather than because of any sex difference per se. The issue of arousal is particularly important, because many studies have shown that the amygdala (a key structure mediating responses to emotionally salient stimuli) is highly sensitive to emotional arousal or intensity, both for aversive stimuli and for pleasant, appetitive stimuli (Calder, Lawrence, & Young, 2001; Davis & Whalen, 2001; Hamann, Ely, Hoffman, & Kilts, 2002). According to this view, the same differences in brain activation would be observed between two groups of men who differed in their arousal level; conversely, if men and women were somehow matched on their levels of elicited arousal, the sex differences in brain activation would be eliminated. An alternative to this arousal hypothesis is the processing mode hypothesis, which proposes that sex differences in brain activation elicited by sexual stimuli arise from differences in cognitive styles or neural pathways recruited by men and women during the processing of sexual stimuli. In this view, men and women should differ in their neural responses to sexual stimuli even after they have been matched on arousal.

Thus our goal was to test these hypotheses by comparing men and women on responses to visual sexual stimuli under conditions where they were equated on elicited arousal. Equating the sexes on arousal is a challenging task, because (once again) males typically respond substantially more strongly to visual sexual stimuli. Matching the sexes on arousal required the careful preselection of visual sexual stimuli that were maximally arousing and minimally aversive to females, through computer-based arousal ratings of hundreds of stimuli by a group of anonymous female raters. In addition, subjects were prescreened to ensure that only subjects who had prior experience with viewing visual sexual stimuli and who found them significantly sexually arousing were included. All subjects were young heterosexual adults.

We examined brain activity with fMRI in 14 men and 14 women while they viewed sexually arousing and neutral photographs. During scanning, subjects passively viewed alternating short blocks (5 different pictures presented over 20 seconds) of four types of photographic stimuli via video goggles: two types of sexually arousing stimuli, including heterosexual couples engaged in sexual activity ("couples" stimuli) and sexually attractive opposite-sex nudes ("opposite-sex" stimuli); and two types of control stimuli, including pleasant scenes depicting nonsexual male–female interaction such as therapeutic massage ("neutral" stimuli) and a fixation cross ("fixation"). Ratings of sexual attractiveness and physical arousal were assessed after scanning. Subjects' ratings of sexual arousal and attractiveness for the stimuli confirmed that we had successfully equated men and women on these measures. Women in fact gave slightly higher ratings than men on both the arousal and attractiveness scales, though not significantly so.

In examining brain activations elicited by the sexual stimuli, we were particularly interested in responses to the couples stimuli, because these stimuli elicited the highest arousal in both groups and allowed us to directly compare female and male responses to the same stimuli. The primary finding was that the amygdala and hypothalamus were more activated in men than in women when participants were viewing the sexually arousing couples stimuli. This can be seen in Figure 9.3a, which shows the regions where men showed greater activation than women for the couples stimuli versus the fixation condition. The group activation maps for the same activation comparison for men and women are shown in Figures 9.3b and 9.3c, respectively (see Figure 9.4 for a three-dimensional rendering of the activations in Figures 9.3b and 9.3c, showing their spatial extent and relation to the rest of the brain). To further test whether the sex differences were related specifically to the sexual aspects of the couples stimuli, we contrasted the activations for the couples stimuli with the closely matched nonsexual neutral stimuli, which controlled for the presence of pleasant social stimuli. Men again showed significantly greater activation in the amygdala and hypothalamus, as well as in the bilateral posterior thalamus and left hippocampus. The greater amygdala activation for men is particularly interesting, because this sex difference had not been reported previously, and it parallels the findings of prior studies with nonhuman animals implicating the amygdala in male but not female sexual appetitive behavior (Everitt, 1990; Newman, 1999).

No areas of greater activation for women than for men were found in our study at the statistical thresholds used ($p < .001$), in line with the results of Karama and colleagues (2002). This absence of greater activations for females fits well with the predicted overall pattern of greater responsiveness of men's brains to visual sexual stimuli. In addition, this finding suggests that women were not engaging in greater cognitive inhibition of sexual arousal or performing some other cognitive regulation of their emotional responses that might account for their lower level of limbic activation in the amygdala and hypothalamus. Individuals have been demonstrated to have the ability to use cognitive strategies to inhibit their emotional responses and corresponding limbic activation (Beauregard et al., 2001) to sexual stimuli—for example, by imagining that they are detached, impassive observers of sexual scenes. Such cognitive regulation activities are typically marked by characteristic increases in activity in brain regions implicated in cognitive control of behavior, including the prefrontal cortex and anterior cingulate cortex.

Although sex differences were observed in specific limbic regions, men and women showed remarkably similar activation patterns across multiple

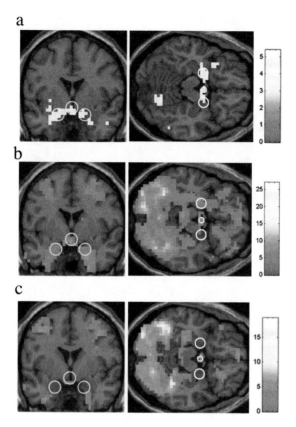

FIGURE 9.3. Results from an fMRI study comparing brain responses of men and women to sexually arousing photographs, showing greater activation for men specifically in the bilateral amygdala and the hypothalamus. Illustrated are brain regions where men showed greater activation than females when viewing sexually arousing photographs versus a control condition in which a fixation cross (+) was presented. The middle circle shows the approximate location of the hypothalamus, whereas the outer two circles indicate the approximate location of the left and right amygdala. Lighter shades on the bars at right indicate larger effects (statistical z-scores). The right hemisphere is on the right of the coronal images. (a) Left: Coronal image showing greater bilateral amygdala and hypothalamic activations for males versus females, for the statistical comparison between sexually arousing stimuli and fixation. Right: Axial view of the same contrast. (b) The areas more active while viewing sexually arousing stimuli versus fixation, for the group of men. (c) The same contrast and views for women. In contrast to the findings for men, there is a lack of significant activity in the bilateral amygdala and the hypothalamus for women in response to sexually arousing photographs. From Hamann, Herman, Nolan, and Wallen (2004). Reprinted by permission of the authors.

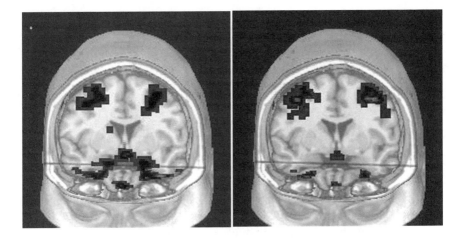

FIGURE 9.4. Three-dimensional rendering of the primary result from the Hamann et al. (2004) study: Greater bilateral amygdala and hypothalamic activations for males (left panel) than for females (right panel), for the statistical comparison between sexually arousing stimuli and fixation in each group. Activations are overlaid on a representative brain to illustrate the spatial relationship between these subcortical structures and the rest of the brain.

brain regions—including ventral striatal regions involved in reward, and cortical regions associated with visual processing, attention, and motor and somatosensory functions (Figure 9.5). This again parallels the findings of Karama and colleagues (2002), who found that most brain activations elicited by visual sexual stimuli were similar for men and women. In light of prior research findings that processing complex, emotionally arousing visual stimuli recruits similar brain activations across several brain areas for men and women (Canli, Zhao, Brewer, Gabrieli, & Cahill, 2000; Kampe, Frith, Dolan, & Frith, 2001; Wager, Phan, Liberzon, & Taylor, 2003), the broad similarities observed between the sexes in response to sexual stimuli are not unexpected. That is, sex differences in brain activation associated with a particular type of emotionally arousing visual stimuli (sexual stimuli) can be conceptualized as being superimposed over a basically similar pattern of brain response to emotionally evocative visual stimuli for men and women.

Overall, the results of our study favored the processing mode hypothesis rather than the arousal hypothesis, because they were obtained when arousal had been equated for men and women, and even when we analyzed a subset of women who had higher arousal than the men. Sexual arousal has multiple psychological and physiological aspects, however, so it remains possible that other aspects of arousal that were not examined might have contributed to the observed sex differences. Other findings, however, suggest that explanations based on simple group differences in arousal are unlikely to explain these find-a

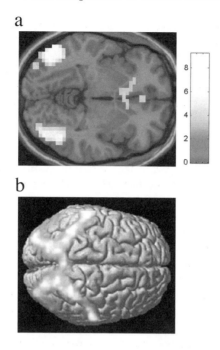

b

FIGURE 9.5. Regions of significant overlap (conjunction) between group activations for males and females. Illustrated are the statistical conjunctions between the activation maps for males and females ($p < .05$ corrected, $\geq = 10$ contiguous voxels), for the couples stimuli versus the neutral, nonsexual stimuli. (a) Axial view ($z = -4$) showing common activation in ventral striatum and occipital cortex. The bar at right indicates maximal z-values. (b) Brain-surface-rendered view of the same map, showing parieto-temporo-occipital and frontal activations spanning regions associated with visual processing, attention, and motor and somatosensory functions. Regions in white surpassed a $p < .05$ corrected threshold. The right hemisphere is on the bottom of the image. From Hamann et al. (2004). Reprinted by permission of the authors.

ings fully. For example, both men and women reported that the couples stimuli (which depicted explicit sexual activity) were more arousing than the opposite-sex nude stimuli. If amygdala activity were only sensitive to arousal level, one would predict that both groups should show either more amygdala activity for the more arousing stimulus type (i.e., the couples stimuli) or an equivalent amount of activity (e.g., if the difference in arousal were not enough to cause a significant change in amygdala activity or a maximal level had already been reached). In fact, when activity in the left amygdala was examined, the response pattern for women fit none of these scenarios: Women showed significantly more amygdala activity for the less arousing opposite-sex stimuli than for the more arousing couples stimuli. Men showed the expected pattern, exhibiting marginally greater amygdala activation for the couples stimuli. These complementary patterns of brain response for men and women clearly pose a challenge to any attempts to explain sex differences in these responses simply in terms of differing levels of sexual arousal. They also indicate that sex differences in brain responses to visual sexual stimuli are modulated by the specific content of the sexually arousing stimuli. Determining which particular properties of the couples stimuli and opposite-sex stimuli lead to these differential brain responses is an important question for further research.

The primary finding of greater amygdala activation for males in response to visual sexual stimuli has subsequently been replicated in two separate studies. Karama and colleagues (S. Karama, personal communication, April 2004) conducted a follow-up study to their 2002 study, using a more conventional fMRI design that involved breaking the original erotic and neutral films into multiple alternating 30-second blocks. With this modified design, which was less subject to low-frequency fMRI noise effects and more sensitive to sex differences in the amygdala, greater activity in the left amygdala was found in males, consistent with the more marked sex difference in the left amygdala found in our (Hamann et al., 2004) study. A second study (Gizewski, Heuel, Karama, Senf, & Forsting, 2004) also used shorter versions of the erotic and neutral films from Karama and colleagues (2002) and found greater activation for men than for women in the left amygdala. As in the Karama and colleagues study, the men in both of these subsequent studies reported higher arousal than the women. Together with the results of our study, these results show that greater amygdala activation for males (particularly in the left amygdala) generalizes to studies using dynamic visual stimuli, and, as expected, to situations where elicited arousal is higher in males than in females.

What might the greater amygdala activation in men correspond to at the psychological level, if not emotional arousal? A leading candidate is motivation, a close relative of arousal. Several studies in humans and nonhuman animals have established that the amygdala plays a critical role in what has been termed "incentive motivation"—that is, the wanting or desire for a reward, as distinct from the pleasure or emotional arousal associated with enjoying the reward (Arana et al., 2003; Gottfried, O'Doherty, & Dolan, 2003). This account would fit well with the behavioral findings described earlier that characterize men as more preoccupied with wanting and desiring visual sexual stimulation, and spending more time and effort seeking such stimuli on the Internet and through other means. In this view, the greater amygdala activation for men reflects a greater appetitive motivation or desire elicited by visual sexual stimuli. If this view is correct, then future neuroimaging studies that assess appetitive motivation—for example, by requiring subjects to expend money or effort to view sexual stimuli—should find a strong relation between this measure of motivation and amygdala activity. Regarding the clinical implications of the Hamann and colleagues (2004) results, a number of sexual disorders such as voyeurism are far more prevalent in men (Gomez, 1991).

The greater amygdala response to visual sexual stimuli and greater appetitive motivation elicited by visual sexual stimuli may contribute to the greater rate of such disorders in males.

Another provocative link between the amygdala and incentive motivation was reported in a structural MRI study of patients who had undergone surgery that removed varying amounts of the amygdala. Sexual drive was positively correlated with the remaining volume of the amygdala: Patients with larger amygdalas remaining after surgery had higher sexual motivation than those who had smaller amygdalas remaining (Baird, Wilson, Bladin, Saling, & Reutens, 2004), and this relationship held for both men and women. It is still unknown, however, whether natural variations in amygdala size in unoperated, healthy individuals are related to sexual motivation or other aspects of sexual behavior. It is interesting to note, however, that the amygdala is larger in men than in women, even when total brain size is taken into account (Goldstein et al., 2001). In summary, the amygdala differs both functionally (i.e., greater responsiveness to visual sexual stimuli in men, as assessed by fMRI) and structurally (i.e., larger size in men, as assessed by structural MRI) between men and women, and both forms of sex differences have been linked to sexual motivation processes.

SEX DIFFERENCES IN NEURAL CORRELATES OF ORGASM

A parallel with the differential roles of the amygdala in male appetitive (precopulatory) versus consummatory (copulatory) sexual responses highlighted in previous animal studies is suggested by a PET study of brain activity in men during consummatory sexual behavior elicited by tactile stimulation by a female partner (Holstege et al., 2003). Relative to a resting baseline, consummatory male sexual behavior (erection and orgasm) elicited decreased activity in only one brain region, the amygdala, bilaterally during erection and in the left amygdala during orgasm. Thus, whereas viewing appetitive sexual stimuli by males in the Hamann and colleagues (2004) study elicited highly localized increases in amygdala activation, consummatory sexual behavior elicited correspondingly focal deactivations in the amygdala. In contrast to the neuroimaging studies of responses to visual sexual stimuli, where no areas of greater activation were found for females, a recent PET study of brain activation during female orgasm (Georgiadis et al., 2004) found activation in the periaqueductal grey (PAG) region for females that had not been found in a previous study of male orgasm (Holstege et al., 2003). The PAG activation for women was of particular interest, because converging evidence from animal studies with cats, rats, and hamsters has demonstrated that the PAG is critical for female reproductive behaviors. Although it was not reported whether the deactivation in the amygdala found previously for males was also observed for females during orgasm, the remaining activations were characterized as being highly similar to those observed previously for males during orgasm, with activations in subcortical regions including the mesodiencephalic junction, lateral putamen, and ventral pallidum, and in all parts of the cerebellum.

In summary, these studies of the neural correlates of consummatory sexual behavior (i.e., orgasm) present a general pattern similar to that found with appetitive visual sexual stimuli: The majority of activated brain regions are the same for both men and women, and the specific regions that do show sex differences in activation parallel the regions that have been implicated in male-specific or female-specific sexual behaviors in nonhuman animals. Further investigation will be required to establish conclusively whether such parallels indeed reflect a conservation of sexually differentiated function in these specific brain regions across species.

To return to the question of the origin of sex differences in human neural response to sexual stimuli, the parallels with nonhuman animals suggest that at least some aspects of sex differences are more likely to stem from evolutionarily conserved neural sex differences between males and females. For example, although it is possible that the activation of the PAG during orgasm in women but not men is attributable to some difference in socialization, this explanation fails to account for why this particular structure should be more active in women. In contrast, the female-specific behavioral functions of this structure that have been identified in nonhuman animals provide a clear basis for understanding why this specific region is more active in women. On the other hand, other sex differences, such as in the specific types of visual stimulus content to which men and women respond maximally, may be heavily influenced by differential socialization and experience.

CONCLUSION AND SUMMARY

The general picture that emerges from these studies is that for most brain regions, men's and women's brain responses during appetitive and consummatory sexual behavior are quite similar. Prominent exceptions to this pattern are found in a handful of subcortical structures regulating emotion, motivation, and physiological response. Remarkably, each of these subcortical structures has also been linked to sex-differentiated sexual behaviors in nonhuman animals. In addition, the amygdala and hypothalamus are also larger in men than in women (Goldstein et al, 2001) and contain high levels of sex hormone receptors (Arnold & Gorski, 1984; Roselli, Klosterman, & Resko, 2001). Thus the localization of human sex differences in functional brain responses to sexual stimuli closely reflects both the location and function of sexually differentiated regions reported in nonhuman animals, as well as the distribution of sex hormone receptors and structural sex differences in the human brain. These parallels suggest a considerable conservation of sex-differentiated reproductive function across mammalian species, and also are consistent with important roles for sex hormones (during both development and maturity) and for structural brain differences in contributing to sex differences in neural responses to sexual stimuli.

LOOKING FORWARD

The studies reviewed here have yielded some provocative findings regarding the neural basis of specific sex differences in human sexual behavior, and suggest a number of avenues for further research. For example, a major unexplored issue concerns the time course of brain responses to sexual stimuli. The activated regions identified in the neuroimaging studies of responses to visual sexual stimuli reviewed here were all based on activations averaged across the presentation of several different visual stimuli (e.g., separate photographs or film images) spanning at least several seconds. Neuroimaging studies using event-related experimental designs, in which the brain responses to individual stimuli can be tracked as they evolve over time, will provide a window into the temporal dynamics of brain responses to sexual stimuli and will allow sex differences in these dynamics to be investigated. Another advantage of analyzing responses to individual stimuli is that individual differences in reactions to stimuli can be taken into account when brain activations are analyzed. For example, the relation between emotional responses to individual stimuli and regional brain activations can be explored. These emotional responses may include a wide variety of measures, including subjective ratings of arousal or attractiveness, as well as physiological measures such as skin conductance response (a measure of autonomic arousal), heart rate, and plethysmography.

An important question concerns whether the greater neural response for men to sexual stimuli is confined to the visual modality. The behavioral sex difference in response to sexual stimuli is strongly tied to the visual modality, and there is little evidence to suggest that men and women differ substantially in their response to auditory sexually arousing stimuli. Evolutionary and sociobiological accounts also have strongly emphasized the visual modality (Buss & Schmidt, 1993; Symons, 1979). A clear question for future research, then, is whether the amygdala and other limbic structures identified in studies of visual sexual stimuli are also active during processing of auditory sexual stimuli (e.g., arousing spoken scripts), and whether men and women differ in their neural responses when stimuli are presented in a nonvisual modality.

In addition, it will be important to assess the effects of individual differences in personality, age, experience, and levels of circulating sex hormones in modulating sex differences in responses to sexual stimuli. Studies have attempted to control for hormonal variations—for example, by testing women at a specific point in the menstrual cycle (e.g., Karama et al., 2002)—but the systematic effects of fluctuations in male and female hormones on brain responses to sexual stimuli have yet to be examined. For example, an event-related potential (ERP) study (Krug, Plihal, Fehm, & Born, 2000) found that

ERP responses to sexual stimuli and other emotional stimuli varied across the menstrual cycle. During the ovulatory phase, the late positive component of the ERP response, which is sensitive to emotional valence, was elevated specifically to sexually arousing stimuli (photographs of opposite-sex nudes), but not to other types of emotionally arousing stimuli (babies) or neutral stimuli (people in everyday situations). These results suggest that changes in circulating hormone levels significantly alter neural responses to sexually arousing stimuli.

As detailed above, sex differences in the neural basis of human sexual behavior can arise from multiple causes, including alterations in brain development, differences in brain morphology, the effects of sex hormones, or different social experiences of men and women. Future research will clarify the contribution of each of these factors to sex differences in sexual behavior, as well as the role of the amygdala and other brain regions in these differential responses. In addition, as more neuroimaging studies begin to investigate these issues, the relative roles of social experience and genetically specified sex differences in shaping the brain's response to sexual stimuli and interactions will gradually become clearer.

ACKNOWLEDGMENTS

This research reported herein was supported by the Center for Behavioral Neuroscience, a Science and Technology Center Program of the National Science Foundation, under Agreement No. IBN-9876754, and by National Institutes of Health Grant No. 1R24MH067314. I thank Kim Wallen, Rebecca Herman, and Carla Harenski for their significant contributions to this research.

REFERENCES

Arana, S. F., Parkinson, J. A., Hinton, E., Holland, A., Owen, A. M., & Roberts, A. C. (2003). Dissociable contributions of the human amygdala and orbitofrontal cortex to incentive motivation and goal selection. *Journal of Neuroscience, 23,* 9632–9638.

Arnold, A. P., & Gorski, R. A. (1984). Gonadal steroid induction of structural sex differences in the central nervous system. *Annual Review of Neuroscience, 7,* 413–442.

Baird, A. D., Wilson, S. J., Bladin, P. F., Saling, M. M., & Reutens, D. C. (2004). The amygdala and sexual drive: Insights from temporal lobe epilepsy surgery. *Annals of Neurology, 55,* 87–96.

Beauregard, M., Levesque, J., & Bourgouin, P. J. (2001). Neural correlates of conscious self-regulation of emotion. *Journal of Neuroscience, 21,* 1–6.

Bradley, M. M., Codispoti, M., Sabatinelli, D., & Lang, P. (2001). Emotion and motivation: II. Sex differences in picture processing. *Emotion, 1,* 300–319.

Buss, D. M., & Schmidt, D. P. (1993). Sexual strategies theory: An evolutionary perspective on human mating. *Psychological Review, 100,* 204–232.

Byrne, D. (1977). Social psychology and the study of sexual behavior. *Personality and Social Psychology Bulletin, 3*, 3–30.

Cahill, L., Uncapher, M., Kilpatrick, L., Alkire, M. T., & Turner, J. (2004). Sex-related hemispheric lateralization of amygdala function in emotionally influenced memory: An FMRI investigation. *Learning and Memory, 11*, 261–266.

Calder, A. J., Lawrence, A. L., & Young, A. W. (2001). Neuropsychology of fear and loathing. *Nature Reviews Neuroscience, 2*, 352–263.

Canli, T., Desmond, J. E., Zhao, Z., & Gabrieli, J. D. E. (2002). Sex differences in the neural basis of emotional memories. *Proceedings of the National Academy of Sciences USA, 99*, 10789–10794.

Canli, T., Zhao, Z., Brewer, J., Gabrieli, J. D. E., & Cahill, L. (2000). Event-related activation in the human amygdala associates with later memory for individual emotional experience. *Journal of Neuroscience, 20*, 1–5.

Davis, M., & Whalen, P. J. (2001). The amygdala: vigilance and emotion. *Molecular Psychiatry, 6*, 12–34.

Everitt, B. J. (1990). Sexual motivation: A neural and behavioral analysis of the mechanisms underlying appetitive and copulatory responses of male rats. *Neuroscience and Biobehavioral Reviews, 14*, 217–232.

Gagnon, J. H. (1977). *Human sexualities.* Glenview, IL: Scott, Foreman.

Gagnon, J. H., & Simon, W. (1973). *Sexual conduct: The social sources of human sexuality.* Chicago: Aldine.

Georgiadis, J. R., Kuipers, R., Nieuwenburg, A., Reinders, S., Pruim, J., van Roon, A., et al. (2004). *Female sexual orgasm: A PET study.* Poster presented at the annual meeting of the Organization for Human Brain Mapping, Budapest, Hungary.

Gizewski, E. R., Heuel, E., Karama, S., Senf, W., & Forsting, M. (2004). *Gender specific cerebral activation during mental rotation test, verb generation and erotic stimuli using fMRI.* Poster presented at the annual meeting of the Organization for Human Brain Mapping, Budapest, Hungary.

Goldstein, J. M., Seidman, J. L., Horton, N. J., Makris, N., Kennedy, D. N., Caviness, V. S., et al. (2001). Normal sexual dimorphism of the adult human brain assessed by *in vivo* magnetic resonance imaging. *Cerebral Cortex, 11*, 490–497.

Gomez, J. (1991). *Psychological and psychiatric problems in men.* New York: Routledge.

Gottfried, J. A., O'Doherty, J., & Dolan, R. J. (2003). Encoding predictive reward value in human amygdala and orbitofrontal cortex. *Science, 301*, 1104–1107.

Gur, R. E., Alsop, D., Glahn, D., Petty, R., Swanson, C. L., Maldjian, J. A., et al. (2000). An fMRI study of sex differences in regional activation to a verbal and spatial task. *Brain and Language, 74*, 157–170.

Hamann, S., & Canli, T. (2004). Individual differences in emotion processing. *Current Opinion in Neurobiology, 14*, 233–238.

Hamann, S. B., Ely, T. D., Hoffman, J. M., & Kilts, C. D. (2002). Ecstasy and agony: Activation of the human amygdala in positive and negative emotion. *Psychological Science, 13*, 135–141.

Hamann, S., Herman, R., Nolan, C., & Wallen, K. (2004). Men and women differ in amygdala response to visual sexual stimuli. *Nature Neuroscience, 7*, 411–416.

Herz, R. S., & Cahill, E. D. (1997). Differential use of sensory information in sexual behavior as a function of gender. *Human Nature, 8*, 275–286.

Holstege, G., Georgiadis, J. R., Paans, A. M. J., Meiners, L. C., van der Graaf, H. C.

E., & Reinders, A. A. T. S. (2003). Brain activation during human male ejaculation. *Journal of Neuroscience, 23*, 9185–9193.

Kampe, K. K., Frith, C. D., Dolan, R. J., & Frith, U. (2001). Reward value of attractiveness and gaze. *Nature, 413*, 589.

Karama, S., Lecours, A. R., Leroux, J.-M., Bourgouin, P., Beaudoin, G., Joubert, S., et al. (2002). Areas of brain activation in males and females during viewing of erotic film excerpts. *Human Brain Mapping, 16*, 1–13.

Kinsey, A., Pomeroy, W., & Martin, C. (1948). *Sexual behavior in the human male.* Philadelphia: Saunders.

Klüver, H., & Bucy, P. C. (1939). Preliminary analysis of functions of the temporal lobes in monkeys. *Archives of Neurology and Psychiatry, 42*, 979–1000.

Krug, R., Plihal, W., Fehm, H. L., & Born, J. (2000). Selective influence of the menstrual cycle on perception of stimuli with reproductive significance: An event-related potential study. *Psychophysiology, 37*, 111–122.

Laumann, E. O., Gagnon, J. H., Michael, R. T., & Michaels, S. (1994). *The social organization of sexuality* Chicago: University of Chicago Press.

Leutmezer, F., Serles, W., Bacher, J., Gröppel, G., Pataraia, E., Aull, S., et al. (1999). Genital automatisms in complex partial seizures. *American Academy of Neurology, 52*, 1188–1191.

Naliboff, B. D., Berman, S., Chang, L., Derbyshire, S. W., Suyenobu, B., Vogt, B. A., et al. (2003). Sex-related differences in IBS patients: Central processing of visceral stimuli. *Gastroenterology, 124*, 1738–1747.

Newman, S. W. (1999). The medial extended amygdala in male reproductive behavior: A node in the mammalian social behavior network. *Annals of the New York Academy of Sciences, 877*, 242–257.

Redoute, J., Stoleru, S., Gregoire, M. C., Costes, N., Cinotti, L., Lavenne, F., et al. (2000). Brain processing of visual sexual stimuli in human males. *Human Brain Mapping, 11*, 162–177.

Roselli, C. E., Klosterman, S., & Resko, J. A. (2001). Anatomic relationships between aromatase and androgen receptor mRNA expression in the hypothalamus and amygdala of adult male cynomolgus monkeys *Journal of Comparative Neurology, 439*, 208–223.

Stoléru, S., Grégoire, M. C., Gérard, D., Decety, J. A., Lafarge, E., Cinotti, L., et al. (1999). Neuroanatomical correlates of visually-evoked sexual arousal in human males. *Archives of Sexual Behavior, 28*, 1–22.

Sumich, A. L., Kumari, V., & Sharma, T. (2003). Neuroimaging of sexual arousal: research and clinical utility. *Hospital Medicine, 64*, 28–33.

Symons, D. (1979). The evolution of human sexuality. Oxford: Oxford University Press.

Terzian, H., & Dalle Ore, G. (1955). Syndrome of Klüver and Bucy reproduced in man by bilateral removal of the temporal lobes. *Neurology, 5*, 373–380.

Trivers, R. L. (1972). Parental investment and sexual selection. In B. Campbell (Ed.), *Sexual selection and the descent of man* (pp. 136–179). Chicago: Aldine.

Wager, T. D., Phan, K. L., Liberzon I., & Taylor S. (2003). Valence gender and lateralization of functional brain anatomy: A meta-analysis of findings from neuroimaging. *NeuroImage, 19*, 513–531.

10

Sex Differences in Brain Functional Magnetic Resonance Imaging Response to Stress

Rajita Sinha

The term "stress" may be defined as a process involving perception, interpretation, response, and adaptation to harmful, threatening, or challenging events (Lazarus & Folkman, 1984). This definition allows for the separate consideration of (1) events that cause stress (internal or external stressful life events); (2) cognitive and affective processes evaluating the event and available coping resources (knowledge, attitudes/beliefs, personality traits, cognitive appraisal, and emotional processing); (3) physiological and neural adaptation to regain homeostasis (in the case of acute stress) or to achieve physiological stability through the process of change (i.e., allostasis, in the case of chronic stress); and (4) behavioral and cognitive responses (coping). These components of stress are influenced by individual differences, resulting from a combination of genetic and environmental factors that play a significant role in determining the vulnerabilities and risk for development of various stress-related physical and psychiatric disorders.

SEX DIFFERENCES IN STRESS RESPONSES

Sexual dimorphism in the stress response is well known. Whereas in rodents the hypothalamic–pituitary–adrenal (HPA) response, as measured by adrenocorticotrophic hormone (ACTH) and cortisol levels, is greater in females than in males (Kitay, 1961; Jones, Brush, & Neame, 1972; Young, 1996), the pic-

203

ture is more complex in humans. In general, across numerous studies, women tend to report higher subjective levels of distress and higher pulse rates, but lower sympathetic arousal and HPA responses to biological and psychological stress, than men do (Kirschbaum, Wust, Faig, & Hellhammer, 1992). There is also some evidence that these differences vary by phase of the menstrual cycle—a finding presumably associated with changing levels of sex steroid hormones. For instance, lower HPA response to psychological stress has been reported in the follicular phase as compared to the luteal phase of the menstrual cycle (Kirschbaum, Kudielka, Gaab, Schommer, & Hellhammer, 1999), and elevated catecholamine responses to stress have been documented in women during the luteal phase of the cycle (Stoney, Davis, & Matthews, 1987).

The differences in psychobiological responses to stress in males and females have led researchers to reconsider the universality of the "fight–flight" response for survival in humans and other species. In a seminal review, Taylor and colleagues (2000) point to emerging evidence indicating that the fight–flight response to stress, marked by increases in sympathetic nervous system activation, is primarily a male response developed in humans and other species out of the necessity to protect against external threat. On the other hand, they cite evidence to suggest that the female response to stress has evolved to maximize the survival of self and offspring. Although the core of the neuroendocrine response in females is similar to that in males, Taylor and colleagues contend that women show lower psychoendocrine responses to stress because their responses to stress involve tending, nurturing, and befriending—functions that are associated with sex hormones (such as oxytocin) and the endogenous opioid system, and not primarily with sympathetic nervous system activation. These ideas constitute a fundamental shift in understanding the psychobiology of stress, and provide an opportunity to conceptualize stress responses on the basis of sex-specific biological and adaptive coping. Such differences may be represented and identifiable in the functional response of the brain to stress.

SEX DIFFERENCES IN PERSONALITY TRAITS, COPING, AND STRESS-RELATED PSYCHIATRIC DISORDERS

Gender differences in personality styles and coping responses have been well documented (see Table 10.1 for a summary of these). In a classic review of research, Maccoby and Jacklin (1974) reported that men are more assertive and dominant than women, and that women are more anxious than men. Feingold (1994) extended these findings in a meta-analysis and reported that men are more assertive and have higher self-esteem, whereas women have higher levels of extraversion, anxiety, trust, and nurturance. On the other

TABLE 10.1. Sex Differences in Factors Influencing Stress Responses

A. Differences in personality traits
   1. Men are more assertive and have higher self-esteem than women.
   2. Women have higher levels of anxiety, trust, extraversion, and nurturance.

B. Differences in stress-related psychopathology
   1. Men have higher rates of externalizing disorders characterized by impulsive, dyscontrolled behaviors, such as substance abuse and antisocial personality disorder.
   2. Women have higher rates of internalizing disorders, including anxiety and depressive disorders.

C. Differences in trauma exposure
   1. Early life stress, particularly childhood sexual abuse, is more common in women than in men.
   2. Childhood abuse increases risk of psychiatric illness in women more than in men.
   3. Men have higher rates of war-related trauma.
   4. Women have higher rates of civilian violence and sexual abuse. Rates of violent victimization and PTSD are higher in women.

D. Differences in biobehavioral responses to stress
   1. Males show greater evidence of "fight–flight" response to stress than women do, with higher levels of sympathetic arousal, blood pressure, catecholamines, and HPA responses, both at baseline and after stress challenge.
   2. Stress response in women is associated with a "tend and befriend" response, with lower sympathetic and HPA response to stress, and with oxytocin, endogenous opioid peptides, and sex steroid hormones regulating the stress response. HPA responses vary as a function of the phase of the menstrual cycle.

E. Differences in coping responses to stress
   1. Men are more likely to respond with instrumental or activity-oriented coping.
   2. Women are more likely to respond by using verbal and self–other directed coping strategies.

Note. PTSD, posttraumatic stress disorder; HPA, hypothalamic–pituitary–adrenal.

hand, no sex differences have been reported in social anxiety, impulsiveness, activity levels, reflectiveness, locus of control, and orderliness. To the extent that these personality traits influence appraisal of life events and the degree to which such events are perceived as threatening/challenging and controllable, they are likely to influence sex differences in stress responses in men and women.

Consistent with these sex differences in personality traits, there are sex differences in the epidemiology of stress-related psychiatric disorders, including personality disorders. Men are prone to "externalizing" disorders characterized by aggressive, dyscontrolled behaviors, such as substance use disorders and antisocial personality disorder. In contrast, women have higher rates of "internalizing" disorders, including anxiety disorders, depression, and borderline personality disorder (Sinha & Rounsaville, 2002; Paris, 2004). Sex differences in the literature on coping strategies provide further confirmation of the "externalizing" and "internalizing" trends, as men tend to respond to stress with instrumental or activity-oriented coping strategies, whereas women report using more passive, self-directed strategies (McCrae & Costa, 1986). Such differences suggest that functional representations of stress appraisal, and behavioral and cognitive responses to stress in the brain, are likely to be sex-specific as well.

There also appear to be some sex differences in physiological and behavioral coping with traumatic and chronic adverse life events. For example, women are more likely than men to develop posttraumatic stress disorder (PTSD) following traumatic events (Weiss, Longhurst, & Mazure, 1999; Widom, 1999). Furthermore, experiences of early trauma, such as physical and childhood sexual abuse, have been found to confer a greater susceptibility to developing psychiatric illness and illicit drug abuse on women than on men (MacMillan et al., 2001). The well-known association between adverse life events and increased risk of major depression is significantly higher in women than in men (Maciejewski, Prigerson, & Mazure, 2001). Early life trauma is associated with an increased HPA reactivity to acute and chronic stressors in women (Heim et al., 2000; Nemeroff, 1996). Women with major depression show greater abnormalities in HPA axis responses as compared to men (Young, 1995; Young & Korszun, 1999). Abnormal cerebrospinal fluid levels of corticotropin-releasing factor and other HPA axis responses, as well as plasma catecholamine regulation, have been reported in traumatized children and adults with or without PTSD (Baker et al., 1999; De Bellis et al., 1994, 1999; Friedman et al., 2001; Heim et al., 2000; Kaufman et al., 1997; Rasmusson et al., 2000, 2001; Yehuda, 1997). These findings indicate that the psychobiological effects of chronic adverse life events confer differential psychiatric disease risk for men and women.

NEURAL ORGANIZATION OF STRESS COMPONENTS

Each of the stress components described previously may be linked to specific and overlapping neural systems that interact in a complex and intricate manner to coordinate the experience and response to stress. A brief, albeit, simplified, overview of the neural organization of the stress components is provided below.

Events that induce a stress response usually produce one or more conditioned or unconditioned emotional reactions, such as fear, anxiety, anger, excitement, pleasure, or sadness. These reactions depend on the specific features of the situation; on personality and trait aspects that contribute to appraisal of the event and availability of coping resources; and on the prior emotional state of the individual. Perception of threat or challenge relies on the brain information-processing circuits, such as the primary sensory projections and sensory association cortices, involved in perceiving external environmental stimuli as well as internally generated cognitive and affective stimuli (McEwen & Stellar, 1993). Appraisal of the event relies on input from the sensory nervous system circuits to the thalamus, insula, and sensory association areas. In addition, the limbic affective processing circuits—including the amygdala and hippocampus, along with subcortical and prefrontal cortical areas, particularly the orbito-frontal and medial prefrontal cortices—contribute to identifying the meaning and significance of events, and to determining stimulus–reward associations (Sinha, 2001). Furthermore, direct input from the thalamus and frontal regions to the amygdala and the limbic affective processing circuits is thought to function as an early warning system, leading to rapid global avoidance and defense responses that are important for the survival of the organism (Gaffan, Murray, & Fabre-Thorpe, 1993; Lovallo, 1997). These circuits also interact with the biological adaptive systems to produce stress-related neuroendocrine responses (McEwen, 1999b). Their interconnections with the ventral and dorsal striatum and prefrontal regions play a key role in approach and avoidance response selection and in the mediation of goal-directed behaviors—functions that are important in cognitive and behavioral coping (Gaffan et al., 1993; Lovallo, 1997; Robbins & Everitt, 1996).

SEX DIFFERENCES IN THE ANATOMY OF CORTICO-LIMBIC EMOTION BRAIN CIRCUITS

Men and women are known to differ in the brain anatomy of regions associated with emotional processing (see Table 10.2 for a summary of these anatomical differences, as well as the differences in response to be discussed later). Men have a larger left planum temporale/anterior sylvian fissure, but women have higher percentages of grey matter in this region (Foundas, Faulhaber, Kulynych, Browning, & Weinberger, 1999; Gur et al., 1999; Kulynych, Vladar, Jones, & Weinberger, 1994). A larger anterior commissure is also seen in females than in males (Allen & Gorski, 1991). Sex differences in the volumes of the anterior hypothalamus, globus pallidus, and putamen have also been reported (Byne et al., 2000; Giedd et al., 1996), and a leftward asymmetry of the inferior parietal lobule has been reported in males as compared to females (Frederikse et al., 2000). Sex differences in cortical regions associated with emotional processing have been noted as well. Women have more grey matter volume in the cingulate cortex, while men show more grey matter volume bilaterally in the mesial temporal lobes and cerebellum (Good et al., 2001). Men are also known to show greater temporal cortex asymmetry as compared to women (Good et al., 2001). Consistent with the anatomical data, higher metabolism has been reported in men versus women in temporo-limbic regions and the cerebellum, and relatively lower metabolism in cingulate regions (Gur et al., 1995). Such sex differences have led researchers to hypothesize that there should be functional differences in emotion processing in men and women as well.

TABLE 10.2. Sex Differences in Brain Morphology and Response to Stress and Emotion

A. Differences in brain morphology
   1. In general, men have larger global volumes of grey and white matter, and also show greater temporal cortex asymmetry.
   2. Women have more grey matter volume in the superior temporal region, inferior frontal region, and cingulate cortex.
   3. Men show increased grey matter volume bilaterally in the mesial temporal lobes and cerebellum.
   4. Women show increased grey matter concentration in the cortical mantle and in parts of the cingulate.

B. Differences in brain response to emotion and emotional memories
   1. Women tend to be more emotionally expressive and to have better episodic emotional memory than men.
   2. Greater lateralization of brain response to emotions is found in men; women show more midline limbic frontal activation in response to emotions.
   3. Emotional memory is predicted by right amygdala activation during encoding in males, but left amygdala activation during encoding in females.
   4. There is more frequent activation of the SCC, thalamus, midbrain, and cerebellum during emotions in females, while males tend to activate the inferior frontal regions and the posterior cortex.
   5. Women show more frequent activation of the basal ganglia during emotions; males show greater clustering of activation in the right striatum.

C. Differences in brain responses to pain and emotional stress
   1. In response to pain stimulation, women show greater activation in the ventromedial PFC, right ACC, and left amygdala, but men show greater activation in the right dorsolateral PFC, insula, and dorsal pons/periaqueductal grey region.
   2. Men show greater pain-induced mu-opioid system activation in limbic regions such as the anterior thalamus, basal ganglia, and amygdala, but women show reduction in mu-opioid system activation in the nucleus accumbens.
   3. During emotional stress experiences, men show activation of medial PFC and ACC, while women show increased activation in SCC and the orbito-frontal cortex.

Note. SCC, subcallosal cingulate cortex; PFC, prefrontal cortex; ACC, anterior cingulate cortex.

SEX DIFFERENCES IN BRAIN FUNCTIONAL RESPONSE TO EMOTIONAL STIMULI

Behavioral studies have shown that women tend to be more emotionally expressive and to have better episodic emotional memory than men (Bradley, Condispoti, Sabatinelli, & Lang, 2001). However, in a meta-analysis of 65 functional neuroimaging studies on emotion, Wager, Phan, Liberzon, and Taylor (2003) did not find evidence of greater brain activation during emotional processing in women as compared to men. Nonetheless, they did report some sex differences: Men showed more lateralized activation in the left inferior frontal cortex, the posterior parietal cortices, and the right striatum, while women tended to show more frequent activation of midline limbic structures, including the subcallosal cingulate cortex, thalamus, basal ganglia, brainstem, and cerebellum.

Interestingly, there is evidence of sex differences in brain activity during encoding of emotional memories as well as retrieval (see review by Hamann & Canli, 2004). In an imaging study using positron emission tomography (PET) (Cahill et al., 2001) and one that used functional magnetic resonance imaging (fMRI) (Canli, Zhao, Brewer, Gabrieli, & Cahill, 2000) findings indicated that amygdala activity at memory encoding predicted later emotional memory performance in both males and females; however, in females the relationship was with the left amygdala, while in males it was with the right amygdala. These data suggest sex differences in the functional specificity of brain activation of regions associated with emotional processing. Bremner and colleagues (2001) also reported sex differences in emotional memory retrieval, with women showing greater activation than men in bilateral posterior hippocampus and cerebellum, but decreased activity in medial prefrontal cortex.

This section and the preceding one have indicated specific sex differences in the structural and functional brain regions associated with emotional processing. These data would support the hypothesis that there are sex differences in the brain's response to stress.

NEUROIMAGING STUDIES OF BRAIN RESPONSES TO STRESS: EFFECTS OF SEX

In one of the first studies examining brain activation during mental stress, Soufer and colleagues (1998) used PET to study brain correlates of mental stress induced by an arithmetic serial subtraction task in healthy volunteers and in individuals with coronary artery disease (CAD). Their findings indicated that in healthy controls, the only region that showed increased activation during the serial subtraction task relative to brain activity during a counting task was the left inferior frontal gyrus. In contrast, individuals with CAD showed greater activation than controls in left parietal cortex (Brodmann's [BA] 39), left anterior cingulate (BA 32), right visual association cortex (BA 18), left fusiform gyrus, and cerebellum. In addition, patients with CAD relative to controls also showed decreases in blood flow in the right thalamus, right superior frontal gyrus (BA 32, 24, 10), and right middle temporal gyrus (BA 21) during mental stress. Soufer and colleagues concluded that such hyperactivation in areas associated with emotional processing among patients with CAD was due to a greater autonomic and emotional response to mental stress among such patients. Although this study only included male subjects, given that there are sex differences in stress responses associated with CAD (Stoney et al., 1987), one may expect that the brain's response to stress in male and female patients with CAD would be sexually dimorphic.

Using PET techniques and mu-opioid receptor radiotracer techniques, Zubieta and colleagues (2003) examined the role of mu-opioid neurotransmission in the regulation of affective states in healthy women. They induced sustained neutral and sad mood by using cued recall of an autobiographical event associated with each of these emotions. Their findings indicated that the sustained sadness was associated with significant deactivation in mu-opioid neurotransmission in the rostral anterior cingulate, ventral pallidum, amygdala, and inferior temporal cortex. Furthermore, the deactivation of mu-opioid neurotransmission was associated with increased negative affect ratings and decreases in positive affect ratings. These data are unique, in that they confirm the involvement of the mu-opioid system in regulation of distress states in women. Although this study did not examine sex differences, Zubieta and colleagues (2002) reported that mu-opioid system activation in response to an intensity-controlled sustained deep tissue pain challenge differed between men and women in the follicular phase of their menstrual cycle. Their findings indicated that men demonstrated larger magnitudes of mu-opioid system activation in the anterior thalamus, ventral basal ganglia, and amygdala as compared to women. Women, on the other hand, showed reduction in mu-opioid system activation in the nucleus accumbens (NA) during pain. The authors cite these findings as consistent with experimental animal studies showing a hyperalgesic response in the NA with blockade of opioid receptors. Thus, at matched levels of pain intensity, men and women differ in the magnitude and direction of response of the mu-opioid system to the stress of physical tissue pain.

In contrast, Naliboff and colleagues (2003) examined brain activity via PET during pain stimulation in response to balloon insertion into the colon during an endoscopy in individuals with irritable bowel syndrome. They reported that during pain relative to rest, women showed greater activation in limbic regions, including the ventromedial prefrontal cortex, right anterior cingulate cortex, and left amygdala, whereas men showed greater activation in the right dorsolateral prefrontal cortex, insula, and dorsal pons/periaqueductal grey region. Once again, these data indicate sex-specific functional responses to the stress of physical pain stimulation.

BRAIN RESPONSES TO EMOTIONAL STRESS: PRELIMINARY EVIDENCE OF SEX DIFFERENCES

In a series of studies, my colleagues and I have been examining the effects of emotional stress on drug craving and relapse in individuals who abuse substances. Emotional stress, or "distress," commonly occurs in situations that are challenging or threatening, and it influences adaptive processes that require self-regulation or "coping" to regain control and attain desired goals (Sinha, 2001). Our initial findings with substance-abusing individuals and healthy volunteers has shown that emotional stress is associated with the subjective experience of multiple negative emotions, such as the experience of anger, sadness, and fear (Sinha, 2001; Sinha, Catapano, & O'Malley, 1999). As difficulties in managing stressful life events and regulation of the emotional distress state are common in a variety of psychiatric illnesses, including addiction, identifying neural circuits associated with emotional distress in humans is of importance to clinical neuroscience. Therefore, using fMRI techniques, we first studied neural circuits underlying emotional stress in drug-naive, healthy individuals (Sinha, Lacadie, Skudlarski, & Wexler, 2004).

Participants in this initial preliminary study were 7 men and 1 woman with a mean age of 33 years ($SD = 5.7$) and educational level of 13.3 years ($SD = 2.3$). Emotional stress was induced via a brief guided imagery and recall method, where subjects were exposed to individualized scripts of stressful life events and neutral relaxing life events. Three personalized stress and three neutral imagery scripts were developed prior to the fMRI session by obtaining specific stimulus and response information for separate stress and neutral events on scene construction questionnaires (for detailed procedures on script development, see Sinha et al., 2003). Subjects rated the level of distress experienced while reporting specific stress situations on a 10-point Likert scale, and only situations rated 8 or above were used for the development of stress scripts. The fMRI session included six scanning trials, with three stress and three neutral trials presented in random order. Each trial was 5.5 minutes long, consisting of a 1.5-minute baseline period, a 2.5-minute guided imagery period, and a 1.5 minute recovery period. Subjects participated in muscle relaxation for 2 minutes between scanning trials.

Before and after each scanning trial, subjects verbally rated their subjective distress and imagery vividness on 10-point Likert scales. A pulse oximeter was attached to each subject's finger to assess pulse rate during each trial. Functional brain images were acquired with an echo planar gradient echo sequence (17 coronal slices perpendicular to the anterior commissure–posterior (AC-PC) line and starting at the frontal poles; TR, 1.5 seconds; TE, 45 milliseconds; flip angle, 85°; 64×64 data matrix; field of view, 20 cm; slice thickness, 6 mm; gap, 1 mm; 220 images per slice). Data acquisition and fMRI image processing were performed according to methods described previously (Wexler et al., 2001). Composite maps were used to compare mean signal change (imagery vs. baseline period) between the stress and the neutral imagery trials at each pixel, with a cluster minimum of 20 adjacent pixels.

Subjective distress ratings indicated moderate increases from baseline during stress trials (stress $M = 4.95$, $SD = 2.45$; neutral $M = -1.25$, $SD = 1.69$; paired $t = 4.29$, $p < .005$). Pulse rate data also indicated significant increases in average pulse rate from baseline during stress trials as compared to neutral trials (stress $M = 3.71$, $SD = 4.14$; neutral $M = -0.83$, $SD = 1.14$; paired $t = 2.93$, $p < .03$). High imagery vividness ratings were achieved both in stress trials ($M = 7.93$, $SD = 1.67$) and in neutral trials ($M = 7.53$, $SD = 1.47$), with no significant differences in vividness ratings across conditions.

Findings indicated increased activation in frontal regions such as the right medial prefrontal regions (BA 8, 9) and ventral anterior cingulate (BA 32) during stress imagery in contrast to the neutral imagery condition ($p < .05$, uncorrected). Furthermore, stress imagery contrasted with neutral imagery also resulted in increased activation ($p < .01$, uncorrected) in specific limbic and midbrain regions, such as the left striatum and thalamic regions, the bi-lateral caudate and putamen, the left hippocampal and parahippocampal regions, and the posterior cingulate (Sinha, Lacadie, Skudlarski, & Wexler, 2004).

To follow up on the Sinha and colleagues (2004) study, voxel-based whole-brain correlation analysis was performed to assess brain regions associ-ated with subjective distress ratings during stress imagery. A significance threshold of $p < .005$ (uncorrected, with a cluster size of 20) was selected for the resulting correlation maps. Findings indicated a significant positive corre-lation between emotional distress and activation in the right caudate and thalamic regions (see Figure 10.1a). A significant inverse correlation between distress ratings and activation of the anterior cingulate and the right insula was also observed (Figure 10.1b).

In this initial study of emotional stress in mostly male healthy volunteers, we found activation of the medial prefrontal regions and the anterior cingulate regions—areas previously associated with modulation of anxiety, self-regulation of emotion, and behavioral self-control (Beauregard, Levesque, & Bourgouin, 2001; Peoples, 2002; Phan, Wager, Taylor, & Liberzon, 2002). Evidence from the correlation analysis showing an inverse association be-

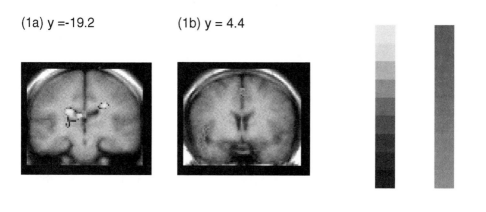

FIGURE 10.1. Voxel-based correlation maps in healthy controls for significant associations during the entire stress imagery period ($p < .005$) between subjective dis-tress ratings and (a) right caudate and thalamic region activation (Talairach coordi-nates: 21, –28, 18); and (b) (inverse correlations) anterior cingulate cortex activation (BA 24) (Talairach coordinates: 1.3, 4.4, 46.6) and right insula activation (Talairach coordinates: –45, 4.4, –5.3). Approximate coordinates (x, y, z) are based on the aver-age center of mass for an activity at a given y-level.

tween the anterior cingulate and distress ratings suggests that increased anterior cingulate activation is associated with reducing/modulating subjective distress. These findings further support the notion that this region is involved in regulating the emotional distress state. In contrast, significant positive association between the right caudate and thalamic regions and subjective distress suggests that these midbrain limbic regions are involved in the subjective experience of distress. This is consistent with preclinical research indicating that expression of distress is associated with stimulation of these limbic regions in laboratory animals undergoing social stress manipulations (Panksepp, Nelson, & Bekkedal, 1997), and in the processing of negative emotions in human neuroimaging studies (George et al., 1995; Phan et al., 2002).

Data from these initial healthy volunteers were also compared to data from 20 treatment-seeking, currently abstinent, cocaine-dependent individuals, to examine the differences in stress response between healthy volunteers and addicted patients (Sinha, Lacadie, Skudlarski, Fulbright, et al., 2005). Although the healthy volunteers and the patients reported similar levels of subjective distress during stress exposure, and also showed similar increases in pulse rate during stress imagery, the patients showed no increase in activation in the anterior cingulate prefrontal region (BA 32), hippocampus, and precentral gyrus during stress exposure, resulting in significant differences in activation of these regions between patients and controls ($p < .01$). This absence of activation during stress suggests hypofunction of fronto-limbic regions important in modulating anxiety and negative emotions in patients with cocaine dependence—a finding that may explain the difficulties in coping with stressful life events often observed in addicted individuals (Sinha, 2001). Interestingly, we have recently shown that cocaine-dependent women show greater activation in the dorsal anterior cingulate (BA 24), middle frontal region (BA 9), inferior frontal region (BA 45), posterior cingulate (BA 31), and insula than do cocaine-dependent men (Li, Kosten, & Sinha, 2005). These findings would suggest that among those with cocaine dependence, women are better able to modulate and regulate distress states than men. However, these results need to be contrasted with those for healthy individuals within each gender, in order to further understand differences in stress response that are due to drug abuse and those that are associated with sexual dimorphism.

In a currently ongoing study (Sinha, Lacadie, & Skudlarski, 2004), we are examining sex differences in emotional stress responses. fMRI brain response data have been obtained on 15 healthy volunteers: 8 men with a mean age of 30.25 ($SD = 7.9$) and 15.5 years of education ($SD = 2.0$); and 7 women with a mean age of 28 ($SD = 8.23$) and 15.6 years of education ($SD = 2.2$). Subjects have participated in two stress and two neutral imagery trials, where they have been exposed to stress and neutral relaxing scripts that were developed by using individualized stress and neutral relaxing events in the manner described previously. fMRI data are being acquired in this study with a 3-tesla Siemens scanner. Functional echo planar imaging sequences are being acquired according to the following parameters: 32 axial slices parallel to the

AC-PC line; TR, 2 seconds; TE, 25 milliseconds; flip angle, 85°; 64 × 64 data matrix; field of view, 220 × 220; slice thickness, 4 mm; gap, 0; 190 measurements.

Subjective ratings of emotional stress, as measured on a 10-point Likert scale, were lower in this study than in the previous study. For men, the mean emotional stress rating was 3.06 (SD = 1.82), while in women it was 2.35 (SD = 1.46). Nonetheless, these ratings were significantly higher than minimal ratings of distress obtained during neutral relaxing imagery ($p < .001$), suggesting that the stress imagery produced reliable although mild increases in subjective distress. One explanation for lower emotional distress ratings could be the higher levels of education and therefore potentially higher adaptive coping skills in this group as compared to the previous group of subjects. There is good evidence to suggest that higher levels of education and a greater knowledge base promote better adaptation and self-regulation of stress (Ray, 2004). On the basis of the lower levels of subjective distress, we expected activation of frontal stress regulation and control regions in this sample, but little activity in subcortical regions associated with the subjective and visceral experience of distress.

Preliminary data analyses contrasting brain activation during stress relative to neutral imagery supported our hypothesis. Results indicated significant activation in the medial prefrontal (BA 8, 9) and the anterior cingulate (BA 32) in men ($p < .05$), whereas women showed significant activation in the medial orbito-frontal region (BA 11) and the subcallosal cingulate gyrus (BA 25) during stress ($p < .05$) (see Figures 10.2a–10.2b), with no significant subcortical limbic activation. These findings, although preliminary, suggest that different frontal brain regions are associated with stress regulation in men and women. The medial prefrontal and the anterior cingulate regions that were activated during stress in men have been associated with emotion regulation, anxiety, and negative affect modulation (see Wager et al., 2003, for a review). Furthermore, the anterior cingulate (BA 32) has been identified as part of the cognitive division of the cingulate gyrus involved in conflict monitoring and response selection (Bush, Luu, & Posner, 2000; Carter & Tiffany, 1999; Kerns et al., 2004), which in the context of stress regulation may signal active or instrumental coping.

In contrast, women showed increased activity in the orbito-frontal cortex and the subcallosal cingulate cortex during stress (see Figure 10.2b). The orbito-frontal cortex is known to be involved in self-regulation of behavior to achieve desired outcomes—specifically, by evaluating the motivational significance of stimuli and by selection of behavior (Rolls, 2000). On the other hand, the subcallosal cingulate cortex (BA 25) has been identified as the affective division of the cingulate gyrus, and women more frequently activate this region during induction of negative mood and sadness (George et al., 1995; Mayberg et al., 1999; Liotti et al., 2000). Interestingly, this region is found to be hypoactive in depressed patients, but subcallosal cingulate activity increases with antidepressant treatment (Brody et al., 1999; Mayberg et al.,

(2a)

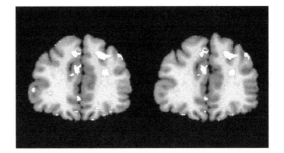

(2b)

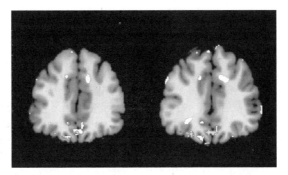

(2c)

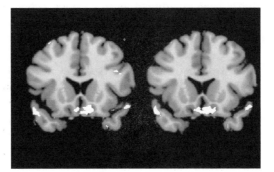

FIGURE 10.2. Significant brain activity during stress imagery in contrast to neutral imagery ($p < .05$) for the following groups: (a) Healthy control men showing increased activity in the medial prefrontal cortex (–2, 35, 39) and the anterior cingulate cortex (–1, 35, 21); (b) healthy control women showing increased activity in the medial orbito-frontal cortex (–3, 35, –8); and (c) healthy control women showing increased activity in the subcallosal cingulate cortex (–3, 11, –10). Talairach coordinates are presented in parentheses, based on the average center of mass for an activity at a given y-coordinate.

2000). Consistent with these previous data, our findings may be interpreted as women directing their attention to the feeling state associated with the distress state rather than planning for required action. Although these findings are preliminary, they are consistent with the findings reported in the earlier section on sex differences in stress regulation and coping. However, there is a clear need to extend these findings further and to examine the association between brain activity and specific stress-related coping strategies more directly.

LOOKING FORWARD

Although numerous studies indicate sex differences in stress responses and in the manifestation of stress-related psychiatric disorders, studies elucidating the underlying brain mechanisms for these differences are rare. This chapter has outlined evidence of sex differences in brain anatomy and responses to emotion and stress experiences. However, this work is in its infancy, and several factors need to be considered to facilitate a better understanding of sex differences in brain stress responses. From a methodological standpoint, there is a clear need to develop and validate stress paradigms that are feasible to implement under the constraints of imaging technology. Thus far, studies have examined early information processing of stress stimuli by using aversive visual stimuli, such as film clips and aversive pictures; autobiographical recall and imagery of stress experiences have also been commonly used. Brain responses to pain stimulation, considered as a specialized example of a stress experience, have been examined with various types of pain stimulation. Although some of the studies using these methods have examined sex differences, the literature can benefit from more information on specific paradigms where sex differences are observed.

There is growing evidence from basic science and clinical studies that gonadal hormones influence brain structure and function in critical ways; as such, they may also play a key role in the sex differences seen in stress responses (for reviews, see McEwen, 1999a, 2001; Steiner, Dunn, & Born, 2003). This research underscores the need to consider the influence of sex hormones and their fluctuations on brain responses to stress. For example, there is some evidence of fluctuation in cortical gamma-aminobutyric acid across the menstrual cycle (Epperson et al., 2002). As discussed by Steiner and colleagues (2003), the sensitivity of various neurotransmitter systems is modulated by sex hormones, with documented effects on mood. Although repeated assessments across the menstrual cycle may be somewhat challenging to implement in neuroimaging studies, the literature could benefit from future studies designed to examine hormonal fluctuations across this cycle, with specific examination of the role of specific gonadal hormones on brain responses to stress.

Finally, as discussed in previous sections of the chapter, there are well-known sex differences in personality traits, coping abilities, adverse life experiences, and the prevalence of stress-related psychiatric disorders. There is also evidence of specific gene–environment interactions influencing stress responses and emotion processing (Barr, Newman, Schwandt, et al., 2004; Caspi et al., 2003; Hariri et al., 2002). Furthermore, recent findings suggest gender-specific associations among specific gene polymorphisms, HPA responses to stress, and vulnerability to anxiety disorders (Barr, Newman, Shannon, et al., 2004; Enoch, Ke, Ferro, Harris, & Goldman, 2003). As research begins to identify brain regions associated with stress experience and regulation, it will be important to examine individual differences in personality, coping, environmental, hormonal, and genetic factors that may explain variations in brain responses to stress. Ultimately, greater knowledge of factors influencing individual responses to stress will permit a more comprehensive understanding of the different ways men and women experience and manage stress, and of their differing vulnerabilities to specific stress-related psychiatric disorders.

ACKNOWLEDGMENTS

Preparation of this chapter was supported by National Institutes of Health (NIH) Grants No. P50-DA16556, No. K02-DA17232, and No. R01-AA13892. I would like to thank the NIH Office of Research on Women's Health for their support of this work. I would also like to thank Cheryl Lacadie, Pawel Skudlarski, and R. Todd Constable for providing technical and administrative support in fMRI data collection and analyses.

REFERENCES

Allen, L. S., & Gorski, R. A. (1991). Sexual dimorphism of the anterior commissure and massa intermedia of the human brain. *Journal of Comparative Neurology, 312*, 97–104.

Baker, D. G., West, S. A., Nicholson, W. E., Ekhator, N. N., Kasckow, J. W., Hill, K. K., et al. (1999). Serial CSF corticotropin-releasing hormone levels and adrenocortical activity in combat veterans with posttraumatic stress disorder. *American Journal of Psychiatry, 156*(4), 585–588.

Barr, C. S., Newman, T. K., Schwandt, M., Shannon, C., Dvoskin, R. L., Lindell, S. G., et al. (2004). Sexual dichotomy of an interaction between transporter gene promoter variant in rhesus macaques. *Proceedings of the National Academy of Sciences USA, 101*(33), 12358–12363.

Barr, C. S., Newman, T. K., Shannon, C., Parker, C., Dvoskin, R. L., Becker, M. L., et al. (2004). Rearing condition and rh5-HTTLPR interact to influence limbic–hypothalamic–pituitary–adrenal axis response to stress in infant macaques. *Biological Psychiatry, 55*, 733–738.

Beauregard, M., Levesque, J., & Bourgouin, P. (2001). Neural correlates of conscious self-regulation of emotion. *Journal of Neuroscience, 21*, 1–6.

Bradley, M. M., Condispoti, M., Sabatinelli, D., & Lang, P. (2001). Emotion and motivation II: sex differences in picture processing. *Emotion, 1*, 300–319.

Bremner, J. D., Soufer, R., McCarthy, G., Delaney, R., Staib, L. H., Duncan, J. S., et al. (2001). Gender differences in cognitive and neural correlates of remembrance of emotional words. *Psychopharmacology Bulletin, 35*, 55–78.

Brody, A. L., Saxena, S., Silverman, D. H., Alborzian, S., Fairbanks, L. A., Phelps, M. E., et al. (1999). Brain metabolic changes in major depressive disorder from pre- to post-treatment with paroxetine. *Psychiatry Research, 91*, 127–139.

Bush, G., Luu, P., & Posner, M. I. (2000). Cognitive and emotional influences in anterior cingulate cortex. *Trends in Cognitive Sciences, 4*(6), 215–222.

Byne, W., Lasco, M. S., Kemether, E., Shinwari, A., Edgar, M. A., Morgello, S., et al. (2000). The interstitial nuclei of the human anterior hypothalamus: An investigation of sexual variation in volume and cell size, number and density. *Brain Research, 856*, 254–258.

Cahill, L., Haier, R. J., White, N. S., Fallon, J., Kilpatrick, L., Lawrence, C., et al. (2001). Sex-related difference in amygdala activity during emotionally influenced memory storage. *Neurobiology of Learning and Memory, 75*, 1–9.

Canli, T., Zhao, Z., Brewer, J., Gabrieli, J. D. E., & Cahill, L. (2000). Event-related activation in the human amygdala associates with later memory for individual emotional experience. *Journal of Neuroscience, 20*, 1–5.

Carter, B. L., & Tiffany, S. T. (1999). Meta-analysis of cue reactivity in addiction research. *Addiction, 94*(3), 327–340.

Caspi, A., Sugden, K., Moffitt, T. E., Taylor, A., Craig, I. W., Harrington, H., et al. (2003). Influence of life stress on depression: Moderation by a polymorphism in the 5-HTT gene. *Science, 301*, 386–389.

De Bellis, M. D., Baum, A. S., Birmaher, B., Keshavan, M. S., Eccard, C. H., Boring, A. M., et al. (1999). A. E. Bennett Research Award. Developmental traumatology: Part I. Biological stress systems. *Biological Psychiatry, 45*(10), 1259–1270.

De Bellis, M. D., Chrousos, G. P., Dorn, L. D., Burke, L., Helmers, K., Kling, M. A., et al. (1994). Hypothalamic–pituitary–adrenal axis dysregulation in sexually abused girls. *Journal of Clinical Endocrinology and Metabolism, 78*(2), 249–255.

Enoch, M., Ke, X., Ferro, E., Harris, C. R., & Goldman, D. (2003). Genetic origins of anxiety in women: A role for a functional catechol-O-methyltransferase polymorphism. *Psychiatric Genetics, 13*(1), 33–41.

Epperson, C. N., Haga, K., Mason, G. F., Sellers, E., Geueorguieva, R., Zhang, W., et al. (2002). Cortical g-aminobutyric acid levels across the menstrual cycle in healthy women and those with premenstrual dysphoric disorder. *Archives of General Psychiatry, 59*, 851–858.

Feingold, A. (1994). Gender differences in personality: A meta-analysis. *Psychological Bulletin, 116*, 429–456.

Foundas, A. L., Faulhaber, J. R., Kulynych, J. J., Browning, C. A., & Weinberger, D. R. (1999). Hemispheric and sex-linked differences in sylvian fissure morphology: A quantitative approach using volumetric magnetic resonance imaging. *Neuropsychiatry, Neuropsychology, and Behavioral Neurology, 12*, 1–10.

Frederikse, M., Lu, A., Aylward, E., Barta, P., Sharma, T., & Pearlson, G. (2000). Sex differences in inferior parietal lobule volume in schizophrenia. *American Journal of Psychiatry, 157*, 422–427.

Friedman, M., McDonagh-Coyle, A., Jalowiec, J., Wang, S., Fournier, D., & McHugo, G. (2001, December). *Neurohormonal findings during treatment of women with PTSD due to childhood sexual abuse (CSA)*. Abstract for the 17th annual meeting of the International Society for Traumatic Stress Studies, New Orleans, LA.

Gaffan, D., Murray, E. A., & Fabre-Thorpe, M. (1993). Interaction of the amygdala with the frontal lobe in reward memory. *European Journal of Neuroscience, 5*(7), 968–975.

George, M. S., Ketter, T. A., Parekh, P. I., Horowitz, B., Herscovitch, P., & Post, R. M. (1995). Brain activity during transient sadness and happiness in healthy women. *American Journal of Psychiatry, 152*(3), 341–351.

Giedd, J. N., Snell, J. W., Lange, N., Rajapakse, J. C., Casey, B. J., Kozuch, P. L., et al. (1996). Quantitative magnetic resonance imaging of human brain development: ages 4–18. *Cerebral Cortex, 6*, 551–560.

Good, C. D., Johnsrude, I., Ashburner, J., Henson, R. N. A., Friston, K. J., & Frackowiak, R. S. J. (2001). Cerebral asymmetry and the effects of sex and handedness on brain structure: A voxel-based morphometric analysis of 465 normal adult human brains. *NeuroImage, 14*, 685–700.

Gur, R. C., Mozley, L. H., Mozley, P. D., Resnick, S. M., Karp, J. S., Alavi, A., et al. (1995). Sex differences in regional cerebral glucose metabolism during a resting state. *Science, 267*, 528–531.

Gur, R. C., Turetsky, B. I., Matsui, M., Yan, M., Bilker, W., Hughett, P., et al. (1999). Sex differences in brain gray and white matter in healthy young adults: Correlations with cognitive performance. *Journal of Neuroscience, 19*, 4065–4072.

Hamann, S., & Canli, T. (2004). Individual differences in emotion processing. *Current Opinion in Neurobiology, 14*, 233–238.

Hariri, A. R., Mattay, V. S., Tessitore, A., Kolachana, B., Fera, F., Goldman, D., et al. (2002). Serotonin transporter genetic variation and the response of the human amygdala. *Science, 297*, 400–403.

Heim, C., Newport, D. J., Heit, S., Graham, Y. P., Wilcox, M., Bonsall, R., et al. (2000). Pituitary–adrenal and autonomic responses to stress in women after sexual and physical abuse in childhood. *Journal of the American Medical Association, 284*(5), 592–597.

Jones, M. T., Brush, F. R., & Neame, R. L. B. (1972). Characteristics of fast feedback control of corticotrophin release by corticosteroids. *Journal of Endocrinology, 55*, 489–497.

Kaufman, J., Birmaher, B., Perel, J., Dahl, R. E., Moreci, P., Nelson, B., et al. (1997). The corticotropin-releasing hormone challenge in depressed abused, depressed nonabused, and normal control children. *Biological Psychiatry, 42*, 669–679.

Kerns, J. G., Cohen, J. D., Macdonald, A. W., III, Cho, R. Y., Stenger, V. A., & Carter, C. S. (2004). Anterior cingulate conflict monitoring and adjustments in control. *Science, 303*, 1023–1026.

Kirschbaum, C., Kudielka, B. M., Gaab, J., Schommer, N. C., & Hellhammer, D. H. (1999). Impact of gender, menstrual cycle phase, and oral contraceptives on the activity of the hypothalamus–pituitary–adrenal axis. *Psychosomatic Medicine, 61*(2), 154–162.

Kirschbaum, C., Wust, S., Faig, H. G., & Hellhammer, D. H. (1992). Heritability of cortisol responses to human-corticotropin releasing factor, ergometry, and psychological stress in humans. *Journal of Clinical Endocrinology and Metabolism, 75*(6), 1526–1530.

Kitay, J. (1961). Sex differences in adrenal cortical secretion in the rat. *Endocrinology, 68*, 818–824.

Kulynych, J. J., Vladar, K., Jones, D. W., & Weinberger, D. R. (1994). Gender differences in the normal lateralization of the supratemporal cortex: MRI surface-rendering morphometry of Heschl's gyrus and the planum temporale. *Cerebral Cortex, 4*, 107–118.

Lazarus, R. S., & Folkman, S. (1984). *Stress, appraisal, and coping*. New York: Springer.

Li, C.-S., Kosten, T. R., & Sinha, R. (2005). Sex differences in brain activation during stress imagery in abstinent cocaine users: A functional magnetic resonance imaging study. *Biological Psychiatry, 57*(5), 487–494.

Liotti, M., Mayberg, H. S., Brannan, S. K., McGinnis, S., Jerabek, P., & Fox, P. T. (2000). Differential limbic–cortical correlates of sadness and anxiety in healthy subjects: Implications for affective disorders. *Biological Psychiatry, 48*, 30–42.

Lovallo, W. R. (1997). *Stress and health: Biological and psychological interactions* (Vol. 1). Thousand Oaks, CA: Sage.

Maccoby, E., & Jacklin, C. N. (1974). *The psychology of sex differences*. Stanford, CA: Stanford University Press.

Maciejewski, P. K., Prigerson, H. G., & Mazure, C. M. (2001). Sex differences in event-related risk for major depression. *Psychological Medicine, 31*(4), 593–604.

MacMillan, H. L., Fleming, J. E., Streiner, D. L., Lin, E., Boyle, M. H., Jamieson, E., et al. (2001). Childhood abuse and lifetime psychopathology in a community sample. *American Journal of Psychiatry, 158*, 1878–1883.

Mayberg, H. S., Brannan, S. K., Tekell, J. L., Silva, J. A., Mahurin, R. K., McGinnis, S., et al. (2000). Regional metabolic effects of fluoxetine in major depression: Serial changes and relationship to clinical response. *Biological Psychiatry, 48*, 830–843.

Mayberg, H. S., Liotti, M., Brannan, S. K., McGinnis, S., Mahurin, R. K., Jerabek, P. A., et al. (1999). Reciprocal limbic-cortical function and negative mood: Converging PET findings in depression and normal sadness. *American Journal of Psychiatry, 156*, 675–682.

McCrae, R. R., & Costa, P. T. (1986). Personality, coping, and coping effectiveness in an adult sample. *Journal of Personality, 54*(2), 385–405.

McEwen, B. S. (1999a). Performance of brain sex differences and structural plasticity of the adult brain. *Proceedings of the National Academy of Sciences USA, 96*, 7128–7130.

McEwen, B. S. (1999b). Stress and hippocampal plasticity. *Annual Review of Neuroscience, 22*, 105–122.

McEwen, B. S. (2001). Invited review. Estrogen's effects on the brain: Multiple sites and molecular mechanisms. *Journal of Applied Physiology, 91*(6), 2785–2801.

McEwen, B. S., & Stellar, E. (1993). Stress and the individual: Mechanisms leading to disease. *Archives of Internal Medicine, 153*, 2093–2101.

Naliboff, B. D., Berman, S. M., Chang, L., Derbyshire, S. W. G., Suyenobu, B., Vogt, B. A., et al. (2003). Sex-related differences in IBS patients: Central processing of visceral stimuli. *Gastroenterology, 124*, 1738–1747.

Nemeroff, C. B. (1996). The corticotropin-releasing factor (CRF) hypothesis of depression: New findings and new directions. *Molecular Psychiatry, 1*, 336–342.

Panksepp, J., Nelson, E., & Bekkedal, M. (1997). Brain systems for the mediation of social separation-distress and social-reward. *Annals of the New York Academy of Sciences, 807,* 78–100.

Paris, J. (2004). Gender differences in personality traits and disorders. *Current Psychiatry Reports, 6,* 71–74.

Peoples, L. L. (2002). Will, anterior cingulate cortex, and addiction. *Science, 296,* 1623–1624.

Phan, K. L., Wager, T., Taylor, S. F., & Liberzon, I. (2002). Functional neuroanatomy of emotion: A meta-ananlysis of emotion activation studies in PET and fMRI. *NeuroImage, 16,* 331–348.

Rasmusson, A., Zimolo, Z., Vasek, J., Lipschitz, D., Mustone, M., Gudmundsen, G., et al. (2001, December). *Increased adrenal DHEA release in premenopausal women with PTSD.* Paper presented at the 17th annual meeting of the International Society for Traumatic Stress Studies, New Orleans, LA.

Rasmusson, A. M., Hauger, R. L., Morgan, C. A. R., Bremner, J. D., Charney, D. S., & Southwick, S. M. (2000). Low baseline and yohimbine-stimulated plasma neuropeptide Y (NPY) in combat-related PTSD. *Biological Psychiatry, 47*(6), 526–539.

Ray, O. (2004). How the mind hurts and heals the body. *American Psychologist, 59*(1), 29–40.

Robbins, T. W., & Everitt, B. J. (1996). Neurobehavioural mechanisms of reward and motivation. *Current Opinion in Neurobiology, 6*(2), 228–236.

Rolls, E. T. (2000). The orbitofrontal cortex and reward. *Cerebral Cortex, 10,* 284–294.

Sinha, R. (2001). How does stress increase risk of drug abuse and relapse? *Psychopharmacology, 158*(4), 343–359.

Sinha, R., Catapano, D., & O'Malley, S. S. (1999). Stress-induced craving and stress responses in cocaine dependent individuals. *Psychopharmacology, 142,* 343–351.

Sinha, R., Lacadie, C., & Skudlarski, P. (2004). [Sex differences in neural responses to emotional stress]. Unpublished raw data.

Sinha, R., Lacadie, C., Skudlarski, P., Fulbright, R. K., Kosten, T. R., Rounsaville, B. J., et al. (in press). Neural activity associated with stress-induced cocaine craving: An fMRI study. *Psychopharmacology.*

Sinha, R., Lacadie, C., Skudlarski, P., & Wexler, B. E. (2004). Neural circuits underlying emotional distress in humans. *Annals of the New York Academy of Sciences, 1032,* 254–257.

Sinha, R., & Rounsaville, B. J. (2002). Sex differences in depressed substance abusers. *Journal of Clinical Psychiatry, 63*(7), 616–627.

Sinha, R., Talih, M., Malison, R., Anderson, G. A., Cooney, N., & Kreek, M. (2003). Hypothalamic–pituitary–adrenal axis and sympatho-adreno-medullary responses during stress-induced and drug cue-induced cocaine craving states. *Psychopharmacology, 170,* 62–72.

Soufer, R., Bremner, J. D., Arrighi, J. A., Cohen, I., Zaret, B. L., Burg, M. M., et al. (1998). Cerebral cortical hyperactivation in response to mental stress in patients with coronary artery disease. *Proceedings of the National Academy of Sciences USA, 95,* 6454–6459.

Steiner, M., Dunn, E., & Born, L. (2003). Hormones and mood: From menarche to menopause and beyond. *Journal of Affective Disorders, 74,* 67–83.

Stoney, C. M., Davis, M. C., & Matthews, K. A. (1987). Sex differences in physiological responses to stress and in coronary heart disease: A causal link? *Psychophysiology, 24*(2), 127–131.

Taylor, S. E., Klein, L. C., Lewis, B. P., Gruenewald, T. L., Gurung, R. A., & Updegraff, J. A. (2000). Biobehavioral responses to stress in females: Tend-and-befriend, not fight-or-flight. *Psychological Review, 107*(3), 411–429.

Wager, T. D., Phan, K. L., Liberzon, I., & Taylor, S. F. (2003). Valence, gender, and lateralization of functional brain anatomy in emotion: A meta-analysis of findings from neuroimaging. *NeuroImage, 19*, 513–531.

Weiss, E. L., Longhurst, J. G., & Mazure, C. M. (1999). Childhood sexual abuse as a risk factor for depression in women: Psychosocial and neurobiological correlates. *American Journal of Psychiatry, 156*(6), 816–828.

Wexler, B. E., Gottschalk, C. H., Fulbright, R. K., Prohovnik, I., Lacadie, C. M., Rounsaville, B. J., et al. (2001). Functional magnetic resonance imaging of cocaine craving. *American Journal of Psychiatry, 158*(1), 86–95.

Widom, C. S. (1999). Posttraumatic stress disorder in abused and neglected children grown up. *American Journal of Psychiatry, 156*(8), 1223–1229.

Yehuda, R. (1997). Sensitization of the hypothalamic–pituitary–adrenal axis in post-traumatic stress disorder. *Annals of the New York Academy of Sciences, 821*, 57–75.

Young, E. A. (1995). Glucocorticoid cascade hypothesis revisited: Role of gonadal steroids. *Depression, 3*, 20–27.

Young, E. A. (1996). Sex differences in response to exogenous corticosterone: A rat model of hypercortisolemia. *Molecular Psychiatry, 1*(4), 313–319.

Young, E. A., & Korszun, A. (1999). Women, stress, and depression: Sex differences in hypothalamic–pituitary–adrenal axis regulation. In E. Leibenluft (Ed.), *Gender differences in mood and anxiety disorders: from bench to bedside* (pp. 31–52). Washington, DC: American Psychiatric Press.

Zubieta, J., Ketter, T. A., Bueller, B. A., Xu, Y., Kilbourn, M. R., Young, E. A., et al. (2003). Regulation of human affective responses by anterior cingulate and limbic μ-opioid transmission. *Archives of General Psychiatry, 60*, 1145–1153.

Zubieta, J., Smith, Y. R., Bueller, J. A., Xu, Y., Kilbourn, M. R., Jewett, D. M., et al. (2002). μ-opioid receptor-mediated antinociceptive responses differ in men and women. *Journal of Neuroscience, 22*, 5100–5107.

IV

Genetic and Neural Analyses of Anxiety-Related Traits

11

Neuroticism as a Genetic Marker for Mood and Anxiety

Nathan A. Gillespie and Nicholas G. Martin

MOOD AND ANXIETY DISORDERS

Almost one in five people will experience a significant mood or anxiety disorder at some stage in life. The lifetime prevalence rates of *Diagnostic and Statistical Manual of Mental Disorders*, third edition, revised (DSM-III-R) mood and anxiety disorders are shown in Table 11.1. As can be seen, the lifetime prevalence of major depression is almost twice as high for females as for males, and this is a robust finding in the literature (Blazer, Kessler, McGonagle, & Swartz, 1994; Breslau, Schultz, & Peterson, 1995; Kendler & Prescott, 1999; Newman, Bland, & Orn, 1988; Parker & Hadzi-Pavlovic, 2001).

Anxiety disorders represent the most common comorbid diagnoses (Sanderson, Beck, & Beck, 1990). Like that of mood disorders, the prevalence of anxiety disorders is higher among females (Kessler et al., 1994). When based on the DSM-III-R, the lifetime prevalence for generalized anxiety disorder (GAD) in the United States is 3.6% for males and 6.6% for females.

In reality, the prevalence rates for mood and anxiety disorders in Table 11.1 are somewhat different, and often these will differ widely even when they are based on structured clinical interviews. Apart from issues of reliability and accuracy of psychiatric classification, the major sources of discrepancy are varying definitions. For instance, Kendler, Neale, Kessler, Heath, and Eaves (1992d) blindly assessed a population-based sample of 1033 same-sex female twin pairs who were administered a structured psychiatric interview contain-

TABLE 11.1. Lifetime Prevalence Rates (%)
of DSM-III-R Mood and Anxiety Disorders

DSM-III-R disorder	Males	Females
Mood disorders		
Major depressive episode	12.7	21.3
Manic episode	1.6	1.7
Dysthymia	4.8	8.0
Any mood disorder	14.7	23.9
Anxiety disorders		
Panic disorder	2.0	5.0
Agoraphobia without panic	3.5	7.0
Social phobia	11.1	15.5
Simple phobia	6.7	15.7
Generalized anxiety disorder	3.6	6.6
Any anxiety disorder	19.2	30.5

Note. Data from Kessler et al. (1994).

ing nine commonly used definitions of major depression. As is shown in Table 11.2, depending on the definition, the lifetime prevalence rates for major depression ranged from 12% to 33%. The broadest criteria (DSM-III, Research Diagnostic Criteria [RDC] probable, and DSM-III-R) have the highest prevalence rates of 31% to 33%. Intermediate criteria (Washington University Criteria [WUC] primary and secondary definite, RDC definite, and the Gershon) have prevalence rates of 20% to 25%. The lowest prevalence rates of 12% to 15% come from diagnoses based on the narrowest definitions

TABLE 11.2. Lifetime Population Prevalence of Major Depression
as a Function of Diagnostic Criteria

Definition	Prevalence	A	C	E
DSM-III	33%	.39	—	.60
RDC (probable)	32%	.39	—	.61
DSM-III-R	31%	.42	—	.58
WUC	25%	.33	—	.64
RDC (definite)	23%	.44	—	.56
Gershon	23%	.45	—	.55
WUC (primary and secondary definite)	20%	.33	—	.64
WUC (probable)	15%	.21	—	.75
WUC (definite)	12%	.24	—	.73

Note. A, C, and E, proportion of variance attributable to additive genetic, shared environmental, and nonshared environmental variance, respectively. RDC, Research Diagnostic Criteria; WUC, Washington University Criteria. Data from Kendler, Neale, Kessler, Heath, and Eaves (1992d).

(WUC probable and definite). Unlike the data for major depression, no data are available that detail the impact of varying definitions on the lifetime population prevalence of anxiety disorders in the United States.

PREVAILING AND ALTERNATIVE TAXONOMIES OF PSYCHOLOGICAL DISTRESS

The *Diagnostic and Statistical Manual of Mental Disorders* (DSM), published by the American Psychiatric Association (1980, 1987, 1994, 2000), remains one of the most popular diagnostic tools for assessing mental disorders. Unfortunately, it is beyond the scope of this chapter to review the limitations of categorical taxonomies; these are reviewed elsewhere (Eysenck, 1986, 1994b; Kirk & Kutchins, 1992; Millon, 1991; Neale, Eaves, & Kendler, 1994, p. 248; Zuckerman, 1999). Categorical models of classification *are* appropriate if the phenotype is indeed discontinuous. For instance, a categorical model would be useful if a psychiatric disorder could be best explained in terms of a single gene of large effect with or without reduced "penetrance" (which is the likelihood that a given gene will result in disease), or perhaps by some form of discrete environmental transmission, such as a bacterium or virus (Eaves, Eysenck, & Martin, 1989).

CONTINUOUS-LIABILITY MODEL

Despite the convenience of using measures with dichotomous outcomes, in reality behaviors and traits of biomedical interest more often represent syndromes of numerous physical, behavioral, and psychiatric symptoms, which are more likely to demonstrate continuous than discrete variation. Although Pearson's work laid much of the foundation for 20th-century statistics (e.g., correlation, regression, and standard deviation), it was Fisher who introduced what is now referred to as the "polygenic model." According to this model, an observed phenotype is caused by a large number of genes or genetic loci, each with small effect, acting additively, and inherited according to strict Mendelian laws.

Polygenic models assume that variation within an observed phenotype is caused in part by segregation of a number of genes with small effect. Therefore, as the number of loci influencing a trait increases, the number of separate phenotypic categories increases, and the overall distribution of classes or categories approaches normality. Superimposed upon this genetic variation are environmental effects, which blur the demarcation between individual classes. This causes the overall distribution to appear continuous. In other words, the distribution can be explained in terms of a continuous variable or "liability," which is determined by genetic *and* environmental factors, thereby making the system multifactorial (Fraser, 1976).

Based on empirical evidence outlined elsewhere (Eaves et al., 1989; Eysenck, 1953; Falconer, 1963), the measures of psychological distress and personality discussed in this chapter assume a continuous-liability distribution. Regardless of whether the data are continuous or ordinal, this model assumes that liability to psychological distress or variation in measures of personality arise from the independent action of a large number of factors, each with small effect, which give rise to a normal distribution of liability (Falconer, 1963). The implicit goal in exploring the genetic etiology of psychological distress is to quantify the genetic and environmental sources of variation in the liability, rather than to focus on the dichotomies or thresholds per se.

A PERSONALITY AND INDIVIDUAL-DIFFERENCES APPROACH

Eysenck argued that the best way to understand mechanisms is to study human individual differences. His chief contribution to psychology was his dimensional model of personality, which presents an alternative to categorical ways, with a quantitative and dimensional representation of human behavior (Eysenck, 1967, 1971b; Eysenck & Rachman, 1965).

Eysenck's theory is based on the Galen–Kant–Wundt scheme, which is strongly rooted in the ancient Greek dimensions of "choleric," "sanguine," "phlegmatic," and "melancholic" humors (Eysenck & Eysenck, 1991). The three orthogonal dimensions of "psychoticism," "extraversion," and "neuroticism," which are independent of intelligence, have consistently emerged as second-order factors or superfactors from large-scale factor-analytic studies (Eysenck, 1971b; Eysenck & Eysenck, 1985, 1991). Each superfactor represents a polygenic and hierarchical phenotype, which forms a continuum based on a number of first-order traits. These traits are empirically derived, are intercorrelated, and in turn give rise to the superfactors above them. The superfactors are based on correlational and factor-analytic methods relying on data from self-report questionnaires, peer and observer ratings, miniature situational studies, experimental psychology, psychological measures, and hormonal and biochemical assays—all of which assume a dynamic and causal aspect that relates behavior to fundamental biological factors (Eysenck, 1971b; Eysenck & Eysenck, 1975, 1985).

Neuroticism

The central focus of this chapter is on neuroticism, and our aim is to demonstrate that individuals with neurotic personalities, in certain environmental circumstances, are highly predisposed to mood and anxiety disorders. An important point is that high scores on neuroticism do not necessarily equate to neurosis. This dimension was originally conceptualized by Eysenck as a quan-

Neuroticism

Anxious Depressed Guilt feelings Low self-esteem
Carefree Irrational Shy Moody Emotional

FIGURE 11.1. Neuroticism and underlying first-order correlated traits. From Eysenck and Eysenck (1985). Copyright 1985 by Eysenck and Eysenck. Adapted by permission.

titative personality trait defined as an individual's vulnerability to various neurotic disorders and psychological distress (Eysenck, 1953, 1967). It is reliably measured by self-report and is highly stable over time (Eysenck & Eysenck, 1991; Gillespie, Evans, Wright, & Martin, 2004; Kirk et al., 2000). In terms of factorial invariance, the same dimension is identifiable in a diverse range of cultures worldwide and across the socioeconomic spectrum (Eysenck & Eysenck, 1983). Moreover, it has emerged in every model of personality based on questionnaire measurement and analyses of ratings of psychiatric symptoms where anxiety and depression have emerged as general dysphoric or negative effect factors (Zuckerman, 1999; Zuckerman, Kuhlman, Joireman, Teta, & Kraft, 1988).

The hierarchical and behavioral consequences of this personality dimension are summarized in Figure 11.1. As with the other dimensions, the first-order traits are measured dimensionally. High scorers are described as anxious, worrying, moody, and frequently depressed (Eysenck & Eysenck, 1991). When high neuroticism is combined with high extraversion, such individuals are likely to be touchy and restless, easily excitable, and even aggressive. Low scorers, on the other hand, are usually calm, even-tempered, controlled, and unworried.

Psychobiology of Neuroticism

Eysenck and Eysenck (1985) argued that neuroticism has a constitutional basis with predictable behavioral consequences. Although he insisted that neurotic disorders can be learned, unlearned, extinguished, and treated with behavioral interventions (Eysenck, 1960; Eysenck & Rachman, 1965), he rejected any behavioral explanation of neuroticism or neurosis that did not acknowledge the underlying biological mechanisms.

Constitutionally, the dimension reflects an inherited lability of the autonomic nervous system (including the amygdala, hippocampus, septum, cingulum, and hypothalamus), which controls autonomic activation and the expression of emotion. Emotional stability–instability is characteristic of the sympathetic–parasympathetic balance within the autonomic nervous system. For this reason, high scores on neuroticism are associated with greater autonomic activation as measured by skin conductance, muscular tension, heart rate, blood pressure, electroencephalogram, and breathing (Eysenck, 1991; Eysenck & Eysenck, 1985).

CLONINGER'S THEORY OF PERSONALITY

In contrast to Eysenck's three-factor model, Cloninger's (1994) revised biosocial model of personality posits seven domains of personality: four temperament domains ("harm avoidance," "novelty seeking," "reward dependence," and "persistence") and three character domains ("self-directedness," "cooperativeness," and "self-transcendence"). All seven of these domains are measured by the Temperament and Character Inventory (TCI; Cloninger, 1994), whereas the first three (harm avoidance, novelty seeking, and reward dependence) are measured by an earlier instrument, the Tridimensional Personality Questionnaire (TPQ; Cloninger, 1986). This section focuses on harm avoidance because, as will be shown, it also demonstrates a very strong phenotypic association with measures of mood and affect.

Harm Avoidance

According to the model, harm avoidance is regulated by serotoninergic cell bodies and reflects variation in the brain's "punishment system" or "behavioral inhibition system," which includes the septo-hippocampal system as well as serotonergic and cholinergic projections (Cloninger, 1987). Individuals high on harm avoidance are characterized as cautious, tense, apprehensive, fearful, inhibited, shy, easily fatigable, and worrying (Cloninger, 1994).

THE OVERLAP AMONG GRAY, EYSENCK, AND CLONINGER

Gray (1986) argued that his dimensions of "anxiety" and "impulsivity" are not necessarily at odds with Eysenck's model of personality, and that his dimensions are at an approximate 45° rotation from Eysenck's dimensions of neuroticism and extraversion (Eysenck & Eysenck, 1985; Gray, 1970). This is illustrated in Figure 11.2, where "anxiety/harm avoidance" runs diagonally across the two-dimensional plane defined by "extraverted" and "neurotic," such that individuals with high harm avoidance fall within the neurotic/introverted quadrant.

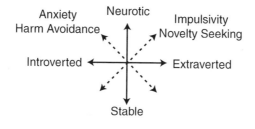

FIGURE 11.2. Relationship between Eysenck's dimensions of neuroticism and introversion, Cloninger's harm avoidance and novelty seeking, and Gray's anxiety and impulsivity. From Eysenck and Eysenck (1985). Copyright 1985 by Eysenck and Eysenck. Adapted by permission.

Of course, the degree of overlap between the various dimensions of personality is an empirical question. Based on a sample of students, Zuckerman and Cloninger (1996) found that Harm Avoidance correlated highly with Neuroticism (0.59) and Extraversion (–0.53). In the same study, the correlation was between EPQ Extraversion and Novelty Seeking (0.44). This was most likely attributable to the fact that the older version of Extraversion contained impulsivity items.

In a factor analysis of Cloninger's and Eysenck's dimensions, Heath, Cloninger, and Martin (1994) concluded that it would be erroneous to assume that they represent "alternative descriptions of the same dimensions of personality." Instead, they suggested that the TPQ and EPQ assess five to six discernible dimensions of genetic variability and at least six dimensions of environmental variability. Slutske and colleagues (1998), in a principal-components analysis of the TPQ and the Eysenck Personality Questionnaire—Revised (EPQ-R; Eysenck & Eysenck, 1991), extracted three higher-order personality dimensions. The first factor, labeled "positive emotionality," had high loadings of TPQ Reward Dependence and EPQ-R Extraversion. TPQ Harm Avoidance and EPQ-R Neuroticism loaded strongly onto the second factor, labeled "negative emotionality."

More recently, an analysis of data from the population-based Australian Twin Registry, using a sample of 3,269 twins ages 18–28 years, has yielded correlations of .58 to .60 for males and females, respectively, between EPQ-R Neuroticism and TPQ Harm Avoidance (Gillespie, Johnstone, Boyce, Heath, & Martin, 2001). High but negative correlations were also found between TPQ Harm Avoidance and EPQ-R Extraversion. These results suggest that harm avoidance does intersect Eysenck's neurotic–introverted quadrant. Indeed, in unpublished analyses using the same twin data, the genetic factors underpinning EPQ-R Neuroticism scores also explained significant proportions of variance in TPQ Harm Avoidance. This is demonstrated by the high additive genetic factor loadings in Table 11.3.

TABLE 11.3. Additive Genetic Factor Loadings Based on a Cholesky Triangular Decomposition of the EPQ-R (Neuroticism, Extraversion, Psychoticism, and Lie) and TPQ (Harm Avoidance, Novelty Seeking, and Reward Dependence) Personality Subscales

	Males (~1250)							Females (~2100)						
	1.	2.	3.	4.	5.	6.	7.	1.	2.	3.	4.	5.	6.	7.
1. Neuroticism	.64							.57						
2. Extraversion	–.20	.67						–.24	.63					
3. Psychoticism	.16	.18	.54					—	.19	.69				
4. Lie	—	–.22	—	.63				—	–.13	–.19	.56			
5. Harm Avoidance	.44	–.36	—	—	.34			.37	–.32	–.15	—	.29		
6. Novelty Seeking	—	.56	.27	–.18	—	–.17		—	.33	.26	–.26	—	.29	
7. Reward Dependence	–.14	.39	–.22	.16	—	—	.32	—	.30	–.23	—	—	—	.47

Note. Nonsignificant loadings are not shown. Data from Gillespie and colleagues (2001).

PREDICTING PSYCHOLOGICAL DISTRESS

Having argued that there is a strong phenotypic association between neuroticism and related constructs such as harm avoidance, the next step is to demonstrate that the same personality dimensions are useful for predicting psychological distress. A chief advantage of the continuous dimensions of personality proposed by Eysenck, Gray, and Cloninger is that they provide a theoretical framework for explaining the biological and social mechanisms of anxiety and mood disorders, as well as a source of testable predictions.

Personality has long been thought to predispose individuals to mood and anxiety disorders (Eysenck, 1953; Eysenck & Rachman, 1965). Eysenck's model predicts that neurotic/introverted individuals, or what he referred to as "dysthymic personalities," are more prone to mood and mood disorders because they condition faster to neurotic responses. In terms of Figure 11.2, individuals who fall within the neurotic/introverted quadrant are more prone to experiencing anxiety, reactive depression, obsessions, phobias, and so on. There are good empirical data to support this prediction. Depressed subjects typically record higher EPQ or EPQ-R Neuroticism and Introversion scores (Corah, 1971; Eysenck, 1971a; Eysenck & Eysenck, 1985; Eysenck & Rachman, 1965; Larsen & Ketelaar, 1991; Maier, Lichtermann, Minges, & Heun, 1992). Other studies have demonstrated a strong phenotypic association between neuroticism and both clinical and symptomatic measures of depression (Berlanga, Heinze, Torres, Apiquian, & Caballero, 1999; Gormley, O'Leary, & Costello, 1999; Hassanyeh, Eccleston, & Davison, 1981; Kerr, Schapira, Roth, & Garside, 1970). The most recent evidence comes from Middeldorp and colleagues, who present their results in Chapter 12 of this volume. They provide compelling evidence, based on data from the population-based Netherlands Twin Register, that there is a significant linear trend linking high neuroticism, low extraversion, and the number of mood and anxiety disorders.

Similarly, harm avoidance is a very good predictor of mood and anxiety disorders and symptoms: premenstrual depression (Freeman, Schweizer, & Rickels, 1995); self-reported depression (Hansenne, Pitchot, Gonzalez Moreno, Machurot, & Ansseau, 1998; Nelson, Cloninger, Przybeck, & Csernansky, 1996; Strakowski, Dunayevich, Keck, & McElroy, 1995; Strakowski, Faedda, Tohen, Goodwin, & Stoll, 1992; Yoshino, Kato, Takeuchi, Ono, & Kitamura, 1994); panic disorder associated with agoraphobia (Saviotti et al., 1991); DSM-III-R Cluster C personality disorders (Ampollini, Marchesi, Signifredi, & Maggini, 1997; Battaglia, Przybeck, Bellodi, & Cloninger, 1996), and other mood and anxiety disorders (Ampollini et al., 1997; Starcevic, Uhlenhuth, Fallon, & Pathak, 1996).

Strong phenotypic associations have been found among extraversion, neuroticism, and symptoms of anxiety (Bachorowski & Newman, 1990; Gershuny & Sher, 1998). Cox, Borger, Taylor, Fuentes, and Ross (1999), in a regression analysis of higher- and lower-order dimensions of the "Big Five" personality dimensions (see Costa & McCrae, 1992) based on 317 undergraduate students, found that higher-order domains of neuroticism and extraversion, as well as the lower-order neuroticism facets of anxiety and self-consciousness, best predict anxiety sensitivity.

What Is the Nature of the Association?

Not only do people with various clinical forms of major depression consistently report higher levels of neuroticism (Fanous, Gardner, Prescott, Cancro, & Kendler, 2002; Kendler, Gardner, & Prescott, 2002; Kendler, Kessler, Neale, Heath, & Eaves, 1993; Kendler, Neale, Kessler, Heath, & Eaves, 1993b; Roberts & Kendler, 1999; Treloar, Martin, Bucholz, Madden, & Heath, 1999), but the association appears to be causal, because neuroticism or neuroticism-like traits can predict future cases of mood and anxiety disorders. Kendler and colleagues (1993b), in a study of 1733 same-sex female twin pairs, found that neuroticism was strongly related to lifetime prevalence of major depression. Neuroticism also predicted the prospective 1-year prevalence of major depression in those who, at time 1, denied previous depressive episodes, and this was not merely because of overlap with prodromal symptoms of major depression.

More evidence for a causal association comes from Kirk and colleagues (2000). As shown in Table 11.4, they found that high scorers on EPQ Neuroticism (Eysenck & Eysenck, 1975; S. B. G. Eysenck, Eysenck, & Barrett, 1985) when compared to low scorers, had significantly higher rates of DSM-IV diag-

TABLE 11.4. Prevalences (%) of DSM-IV Diagnoses for a Sample of Female and Male Twins Selected on the Basis of Extreme EPQ Neuroticism Scores (Obtained on Average 10 Years Prior to Formal Diagnoses)

DSM-IV diagnosis	Females				Males			
	Deciles				Deciles			
	1 & 2 (n = 852)	9 & 10 (n = 676)	OR	p	1 & 2 (n = 495)	9 & 10 (n = 447)	OR	p
Depression	14.0	41.1	2.9	***	10.9	32.7	3.0	***
Dysthymia	0.2	1.9	9.5	***	0.0	0.4	—	.14
OCD	1.4	9.2	6.4	***	1.6	11.0	6.9	***
Social phobia	2.1	11.4	5.4	***	1.6	12.5	7.8	***
GAD	1.0	1.6	1.5	.33	0.0	1.8	—	**
Panic w/o agoraphobia	1.3	4.1	3.2	***	0.4	2.9	7.2	**
Panic + agoraphobia	0.5	2.4	4.8	***	0.0	2.7	—	**
Agoraphobia w/o panic	0.7	4.1	5.9	***	0.0	1.3	3.2	.12

Note. OR, odds ratio. Data from Kirk et al. (2000).
$*p < .05$; $**p < .01$; $***p < .001$.

noses of major depression, dysthymia, obsessive–compulsive disorder (OCD), panic disorder with or without agoraphobia, agoraphobia without panic disorder, social phobia, and GAD. Most interestingly, selection was based on the 12-item short-scale Neuroticism questionnaire given, on average, 10 years prior to the formal DSM-IV diagnoses' being made.

THE GENETIC EPIDEMIOLOGY OF PSYCHOLOGICAL DISTRESS AND PERSONALITY

The next step is to explain this relationship more precisely in terms of genetic and environmental effects. The branch of science referred to as "behavior genetics" is distinct from fields such as sociobiology or evolutionary psychology, because it focuses on the role of genetic and environmental influences as contributors to individual differences. The chief advantage of this approach is that it permits researchers to generate and test explicit hypotheses regarding the genetic and environmental etiology of complex behaviors.

Genetic Epidemiology of Major Depression

Evidence for the genetic contribution to major depression is compelling and comes from a variety of study designs, many of which rely on large population-based twin registries (Bierut et al., 1999; Kendler, Gardner, & Prescott, 1998; Kendler, Heath, Martin, & Eaves, 1986, 1987; Kendler, Karkowski, Corey, & Neale, 1998; Kendler, Neale, Kessler, Heath, & Eaves,

1992a, 1993a; Kendler, Pedersen, Neale, & Mathe, 1995; Kendler & Prescott, 1999; Kendler et al., 1994; Lyons et al., 1998; McGuffin, Katz, Watkins, & Rutherford, 1996; Silberg et al., 1999; Tambs, 1991). A significant genetic component is consistently found, regardless of whether the analyses are based on self-report or continuous symptom counts (Kendler et al., 1986, 1987, 1994; Tambs, 1991), on clinical categorical diagnoses (Bierut et al., 1999; Kendler et al., 1992a; Kendler, Pedersen, et al., 1995; Kendler & Prescott, 1999; Kendler, Walters, et al., 1995; Lyons et al., 1998; McGuffin et al., 1996; Silberg et al., 1999), or hospital or clinical samples (Kendler, Pedersen, Johnson, Neale, & Mathe, 1993; Kendler, Pedersen, et al., 1995; McGuffin et al., 1996).

In the same way that lifetime prevalence estimates change as a function of varying definition, the estimates of environmental and genetic variance underpinning variation in major depression also vary. Table 11.2 also includes standardized genetic and environmental variance components under the best-fitting models for twin pair resemblance, as a function of the particular diagnostic systems. For all nine definitions, there was no evidence to support the contribution of shared environmental or cultural effects in the etiology of major depression. Instead, family aggregation (i.e., the degree to which siblings and genetically related family members are more or less alike) could be entirely explained by significant but moderate proportions of additive genetic variance. With the exception of the WUC, which exclude secondary cases, the magnitude of genetic influence appears to be similar regardless of whether depression is broadly or narrowly defined. In other words, for seven of the definitions, the genetic contribution to major depression ranged from 33% to 45%, whereas for the two definitions that were restricted to only primary cases of major depression, the genetic contribution was much lower (from 21% to 24%).

Despite the inherent limitations of meta-analysis, the least of which is the heterogeneity of samples (see Eysenck, 1994a, 1995), Sullivan, Neale, and Kendler (2000) have reviewed the literature that has explored the sources of familial aggregation for major depression. In their meta-analysis, six twin studies met the authors' inclusion criteria, which included more than 21,000 subjects who had received the DSM-III-R interview for major depression (Bierut et al., 1999; Kendler, Pedersen, et al., 1995; Kendler & Prescott, 1999; Lyons et al., 1998; McGuffin et al., 1996).

Equating the response thresholds for opposite-sex dizygotic twin pairs provided a poor fit to the data, which is indicative of significant sex differences in the prevalence previously mentioned. Yet, despite significant sex difference in prevalence, the estimates of genetic and environmental variance across sex as well as between clinical and nonclinical samples could be equated. In terms of the liability to major depression, the best-fitting model estimated that additive genetic effects explained 37% of the variance in major depression, while the remaining variance was explained entirely by aspects of the environment that were unshared between siblings. Again, there was no evidence of cultural or shared environmental effects. In other words, there is nothing to suggest that variation in vulnerability to major depression is environmentally transmitted from parents to offspring or influenced by common environmental factors shared within families. Rather, the most salient features of the environment are aspects that are unique to twins, and a proportion of this variance must also include measurement error.

Genetic Epidemiology of Anxiety Disorders

Evidence for a genetic contribution to anxiety disorders is equally compelling and also comes from a variety of study designs (Chantarujikapong et al., 2001; Hettema, Prescott, & Kendler, 2001; Hudson et al., 2003; Kendler, Neale, Kessler, Heath, & Eaves, 1992b, 1992c; Kendler, Walters, et al., 1995; Koenen et al., 2002; Mendlewicz, Papadimitriou, & Wilmotte, 1993; Noyes, Clarkson, Crowe, Yates, & McChesney, 1987; Scherrer et al., 2000; Skre, Onstad, Torgersen, Lygren, & Kringlen, 1993; Sullivan, Kovalenko, York, Prescott, & Kendler, 2003; Torgersen, 1983).

Hettema, Neale, and Kendler (2001) meta-analyzed data from family and twin studies of panic disorder, GAD, phobias, and OCD. Their results based on the twin studies are summarized in Table 11.5. Three twin studies

TABLE 11.5. Summary of Population-Based Twin Studies that Have Investigated the Genetic (A) and Environmental (C/E) Etiology of Anxiety Disorders

| Diagnosis | Sex | Components of variance | | |
		A	C	E
DSM-III-R GAD	Male	.32	—	.68
DSM-III-R GAD	Female	.32	.17	.51
DSM-III-R panic disorder[a]	Female	.37	—	.63
DSM-III-R panic disorder[a]	Male	.43	—	.57
DSM-III social phobia	Female	.30	—	.70
DSM-III agoraphobia	Female	.39	—	.61
DSM-III simple phobia, animal	Female	.32	—	.68
DSM-III simple phobia, situational	Female	—	.27	.73
DSM-III simple phobia, medical	Female	—	.32	.68
DSM-III social phobia	Male	.20	—	.80
DSM-III agoraphobia	Male	.37	—	.63
DSM-III simple phobia, animal	Male	.35	—	.65
DSM-III simple phobia, situational	Male	.25	—	.75
DSM-III simple phobia, medical	Male	.28	—	.72

Note. A, C, and E, proportions of variance attributable to additive genetic, shared environmental, and nonshared environmental effects, respectively. Best-fitting final models only are shown. From Hettema, Neale, and Kendler (2001). Copyright 2001 by the American Psychiatric Association. Adapted by permission.

that included almost 13,000 subjects (Hettema, Prescott, & Kendler, 2001; Scherrer et al., 2000; Skre et al., 1993) met the author's inclusion criteria, but only two of them provided estimates of genetic and environmental heritability. Data from the two larger studies by Scherrer and colleagues (*n* = 6724) and Hettema and colleagues (*n* = 6200) were combined; the GAD definition of 1 month's minimum duration was used. The best-fitting model for GAD estimated that 32% (95% confidence interval = 24–39%) of the variance in GAD was best explained by additive genetic effects, and that the same genes predisposed men and women alike to GAD.

There were important sex differences, and unlike the genetics of major depression, there was evidence that shared environmental or cultural effects contributed to 17% of the variation in male GAD. This was also in contrast to the two twin studies examining panic disorder. Meta-analysis of results based on the two community samples revealed that the model parameters could be combined across sex. Under the best-fitting models, additive genetic effects explained 43% of the variance, while the remaining variance was entirely attributable to aspects of the environment that were unshared between siblings.

Genetic Epidemiology of Personality

Evidence for the genetic contributions to individual differences in adult personality comes from studies of twin pairs reared together (Eaves & Young, 1981; Loehlin & Nichols, 1976; Rose & Kaprio, 1988; Rose, Kaprio, Williams, Viken, & Obremski, 1990; Rose, Koskenvuo, Kaprio, Sarna, & Langinvainio, 1988); separated twin pairs (Bouchard, Lykken, McGue, Segal, & Tellegen, 1990; Pedersen, Plomin, McClearn, & Friberg, 1988; Shields, 1962; Tellegen et al., 1988); nontwin adoptees and their biological and adoptive families (Loehlin, 1982, 1985; Loehlin, Horn, & Willerman, 1981; Scarr, Webber, Weinberg, & Wittig, 1981); and twin pairs reared together and their relatives—parents, siblings, spouses, and adult children (Eaves, 1978; Eaves, Heath, Neale, Hewitt, & Martin, 1998; Lake, Eaves, Maes, Heath, & Martin, 1999; Price, Vandenberg, Iyer, & Williams, 1982). Although a variety of assessment instruments have been used in different studies, a core of Extraversion and Neuroticism items from the Eysenck personality questionnaires (the Maudsley Medical Questionnaire, Maudsley Personality Inventory, Eysenck Personality Inventory, EPQ, and EPQ-R), or equivalent items, have been used in most studies.

Among the numerous reports based on twin data that have examined the heritability of neuroticism and extraversion, nearly all have arrived at genetic estimates in the vicinity of 50% (Eaves & Eysenck, 1975; Eaves et al., 1998, 1999; Fanous et al., 2002; Floderus-Myrhed, Pedersen, & Rasmuson, 1980; Heath et al., 1997; Jang, Livesley, & Vernon, 1996; Jardine, Martin, & Henderson, 1984; Jinks & Fulker, 1970; Kendler, Neale, Kessler, Heath, & Eaves, 1993; Macaskill, Hopper, White, & Hill, 1994; Martin, Eaves, & Fulker, 1979; Pedersen et al., 1988; Rose et al., 1988; Saudino,

Pedersen, Lichtenstein, McClearn, & Plomin, 1997; Viken, Rose, Kaprio, & Koskenvuo, 1994).

More recently, population-based twin studies have begun exploring the genetic epidemiology of other personality dimensions, such as Cloninger's (1994) dimensions of temperament and character, and the five-factor model of personality proposed by Costa and McCrae (1992). Familial aggregation for Cloninger's dimension of harm avoidance, which is closely related to Eysenck's neuroticism, can be almost entirely explained by genetic effects (Cloninger et al., 1998; Heath et al., 1994; Page & Martin, 1998). Despite theoretical debate over the relationship or overlap between Eysenck's dimension of psychoticism and Costa and McCrae's dimensions of openness, agreeableness, and conscientiousness, the two dimensions of extraversion and neuroticism in the Big Five are closely related to the same dimensions in the Eysenckian model (Costa & McCrae, 1995).

Sources of Covariance among Neuroticism, Mood Disorders, and Anxiety Disorders

The phenotypic association between measures of psychological distress and personality, including the evidence for significant heritability in each, raises the question of whether the observed correlations reflect common genetic or environmental diatheses, or whether there are genetic or environmental effects that are unique to each phenotype and condition.

Based on data from the Australian Twin Registry, Jardine and colleagues (1984) examined the covariance between the symptoms of anxiety and depression, using a shortened version of the Delusion Symptoms States Inventory (Bedford & Deary, 1997; Foulds & Bedford, 1975) as well as the Neuroticism scale from the EPQ (Eysenck & Eysenck, 1975). Their results revealed that the phenotypic covariation between the two measures could be best explained by a single genetic factor common to both measures. There was no evidence for genetic factors specific to one measure and having no influence on the other. In a longitudinal design based on 1733 same-sex female twin pairs, Kendler and colleagues (1993b) have estimated that the proportion in the observed correlation between neuroticism and the liability to major depression that could be explained by a shared genetic risk was approximately 70%. In the same study, extraversion was unrelated to lifetime or 1-year prevalence of major depression.

Using the same data from the study by Jardine and colleagues (1984), Kendler and colleagues (1986) showed that the covariation between the symptoms of anxiety and depression is influenced by the same genes, but that the syndromes are differentiated by unique environment stressors. Although the covariance appears to best be explained by a single underlying continuum of liability, Neale and Kendler (1995) have tested a number of alternative but more complex models that could also explain the association between major depression and GAD. These include (1) random multiformity, in which affective status on one disorder abruptly increases risk for the second; (2) extreme multiformity, where only extreme cases have an abruptly increased risk for the second disorder; (3) three independent disorders, in which excess comorbid cases are due to a separate, third disorder; (4) correlated liabilities, where the risk factors for the two disorders correlate; and (5) direct causality, where the liability for one disorder is a cause of the other disorder. When based on a large population-based sample of 2,163 female twins, their results were unfortunately equivocal, with several models providing comparable fits to the data. Less equivocal, however, was the conclusion that comorbidity is best represented by two correlated liability distributions, and that a model of alternative forms of a single dimension of liability provides a better fit when compared to a model of three independent disorders (i.e., major depression, GAD, and major depression with GAD).

Bivariate analyses based on adolescent populations have also supported Kendler and colleagues' (1986) "same genes, different environment" hypothesis (Eley, 1999; Eley & Stevenson, 1999a, 1999b). These findings have also been replicated when based on DSM-III and DSM-III-R diagnoses of major depression and GAD (Kendler, 1996; Kendler et al., 1992c, 1993b; Kendler, Walters, et al., 1995), and altering the diagnostic criteria does not change the overall picture. The genetic covariance between major depression and GAD is consistent, regardless of whether or not the diagnostic hierarchies for GAD include mood or psychotic disorders, or whether the minimum duration of illness is reduced from 6 months to 1 month (Kendler et al., 1992c).

CONCLUSIONS

Identification of the genes predisposing individuals to anxiety disorders and depression would be a major breakthrough in psychiatric genetics and would reset the research agenda both in academic psychiatry and in the pharmaceutical industry. The first step in this process is conducting replicated linkage studies to provide a firm foundation for fine mapping and gene identification. Ultimately, we hope that this work will lead to a more comprehensive understanding of mood and anxiety disorders, and at the same time improve the treatment of some of society's most burdensome diseases.

LOOKING FORWARD

Despite the knowledge that heredity plays an important role in personality, mood, and anxiety, locating the quantitative trait loci for these complex traits and for disorders linked to them has proved difficult, although there have been some successes—for example, Crohn's disease (Low et al., 2004; Peltekova et al., 2004; Stoll et al., 2004), schizophrenia (Berrettini, 2004; O'Donovan, Williams, & Owen, 2003; Riley, 2004), and asthma (Cookson,

2002; Cookson & Moffatt, 2002; Halapi & Hakonarson, 2004; Wills-Karp & Ewart, 2004).

Among a number of genes, those controlling serotonin (5-HT) remain strong candidates. Owens and Nemeroff (1994), in their review, have shown considerable evidence to support the hypothesis that there are significant differences in the serotonergic systems of patients with and without major depression. Based on Lesch and colleagues' (1996) finding that the short allele of the serotonin transporter gene (*5-HTTLPR*) reduces the transcriptional efficiency, Caspi and colleagues (2003) have since reported that variation in this polymorphism moderates the influence of stressful life events on major depression. However, replication has proven difficult (see Gillespie, Whitfield, Williams, Heath, & Martin, 2005). In terms of personality, Sen, Burmeister, and Ghosh (2004) have reported a highly significant association between *5-HTTLPR* and NEO Personality Inventory Neuroticism, but they found no association with TCI/TPQ Harm Avoidance or with any other anxiety-related personality traits, and EPQ Neuroticism was not included in the analyses. Lesch and Canli (Chapter 13, this volume) show how individual differences in anxiety-related personality traits correlate with genetic variations in the *5-HTTLPR* pathway, specifically with a functional C-1019G single-nucleotide polymorphism in the transcriptional control region of the 5-HT_{1A} receptor gene.

Genome-wide linkage analyses of neuroticism with anxiety and depression in England (Fullerton et al., 2003), Iceland (Thorgeirsson et al., 2003), and the United States (Abkevich et al., 2003; Holmans et al., 2004; Zubenko et al., 2003) are beginning to yield converging results. These studies also highlight the need for replication before fine mapping can begin. Other studies using the "extremely discordant and concordant" sibling pairs design are underway in Australia (Kirk et al., 2000), the Netherlands (Boomsma et al., 2000), and England (Sham et al., 2000), and results will soon be appearing. If the examples of schizophrenia and bipolar disorder are guides (see Levinson, Levinson, Segurado, & Lewis, 2003; Lewis et al., 2003; Segurado et al., 2003), truth will emerge not from any one study, but from careful meta-analysis of a large number of these very large studies.

ACKNOWLEDGMENTS

This work was supported by National Institutes of Health Grants No. AA07535, No. AA07728, No. AA10249, and No. AA11998, and by National Health and Medical Research Council (NHMRC, Australia) Grants No. 941177 and No. 971232.

REFERENCES

Abkevich, V., Camp, N. J., Hensel, C. H., Neff, C. D., Russell, D. L., Hughes, D. C., et al. (2003). Predisposition locus for major depression at chromosome 12q22–12q23.2. *American Journal of Human Genetics, 73*(6), 1271–1281.

American Psychiatric Association. (1980). *Diagnostic and statistical manual of mental disorders* (3rd ed.). Washington, DC: Author.

American Psychiatric Association. (1987). *Diagnostic and statistical manual of mental disorders* (3rd ed., rev.). Washington, DC: Author.

American Psychiatric Association. (1994). *Diagnostic and statistical manual of mental disorders* (4th ed.). Washington, DC: Author.

American Psychiatric Association. (2000). *Diagnostic and statistical manual of mental disorders* (4th ed., text rev.). Washington, DC: Author.

Ampollini, P., Marchesi, C., Signifredi, R., & Maggini, C. (1997). Temperament and personality features in panic disorder with or without comorbid mood disorders. *Acta Psychiatrica Scandinavica, 95*(5), 420–423.

Bachorowski, J. A., & Newman, J. P. (1990). Impulsive motor behavior: Effects of personality and goal salience. *Journal of Personality and Social Psychology, 58*(3), 512–518.

Battaglia, M., Przybeck, T. R., Bellodi, L., & Cloninger, C. R. (1996). Temperament dimensions explain the comorbidity of psychiatric disorders. *Comprehensive Psychiatry, 37*(4), 292–298.

Bedford, A., & Deary, I. J. (1997). The personal disturbance scale (DSSI/SAD) development, use and structure. *Personality and Individual Differences, 22*(4), 493–510.

Berlanga, C., Heinze, G., Torres, M., Apiquian, R., & Caballero, A. (1999). Personality and clinical predictors of recurrence of depression. *Psychiatric Services, 50*(3), 376–380.

Berrettini, W. (2004). Bipolar disorder and schizophrenia: Convergent molecular data. *Neuromolecular Medicine, 5*(1), 109–117.

Bierut, L. J., Heath, A. C., Bucholz, K. K., Dinwiddie, S. H., Madden, P. A., Statham, D. J., et al. (1999). Major depressive disorder in a community-based twin sample: Are there different genetic and environmental contributions for men and women? *Archives of General Psychiatry, 56*(6), 557–563.

Blazer, D. G., Kessler, R. C., McGonagle, K. A., & Swartz, M. S. (1994). The prevalence and distribution of major depression in a national community sample: The National Comorbidity Survey. *American Journal of Psychiatry, 151*(7), 979–986.

Boomsma, D. I., Beem, A. L., van den Berg, M., Dolan, C. V., Koopmans, J. R., Vink, J. M., et al. (2000). Netherlands Twin Family Study of Anxious Depression (NETSAD). *Twin Research, 3*(4), 323–334.

Bouchard, T. J., Jr., Lykken, D. T., McGue, M., Segal, N. L., & Tellegen, A. (1990). Sources of human psychological differences: The Minnesota Study of Twins Reared Apart. *Science, 250,* 223–228.

Breslau, N., Schultz, L., & Peterson, E. (1995). Sex differences in depression: A role for preexisting anxiety. *Psychiatry Research, 58*(1), 1–12.

Caspi, A., Sugden, K., Moffitt, T. E., Taylor, A., Craig, I. W., Harrington, H., et al. (2003). Influence of life stress on depression: Moderation by a polymorphism in the 5–HTT gene. *Science, 301,* 386–389.

Chantarujikapong, S. I., Scherrer, J. F., Xian, H., Eisen, S. A., Lyons, M. J., Goldberg, J., et al. (2001). A twin study of generalized anxiety disorder symptoms, panic disorder symptoms and post-traumatic stress disorder in men. *Psychiatry Research, 103*(2–3), 133–145.

Cloninger, C. R. (1986). A unified biosocial theory of personality and its role in the development of anxiety states. *Psychiatric Developments, 4*(3), 167–226.

Cloninger, C. R. (1987). A systematic method for clinical description and classification of personality variants: A proposal. *Archives of General Psychiatry, 44*(6), 573–588.

Cloninger, C. R. (1994). *The Temperament and Character Inventory (TCI): A guide to its development and use.* St. Louis, MO: Centre for Psychobiology of Personality, Washington University.

Cloninger, C. R., Van Eerdewegh, P., Goate, A., Edenberg, H. J., Blangero, J., Hesselbrock, V., et al. (1998). Anxiety proneness linked to epistatic loci in genome scan of human personality traits. *American Journal of Medical Genetics, 81*(4), 313–317.

Cookson, W. (2002). Genetics and genomics of asthma and allergic diseases. *Immunological Reviews, 190,* 195–206.

Cookson, W. O., & Moffatt, M. F. (2002). The genetics of atopic dermatitis. *Current Opinion in Allergy and Clinical Immunology, 2*(5), 383–387.

Corah, N. L. (1971). Neuroticism and extraversion in the MMPI: Empirical validation and exploration. In H. J. Eysenck (Ed.), *Readings in introversion and extraversion: Fields of application* (Vol. 2, pp. 232–240). London: Staples Press.

Costa, P. T., Jr., & McCrae, R. R. (1992). *Revised NEO Personality Inventory (NEO PI-R) and NEO Five-Factor Inventory (NEO FFI) professional manual.* Odessa, FL: Psychological Assessment Resources.

Costa, P. T., Jr., & McCrae, R. R. (1995). Primary traits of Eysenck's P-E-N system: Three- and five-factor solutions. *Journal of Personality and Social Psychology, 69*(2), 308–317.

Cox, B. J., Borger, S. C., Taylor, S., Fuentes, K., & Ross, L. M. (1999). Anxiety sensitivity and the five-factor model of personality. *Behaviour Research and Therapy, 37*(7), 633–641.

Eaves, L. J. (1978). Twins as a basis for the causal analysis of human personality. *Progress in Clinical and Biological Research, 24A,* 151–174.

Eaves, L. J., & Eysenck, H. J. (1975). The nature of extraversion: A genetical analysis. *Journal of Personality and Social Psychology, 32*(1), 102–112.

Eaves, L. J., Eysenck, H. J., & Martin, N. G. (1989). *Genes, culture, and personality: An empirical approach.* London: Academic Press.

Eaves, L. J., Heath, A., Martin, N., Maes, H., Neale, M., Kendler, K., et al. (1999). Comparing the biological and cultural inheritance of personality and social attitudes in the Virginia 30,000 study of twins and their relatives. *Twin Research, 2*(2), 62–80.

Eaves, L. J., Heath, A. C., Neale, M. C., Hewitt, J. K., & Martin, N. G. (1998). Sex differences and non-additivity in the effects of genes on personality. *Twin Research, 1*(3), 131–137.

Eaves, L. J., & Young, P. A. (1981). Genetic theory and personality differences. In R. Lynn (Ed.), *Dimensions of personality* (pp. 129–180). Oxford: Pergamon Press.

Eley, T. C. (1999). Behavioral genetics as a tool for developmental psychology: Anxiety and depression in children and adolescents. *Clinical Child and Family Psychology Review, 2*(1), 21–36.

Eley, T. C., & Stevenson, J. (1999a). Exploring the covariation between anxiety and depression symptoms: A genetic analysis of the effects of age and sex. *Journal of Child Psychology and Psychiatry, 40*(8), 1273–1282.

Eley, T. C., & Stevenson, J. (1999b). Using genetic analyses to clarify the distinction between depressive and anxious symptoms in children. *Journal of Abnormal Child Psychology, 27*(2), 105–114.

Eysenck, H. J. (1953). *The structure of human personality*. London: Methuen.

Eysenck, H. J. (1960). *Behavior therapy and the neuroses*. New York: Pergamon Press.

Eysenck, H. J. (1967). *The biological basis of personality*. Springfield, IL: Thomas.

Eysenck, H. J. (1971a). The differentiation between normal and various neurotic groups on the Maudsley Personality Inventory. In H. J. Eysenck (Ed.), *Readings in introversion and extraversion: Fields of application* (Vol. 2, pp. 220–230). London: Staples Press.

Eysenck, H. J. (1971b). Relation between intelligence and personality. *Perceptual and Motor Skills, 32*, 637–638.

Eysenck, H. J. (1986). A critique of contemporary classification and diagnosis. In T. Millon & G. L. Klerman (Eds.), *Contemporary directions in psychopathology: Toward the DSM-IV* (pp. 73–98). New York: Guilford Press.

Eysenck, H. J. (1991). *Smoking, stress, and personality: Psychosocial factors in the prevention of cancer and coronary heart disease*. New York: Springer-Verlag.

Eysenck, H. J. (1994a). Meta-analysis and its problems. *British Medical Journal, 309*, 789–792.

Eysenck, H. J. (1994b). Normality–abnormality and the three-factor model of personality. In S. Strack & M. Lor (Eds.), *Differentiating normal and abnormal personality* (pp. 3–25). New York: Springer.

Eysenck, H. J. (1995). Meta-analysis of best-evidence synthesis? *Journal of Evaluation in Clinical Practice, 1*(1), 29–36.

Eysenck, H. J., & Eysenck, M. W. (1985). *Personality and individual differences: A natural science approach*. New York: Plenum Press.

Eysenck, H. J., & Eysenck, S. B. G. (1975). *Manual for the Eysenck Personality Questionnaire (Adult and Junior)*. San Diego, CA: Digits.

Eysenck, H. J., & Eysenck, S. B. G. (1983). The cross-cultural study of personality. In C. D. Spielberger & J. N. Butcher (Eds.), *Advances in personality assessment* (Vol. 2, pp. 41–69). Hillsdale, NJ: Erlbaum.

Eysenck, H. J., & Eysenck, S. B. G. (1991). *Manual of the Eysenck Personality Scales (EPS Adult)*. London: Hodder & Stoughton.

Eysenck, H. J., & Rachman, S. (1965). *The causes and cures of neurosis: An introduction to modern behaviour therapy based on learning theory and the principles of conditioning*. London: Routledge & Kegan Paul.

Eysenck, S. B. G., Eysenck, H. J., & Barrett, P. (1985). A revised version of the Psychoticism scale. *Personality and Individual Differences, 6*(1), 21–30.

Falconer, D. S. (1963). Quantitative inheritance. In W. J. Burdette (Ed.), *Methodology in mammalian genetics* (pp. 193–216). San Francisco: Holden-Day.

Fanous, A., Gardner, C. O., Prescott, C. A., Cancro, R., & Kendler, K. S. (2002). Neuroticism, major depression and gender: A population-based twin study. *Psychological Medicine, 32*(4), 719–728.

Floderus-Myrhed, B., Pedersen, N., & Rasmuson, I. (1980). Assessment of heritability for personality, based on a short-form of the Eysenck Personality Inventory: A study of 12,898 twin pairs. *Behavior Genetics, 10*(2), 153–162.

Foulds, G. A., & Bedford, A. (1975). Hierarchy of classes of personal illness. *Psychological Medicine, 5*, 181–202.

Fraser, F. C. (1976). The multifactorial/threshold concept: Uses and misuses. *Teratology, 14*(3), 267–280.

Freeman, E. W., Schweizer, E., & Rickels, K. (1995). Personality factors in women with premenstrual syndrome. *Psychosomatic Medicine, 57*(5), 453–459.

Fullerton, J., Cubin, M., Tiwari, H., Wang, C., Bomhra, A., Davidson, S., et al. (2003). Linkage analysis of extremely discordant and concordant sibling pairs identifies quantitative-trait loci that influence variation in the human personality trait neuroticism. *American Journal of Human Genetics, 72*(4), 879–890.

Gershuny, B. S., & Sher, K. J. (1998). The relation between personality and anxiety: Findings from a 3-year prospective study. *Journal of Abnormal Psychology, 107*(2), 252–262.

Gillespie, N. A., Evans, D. E., Wright, M. M., & Martin, N. G. (2004). Genetic simplex modeling of Eysenck's dimensions of personality in a sample of young Australian twins. *Twin Research, 7*, 637–648.

Gillespie, N. A., Whitfield, J. B., Williams, B., Heath, A. C., & Martin, N. G. (2005). The relationship between stressful life events, the serotonin transporter (5–HTTLPR) genotype and major depression. *Psychological Medicine, 35*, 101–111.

Gormley, N., O'Leary, D., & Costello, F. (1999). First admissions for depression: Is the 'no-treatment interval' a critical predictor of time to remission? *Journal of Affective Disorders, 54*(1–2), 49–54.

Gray, J. A. (1970). The psychophysiological basis of introversion–extraversion. *Behaviour Research and Therapy, 8*, 249–266.

Gray, J. A. (1986). Discussion arising from: Cloninger, C. R. A unified biosocial theory of personality and its role in the development of anxiety states. *Psychiatric Developments, 3*, 167–226.

Halapi, E., & Hakonarson, H. (2004). Recent development in genomic and proteomic research for asthma. *Current Opinion in Pulmonary Medicine, 10*(1), 22–30.

Hansenne, M., Pitchot, W., Gonzalez Moreno, A., Machurot, P. Y., & Ansseau, M. (1998). The Tridimensional Personality Questionnaire (TPQ) and depression. *European Psychiatry, 13*(2), 101–103.

Hassanyeh, F., Eccleston, D., & Davison, K. (1981). Rating of anxiety, depression and vulnerability: The development of a new rating scale (the Anxiety and Depression Scale). *Acta Psychiatrica Scandinavica, 64*(4), 301–313.

Heath, A. C., Bucholz, K. K., Madden, P. A., Dinwiddie, S. H., Slutske, W. S., Bierut, L. J., et al. (1997). Genetic and environmental contributions to alcohol dependence risk in a national twin sample: Consistency of findings in women and men. *Psychological Medicine, 27*(6), 1381–1396.

Heath, A. C., Cloninger, C. R., & Martin, N. G. (1994). Testing a model for the genetic structure of personality: A comparison of the personality systems of Cloninger and Eysenck. *Journal of Personality and Social Psychology, 66*(4), 762–775.

Hettema, J. M., Neale, M. C., & Kendler, K. S. (2001). A review and meta-analysis of the genetic epidemiology of anxiety disorders. *American Journal of Psychiatry, 158*(10), 1568–1578.

Holmans, P., Zubenko, G. S., Crowe, R. R., DePaulo, J. R., Jr., Scheftner, W. A., Weissman, M. M., et al. (2004). Genomewide significant linkage to recurrent, early-onset major depressive disorder on chromosome 15q. *American Journal of Human Genetics, 74*(6), 1154–1167.

Hudson, J. I., Mangweth, B., Pope, H. G., Jr., De Col, C., Hausmann, A., Gutweniger, S., et al. (2003). Family study of affective spectrum disorder. *Archives of General Psychiatry, 60*(2), 170–177.

Jang, K. L., Livesley, W. J., & Vernon, P. A. (1996). Heritability of the Big Five personality dimensions and their facets: A twin study. *Journal of Personality, 64*(3), 577–591.

Jardine, R., Martin, N. G., & Henderson, A. S. (1984). Genetic covariation between neuroticism and the symptoms of anxiety and depression. *Genetic Epidemiology, 1*(2), 89–107.

Jinks, J. L., & Fulker, D. W. (1970). Comparison of the biometrical, genetical, MAVA, and classical approaches to the analysis of human behavior. *Psychological Bulletin, 73*(5), 311–349.

Kendler, K. S. (1996). Major depression and generalised anxiety disorder: Same genes, (partly) different environments—revisited. *British Journal of Psychiatry Supplements, 30*, 68–75.

Kendler, K. S., Gardner, C. O., & Prescott, C. A. (1998). A population-based twin study of self-esteem and gender. *Psychological Medicine, 28*(6), 1403–1409.

Kendler, K. S., Gardner, C. O., & Prescott, C. A. (2002). Toward a comprehensive developmental model for major depression in women. *American Journal of Psychiatry, 159*(7), 1133–1145.

Kendler, K. S., Heath, A. C., Martin, N. G., & Eaves, L. J. (1986). Symptoms of anxiety and depression in a volunteer twin population: The etiologic role of genetic and environmental factors. *Archives of General Psychiatry, 43*(3), 213–221.

Kendler, K. S., Heath, A. C., Martin, N. G., & Eaves, L. J. (1987). Symptoms of anxiety and symptoms of depression: Same genes, different environments? *Archives of General Psychiatry, 44*(5), 451–457.

Kendler, K. S., Karkowski, L. M., Corey, L. A., & Neale, M. C. (1998). Longitudinal population-based twin study of retrospectively reported premenstrual symptoms and lifetime major depression. *American Journal of Psychiatry, 155*(9), 1234–1240.

Kendler, K. S., Kessler, R. C., Neale, M. C., Heath, A. C., & Eaves, L. J. (1993). The prediction of major depression in women: Toward an integrated etiologic model. *American Journal of Psychiatry, 150*(8), 1139–1148.

Kendler, K. S., Neale, M. C., Kessler, R. C., Heath, A. C., & Eaves, L. J. (1992a). Familial influences on the clinical characteristics of major depression: A twin study. *Acta Psychiatrica Scandinavica, 86*(5), 371–378.

Kendler, K. S., Neale, M. C., Kessler, R. C., Heath, A. C., & Eaves, L. J. (1992b). Generalized anxiety disorder in women: A population-based twin study. *Archives of General Psychiatry, 49*(4), 267–272.

Kendler, K. S., Neale, M. C., Kessler, R. C., Heath, A. C., & Eaves, L. J. (1992c). Major depression and generalized anxiety disorder: Same genes, (partly) different environments? *Archives of General Psychiatry, 49*(9), 716–722.

Kendler, K. S., Neale, M. C., Kessler, R. C., Heath, A. C., & Eaves, L. J. (1992d). A population-based twin study of major depression in women: The impact of varying definitions of illness. *Archives of General Psychiatry, 49*(4), 257–266.

Kendler, K. S., Neale, M. C., Kessler, R. C., Heath, A. C., & Eaves, L. J. (1993a). The lifetime history of major depression in women: Reliability of diagnosis and heritability. *Archives of General Psychiatry, 50*(11), 863–870.

Kendler, K. S., Neale, M. C., Kessler, R. C., Heath, A. C., & Eaves, L. J. (1993b). A longitudinal twin study of personality and major depression in women. *Archives of General Psychiatry, 50*(11), 853–862.

Kendler, K. S., Pedersen, N. L., Johnson, L., Neale, M. C., & Mathe, A. A. (1993). A pilot Swedish twin study of affective illness, including hospital- and population-ascertained subsamples. *Archives of General Psychiatry, 50*(9), 699–700.

Kendler, K. S., Pedersen, N. L., Neale, M. C., & Mathe, A. A. (1995). A pilot Swedish twin study of affective illness including hospital- and population-ascertained subsamples: Results of model fitting. *Behavior Genetics, 25*(3), 217–232.

Kendler, K. S., & Prescott, C. A. (1999). A population-based twin study of lifetime major depression in men and women. *Archives of General Psychiatry, 56*(1), 39–44.

Kendler, K. S., Walters, E. E., Neale, M. C., Kessler, R. C., Heath, A. C., & Eaves, L. J. (1995). The structure of the genetic and environmental risk factors for six major psychiatric disorders in women: Phobia, generalized anxiety disorder, panic disorder, bulimia, major depression, and alcoholism. *Archives of General Psychiatry, 52*(5), 374–383.

Kendler, K. S., Walters, E. E., Truett, K. R., Heath, A. C., Neale, M. C., Martin, N. G., et al. (1994). Sources of individual differences in depressive symptoms: Analysis of two samples of twins and their families. *American Journal of Psychiatry, 151*(11), 1605–1614.

Kerr, T. A., Schapira, K., Roth, M., & Garside, R. F. (1970). The relationship between the Maudsley Personality Inventory and the course of affective disorders. *British Journal of Psychiatry, 116*, 11–19.

Kessler, R. C., McGonagle, K. A., Zhao, S., Nelson, C. B., Hughes, M., Eshleman, S., et al. (1994). Lifetime and 12–month prevalence of DSM-III-R psychiatric disorders in the United States: Results from the National Comorbidity Survey. *Archives of General Psychiatry, 51*(1), 8–19.

Kirk, K. M., Birley, A. J., Statham, D. J., Haddon, B., Lake, R. I., Andrews, J. G., et al. (2000). Anxiety and depression in twin and sib pairs extremely discordant and concordant for neuroticism: Prodromus to a linkage study. *Twin Research, 3*(4), 299–309.

Kirk, S. A., & Kutchins, H. (1992). *The selling of DSM: The rhetoric of science in psychiatry*. New York: Aldine de Gruyter.

Koenen, K. C., Harley, R., Lyons, M. J., Wolfe, J., Simpson, J. C., Goldberg, J., et al. (2002). A twin registry study of familial and individual risk factors for trauma exposure and posttraumatic stress disorder. *Journal of Nervous and Mental Disease, 190*(4), 209–218.

Lake, R. I. E., Eaves, L. J., Maes, H. M., Heath, A. C., & Martin, N. G. (1999). Further evidence against the environmental transmission of individual differences in neuroticism from a collaborative study of 45850 twins and relatives on two continents. *Behavior Genetics, 30*, 223–233.

Larsen, R. J., & Ketelaar, T. (1991). Personality and susceptibility to positive and negative emotional states. *Journal of Personality and Social Psychology, 61*(1), 132–140.

Lesch, K. P., Bengel, D., Heils, A., Sabol, S. Z., Greenberg, B. D., Petri, S., et al. (1996). Association of anxiety-related traits with a polymorphism in the serotonin transporter gene regulatory region. *Science, 274*, 1527–1531.

Levinson, D. F., Levinson, M. D., Segurado, R., & Lewis, C. M. (2003). Genome scan meta-analysis of schizophrenia and bipolar disorder: Part I. Methods and power analysis. *American Journal of Human Genetics, 73*(1), 17–33.

Lewis, C. M., Levinson, D. F., Wise, L. H., DeLisi, L. E., Straub, R. E., Hovatta, I., et al. (2003). Genome scan meta-analysis of schizophrenia and bipolar disorder: Part II. Schizophrenia. *American Journal of Human Genetics, 73*(1), 34–48.

Loehlin, J. C. (1982). Are personality traits differentially heritable? *Behavior Genetics, 12*(4), 417–428.

Loehlin, J. C. (1985). Fitting heredity–environment models jointly to twin and adoption data from the California Psychological Inventory. *Behavior Genetics, 15*(3), 199–221.

Loehlin, J. C., Horn, J. M., & Willerman, L. (1981). Personality resemblance in adoptive families. *Behavior Genetics, 11*(4), 309–330.

Loehlin, J. C., & Nichols, R. C. (1976). *Heredity, environment and personality: A study of 850 sets of twins.* Austin: University of Texas Press.

Low, J. H., Williams, F. A., Yang, X., Cullen, S., Colley, J., Ling, K. L., et al. (2004). Inflammatory bowel disease is linked to 19p13 and associated with ICAM-1. *Inflammatory Bowel Disease, 10*(3), 173–181.

Lyons, M. J., Eisen, S. A., Goldberg, J., True, W., Lin, N., Meyer, J. M., et al. (1998). A registry-based twin study of depression in men. *Archives of General Psychiatry, 55*(5), 468–472.

Macaskill, G. T., Hopper, J. L., White, V., & Hill, D. J. (1994). Genetic and environmental variation in Eysenck Personality Questionnaire scales measured on Australian adolescent twins. *Behavior Genetics, 24*(6), 481–491.

Maier, W., Lichtermann, D., Minges, J., & Heun, R. (1992). Personality traits in subjects at risk for unipolar major depression: A family study perspective. *Journal of Affective Disorders, 24*(3), 153–163.

Martin, N. G., Eaves, L. J., & Fulker, D. W. (1979). The genetical relationship of impulsiveness and sensation seeking to Eysenck's personality dimensions. *Acta Geneticae Medicae et Gemellologiae (Roma), 28*(3), 197–210.

McGuffin, P., Katz, R., Watkins, S., & Rutherford, J. (1996). A hospital-based twin register of the heritability of DSM-IV unipolar depression. *Archives of General Psychiatry, 53*(2), 129–136.

Mendlewicz, J., Papadimitriou, G. N., & Wilmotte, J. (1993). Family study of panic disorder: Comparison with generalized anxiety disorder, major depression and normal subjects. *Psychiatric Genetics, 3*, 73–78.

Millon, T. (1991). Classification in psychopathology: Rationale, alternatives and standards. *Journal of Abnormal Psychology, 100*, 245–261.

Neale, M. C., Eaves, L. J., & Kendler, K. S. (1994). The power of the classical twin study to resolve variation in threshold traits. *Behavior Genetics, 24*(3), 239–258.

Neale, M. C., & Kendler, K. S. (1995). Models of comorbidity for multifactorial disorders. *American Journal of Human Genetics, 57*(4), 935–953.

Nelson, E. C., Cloninger, C. R., Przybeck, T. R., & Csernansky, J. G. (1996). Platelet serotonergic markers and Tridimensional Personality Questionnaire measures in a clinical sample. *Biological Psychiatry, 40*(4), 271–278.

Newman, S. C., Bland, R. C., & Orn, H. (1988). Morbidity risk of psychiatric disorders. *Acta Psychiatrica Scandinavica, 338*(Suppl.), 50–56.

Noyes, R., Jr., Clarkson, C., Crowe, R. R., Yates, W. R., & McChesney, C. M. (1987). A family study of generalized anxiety disorder. *American Journal of Psychiatry, 144*(8), 1019–1024.

O'Donovan, M. C., Williams, N. M., & Owen, M. J. (2003). Recent advances in the genetics of schizophrenia. *Human Molecular Genetics, 12*(Spec. No. 2), R125–R133.

Owens, M. J., & Nemeroff, C. B. (1994). Role of serotonin in the pathophysiology of depression: Focus on the serotonin transporter. *Clinical Chemistry, 40*(2), 288–295.

Page, A. C., & Martin, N. G. (1998). Testing a genetic structure of blood–injury–injection fears. *American Journal of Medical Genetics, 81*(5), 377–384.

Parker, G., & Hadzi-Pavlovic, D. (2001). Is any female preponderance in depression secondary to a primary female preponderance in anxiety disorders? *Acta Psychiatrica Scandinavica, 103*(4), 252–256.

Pedersen, N. L., Plomin, R., McClearn, G. E., & Friberg, L. (1988). Neuroticism, extraversion, and related traits in adult twins reared apart and reared together. *Journal of Personality and Social Psychology, 55*(6), 950–957.

Peltekova, V. D., Wintle, R. F., Rubin, L. A., Amos, C. I., Huang, Q., Gu, X., et al. (2004). Functional variants of OCTN cation transporter genes are associated with Crohn disease. *Nature Genetics, 36*(5), 471–475.

Price, R. A., Vandenberg, S. G., Iyer, H., & Williams, J. S. (1982). Components of variation in normal personality. *Journal of Personality and Social Psychology, 42*, 328–340.

Riley, B. (2004). Linkage studies of schizophrenia. *Neurotoxicity Research, 6*(1), 17–34.

Roberts, S. B., & Kendler, K. S. (1999). Neuroticism and self-esteem as indices of the vulnerability to major depression in women. *Psychological Medicine, 29*(5), 1101–1109.

Rose, R. J., & Kaprio, J. (1988). Frequency of social contact and intrapair resemblance of adult monozygotic cotwins—or does shared experience influence personality after all? *Behavior Genetics, 18*(3), 309–328.

Rose, R. J., Kaprio, J., Williams, C. J., Viken, R., & Obremski, K. (1990). Social contact and sibling similarity: Facts, issues, and red herrings. *Behavior Genetics, 20*(6), 763–778.

Rose, R. J., Koskenvuo, M., Kaprio, J., Sarna, S., & Langinvainio, H. (1988). Shared genes, shared experiences, and similarity of personality: Data from 14,288 adult Finnish co-twins. *Journal of Personality and Social Psychology, 54*(1), 161–171.

Sanderson, W. C., Beck, A. T., & Beck, J. (1990). Syndrome comorbidity in patients with major depression or dysthymia: Prevalence and temporal relationships. *American Journal of Psychiatry, 147*(8), 1025–1028.

Saudino, K. J., Pedersen, N. L., Lichtenstein, P., McClearn, G. E., & Plomin, R. (1997). Can personality explain genetic influences on life events? *Journal of Personality and Social Psychology, 72*(1), 196–206.

Saviotti, F. M., Grandi, S., Savron, G., Ermentini, R., Bartolucci, G., Conti, S., et al. (1991). Characterological traits of recovered patients with panic disorder and agoraphobia. *Journal of Affective Disorders, 23*(3), 113–117.

Scarr, S., Webber, P. L., Weinberg, R. A., & Wittig, M. A. (1981). Personality resemblance among adolescents and their parents in biologically related and adoptive families. *Progress in Clinical and Biological Research, 69*(Pt. B), 99–120.

Scherrer, J. F., True, W. R., Xian, H., Lyons, M. J., Eisen, S. A., Goldberg, J., et al. (2000). Evidence for genetic influences common and specific to symptoms of generalized anxiety and panic. *Journal of Affective Disorders, 57*(1–3), 25–35.

Segurado, R., Detera-Wadleigh, S. D., Levinson, D. F., Lewis, C. M., Gill, M., Nurnberger, J. I., Jr., et al. (2003). Genome scan meta-analysis of schizophrenia and bipolar disorder: Part III. Bipolar disorder. *American Journal of Human Genetics, 73*(1), 49–62.

Sen, S., Burmeister, M., & Ghosh, D. (2004). Meta-analysis of the association between a serotonin transporter promoter polymorphism (5–HTTLPR) and anxiety-related personality traits. *American Journal of Medical Genetics, 127B*(1), 85–89.

Sham, P. C., Sterne, A., Purcell, S., Cherny, S., Webster, M., Rijsdijk, F., et al. (2000). GENESiS: Creating a composite index of the vulnerability to anxiety and depression in a community-based sample of siblings. *Twin Research, 3*(4), 316–322.

Shields, J. (1962). *Monozygotic twins.* Oxford: Oxford University Press.

Silberg, J., Pickles, A., Rutter, M., Hewitt, J., Simonoff, E., Maes, H., et al. (1999). The influence of genetic factors and life stress on depression among adolescent girls. *Archives of General Psychiatry, 56*(3), 225–232.

Skre, I., Onstad, S., Torgersen, S., Lygren, S., & Kringlen, E. (1993). A twin study of DSM-III-R anxiety disorders. *Acta Psychiatrica Scandinavica, 88*(2), 85–92.

Slutske, W. S., Heath, A. C., Madden, P. A. F., Bucholz, K. K., Dinwiddie, S. H., Dunne, M. P., et al. (1998). *Personality and the common genetic risk for conduct disorder and alcohol dependence.* Paper presented at the 28th annual meeting of the Behavior Genetics Association, Stockholm, Sweden.

Starcevic, V., Uhlenhuth, E. H., Fallon, S., & Pathak, D. (1996). Personality dimensions in panic disorder and generalized anxiety disorder. *Journal of Affective Disorders, 37*(2–3), 75–79.

Stoll, M., Corneliussen, B., Costello, C. M., Waetzig, G. H., Mellgard, B., Koch, W. A., et al. (2004). Genetic variation in DLG5 is associated with inflammatory bowel disease. *Nature Genetics, 36*(5), 476–480.

Strakowski, S. M., Dunayevich, E., Keck, P. E., Jr., & McElroy, S. L. (1995). Affective state dependence of the Tridimensional Personality Questionnaire. *Psychiatry Research, 57*(3), 209–214.

Strakowski, S. M., Faedda, G. L., Tohen, M., Goodwin, D. C., & Stoll, A. L. (1992). Possible affective-state dependence of the Tridimensional Personality Questionnaire in first-episode psychosis. *Psychiatry Research, 41*(3), 215–226.

Sullivan, P. F., Kovalenko, P., York, T. P., Prescott, C. A., & Kendler, K. S. (2003). Fatigue in a community sample of twins. *Psychological Medicine, 33*(2), 263–281.

Sullivan, P. F., Neale, M. C., & Kendler, K. S. (2000). Genetic epidemiology of major depression: Review and meta-analysis. *American Journal of Psychiatry, 157*(10), 1552–1562.

Tambs, K. (1991). Transmission of symptoms of anxiety and depression in nuclear families. *Journal of Affective Disorders, 21*(2), 117–126.

Tellegen, A., Lykken, D. T., Bouchard, T. J., Jr., Wilcox, K. J., Segal, N. L., & Rich, S. (1988). Personality similarity in twins reared apart and together. *Journal of Personality and Social Psychology, 54*(6), 1031–1039.

Thorgeirsson, T. E., Oskarsson, H., Desnica, N., Kostic, J. P., Stefansson, J. G., Kolbeinsson, H., et al. (2003). Anxiety with panic disorder linked to chromosome 9q in Iceland. *American Journal of Human Genetics, 72*(5), 1221–1230.

Torgersen, S. (1983). Genetic factors in anxiety disorders. *Archives of General Psychiatry, 40*(10), 1085–1089.

Treloar, S. A., Martin, N. G., Bucholz, K. K., Madden, P. A., & Heath, A. C. (1999).

Genetic influences on post-natal depressive symptoms: Findings from an Australian twin sample. *Psychological Medicine, 29*(3), 645–654.

Viken, R. J., Rose, R. J., Kaprio, J., & Koskenvuo, M. (1994). A developmental genetic analysis of adult personality: Extraversion and neuroticism from 18 to 59 years of age. *Journal of Personality and Social Psychology, 66*(4), 722–730.

Wills-Karp, M., & Ewart, S. L. (2004). Time to draw breath: Asthma-susceptibility genes are identified. *Nature Reviews Genetics, 5*(5), 376–387.

Yoshino, A., Kato, M., Takeuchi, M., Ono, Y., & Kitamura, T. (1994). Examination of the tridimensional personality hypothesis of alcoholism using empirically multivariate typology. *Clinical and Experimental Research, 18*(5), 1121–1124.

Zubenko, G. S., Maher, B., Hughes, H. B., III, Zubenko, W. N., Stiffler, J. S., Kaplan, B. B., et al. (2003). Genome-wide linkage survey for genetic loci that influence the development of depressive disorders in families with recurrent, early-onset, major depression. *American Journal of Medical Genetics, 123B*(1), 1–18.

Zuckerman, M. (1999). *Vulnerability to psychopathology: A biosocial model.* Washington, DC: American Psychological Association.

Zuckerman, M., & Cloninger, C. R. (1996). Relationships between Cloninger's, Zuckerman's, and Eysenck's dimensions of personality. *Personality and Individual Differences, 21*(2), 283–285.

Zuckerman, M., Kuhlman, D. M., Joireman, J., Teta, P., & Kraft, M. (1988). What lies beyond E and N?: Factor analyses of scales believed to measure basic dimensions of personality. *Journal of Personality and Social Psychology, 54*, 96–107.

12

The Association of Personality with Anxious and Depressive Psychopathology

Christel M. Middeldorp, Danielle C. Cath, Mireille van den Berg, A. Leo Beem, Richard van Dyck, and Dorret I. Boomsma

The questions of to what extent and in which ways personality dimensions are associated with anxious and depressive psychopathology are still unresolved. Most research has focused on "neuroticism" and "extraversion," or traits related to these personality dimensions. Neuroticism was originally described as reflecting emotional instability and anxiety proneness (Eysenck & Rachman, 1965). This trait was hypothesized to be related to the "visceral brain," more often called the "limbic system," which was supposed to regulate emotional expression and to control autonomic responses. According to Eysenck (1967), neurotic subjects are characterized by higher levels of autonomic activity (or reactivity), mediated by the visceral brain.

Extraversion was described as reflecting sociability, liveliness, impulsivity, and the level of ease and pleasure felt in the company of others (Eysenck & Rachman, 1965). The last-mentioned trait was theorized to be related to the ascending reticular activating system, with a higher level of arousal in introverts and a higher level of inhibition in extraverts (Eysenck, 1967). A wide range of electrophysiological and other psychophysiological studies confirmed this hypothesis (Stelmack, 1981).

Cloninger (1986) proposed that "harm avoidance," an anxiety-related trait, is positioned between neuroticism and extraversion. This positioning was confirmed by a strong positive correlation with neuroticism ($r = .63$) and a strong negative correlation with extraversion ($r = -.55$), as measured with the Eysenck Personality Questionnaire (EPQ) (see Heath, Cloninger, & Martin, 1994).

Two dimensions that are related to neuroticism and extraversion are "positive affectivity" and "negative affectivity." Negative affectivity is a general dimension of subjective distress and unpleasurable engagement, whereas positive affectivity reflects the extent to which a person feels enthusiastic, active, and alert (Watson, Clark, & Tellegen, 1988). There is general consensus that individuals scoring high on neuroticism exhibit negative affectivity (Shankman & Klein, 2003). Therefore, "negative affectivity" and "neuroticism" are often used interchangeably in the literature. However, this does not hold for the relation between extraversion and positive affectivity. Since extraversion does not only measure positive affectivity, but also impulsivity and sociability, this dimension encompasses more than positive affectivity only (Clark, Watson, & Mineka, 1994).

A further personality trait is "sensation seeking," which was considered to be a measure of the impulsivity and sociability parts of Eysenck's broader extraversion dimension and to be independent of neuroticism (Zuckerman, 1979). Zuckerman (1979) defined this trait as "the need for varied, novel, and complex sensations and experiences and the willingness to take physical and social risks for the sake of such experience" (p. 10). Sensation seeking was also supposed to be related to an individual's level of arousal. Different studies investigating the relation between sensation seeking and Eysenck's personality dimensions found correlations between extraversion and sensation seeking from .09 to .42 in men and from .11 to .44 in women (Zuckerman, 1979). The correlations of neuroticism and sensation seeking were nonsignificant (Zuckerman, 1979).

Several hypotheses regarding the relationships of these personality dimensions to anxious and/or depressive psychopathology have been put forward. Eysenck and Rachman (1965) hypothesized that subjects with symptoms of anxiety and/or depression would be high in neuroticism and low in extraversion. Gray (1982) suggested that these two dimensions could be combined into one trait, reflecting the level of activity in the behavioral inhibition system and indicating a person's vulnerability for anxiety and depression. This led to the harm avoidance dimension (Cloninger, 1986). Clark and Watson (1991) developed the tripartite model, which agrees with Eysenck's model that negative affectivity is a risk factor for both anxiety and depression. However, according to the tripartite model, low positive affectivity is related to depression only, whereas autonomic hyperarousal (e.g., racing heart, trembling, shortness of breath, dizziness) is related to anxiety. Finally, sensation seeking was hypothesized to be unrelated to depression and anxiety disorders, since it is not associated with neuroticism (Zuckerman, 1979).

Research so far has confirmed that negative affectivity/neuroticism is related to both depression and anxiety (for reviews, see Bienvenu & Stein, 2003; Clark et al., 1994; Shankman & Klein, 2003). This also applies to harm avoidance (Brown, Svrakic, Przybeck, & Cloninger, 1992; Cloninger, 2002;

Shankman & Klein, 2003). Results have been contradictory concerning the association between low positive affectivity/extraversion and depression or anxiety disorders (see Shankman & Klein, 2003, for a review). A possible source of confounding, which is not taken into account in most studies, is the highly prevalent comorbidity between anxiety and depression. If, for example, high neuroticism is a risk factor for both anxiety and depression, but low extraversion only for depression (as supposed in the tripartite model), it may be hypothesized that subjects with pure anxiety disorders are only high in neuroticism, while subjects with both anxiety and depression are low in extraversion as well. As a consequence, whether or not a study focusing on anxiety observes that low extraversion is related to anxiety will depend on the number of subjects with comorbid anxiety and depression. This is just one example of how comorbidity may modify the association between personality and psychopathology.

Several approaches can be used to take comorbidity into account when investigators are examining the association between personality and psychopathology. One way is to study subjects with the pure disorders separately from the subjects with the comorbid condition. Another possibility is to compare the mean scores on personality dimensions of normal controls and affected subjects while correcting for comorbid disease. For example, in an analysis of variance (ANOVA) or a regression analysis, all disorders can be included in one model. Finally, factor analyses or structural equation modeling can be used to investigate the etiology of the correlation between measures of personality and anxious or depressive psychopathology.

In all studies taking these approaches, neuroticism was related to major depression and anxiety disorders (Bienvenu et al., 2001; Brown, Chorpita, & Barlow, 1998; de Graaf, Bijl, ten Have, Beekman, & Vollebergh, 2004; Johnson, Turner, & Iwata, 2003; Krueger, McGue, & Iacono, 2001; Trull & Sher, 1994). In addition, all studies except one (Johnson et al., 2003) found a relation between low extraversion and one or more of the anxiety disorders, although results were not always consistent on the level of specific diagnoses (Bienvenu et al., 2001; Brown et al., 1998; Trull & Sher, 1994). Results were contradictory regarding the relation between low extraversion and major depression. Brown and colleagues (1998) and Trull and Sher (1994) did find an association, whereas Bienvenu and colleagues (2001) and Johnson and colleagues (2003) did not. Krueger and colleagues (2001) found that internalization—a factor on which depression and anxiety disorders loaded—correlated negatively with positive emotionality in women, but not in men. These studies also revealed that comorbidity between anxiety and depression is associated with neuroticism (Andrews, Slade, & Issakidis, 2002; Bienvenu et al., 2001; de Graaf et al., 2004) and, to a limited extent, with low extraversion (Bienvenu et al., 2001). Andrews and colleagues (2002) even found a linear relationship between neuroticism and the number of disorders. To summarize, studies that take comorbidity into account find in general that high neuroticism and low extraversion are related to depression as well as anxiety; this is in agreement with Eysenck's theory and in contradiction to the tripartite model.

The association between sensation seeking and anxious or depressive psychopathology has been studied far less often, and results are contradictory. To our knowledge, no previous studies have investigated this relation while taking comorbidity into account. Zuckerman (1979) concluded that although there is no association between sensation seeking and depression or general trait anxiety, sensation seeking could be negatively related to fearfulness of more specific types. However, in two recent studies, low levels of sensation seeking appeared to be related to major depression (Carton, Morand, Bungenera, & Jouvent, 1995; Farmer et al., 2001).

In this chapter, we describe two studies that investigated the relationship between the personality dimensions of neuroticism, extraversion, and sensation seeking on the one hand, and anxiety and depression on the other. In both studies, comorbidity was taken into account. The goals of these studies were to test whether Eysenck's model or the tripartite model best describes the data, and to test the extent to which sensation seeking is related to anxious and depressive psychopathology. The latter issue is interesting, because Zuckerman (1979) based his hypothesis that sensation seeking is not associated to anxiety and depression on the absence of a correlation between neuroticism and sensation seeking. However, as he also acknowledged, sensation seeking is correlated with extraversion. Since low extraversion may be related to anxiety and depression, this could be the case for sensation seeking as well.

The first study was based on self-report questionnaire data of personality and psychopathology from twins and their siblings registered in the Netherlands Twin Register (NTR). In 1991, 1993, and 1997, a survey was sent to twins; in 1997, their siblings were also approached. These three waves were combined for the analyses, in order to obtain one of the largest samples so far used to investigate the association of neuroticism, extraversion, and sensation seeking with symptoms of anxiety and depression. Correlations were calculated within and between the personality and psychopathology dimensions. Furthermore, to take comorbidity into account, subjects were divided into cases and normal controls on the measures of anxiety and depression, with the 95th percentile used as a cutoff score. Next, the mean scores on the personality measures of the pure cases and the comorbid cases were compared with the means of the normal controls.

In the second study, data from a diagnostic psychiatric interview administered to a selected sample of twins and their siblings were analyzed. Scores on neuroticism, extraversion, and sensation seeking were compared between subjects without psychopathology and subjects with depression or an anxiety disorder defined according to the *Diagnostic and Statistical Manual of Mental Disorders*, fouth edition (DSM-IV; American Psychiatric Association, 1994). This analysis was performed while correcting for comorbidity, by comparing the means between normal controls and affected subjects with all disorders included in the same model. Finally, mean personality scores were compared between subjects with zero, one, two, or three or more disorders. The two studies are described separately, followed by an overall discussion.

STUDY I: THE ASSOCIATION OF PERSONALITY WITH ANXIOUS AND DEPRESSIVE PSYCHOPATHOLOGY MEASURED DIMENSIONALLY

The first study was part of an ongoing longitudinal survey study of the NTR, which has assessed families with adolescent and adult twins roughly every 2 years since 1991. Sample selection and response rates are described in detail in Boomsma and colleagues (2002). Each survey was sent to the twins and additional family members—namely, parents in 1991 and 1993, parents and siblings in 1995, and siblings in 1997. Each survey, with the exception of the 1995 wave, collected information on personality and psychopathology. For this study, data from twins and siblings from the 1991, 1993, and 1997 surveys were used. In these years, questionnaires were returned at least once by 2,825 male and 3,636 female twins, and 668 brothers and 840 sisters, from 3,349 families. Forty-two percent of the subjects participated two or three times, and 58% participated once. The mean ages of the subjects at the time of the three waves were 18, 20, and 27 years, with standard deviations 2.3, 8.4, and 10.5 years, respectively.

On all three occasions, sensation seeking was measured with the Dutch translation of the Zuckerman Sensation Seeking Scale (Feij & van Zuilen, 1984; Zuckerman, 1971). Neuroticism, extraversion, and somatic anxiety were measured with the Amsterdamse Biografische Vragenlijst (ABV; Wilde, 1970). The ABV Neuroticism and Extraversion scales are very similar to those of the EPQ (Eysenck & Eysenck, 1964). Somatic anxiety is measured with items such as "Do you often have a headache?" and "Do you have heart palpitations?" Anxiety was measured with the Dutch translation of the Spielberger State–Trait Anxiety Inventory—Trait version (STAI; Spielberger, Gorsuch, & Lushene, 1970; Van der Ploeg, Defares, & Spielberger, 1979). Depression was measured with two different inventories in the three surveys. In 1991, the Anxious/Depressed symptom scale of the Young Adult Self-Report (YASR; Achenbach, 1990; Verhulst, van Ende, & Koot, 1997) was used; in 1993, the 13-item version of the Beck Depression Inventory (BDI; Beck, Rial, & Rickels, 1974) was used; and in 1997, both instruments were used.

For all personality and psychopathology measures, normalized scores were calculated according to Blom's (1958) methods, so that we could compare the scores across scales and time. These scores were averaged over time when a subject had participated more than once in the survey study. Figures 12.1a to 12.1g show the distributions of the mean normalized scores for neu-

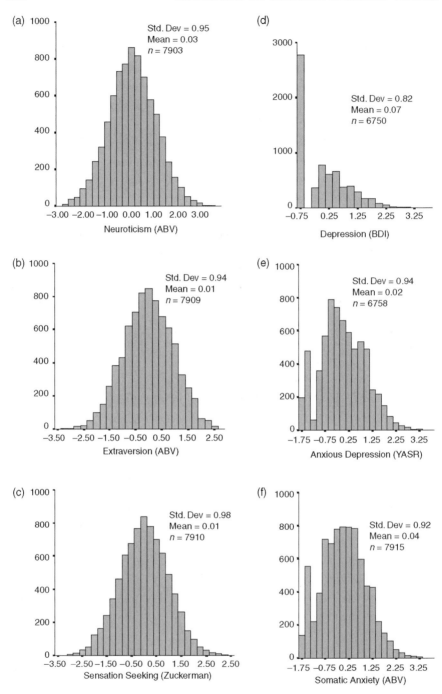

FIGURE 12.1. Distributions of personality and psychopathology normalized scores and genetic factor scores.

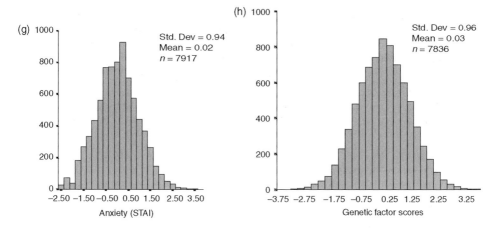

FIGURE 12.1. *(continued)*

roticism, extraversion, sensation seeking, depression, anxious depression, somatic anxiety, and anxiety, respectively. All variables were more or less normally distributed, with the exception of the depression scores.

Mean scores were compared between sexes with student's *t*-test. All
dimensions differed significantly (*p* < .0001) between men and women, with
men scoring lower on neuroticism and all psychopathology measures, and
higher on extraversion and sensation seeking (Table 12.1).

Pearson correlations were calculated within and between the personality
and psychopathology dimensions for men and women separately. The correlations within and between the personality and psychopathology dimensions
were all significant at the level of alpha < .01 (Table 12.2). It is clear that mea-

**TABLE 12.1. Mean Raw and Normalized Scores and Standard Deviations
for Neuroticism, Extraversion, Sensation Seeking (Total Score), Beck
Depression Inventory, Anxious Depression, Somatic Anxiety, and Anxiety
for Men and Women**

	Men		Women	
	Raw (*SD*)	Normalized (*SD*)	Raw (*SD*)	Normalized (*SD*)
Neuroticism	46.59 (21.34)	−0.19 (0.92)	55.18 (23.38)	0.19 (0.94)
Extraversion	60.77 (15.32)	0.03 (0.96)	59.88 (15.16)	−0.05 (0.93)
Sensation seeking	11.74 (1.75)	0.33 (0.91)	10.59 (1.91)	−0.24 (0.95)
Depression	1.30 (2.21)	−0.07 (0.77)	1.98 (2.84)	0.17 (0.85)
Anxious depression	3.77 (3.57)	−0.22 (0.86)	5.65 (4.59)	0.20 (0.96)
Somatic anxiety	17.55 (4.71)	−0.10 (0.87)	18.85 (5.43)	0.14 (0.94)
Anxiety	31.90 (7.50)	−0.13 (0.91)	34.27 (8.59)	0.15 (0.95)

TABLE 12.2. Correlations for Neuroticism, Extraversion, Total Score on Sensation Seeking, Beck Depression Inventory, Somatic Anxiety, Anxious Depression, and Anxiety for Men (Upper Diagonal) and Women (Lower Diagonal)

	Neu	Ext	SSS	BDI	AD	SoA	Anx
Neu		−.22	.19	.53	.60	.59	.69
Ext	−.22		.36	−.18	−.23	−.12	−.24
SSS	.18	.31		.08	.08	.17	.13
BDI	.58	−.20	.08		.48	.40	.58
AD	.70	−.27	.10	.56		.42	.61
SoA	.61	−.19	.13	.46	.48		.47
Anx	.75	−.22	.14	.65	.71	.53	

Note. Neu, neuroticism; Ext, extraversion; SSS, sensation seeking (total score); BDI, Beck Depression Inventory; AD, anxious depression; SoA, somatic anxiety; Anx, anxiety.

sures of anxiety and depression were highly correlated. Moderate correlations were seen within the personality measures, with a negative correlation between neuroticism and extraversion. Regarding the relation between personality and psychopathology, neuroticism showed high correlations with anxiety as well as depression, while extraversion was (to a lesser extent) negatively correlated with these symptoms. Sensation seeking did not appear to be related to any of these measures, and especially not to depression. Finally, these conclusions were very similar for men and women, with no differences in the size of the correlations.

Correlations among the psychopathology measures were high, and it was possible that the correlations between the personality measures of neuroticism and extraversion and all the psychopathology measures were due to just one of the psychopathology dimensions. Therefore, for the four psychopathology measures (depression [BDI], anxious depression [YASR], somatic anxiety [ABV], and anxiety [STAI]), the population was divided into cases and normal controls, with the 95th percentile as a cutoff score. Cases were further divided into subjects with pure "disorders" and with comorbid conditions. This led to 15 groups of cases, as summarized in Table 12.3 (e.g., one group with cases of pure depression, one group of cases with depression and somatic anxiety, etc.). Since subjects had to have a score on all four instruments to be categorized in one of the groups, 2416 subjects were excluded from this analysis. In a multivariate analysis of variance (MANOVA), personality scores for each group of cases were compared with those for the normal controls. Table 12.3 shows that all groups of cases had significantly higher neuroticism scores than the normal controls ($p < .0001$), and that almost all groups of cases had significantly lower extraversion scores ($p < .0001$ or $p < .001$), whereas just one group scored significantly higher on sensation seeking ($p < .05$).

TABLE 12.3. Mean Scores and Standard Deviations for Neuroticism, Extraversion, and Sensation Seeking (Total Score) for the Nondisordered Controls and the 14 Groups of Cases with Scores above the 95th Percentile on Depression, Anxious Depression, Somatic Anxiety, and/or Anxiety

	n	Neu (SD)	Ext (SD)	SSS (SD)
Controls	4994	-0.16 (0.83)	0.05 (0.92)	-0.03 (0.96)
BDI	90	0.86 (0.56)***	-0.31 (0.93)***	0.02 (0.93)
AD	95	1.09 (0.58)***	-0.46 (1.03)***	0.09 (1.05)
SoA	98	1.01 (0.71)***	-0.20 (0.96)**	-0.07 (1.07)
Anx	35	1.33 (0.53)***	-0.54 (0.97)***	-0.05 (0.93)
BDI + AD	14	1.41 (0.41)***	-0.86 (0.86)***	0.07 (0.73)
BDI + SoA	17	1.01 (0.51)***	-0.59 (0.97)**	0.19 (1.22)
BDI + Anx	25	1.48 (0.45)***	-0.23 (0.84)	-0.27 (1.04)
AD + SoA	9	1.40 (0.55)***	-0.37 (0.79)	0.37 (0.58)
AD + Anx	41	1.72 (0.49)***	-0.50 (0.81)***	0.28 (0.91)*
SoA + Anx	14	1.74 (0.50)***	-0.64 (0.94)**	-0.26 (1.20)
BDI + AD + SoA	11	1.40 (0.56)***	-0.96 (0.99)***	-0.08 (1.23)
BDI + AD + Anx	39	1.72 (0.62)***	-0.75 (0.92)***	0.01 (0.94)
BDI + SoA + Anx	18	1.82 (0.55)***	-0.87 (0.91)***	0.32 (0.98)
AD + SoA + Anx	10	1.93 (0.25)***	-0.33 (0.40)	-0.20 (1.03)
BDI + AD + SoA + Anx	43	2.11 (0.48)***	-0.89 (0.91)***	-0.01 (0.96)

Note. Abbreviations as in Table 12.2.
*$p < .05$ versus controls; **$p < .001$ versus controls; *** $p < .0001$ versus controls.

STUDY II: THE ASSOCIATION OF PERSONALITY WITH PSYCHOPATHOLOGY CATEGORIZED ACCORDING TO DSM-IV DIAGNOSES

In 1998, we performed a selection to obtain a subsample of twin families that would be informative for a linkage study to localize the genes underlying the susceptibility to anxiety and depression. The selection strategy was based on the recommendation of Eaves and Meyer (1994) and Risch and Zhang (1995) to select sibling pairs for genotyping with extreme scores (high–high, low–low, low–high, or high–low) on a quantitative scale of interest. Simulation studies have shown the optimal selection percentages for linkage analysis in sibling pairs from random samples (Dolan & Boomsma, 1998). Concordant sibling pairs were selected when both had scores in the top 12% or in the bottom 12% of the phenotypic distribution. For discordant pairs, an "asymmetrical" criterion appeared to be optimal. Discordant sibling pairs were selected if one sibling had a score in the top 25% and the other in the bottom 20%, or if one had a score in the top 20% and the other in the bottom 25%. The quantitative scale used for the selection consisted of a genetic factor score expressing a subject's genetic susceptibility to "anxious depression." The formula to calculate these factor scores was derived from a multivariate genetic analysis on the anxiety, depression, neuroticism, and somatic anxiety data collected for twins and their siblings in 1991, 1993, and 1997. This analysis revealed that covariances for these traits could be fully attributed to a common genetic factor (Boomsma et al., 2000). The value of this common genetic factor could be estimated for each individual by using the individual scores on the traits and the factor loadings on the common genetic factor. Since the factor loadings on the common genetic factor were different for males and females, the formulas to estimate the genetic factor score were different for males and females. Furthermore, genetic factor scores depended on whether the BDI or the YASR depression scale was used in the construction. For example, this was the formula for males when the score on the YASR was used: Genetic factor score = 0.144 × anxiety + 0.117 × neuroticism + 0.039 × somatic anxiety + d.064 × depression (YASR). More detailed information on how the factor scores were calculated is provided elsewhere (Boomsma et al., 2000). The correlation between the factor scores calculated with the score on the BDI and the score on the YASR in the 1997 survey was .98.

A factor score could be calculated for 7,836 twins and siblings who participated at least once in the 1991, 1993, or 1997 survey (see Figure 12.1h). Subjects who missed one or more of the inventories that measured neuroticism, anxiety, somatic anxiety, or depression were excluded. Based on these factor scores, 561 families were selected in which both members of a sibling pair had extreme factor scores. All members of the selected families, regardless of their genetic factor scores, were asked to provide a buccal swab for DNA isolation. Twins and siblings in these families were also asked to participate in a diagnostic psychiatric interview. For example, in monozygotic twin pairs in which one (or both) of the twins formed an extreme pair with an additional sibling, both the twins and the additional sibling were invited to take part in the study. Finally, a subsample of concordant and discordant monozygotic twins and seven unselected families participated in the interview. In 143 families, not all family members were approached. Eventually, 332 male and 504 female twins, and 193 brothers and 227 sisters, from 479 families were interviewed. One hundred and seven subjects were not available (e.g., because the phone was not answered several times), and 154 subjects refused to participate.

Table 12.4 shows the consequences of the selection on the distribution of the factor scores on an individual level. Eighty percent of the interviewed subjects had extreme scores (i.e., above the 75th or below the 25th percentile of the total population). Subjects who refused to participate had less extreme scores than the subjects who participated, whereas subjects who were not available for the interview had more extreme scores. For 17 twins and siblings, no genetic factor score was available. They were asked to participate in the interview because they were family members of an extreme-scoring sibling

TABLE 12.4. Interview Participation and Factor Scores

	Not approached (n/%)	Participated (n/%)	Refused participation (n/%)	Respondent not available (n/%)
fs ≥ 75th %	1803 (28.5%)	460 (37.1%)	45 (29.4%)	52 (48.6%)
fs ≤ 25th %	1671 (26.4%)	480 (38.7%)	70 (45.8%)	34 (31.8%)
fs between 25th % and 75th %	2808 (44.3%)	256 (20.6%)	31 (20.3%)	20 (18.7%)
fs ≥ 75th % and ≤ 25th %	54 (0.9%)	44 (3.5%)	7 (4.6%)	1 (0.9%)
Total	6336 (100%)	1240 (100%)[a]	153 (100%)[b]	107 (100%)

Note. Factor scores (fs) were calculated in 1991, 1993, and 1997. A subject was assigned to a group on the basis of his or her lowest or highest score on these three occasions. Subjects who scored above the 75th percentile on one occasion and below the 25th percentile on another were classified in a separate group.
[a]For 16 twins and siblings who participated in the CIDI, a factor score is missing; [b]For one subject who refused to participate, a factor score is missing.

pair. Twelve of them had not returned a questionnaire. Five participants had filled out a questionnaire, but missed items on the scales used to calculate the factor scores. Mean age of the participants at the time of the interview was 28.3 years.

Correlations within and between the personality and psychopathology dimensions were somewhat higher in the selected sample than in the total population. The highest correlations in the selected population were found between neuroticism and anxiety—namely, .80 in men and .84 in women. In the total population, these correlations were .69 and .75, respectively.

During the telephone interview, the following sections from the lifetime computerized version of the Composite International Diagnostic Interview (CIDI; World Health Organization, 1992) were administered to obtain lifetime DSM-IV diagnoses (American Psychiatric Association, 1994): Demographics (Sections A); Social Phobia, Agoraphobia, Panic Disorder, and Generalized Anxiety Disorder (D33 and further); Depression and Dysthymia (E); Mania Screen and Bipolar Affective Disorder (F); and Obsessive–Compulsive Disorder (K1–K22). The CIDI is a fully standardized diagnostic interview. No information on the reliability and validity of the Dutch version of the CIDI is available, but good reliability and validity have been reported for the American CIDI (Andrews & Peters, 1998). All interviewers were trained by the Dutch World Health Organization training center. The interviews were taped, and a trained clinician (C. M. M.) reviewed 126 interviews (10%) to check whether the interviewers had administered the CIDI appropriately. This appeared to be the case. However, it was apparent that questions regarding age of onset and age of recency were not reliably answered, because of comments made by the subjects such as "I have to guess" or "I do not know; I suppose I was around __ years of age." This was also the case with respect to the number of episodes reported in major depression.

According to the diagnostic algorithm as obtained with the CIDI, subjects could be classified into one of three categories: "not affected," "affected," or "fulfilling the positive criteria, but not the exclusion criteria." The third category consisted of subjects with more than one anxiety disorder, subjects who exhibited symptoms of generalized anxiety disorder exclusively during a depressive episode, and subjects who fulfilled the criteria for an anxiety disorder but did not seek help for their symptoms. Subjects in this category were classified as "affected."

We analyzed data on major depression, dysthymia, generalized anxiety disorder, social phobia, panic disorder with or without agoraphobia, and agoraphobia without a history of panic disorder. Subjects with one of the latter three diagnoses were considered as one group, which is further referred to as "panic/agoraphobia." Subjects with bipolar disorder and/or obsessive–compulsive disorder without any other condition were excluded from the analyses ($n = 8$). Table 12.5 shows the number of subjects with no, one, two, three, four, or five diagnoses and the distribution of the disorders in these groups. Comorbidity was very common, especially in women or when an anxiety disorder was present.

MANOVAs were performed with the mean scores on the personality dimensions as dependent variables. In the first analysis, the diagnoses of major

TABLE 12.5. Frequency of the Number of Disorders in Men and in Women, with Specifications of Which Diagnoses Were Made

n disorders	Total (%)[a]	MDD (%)	Dys (%)	GAD (%)	Panic (%)	Social P (%)
Men						
0	454 (87.2)					
1	45 (8.6)	28 (5.4)	0	4 (0.8)	7 (1.3)	6 (1.1)
2	16 (3.1)	14 (2.7)	0	10 (1.9)	4 (0.8)	4 (0.8)
3	6 (1.1)	6 (1.1)	3 (0.6)	4 (0.8)	3 (0.6)	2 (0.4)
Total n men	521	48 (9.2)	3 (0.6)	18 (3.4)	14 (2.7)	12 (2.3)
Women						
0	532 (73.3)					
1	108 (14.8)	67 (9.2)	2 (0.3)	8 (1.1)	20 (2.7)	11 (1.5)
2	49 (6.7)	40 (5.5)	8 (1.1)	18 (2.5)	20 (2.7)	12 (1.6)
3	28 (3.8)	27 (3.7)	7 (1.0)	19 (2.6)	18 (2.5)	13 (1.8)
4	8 (1.1)	7 (1.0)	6 (0.8)	7 (1.0)	6 (0.8)	6 (0.8)
5	2 (0.3)	2 (0.3)	2 (0.3)	2 (0.3)	2 (0.3)	2 (0.3)
Total n women	727	143 (19.6)	25 (3.4)	54 (7.4)	66 (9.1)	44 (6.0)

Note. MDD, major depression; Dys, dysthymia; GAD, generalized anxiety disorder; Social P, social phobia.
[a]Percentages were always calculated from the total group of men ($n = 521$) or women ($n = 727$).

depression, dysthymia, social phobia, generalized anxiety disorder, or panic/agoraphobia constituted the independent variables. By including these variables in the model at the same time, we could control for comorbidity. The MANOVA showed that mean scores on the personality and psychopathology measures differed significantly between unaffected subjects and subjects with a diagnosis of major depression, social phobia, generalized anxiety disorder, or panic/agoraphobia ($p < .0005$) (Table 12.6). Only the scores of subjects diagnosed with dysthymia were not significantly different from those of the group without a disorder, although their scores were the same as or even higher than those of the other subjects with depression or an anxiety disorder. Interaction between variables was not included in the analysis, because power was too low to detect significant effects. Considering the results in more detail, the univariate tests demonstrated that subjects diagnosed with major depression, social phobia, generalized anxiety disorder, or panic/agoraphobia all differed significantly from the subjects without a disorder in their scores on neuroticism ($p \sim .005$). With regard to extraversion, only the subjects with social phobia or panic/agoraphobia showed decreased scores in comparison with the normal group ($p < .05$). On sensation seeking, subjects with diagnoses did not differ from normal controls.

TABLE 12.6. Mean Scores and Standard Deviations on Psychopathology and Personality Measures for Men and Women, with or without a DSM-IV Diagnosis of a Mood or Anxiety Disorder

	No diagnoses	MDD	Dys	GAD	Panic	Social P
Men						
BDI (*SD*)	−0.16 (0.72)	0.91 (0.97)	1.81 (0.91)	0.94 (0.96)	0.71 (0.78)	1.01 (1.28)
AD (*SD*)	−0.30 (0.88)	0.75 (0.91)	1.33 (0.07)	0.97 (0.57)	0.17 (1.33)	0.69 (0.80)
SoA (*SD*)	−0.26 (0.89)	0.58 (0.85)	0.89 (0.72)	0.81 (0.75)	0.35 (0.70)	0.82 (1.03)
Anx (*SD*)	−0.33 (1.00)	0.87 (1.09)	1.78 (0.23)	1.30 (0.61)	0.70 (0.87)	1.01 (1.36)
Neu (*SD*)	−0.40 (1.03)	0.75 (1.11)	1.50 (0.95)	1.06 (0.63)	0.35 (1.22)	1.16 (1.06)
Ext (*SD*)	0.14 (1.00)	−0.04 (1.26)	−0.95 (0.70)	0.03 (1.30)	−0.54 (0.88)	−0.48 (1.02)
SSS (*SD*)	0.26 (0.89)	0.32 (0.90)	0.42 (0.37)	0.53 (0.94)	−0.31 (0.78)	0.31 (0.89)
Women						
BDI (*SD*)	−0.01 (0.79)	0.92 (0.96)	1.63 (0.99)	1.29 (0.81)	0.76 (0.88)	1.00 (0.87)
AD (*SD*)	−0.06 (0.92)	0.96 (0.98)	1.43 (0.90)	1.28 (0.86)	0.99 (0.99)	1.38 (0.80)
SoA (*SD*)	−0.08 (0.93)	0.69 (1.05)	1.10 (1.06)	0.78 (1.04)	0.93 (0.92)	0.92 (0.95)
Anx (*SD*)	−0.17 (1.01)	0.92 (1.00)	1.68 (0.98)	1.39 (0.88)	0.91 (0.94)	1.20 (0.90)
Neu (*SD*)	−0.17 (1.03)	0.87 (0.97)	1.36 (0.99)	1.24 (0.91)	0.92 (0.88)	1.11 (0.86)
Ext (*SD*)	−0.03 (0.91)	−0.37 (0.90)	−0.82 (1.00)	−0.66 (0.88)	−0.44 (0.89)	−0.69 (0.74)
SSS (*SD*)	−0.41 (0.96)	−0.39 (0.97)	−0.55 (1.10)	−0.56 (0.96)	−0.32 (0.95)	−0.25 (0.90)

Note. Abbreviations as in Tables 12.2 and 12.5.

A second MANOVA, with the personality dimensions as independent variables and with the number of CIDI diagnoses as independent variable (zero, one, two, or three or more) did also reach significance ($p < .0001$) (Table 12.7). The univariate tests showed that neuroticism and extraversion, but not sensation seeking, were significantly different among the four groups of subjects. Figure 12.2 shows a positive relation between neuroticism and the number of disorders, and a negative relation between extraversion and the number of disorders.

DISCUSSION

We have presented results from two studies, which aimed to explore whether Eysenck's model or the tripartite model best describes the relation of neuroticism and extraversion to depressive and anxious psychopathology. Both models hypothesize that anxiety and depression are related to high neuroticism. Eysenck theorized that depression and anxiety are both also related to low extraversion. The tripartite model, on the other hand, hypothesizes that

TABLE 12.7. Mean Scores and Standard Deviations on Psychopathology and Personality Measures for Men and Women with Zero, One, Two, or Three or More Disorders

	Zero	One	Two	Three or more
Men				
BDI (*SD*)	−0.16 (0.72)	0.71 (0.91)	1.15 (1.00)	0.90 (0.90)
AD (*SD*)	−0.30 (0.88)	0.45 (1.01)	0.83 (0.92)	0.91 (0.66)
SoA (*SD*)	−0.26 (0.89)	0.39 (0.93)	0.83 (0.73)	0.75 (0.52)
Anx (*SD*)	−0.33 (1.00)	0.51 (1.14)	1.29 (0.81)	1.32 (0.47)
Neu (*SD*)	−0.40 (1.03)	0.43 (1.16)	1.24 (0.78)	1.03 (0.81)
Ext (*SD*)	0.14 (1.00)	−0.26 (1.31)	0.15 (1.19)	0.12 (1.12)
SSS (*SD*)	0.26 (0.89)	0.04 (0.85)	0.64 (1.10)	0.26 (0.46)
Women				
BDI (*SD*)	−0.01 (0.79)	0.66 (0.93)	0.93 (1.02)	1.33 (0.72)
AD (*SD*)	−0.06 (0.92)	0.74 (1.01)	1.14 (0.91)	1.38 (0.81)
SoA (*SD*)	−0.08 (0.93)	0.53 (0.98)	0.86 (1.01)	1.00 (0.99)
Anx (*SD*)	−0.17 (1.01)	0.65 (0.94)	0.93 (1.02)	1.47 (0.79)
Neu (*SD*)	−0.17 (1.03)	0.70 (0.98)	0.88 (0.91)	1.31 (0.81)
Ext (*SD*)	−0.03 (0.91)	−0.28 (0.94)	−0.40 (0.73)	−0.42 (0.92)
SSS (*SD*)	−0.41 (0.96)	−0.28 (0.93)	−0.75 (0.87)	−0.47 (1.02)

Note. Abbreviations as in Table 12.2.

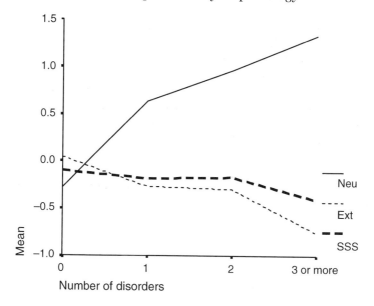

FIGURE 12.2. Relation between number of disorders and scores on neuroticism (Neu), extraversion (Ext), and sensation seeking (SSS).

depression, but not anxiety, is related to low positive affectivity, whereas anxiety is related to symptoms of autonomic hyperarousal. A second goal was to examine the relation of sensation seeking to anxious and depressive psychopathology. The analyses clearly showed that neuroticism is highly correlated with all measures of anxiety and depression. Low extraversion is also related to anxiety and depression, but to a lesser extent. Sensation seeking is not associated with anxiety and/or depression. In Study I, subjects with a score above the 95th percentile on anxious depression and anxiety had significantly higher sensation-seeking scores than normal controls ($p < .05$). This may simply reflect a consequence of multiple testing. The results support Eysenck's theory that depressive and/or anxious subjects score high on neuroticism and low on extraversion, as well as Zuckerman's hypothesis that sensation seeking, although weakly correlated with extraversion, is not related to anxiety and/or depression. These results thus suggest that the tripartite model can be rejected.

In all analyses, comorbidity between depression and anxiety was considered. In the first study, we used a cutoff score of the 95th percentile on the psychopathology questionnaires to divide subjects into groups consisting of normal controls, subjects with pure "disorders," and subjects with comorbid "disorders." Differences in personality measures with the normal controls were tested separately for all affected groups. In the second study, comorbidity was controlled for by including all disorders in the model, when personality scores were compared between subjects with and without a disorder. Finally, the effect of comorbidity was directly investigated by analyzing the association between personality and the number of disorders. All analyses showed very similar results, although in the first study the division between the groups of affected and unaffected is based on self-report questionnaires and not on clinical criteria. The STAI, for example, has been shown not to assess anxiety only, but also depression and general negative affect (Bieling, Antony, & Swinson, 1998; Kennedy, Schwab, Morris, & Beldia, 2001). In our own sample, all four questionnaires (the BDI, the YASR, the STAI, and the ABV subscale for somatic anxiety) do not seem to distinguish between disorders (Table 12.6). Furthermore, the ABV subscale for somatic anxiety and the STAI—Trait version ask subjects to indicate how they generally feel, and the YASR asks about the last 6 months. Therefore, it is questionable whether state is measured with these questionnaires. However, the results are remarkably the same as the results of Study II. First, the relationship to the personality dimensions was the same for anxiety and depression measured either dimensionally or categorically. Second, neuroticism scores were higher and extraversion scores were lower when subjects suffered from more than one disorder.

Some results deserve further attention. In Study II, dysthymia was the only disorder that was not associated with neuroticism, although the neuroticism scores of subjects with dysthymia were comparable to those of the other groups diagnosed with a psychiatric disorder. This result might be a consequence of the low prevalence of dysthymia. Another explanation could be that the high neuroticism scores of subjects with dysthymia were due to comorbid disorders, since most of them also had another diagnosis—mainly major depression. This appears in accordance with Klein and Santiago's (2003) argument that the distinction between dysthymia and chronic depression is not meaningful. To our knowledge, there are no studies that have investigated the relation between neuroticism and dysthymia as a separate disorder while taking comorbidity into account.

Another interesting point is that in the first analysis of Study II, low extraversion only seemed related to social phobia and panic/agoraphobia and not to the other disorders, whereas this did not appear to be the case in Study I or in the second part of Study II. This might be due to a lack of power, since the trend was clearly the same for all disorders (Table 12.6). However, in other studies that took comorbidity into account, low extraversion did not appear to be associated with all disorders either. One of the studies found that low extraversion was related to social phobia and agoraphobia, but not to panic disorder and major depression (Bienvenu et al., 2001). Another study found that low extraversion was related to social phobia and major depression, but not to generalized anxiety disorder and panic disorder and/or agoraphobia (Brown et al., 1998). An explanation for these somewhat divergent findings could be that whereas neuroticism seems to be an independent risk factor, extraversion may interact with other risk factors—for example, life events. In other words, subjects who score high on extraversion may be less sensitive to the effect of life events, or subjects with high extraversion may be less prone to adverse events that are associated with these disorders. For example, an extraverted, highly social individual may be at lower risk for a divorce. A recent study investigated the opposite of the latter hypothesis for sensation seeking, life events, and depression (Farmer et al., 2001). They hypothesized that subjects with high levels of sensation seeking might be more at risk for adverse events (which are related to major depression) because of their accident-prone behavior. This did not appear to be the case. However, this seems a promising direction of research. Interaction effects could lead to conflicting results, as in the case of the relation with low extraversion. When the group of affected subjects includes a relatively high number of patients who have experienced adverse effects and get a disorder because they are also low in extraversion, a relationship between extraversion and the disorder will be found. When, on the opposite, the group of affected subjects consists mainly of highly neurotic patients who already have a high risk of developing a psychiatric disorder, the relationship may be missed. This might explain why in our study low extraversion did not seem to be associated with all of the disorders we examined, while extraversion scores were found to decrease with the number of disorders. Subjects with comorbidity are probably more vulnerable to disorders (e.g., because of high neuroticism scores in combination with low extraversion scores) than subjects with a pure disorder.

The finding that sensation seeking is not related to anxiety and depression, but is weakly correlated to extraversion, is consistent with the view (which emerged after the development of the first version of the EPQ and the ABV) that impulsivity may reflect a third personality dimension independent of extraversion and neuroticism (Clark et al., 1994; Zuckerman, 1994).

Concerning the etiology of depression and anxiety, the linear relation between neuroticism and low extraversion on the one hand, and the number of disorders on the other, links nicely to the hypothesis that anxiety and depression are polygenic disorders with a partly shared common genetic background (Gray & McNaughton, 2000; Jardine, Martin, & Henderson, 1984; Kendler et al., 1995; Kendler, Neale, Kessler, Heath, & Eaves, 1993). The higher an individual's neuroticism score, and perhaps the lower the person's score on extraversion, the more genes the individual probably has that increase the vulnerability for depression and/or anxiety. This might also explain part of the comorbidity, as Bienvenu and colleagues (2001) have already suggested, because subjects scoring high on neuroticism and low on extraversion have an increased chance to have depression or an anxiety disorder—and, as a consequence, have a higher chance to have both disorders as well.

In addition, in both studies (although this was not formally tested), the relation between the personality dimensions and anxious or depressive psychopathology appeared to be the same for men and women. This signifies that the higher prevalence rates for anxiety and depression in women are more likely to be explained by the higher neuroticism scores than by a different etiological background for anxiety and depression. This is confirmed by Goodwin and Gotlib (2004), who found that higher neuroticism scores in women might explain the gender difference in prevalence of major depression. The question of why women have higher neuroticism scores than men remains.

To conclude, high neuroticism and low extraversion are related to anxiety and depression, even when comorbidity between these disorders is taken into account. Sensation seeking seems an independent personality dimension, which is not associated with anxious and depressive psychopathology.

LOOKING FORWARD

The question of how to define psychiatric phenotypes has become more and more important during the last decades. This is partly induced by the realization that DSM categories cannot double as phenotypes when investigators are trying to discover robust genetic markers (Charney et al., 2002). The effect of a gene can, for instance, be missed when this gene leads to a pattern of symptoms that differs from a disorder as defined by the DSM-IV (for an illustration of this problem, see Hudziak, 2002). Considering the association of neuroticism and extraversion with anxious or depressive psychopathology, we would recommend that future gene-finding studies include these traits, in addition to specific disorders. The definitions of these traits are not fully etiologically based either, although neuroticism was originally hypothesized to be related to the visceral brain and extraversion to the ascending reticular arousal system (Eysenck, 1967). However, the Neuroticism and Extraversion scales consist of a broad spectrum of symptoms correlated with the more narrowly defined DSM-IV depression and anxiety disorders. A quantitative trait locus (QTL) responsible for a certain pattern of symptoms, which is not classified as a disorder according to the DSM-IV, might be detected when neuroticism and extraversion are investigated. Especially when these traits are analyzed simultaneously, an increase in statistical power for QTL detection might be realized (e.g., Boomsma & Dolan, 1998; Marlow et al., 2003). Furthermore, analyses of continuous traits such as neuroticism and extraversion have higher power to detect QTL effects than analyses of dichotomous traits such as depression. The demonstration of a relation between these personality traits and depression and anxiety forms a promising start for investigating whether genes that influence neuroticism and extraversion are also associated with anxious or depressive psychopathology. If candidate genes can be identified, it even becomes possible to examine what kinds of symptoms distinguish subjects with particular variants of those genes from other subjects. Ultimately, this strategy could lead to a more etiologically based classification system.

ACKNOWLEDGMENTS

The research reported in this chapter was supported by the Netherlands Organization for Scientific Research (NWO/ZonMW; Grant Nos. 940-37-024, 904-61-090, 575-25-006).

REFERENCES

Achenbach, T. M. (1990). *The Young Adult Self Report.* Burlington: University of Vermont, Dept of Psychiatry.

American Psychiatric Association. (1994). *Diagnostic and statistical manual of mental disorders* (4th ed.). Washington DC: Author.

Andrews, G., & Peters, L. (1998). The psychometric properties of the Composite International Diagnostic Interview. *Social Psychiatry and Psychiatric Epidemiology, 33,* 80–88.

Andrews, G., Slade, T., & Issakidis, C. (2002). Deconstructing current comorbidity: Data from the Australian National Survey of Mental Health and Well-Being. *British Journal of Psychiatry, 181,* 306–314.

Beck, A. T., Rial, W. Y., & Rickels, K. (1974). Short form of depression inventory: Cross-validation. *Psychological Reports, 34,* 1184–1186.

Bieling, P. J., Antony, M. M., & Swinson, R. P. (1998). The State–Trait Anxiety Inventory, Trait version: Structure and content re-examined. *Behaviour Research and Therapy, 36,* 777–788.

Bienvenu, O. J., Brown, C., Samuels, J. F., Liang, K. Y., Costa, P. T., Eaton, W. W., et al. (2001). Normal personality traits and comorbidity among phobic, panic and major depressive disorders. *Psychiatry Research, 102,* 73–85.

Bienvenu, O. J., & Stein, M. B. (2003). Personality and anxiety disorders: A review. *Journal of Personality Disorders, 17,* 139–151.

Blom, G. (1958). *Statistical estimates and transformed beta variables.* New York: Wiley.

Boomsma, D. I., Beem, A. L., van den, B. M., Dolan, C. V., Koopmans, J. R., Vink, J. M., et al. (2000). Netherlands Twin Family Study of Anxious Depression (NETSAD). *Twin Research, 3,* 323–334.

Boomsma, D. I., & Dolan, C. V. (1998). A comparison of power to detect a QTL in sib-pair data using multivariate phenotypes, mean phenotypes, and factor scores. *Behavior Genetics, 28,* 329–340.

Boomsma, D. I., Vink, J. M., Van Beijsterveldt, T. C., de Geus, E. J., Beem, A. L., Mulder, E. J., et al. (2002). Netherlands Twin Register: a focus on longitudinal research. *Twin Research, 5,* 401–406.

Brown, S. L., Svrakic, D. M., Przybeck, T. R., & Cloninger, C. R. (1992). The relationship of personality to mood and anxiety states: A dimensional approach. *Journal of Psychiatric Research, 26,* 197–211.

Brown, T. A., Chorpita, B. F., & Barlow, D. H. (1998). Structural relationships among dimensions of the DSM-IV anxiety and mood disorders and dimensions of negative affect, positive affect, and autonomic arousal. *Journal of Abnormal Psychology, 107,* 179–192.

Carton, S., Morand, P., Bungenera, C., & Jouvent, R. (1995). Sensation-seeking and emotional disturbances in depression: Relationships and evolution. *Journal of Affective Disorders, 34,* 219–225.

Charney, D. S., Barlow, D. H., Botteron, K., Cohen, J. D., Goldman, D., Gur, R. E., et al. (2002). Neuroscience research agenda to guide development of a patho-physiologically based classification system. In D. J. Kupfer, M. B. First, & D. A. Regier (Eds.), *A research agenda for DSM-V* (pp. 31–83). Washington, DC: American Psychiatric Association.

Clark, L. A., & Watson, D. (1991). Tripartite model of anxiety and depression: Psychometric evidence and taxonomic implications. *Journal of Abnormal Psychology, 100,* 316–336.

Clark, L. A., Watson, D., & Mineka, S. (1994). Temperament, personality, and the mood and anxiety disorders. *Journal of Abnormal Psychology, 103,* 103–116.

Cloninger, C. R. (1986). A unified biosocial theory of personality and its role in the development of anxiety states. *Psychiatric Developments, 4,* 167–226.

Cloninger, C. R. (2002). Relevance of normal personality for psychiatrists. In J. Benjamin, R. P. Ebstein, & R. H. Belmaker (Eds.), *Molecular genetics and the human personality* (pp. 33–42). Washington, DC: American Psychiatric Press.

de Graaf, R., Bijl, R. V., ten Have, M., Beekman, A. T., & Vollebergh, W. A. (2004). Rapid onset of comorbidity of common mental disorders: Findings from the Netherlands Mental Health Survey and Incidence Study (NEMESIS). *Acta Psychiatrica Scandinavica, 109,* 55–63.

Dolan, C. V., & Boomsma, D. I. (1998). Optimal selection of sib pairs from random samples for linkage analysis of a QTL using the EDAC test. *Behavior Genetics, 28,* 197–206.

Eaves, L., & Meyer, J. (1994). Locating human quantitative trait loci: Guidelines for the selection of sibling pairs for genotyping. *Behavior Genetics, 24,* 443–455.

Eysenck, H. J. (1967). *The biological basis of personality.* Springfield, IL: Thomas.

Eysenck, H. J., & Eysenck, S. B. G. (1964). *Eysenck Personality Inventory.* San Diego, CA: Educational Industrial Testing Service.

Eysenck, H. J., & Rachman, S. (1965). *The causes and cures of neurosis.* San Diego, CA: Knapp.

Farmer, A., Redman, K., Harris, T., Mahmood, A., Sadler, S., & McGuffin, P. (2001). Sensation-seeking, life events and depression. The Cardiff Depression Study. *British Journal of Psychiatry, 178,* 549–552.

Feij, J. A., & van Zuilen, R. W. (1984). *Handleiding bij de spanningsbehoeftelijst (SBL).* Lisse, The Netherlands: Swets & Zeitlinger.

Goodwin, R. D., & Gotlib, I. H. (2004). Gender differences in depression: The role of personality factors. *Psychiatry Research, 126,* 135–142.

Gray, J. A. (1982). *The neuropsychology of anxiety: An enquiry into the functions of the septo-hippocampal system.* Oxford: Oxford University Press.

Gray, J. A., & McNaughton, N. (2000). *The neuropsychology of anxiety: An enquiry into the functions of the septo-hippocampal system* (2nd ed.). Oxford: Oxford University Press.

Heath, A. C., Cloninger, C. R., & Martin, N. G. (1994). Testing a model for the genetic structure of personality: A comparison of the personality systems of Cloninger and Eysenck. *Journal of Personality and Social Psychology, 66,* 762–775.

Hudziak, J. J. (2002). Importance of phenotype definition in genetic studies of child psychopathology. In J. E. Helzer & J. J. Hudziak (Eds.), *Defining psychopatholo-*

gy in the 21st century: DSM-V and beyond (pp. 211–230). Washington, DC: American Psychiatric Press.

Jardine, R., Martin, N. G., & Henderson, A. S. (1984). Genetic covariation between neuroticism and the symptoms of anxiety and depression. *Genetic Epidemiology, 1,* 89–107.

Johnson, S. L., Turner, R. J., & Iwata, N. (2003). BIS/BAS levels and psychiatric disorder: An epidemiological study. *Journal of Psychopathology and Behavioral Assessment, 25,* 25–36.

Kendler, K. S., Neale, M. C., Kessler, R. C., Heath, A. C., & Eaves, L. J. (1993). A longitudinal twin study of personality and major depression in women. *Archives of General Psychiatry, 50,* 853–862.

Kendler, K. S., Walters, E. E., Neale, M. C., Kessler, R. C., Heath, A. C., & Eaves, L. J. (1995). The structure of the genetic and environmental risk factors for six major psychiatric disorders in women: Phobia, generalized anxiety disorder, panic disorder, bulimia, major depression, and alcoholism. *Archives of General Psychiatry, 52,* 374–383.

Kennedy, B. L., Schwab, J. J., Morris, R. L., & Beldia, G. (2001). Assessment of state and trait anxiety in subjects with anxiety and depressive disorders. *Psychiatric Quarterly, 72,* 263–276.

Klein, D. N., & Santiago, N. J. (2003). Dysthymia and chronic depression: Introduction, classification, risk factors, and course. *Journal of Clinical Psychology, 59,* 807–816.

Krueger, R. F., McGue, M., & Iacono, W. G. (2001). The higher-order structure of common DSM mental disorders: Internalization, externalization, and their connections to personality. *Personality and Individual Differences, 30,* 1245–1259.

Marlow, A. J., Fisher, S. E., Francks, C., MacPhie, I. L., Cherny, S. S., Richardson, A. J., et al. (2003). Use of multivariate linkage analysis for dissection of a complex cognitive trait. *American Journal of Human Genetics, 72,* 561–570.

Risch, N., & Zhang, H. (1995). Extreme discordant sib pairs for mapping quantitative trait loci in humans. *Science, 268,* 1584–1589.

Shankman, S. A., & Klein, D. N. (2003). The relation between depression and anxiety: An evaluation of the tripartite, approach–withdrawal and valence–arousal models. *Clinical Psychology Review, 23,* 605–637.

Spielberger, C. D., Gorsuch, R. L., & Lushene, R. E. (1970). *STAI: Manual for the State–Trait Anxiety Inventory.* Palo Alto, CA: Consulting Psychologists Press.

Stelmack, R. M. (1981). The psychophysiology of extraversion and neuroticism. In H. J. Eysenck (Ed.), *A model for personality* (pp. 38–64). Berlin: Springer-Verlag.

Trull, T. J., & Sher, K. J. (1994). Relationship between the five-factor model of personality and Axis I disorders in a nonclinical sample. *Journal of Abnormal Psychology, 103,* 350–360.

Van der Ploeg, H., Defares, P. B., & Spielberger, C. D. (1979). *Zelfbeoordelingsvragenslijst STAI, versie DY-1 en DY-2.* Lisse, The Nertherlands: Swets & Zeitlinger.

Verhulst, F. C., van Ende, J., & Koot, H. M. (1997). *Handleiding voor de Youth Self Report.* Rotterdam: Afdeling Kinderen Jeugdpsychiatrie, Sophia Kinderziekenhuis/Academisch Ziekenhuis Rotterdam/Erasmus Universiteit Rotterdam.

Watson, D., Clark, L. A., & Tellegen, A. (1988). Development and validation of brief measures of positive and negative affect: The PANAS scales. *Journal of Personality and Social Psychology, 54,* 1063–1070.

Wilde, G. J. S. (1970). *Neurotische labiliteit gemeten volgens de vragenlijstmethode [The questionnaire method as a means of measuring neurotic instability]*. Amsterdam: Van Rossen.

World Health Organization. (1992). *Composite International Diagnostic Interview (Version 2.1)*. Geneva: Author.

Zuckerman, M. (1971). Dimensions of sensation seeking. *Journal of Consulting and Clinical Psychology, 36,* 45–52.

Zuckerman, M. (1979). *Sensation seeking: Beyond the level of optimal arousal.* New York: Wiley.

Zuckerman, M. (1994). *Behavioral expressions and biosocial bases of sensation seeking.* New York: Cambridge University Press.

13

5-HT$_{1A}$ Receptor and Anxiety-Related Traits

PHARMACOLOGY, GENETICS, AND IMAGING

Klaus-Peter Lesch and Turhan Canli

Brain serotonin (5-HT) has been implicated in a number of physiological processes and pathological conditions. These effects are mediated by at least 14 different 5-HT receptors. Although multiple lines of evidence implicate the 5-HT$_{1A}$ receptor in the pathophysiology of anxiety disorders and depression, as well as in the mechanism of action of anxiolytics and antidepressants, its relevance to the therapeutic effectiveness of these drugs has been a matter of considerable debate (Griebel, 1995; Hensler, 2003; Hjorth et al., 2000; Lesch, Zeng, Reif, & Gutknecht, 2003).

The physiological properties of 5-HT$_{1A}$ receptors are amazingly complex. 5-HT$_{1A}$ receptors operate both as somatodendritic autoreceptors and as postsynaptic receptors. Somatodendritic 5-HT$_{1A}$ autoreceptors are predominantly located on 5-HT neurons and dendrites in the brainstem raphe complex. Their activation by 5-HT or 5-HT$_{1A}$ agonists decreases the firing rate of serotonergic neurons and subsequently reduces the synthesis, turnover, and release of 5-HT from nerve terminals in all projection areas. Postsynaptic 5-HT$_{1A}$ receptors are widely distributed in forebrain regions that receive serotonergic input, notably in the cortex, hippocampus, septum, amygdala, and hypothalamus. Their activation results in membrane hyperpolarization and decreased neuronal excitability. 5-HT$_{1A}$ receptors decrease adenylyl cyclase activity via inhibitory G proteins, and hippocampal heteroceptors mediate neuronal inhibition by acting on G-protein-regulated inwardly rectifying potassium (GIRK) channels. Physiological responses depend upon the function of the target cells (e.g., hypothermia, activation of the hypothalamic pituitary adrenocortical system) (Hamon et al., 1990). Moreover, 5-HT$_{1A}$ receptor expression is modulated by steroid hormones, and 5-HT$_{1A}$-mediated signaling is an important regulator of gene expression, both through its coupling to G proteins that inhibit adenylyl cyclase and through modulation of GIRK2 channels.

The effects of 5-HT$_{1A}$ receptor-selective agents, such as the agonist 8-hydroxy-2-(di-n-propylamino) tetralin (8-OH-DPAT), and the partial agonists ipsapirone and gepirone, have been extensively studied in rodents (De Vry, 1995). Both agonists and partial agonists induce a dose-dependent anxiolytic effect that correlates with the inhibition of serotonergic neuron firing, the decrease of 5-HT release, and the reduction of 5-HT signaling at postsynaptic target receptors. Blockade of the negative feedback by selective 5-HT$_{1A}$ receptor antagonists, such as WAY 100635, increases firing of the serotonergic neurons but exerts no obvious effects on 5-HT neurotransmission or behavior (Olivier, Soudijn, & van Wijngaarden, 1999), while the combination with selective 5-HT reuptake inhibitors (SSRIs) augments increases in 5-HT levels in terminal regions.

The converging lines of evidence that 5-HT$_{1A}$ receptor dysfunction is involved in mood and anxiety disorders have also stimulated studies in mice with genetically modified 5-HT$_{1A}$ receptor function. As anticipated, mice with a targeted inactivation of the 5-HT$_{1A}$ receptor gene display a spontaneous phenotype that is associated with a gender-modulated and gene-dose-dependent increase of anxiety-related behavior and stress reactivity in several conflict paradigms (Lesch et al., 2003; Toth, 2003). Activation of presynaptic 5-HT$_{1A}$ receptors provides the brain with an autoinhibitory feedback system controlling 5-HT neurotransmission. Thus enhanced anxiety-related behavior is most likely to represent a consequence of increased terminal 5-HT availability resulting from the lack of or reduction in presynaptic somatodendritic 5-HT$_{1A}$ autoreceptor negative feedback function (Lesch & Mössner, 1999).

This mechanism is also consistent with recent theoretical models of fear and anxiety that are primarily based upon pharmacologically derived data. The cumulative reduction in serotonergic impulse flow to septo-hippocampal and other limbic and cortical areas involved in the control of anxiety is believed to explain the anxiolytic effects of ligands with selective affinity for the 5-HT$_{1A}$ receptor in some animal models of anxiety-related behavior. This notion is based in part on evidence that 5-HT$_{1A}$ agonists (e.g., 8-OH-DPAT) and antagonists (e.g., WAY 100635) have anxiolytic or anxiogenic effects, respectively. However, to complicate matters further, 8-OH-DPAT has anxiolytic effects when injected in the raphe nucleus, whereas it is anxiogenic when applied to the hippocampus. Thus stimulation of postsynaptic 5-HT$_{1A}$ receptors has been proposed to elicit anxiogenic effects, while activation of 5-HT$_{1A}$ autoreceptors is thought to induce anxiolytic effects via suppression of serotonergic neuronal firing, resulting in attenuated 5-HT release in limbic terminal fields.

ALLELIC VARIATION OF 5-HT$_{1A}$ RECEPTOR FUNCTION

The 5-HT$_{1A}$ receptor is encoded by an intronless gene (*HTR1A*) located on human chromosome 5q12.3. Several rare missense polymorphisms, including the Gly22Ser variant (which results in altered agonist-elicited downregulation), have been found within the protein coding of *HTR1A*. Moreover, Lemonde and colleagues (2003) reported a functional C-1019G single-nucleotide polymorphism (SNP) in the transcriptional control region of *HTR1A* (*HTR1A-1019*), and they demonstrated in *in vitro* experiments that the G variant displays differential binding efficiency of the repressor–enhancer-type transcriptional regulator NUDR/DEAF-1. NUDR/DEAF-1 is coexpressed with both pre- and postsynaptic 5-HT$_{1A}$ receptors, but its regulation of *HTR1A* transcription may differ in presynaptic raphe versus postsynaptic target cells (Lemonde et al., 2003).

The role of the *HTR1A-1019* polymorphism in the modulation of individual differences in personality traits was evaluated by a population genetic study of a sample of healthy volunteers (Strobel et al., 2003). It was predicted that the *HTR1A-1019* genotype would be associated with scores on measures of personality traits related to anxiety and depression, particularly with the Neuroticism and Harm Avoidance subscales of the Revised NEO Personality Inventory (NEO PI-R; Costa & McCrae 1992) and the Tridimensional Personality Questionnaire (TPQ; Cloninger, Svrakic, & Przybeck, 1993), respectively.

There was a significant effect of *HTR1A-1019* SNP on NEO PI-R Neuroticism: Carriers of the G allele obtained higher Neuroticism scores than noncarriers (see Figure 13.1). Subsequent analyses revealed that the effect of *HTR1A-1019* SNP on Neuroticism was primarily due to associations of this polymorphism with N1 Anxiety and with N3 Depression, whereas no significant associations with the other Neuroticism facets were detected. Because anxiety-like behavior was apparent not only in Htr1a–/– null mutant mice but also in heterozygous Htr1a+/– mice, indicating that a partial receptor deficit is sufficient to cause the behavioral phenotype (Toth, 2003), the sample was dichotomized according to absence (G–) versus presence (G+) of the G allele. Subsequent analyses focusing on the discriminant validity of the finding of higher Neuroticism scores in carriers of the *HTR1A-1019* G allele did not show association with the other NEO PI-R domain scales, Extraversion, Openness, Agreeableness, and Conscientiousness. Regarding convergent validity, a significant effect of the *HTR1A-1019* SNP was detected in carriers of the G allele exhibiting higher TPQ Harm Avoidance scores. These results suggest that allelic variation in 5-HT$_{1A}$ receptor expression modulates individual differences in anxiety- and depression-related personality traits, and they further support the evidence that implicates the 5-HT$_{1A}$ receptor in the pathophysiology of anxiety and depression.

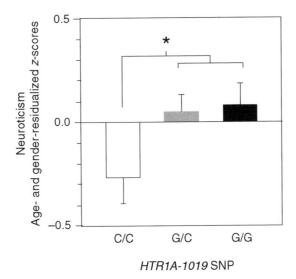

FIGURE 13.1. Effect of the *HTR1A-1019* polymorphism in the modulation of NEO PI-R Neuroticism. Carriers of the G allele (*n* = 225) exhibited significantly higher age- and gender-residualized Neuroticism *z*-scores than individuals homozygous for the C variant (*n* = 59). Adapted from Strobel et al. (2003).

5-HT$_{1A}$ RECEPTORS IN ANXIETY DISORDERS AND DEPRESSION

Although results have differed widely across studies, 5-HT$_{1A}$ receptors have been implicated in both depression and anxiety disorders. Early drug challenge studies had revealed an attenuation of 5-HT$_{1A}$ receptor-induced hypothermic and neuroendocrine responses in patients with depression and panic disorder (PD), reflecting dysfunction of both pre- and postsynaptic 5-HT$_{1A}$ receptors (Lesch, Mayer, et al., 1990; Lesch et al., 1992). A postmortem study also found decreased 5-HT$_{1A}$ receptor messenger RNA (mRNA) expression and ligand binding in the raphe and hippocampus, but not in dorsal or anterior prefrontal cortical areas, in brains of depressed persons who committed suicide (Cheetham, Crompton, Katona, & Horton, 1990); these findings seem to correlate well with an attenuation of 5-HT$_{1A}$ receptor-mediated hypothermic and neuroendocrine responses (Lesch, Mayer, et al., 1990), and may thus support the notion of dysfunctional pre- and postsynaptic 5-HT$_{1A}$ receptors. Likewise, a decrease in 5-HT$_{1A}$ ligand binding elicited by positron emission tomography (PET) has been shown in forebrain areas such as the medial temporal lobe, as well as in the raphe of depressed patients (Drevets et al., 1999; Sargent et al., 2000). Investigations using 5-HT$_{1A}$ receptor challenge and PET imaging revealed similar deficiencies in PD (Lesch et al., 1992; Neumeister et al., 2004).

Hippocampal 5-HT$_{1A}$ receptor expression is under tonic inhibition by corticosteroid receptor stimulation. Both glucocorticoid administration and chronic stress (a concomitant pathophysiological factor in mood disorders) have also been demonstrated to result in down-regulation of 5-HT$_{1A}$ receptor density and mRNA levels in the hippocampus in the animal model (Flügge, 1995; Lopez, Chalmers, Little, & Watson, 1998; Wissink, Meijer, Pearce, van der Burg, & van der Saag, 2000). In contrast, 5-HT$_{1A}$ receptors in the raphe seem insensitive to circulating corticosteroids (Chalmers, Kwak, Mansour, Akil, & Watson, 1993). Abnormal 5-HT$_{1A}$ receptor expression in this structure may instead reflect neuromorphological abnormalities that affect 5-HT$_{1A}$ receptor number.

Although initial association studies of the *HTR1A* variations produced ambiguous results in mood disorders (Arias et al., 2002; Nishiguchi et al., 2002), Lemonde and colleagues (2003) also showed that the G variant of the *HTR1A-1019* polymorphism is associated with severe depression and suicidality. Given the considerable comorbidity of depression and anxiety, as well as associations of the G variant with anxiety- and depression-related personality traits—particularly with higher scores on NEO Neuroticism and TPQ Harm Avoidance (Rothe et al., 2004; Strobel et al., 2003)—relevance of the *HTR1A-1019* polymorphism in anxiety disorders such as PD is plausible.

PD typically has its onset between late adolescence and the mid-30s. Panic attacks are sudden, appear to be unprovoked, and are often disabling. They may include intense fear, fear of dying, or a sense that something unimaginably horrible is about to occur and one is powerless to prevent it. Discomfort may be accompanied by several physiological symptoms, including palpitations, chest pain, choking sensations, sweating, trembling or shaking, dizziness, lightheadedness or nausea, flushes or chills, and/or tingling or numbness in the hands. Other manifestations may include fear of losing control and doing something embarrassing, dreamlike sensations, or perceptual distortions. A panic attack typically lasts several minutes to hours and may be one of the most distressing experiences a person may experience. Panic attacks are followed by persistent concerns about having additional attacks, worry about the implications of the attack or its consequences, and significant changes in behavior related to the attacks.

After one or repeated panic attacks—for instance, while driving, shopping in a crowded store, or riding in an elevator—patients may develop an irrational fear, or phobia, about these situations and begin to avoid them. Ultimately, the pattern of avoidance and level of anxiety about another attack may reach a point where a patient with PD may be unable to drive or even to leave home. At this stage, PD is complicated by agoraphobia. The first attacks are frequently triggered by physical illnesses, psychosocial stress, or certain drug treatments or drugs of abuse that increase activity of the neural systems involved in fear and anxiety responses. Although a considerable genetic component contributes to the susceptibility to PD (for a review, see Lesch, 2003), attacks can be pharmacologically precipitated by carbon dioxide, caffeine, lactate, cholecystokinin tetrapeptide, and serotonergic compounds (Lesch et al., 1992).

GENETICS OF PANIC DISORDER
AND THE *HTR1A-1019* POLYMORPHISM

Two complete genome-wide linkage scans for PD liability genes have been published (Crowe, Goedken, Samuelson, Wilson, & Nelson, 2001; Knowles et al., 1998). Although none of the findings reached a level of statistical confidence according to stringent criteria, a region suggestive of a susceptibility locus for PD on chromosome 7p15 was independently identified in both studies. Crowe and colleagues (2001) detected the highest lod score of 2.23 at the D7S2846 locus, located at 57.8 cM on chromosome 7, in a region that lies within 15 cM from the D7S435 locus reported by Knowles and colleagues (1998). Linkage to numerous other markers over a substantial proportion of the human genome had previously been excluded under various parametric models in different sets of pedigrees (for a review, see Lesch, 2003). Some of the conflicting results of linkage analyses in PD may be ascribed to methodological differences in family ascertainment, phenotype definition, diagnostic assessment, and approaches data analysis. It is even more likely that they represent true etiological differences due to locus heterogeneity. Susceptibility to PD may thus be influenced either by an incompletely penetrant major gene in some families or by multiple genes of weak and varying effect in others. Since evidence for a genetic liability in PD is persuasive, a small number of putative vulnerability genes—including the genes for γ-aminobutyric acid-A, dopamine D2 and D4, cholecystokinin B, and adenosine A1 and A2a receptors, as well as those for the 5-HT transporter and monoamine oxidase A—have been assessed in association studies (Lesch, 2003).

Since several preclinical and clinical studies also implicate the 5-HT$_{1A}$ receptor in the pathogenesis of PD, the impact of *HTR1A-1019* polymorphism was investigated by means of an association analysis in a cohort of 134 patients with PD (Rothe et al., 2004). Only a trend toward association in genotype and allele frequency between patients with PD and control subjects was observed. Significant differences were also not seen when men and women were analyzed separately. In the subgroup of patients with PD and agoraphobia, however, an association with a significant excess of the G/G genotype and the G allele of the *HTR1A-1019* SNP as compared to controls was detected (Figure 13.2).

These findings are consistent with the reports that the G allele is associated with both major depression and depression-related personality traits in healthy volunteers (Lemonde et al., 2003; Strobel et al., 2003), since approximately 30% of patients had secondary major depression and the association was only observed in the subgroup of patients with agoraphobia. In fact, comorbidity between depression and agoraphobia is a clinically well-

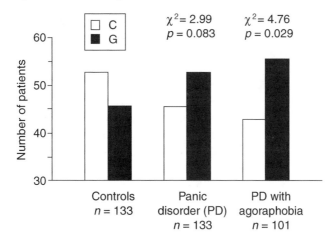

FIGURE 13.2. Allele frequencies of the *HTR1A-1019* polymorphism in patients with PD and controls. Adapted from Rothe et al. (2004).

described phenomenon; it is considerably higher than between the comorbidity depression and other phobias, and is influenced by both genetic and individual environmental factors (Kendler, Neale, Kessler, Heath, & Eaves, 1993). Nevertheless, future studies with independent, larger, and family-based designs are desiderata.

In summary, the Rothe and colleagues (2004) results suggest that the *HTR1A-1019* polymorphism contributes to the pathogenesis of agoraphobia in PD, and they further support a role of the 5-HT$_{1A}$ in anxiety. This notion has recently been underscored by Huang and colleagues (2004), who reported an association of the *HTR1A-1019* SNP with PD as well as with schizophrenia and substance use disorders. It remains to be discussed whether therapeutic responses to serotonergic agents are influenced by this *HTR1A* variation.

PHARMACOGENETICS OF 5-HT$_{1A}$ RECEPTORS

Because the detailed mechanisms of antidepressant responses continue to be enigmatic, studies have shifted their focus from adaptive changes in neurotransmitter release, uptake, and metabolism to modulation of gene expression, synaptic plasticity, neurogenesis, and neuronal survival (Lesch, 2001; Santarelli et al., 2003). Treatment response to serotonergic antidepressant and anxiolytic drugs, such as prototypical tricyclics (e.g., clomipramine) and the SSRIs (e.g., fluvoxamine, paroxetine, citalopram, and sertraline), is influenced by genetic factors and depends on the structure or functional expression of various gene products that mediate serotonergic signaling. Although treatment response is believed to involve both genetic and environmental factors, the contribution of an individual gene to drug response is likely to be modest. However, interactions between different genes may result in a dramatic modification of drug response (additive, nonadditive, or multiplicative gene effects). The challenge faced by research into the genetic basis of drug response is to identify genes with relatively small effects against a background of substantial genetic and environmental variation.

Intriguingly, down-regulation and hyporesponsivity of 5-HT$_{1A}$ receptors in patients with major depression are not reversed by antidepressant drug treatment (Lesch, Disselkamp-Tietze, & Schmidtke, 1990; Lesch, Hoh, Schulte, Osterheider, & Muller, 1991; Sargent et al., 2000), raising the possibility that low receptor function is a trait feature and therefore a pathogenetic mechanism of the disease. While deficits in hippocampal 5-HT$_{1A}$ receptor function may contribute to the cognitive abnormalities associated with mood disorders, recent work suggests that activation of this receptor stimulates neurogenesis in the dentate gyrus of the hippocampus. By using both a mouse model with a targeted ablation of the 5-HT$_{1A}$ receptor and radiological methods, Santarelli and colleagues (2003) have provided persuasive evidence that 5-HT$_{1A}$-activated hippocampal neurogenesis is essentially required for the behavioral effects of long-term antidepressant treatment with SSRIs.

Since a given genetic predisposition, such as allelic variation in 5-HT$_{1A}$ function, increases susceptibility to anxious or depressive features as well as depression and PD, it may also lead to less favorable antidepressant responses in patients affected by mood disorders. Preliminary evidence that allelic variation of 5-HT$_{1A}$ receptor expression influences the response to antidepressant treatment is now provided by two independent studies. Serretti and colleagues (2004) assessed the severity of depressive symptoms in 151 patients with major depression and 111 patients with bipolar disorder before and following 6 weeks of treatment with the SSRI fluvoxamine; they demonstrated that in bipolar disorder, but not in unipolar depression, patients homozygous for the C variant of the *HTR1A-1019* polymorphism showed a better response than carriers of the G allele did. Interestingly, the results failed to reveal an interaction between the *HTR1A-1019* SNP and a previously reported effect of a functional gene variant of the 5-HT transporter. Lemonde, Du, Bakish, Hrdina, and Albert (2004) also reported that antidepressant response to the SSRI fluoxetine, the norepinephrine reuptake inhibitor nefadozone, and the 5-HT$_{1A}$ agonist flibanserin, which desensitize the 5-HT$_{1A}$ autoreceptor as one of their mechanisms of action, was associated with *HTR1A-1019* polymorphism in 118 depressed patients. Patients homozygous for the G variant of the *HTR1A-1019* polymorphism improved significantly less on flibanserin, and in pooled antidepressant treatment groups they were twice as likely to be nonresponders as those with the C/C genotype. These findings further corroborate the hypothesis that genetic variations in *HTR1A* may not only predispose people to psychiatric disorders, but may also contribute to individual differences in responsiveness to antidepressant treatment.

Taken together, these findings indicate that allelic variation in 5-HT$_{1A}$ receptor expression seems to play a critical role in the development and modulation of individual differences in anxiety- and depression-related personality traits, as well as in the pathophysiology of anxiety disorders and syndromal dimensions of depression, psychosis, and substance abuse. Evidence that this polymorphism also influences therapeutic responses to serotonergic agents may have implications for tailoring individual antidepressant or anxiolytic treatment.

5-HT$_{1A}$ RECEPTOR KNOCKOUT AND ANXIETY

The converging lines of evidence that 5-HT$_{1A}$ receptor deficiency or dysfunction is involved in depression and anxiety disorders led to the genetic inactivation of this receptor in mice (for reviews, see Lesch, 2005; Lesch et al., 2003). Htr1a knockout (KO) mice show a complete lack of ligand binding to brain 5-HT$_{1A}$ receptors in null-mutant Htr1a–/– mice, with intermediate binding in the heterozygote Htr1a+/– mice. Importantly, a similar behavioral phenotype characterized by increased anxiety-related behavior and stress reactivity in several avoidance and behavioral despair paradigms was observed in three different KO mouse strains (Lesch & Mössner, 1999).

Htr1a KO mice consistently display a spontaneous phenotype that is associated with a gender-modulated and gene-/dose-dependent increase of anxiety-related behaviors (Heisler et al., 1998; Parks, Robinson, Sibille, Shenk, & Toth, 1998; Ramboz et al., 1998). With the exception of an enhanced sensitivity of terminal 5-HT$_{1B}$ receptors, no major neuroadaptational changes were detected. Worthy of note is that this behavioral phenotype was observed in several strains of mice into which the mutation was bred (mice of Swiss–Webster [SW], C57BL/6J, and 129/SV backgrounds), substantiating the assumption that this behavior is an authentic consequence of reduced or absent 5-HT$_{1A}$ receptors. Although all investigators used open-field exploratory behavior as a model for assessing anxiety, two groups confirmed that Htr1a KO mice had increased anxiety by using other models—either the elevated zero maze or elevated plus maze test (Heisler et al., 1998; Ramboz et al., 1998). These ethologically based conflict models test fear- and anxiety-related behaviors by placing the natural tendencies for rodents to prefer enclosed, dark spaces in conflict with their interest in exploring novel environments.

Activation of presynaptic 5-HT$_{1A}$ receptors provides the brain with an autoinhibitory feedback system controlling 5-HT neurotransmission. Thus enhanced anxiety-related behavior is most likely to represent a consequence of increased terminal 5-HT availability resulting from the lack or reduction in presynaptic somatodendritic 5-HT$_{1A}$ autoreceptor negative feedback function (Lesch & Mössner, 1999). Although extracellular 5-HT concentrations and 5-HT turnover appear to be unchanged in the brains of Htr1a KO mice with a

SW or 129/SV background, indirect evidence for increased presynaptic serotonergic activity resulting in elevated synaptic 5-HT concentrations is provided by the compensatory up-regulation of terminal 5-HT release-inhibiting
5-HT$_{1B}$ receptors (Olivier et al., 2001; Toth, 2003). In contrast to Htr1a KO
mice with a SW or 129/SV background, extracellular 5-HT concentrations
were significantly elevated in mutant C57BL/6 mice in the frontal cortex and
hippocampus (Parsons, Kerr, & Tecott, 2001). This may reflect a lack of compensatory changes in 5-HT$_{1B}$ receptors, and is consistent with findings that
C57BL/6 mice are more aggressive and susceptible to drugs of abuse than
many other strains.

Several studies addressed electrophysiological properties of both presynaptic serotonergic neurons and postsynaptic hippocampal neurons in
Htr1a KO mice. A robust increase in the mean firing rate in dorsal raphe neurons was reported, although a considerable number of neurons were firing in
their normal range, and 5-HT release was not altered (Richer, Hen, & Blier,
2002). Moreover, mutant mice showed an absence of paired-pulse inhibition
in the CA1 region and lack of paired-pulse facilitation in the dentate gyrus,
suggesting altered hippocampal excitability and impaired plasticity of the hippocampal network, with consequences for cognition, learning, and memory
(Sibille, Pavlides, Benke, & Toth, 2000).

Since avoidance induced by conflict and fear is only one dimension of
anxiety-related responses, other components—including autonomic systems
activation, responsiveness to stress, 5-HT dynamics, and neuronal excitability
in limbic circuitries—appear to be involved in fear and anxiety. As a facet
of anxiety-like behavior, Htr1a KO mice show genotype-dependent and
background-strain-unrelated increase in stress reactivity in two paradigms of
behavioral despair, the forced swim and tail suspension tests. Autonomic
manifestations of anxiety and stress responsiveness in a novel environment or
during exposure to other stressors (increased heart rate and body temperature,
as well as attenuated release of corticosterone) are also characteristic of
Htr1a KO mice (Groenink et al., 2003). The reduced immobility in stress–
antidepressant test models is due either to an increased serotonergic tone
resulting from the compromised 5-HT$_{1A}$ autoreceptor-dependent negative
feedback regulation or to enhanced dopamine and norepinephrine function,
because it is reversed by pretreatment with a-methyl-*para*-tyrosine, but not by
para-chlorophenylalanine (Mayorga et al., 2001).

Although the behavior of Htr1a KO mice in various stress-related paradigms is more consistent with increased emotionality, their behavior essentially corresponds to the performance of rodents treated with antidepressants.
The role of 5-HT$_{1A}$ receptors in the therapeutic action of antidepressant drugs
has attracted extraordinary interest; however, there is substantial conflicting
evidence regarding the involvement of other serotonergic receptor subtypes
and neurotransmitter systems or neurocircuits that interact with 5-HT neurotransmission. Electrophysiological studies in rats indicate that each class of
antidepressants enhances 5-HT neurotransmission via differential adaptive

changes in the 5-HT$_{1A}$ receptor-modulated negative feedback regulation—changes that eventually lead to an overall increase of terminal 5-HT (for a review, see Blier & Ward, 2003)—and desensitization of 5-HT$_{1A}$ responsivity following antidepressant treatment has been demonstrated in rodents and humans (Lerer et al., 1999; Lesch et al., 1991; Sargent et al., 2000). The neuroadaptive mechanisms of antidepressant action of tricyclics or SSRIs are exceedingly complex. As the onset of clinical improvement commonly takes 2–3 weeks or more after initiation of antidepressant drug administration, progressive functional desensitization of pre- and postsynaptic serotonergic receptors (including 5-HT$_{1A}$, 5-HT$_{1B}$, and 5-HT$_{2A}$), which is set off by blockade of the 5-HT transporter, has been implicated in these delayed therapeutic effects. In conclusion, the phenotypic similarity between anxiety-related behavior and stress reactivity in humans and Htr1a KO mice powerfully validates the practicability of genetically manipulated animal models.

Since the 5-HT$_{1A}$ receptor is expressed in different brain subsystems, it is of interest to clarify whether pre- or postsynaptic receptors are required to maintain normal expression of anxiety-related behavior in mice. With an elegant conditional rescue approach, Gross and colleagues (Gross & Hen, 2004; Gross et al., 2002) illustrated that expression of the 5-HT$_{1A}$ receptor in the hippocampus and cortex, but not in the raphe nuclei, is required to rescue the behavioral phenotype in Htr1a KO mice. The findings indicate that deletion of the 5-HT$_{1A}$ receptor in mice (specifically in forebrain structures) results in a robust anxiety-related phenotype, and that this phenotype in Htr1a KO mice is caused by the absence of the receptor during a critical period of postnatal development, whereas inactivation of 5-HT$_{1A}$ in adulthood does not affect anxiety. Even more importantly, the findings further support the notion of a central role for 5-HT in the early development of neurocircuits mediating emotion (Di Pino, Mössner, Lesch, Lauder, & Persico, 2004; Lesch et al., 2003). Although there is converging evidence that the 5-HT$_{1A}$ receptor mediates anxiety-related behavior, the neurodevelopmental mechanisms that render Htr1a KO mice more anxious are highly complex, and their details remain to be elucidated.

MOLECULAR AND FUNCTIONAL IMAGING OF THE 5-HT$_{1A}$ RECEPTOR

While 5-HT$_{1A}$ receptors display high density in the limbic and cortical regions critically involved in mood regulation, PET studies have reported reduced 5-HT$_{1A}$ receptor binding in these regions in patients with major depression (Bhagwagar, Rabiner, Sargent, Grasby, & Cowen, 2004; Drevets et al., 1999; Sargent et al., 2000) and PD (Neumeister et al., 2004).

Quite unexpectedly, Huang and colleagues (2004) demonstrated that 5-HT$_{1A}$ receptor binding in prefrontal cortex of persons who committed suicide was not associated with the *HTR1A-1019* genotype, suggesting that 5-HT$_{1A}$ receptor availability in the mature brain is modulated by factors that obscure effects of gene regulatory mechanisms on its expression. Furthermore, it remains unclear whether allelic variation of 5-HT$_{1A}$ receptor function is equally operative at both the somatodendritic autoreceptor and the post-synaptic receptor levels. Since the physiological and genetic determinants controlling 5-HT$_{1A}$ receptor expression and function are largely unknown, David and colleagues (2005) studied the influence of *HTR1A-1019* SNP and a repeat length variation in the 5-HT transporter gene (the 5-HT transporter gene-linked polymorphic region, or *5-HTTLPR*) on 5-HT$_{1A}$ receptor expression in the living human brain, using the 5-HT$_{1A}$-selective PET ligand [^{11}C]WAY 100635. Higher scores in anxiety-related traits were associated with the short variant of the *5-HTTLPR*, which results in low 5-HT uptake function (Lesch et al., 1996). Whereas the *HTR1A-1019* SNP did not show any significant effects on ligand binding, 5-HT$_{1A}$ receptor binding potential values were lower in all brain regions in subjects homo- and heterozygous for the *5-HTTLPR* short variant, compared with subjects homozygous for the long variant.

The findings demonstrate regulatory effects of the 5-HT transporter on the 5-HT$_{1A}$ receptor, a functionally related but distinct mediator of serotonergic neurotransmission. Mechanistically, the lower transcriptional efficiency associated with the short variant of the *5-HTTLPR* may lead to decreased 5-HT transporter function, which may lead to a lifelong increase in 5-HT tone, which in turn may desensitize and down-regulate 5-HT$_{1A}$ receptors. On the other hand, the lack of an effect of the *HTR1A-1019* SNP—together with findings from postmortem brain, pharmacological challenge, and imaging studies consistently demonstrating low pre- and postsynaptic 5-HT$_{1A}$ receptor expression and function—rules out the hypothesis that depressed and/or suicidal patients with this polymorphism would show increased 5-HT$_{1A}$ autoreceptor expression in the raphe, thus mediating increased inhibition of serotonergic neurons (Lemonde et al., 2003).

The association of the *5-HTTLPR* short variant with reduced 5-HT$_{1A}$ receptor binding potential is consistent with studies in mice deficient for the 5-HT transporter. In 5-HT transporter KO mice, lack of 5-HT clearance results in a persistent 7- to 13-fold increase of 5-HT concentrations in the extracellular space as assessed by *in vivo* microdialysis in different brain regions—including prefrontal cortex, striatum, nucleus accumbens, and substantia nigra (Fabre et al., 2000; Shen et al., 2004)—whereas overall concentrations of brain tissue 5-HT are markedly reduced (Bengel et al., 1998). This altered central 5-HT homeostasis results in differential regulation of pre- and postsynaptic 5-HT receptors. Excess of extracellular 5-HT activates the negative autoinhibitory feedback and reduces cellular 5-HT availability by stimulating 5-HT$_{1A}$ receptors, which leads to their desensitization and downregulation in the midbrain raphe complex, and to a lesser extent in the hypothalamus, septum, and amygdala, but not in the frontal cortex and hippocampus (Fabre et al., 2000; Li, Wichems, Heils, Lesch, & Murphy, 2000). Although postsynaptic 5-HT$_{1A}$ receptors appear to be largely unchanged in the frontal cortex and hippocampus, indirect evidence for decreased presynaptic serotonergic activity but reduced 5-HT clearance resulting in elevated synaptic 5-HT concentrations is provided by compensatory alterations in 5-HT synthesis and turnover—down-regulation of terminal 5-HT release-inhibiting 5-HT$_{1B}$ receptors (Fabre et al., 2000). Partial down-regulation of postsynaptic 5-HT$_{1A}$ receptors in some forebrain regions, but a several-fold increase in extracellular 5-HT concentrations in 5-HT transporter KO mice, could therefore cause excess net activation of postsynaptic 5-HT$_{1A}$ receptors, resulting in increased anxiety-like behavior and its reversal by the 5-HT$_{1A}$ receptor antagonist WAY 100635 (Holmes, Yang, Lesch, Crawley, & Murphy, 2003).

Taken together, these findings add to an emerging picture that allelic variation in 5-HT transporter function, but not the 5-HT$_{1A}$ receptor gene, regulates 5-HT$_{1A}$ receptor availability in humans and thus offers a plausible physiological mechanism underlying the association among 5-HT transporter gene variation, personality, behavioral traits, and affective states. The findings also underscore the potential utility of mouse–human experimental parallels for the understanding of genetic effects on human brain function.

In order to have another look at the effect of the *HTR1A-1019* and *5-HTTLPR* genotypes on 5-HT$_{1A}$ receptor responsivity *in vivo*, we used the pharmacological challenge approach to examine hypothermic and neuroendocrine responses to the selective 5-HT$_{1A}$ receptor ligand ipsapirone (IPS) in 27 healthy subjects, who received either 0.3 mg/kg of IPS or a placebo under double-blind, random-assignment conditions. Regarding the *HTR1A-1019* polymorphism, 5-HT$_{1A}$ receptor-mediated thermoregulatory responses, $F(2, 24) = 0.06$, $p = .93$; adrenocorticotropic hormone (ACTH) responses, $F(2, 24) = 0.67$, $p = .52$; and cortisol responses, $F(2, 24) = 0.00$, $p = .99$, to IPS revealed no significant difference between genotypes and pre- or postsynaptic 5-HT$_{1A}$ function (Figure 13.3A). Although 5-HT$_{1A}$ receptor-mediated thermoregulatory responses, $F(1, 25) = 1.42$, $p = .25$, and cortisol responses, $F(1, 25) = 1.09$, $p = .31$, to IPS revealed no robust difference between the *5-HTTLPR* l/l and l/s genotypes (the s/s genotype was not observed in this cohort), IPS-induced ACTH release, $F(2, 24) = 4.67$, $p = .04$, was significantly lower in individuals heterozygous for the *5-HTTLPR* short variant (Figure 13.3B). Since the ACTH response may be considered a direct response to postsynaptic 5-HT$_{1A}$ receptor activation, these results provide further support for the notion that 5-HT$_{1A}$ receptor expression and responsivity in the adult brain is influenced by allelic variation of 5-HT transporter function but not by the *HTR1A-1019* genotype.

Genetic influences on behavior may be 10-fold more sensitively studied by using measures of brain-based endophenotypes than by using traditional measures of behavior, such as self-report questionnaire data (Hamer, 2002). This remarkable increase in sensitivity is due to the fact that neural circuits mediate the genetic effects on behavior through cognitive processes that they

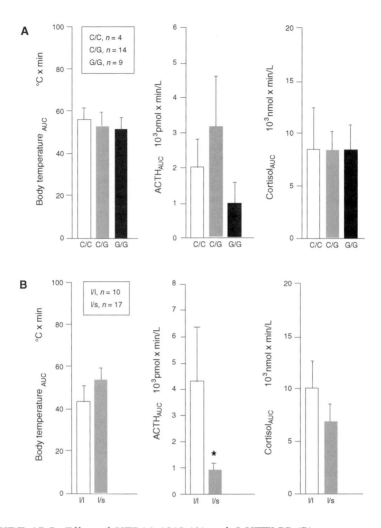

FIGURE 13.3. Effect of *HTR1A-1019* (A) and *5-HTTLPR* (B) genotypes on pre- and postsynaptic 5-HT$_{1A}$ receptor responsivity *in vivo*. Hypothermic and neuroendocrine responses to the selective 5-HT$_{1A}$ receptor ligand ipsapirone (IPS) were examined in 27 healthy subjects. IPS tests were conducted at rest in bed, and the subjects, who were familiar with the investigative setting, remained awake throughout the study. Each subject received 0.3 mg/kg IPS hydrochloride or identical placebo tablets orally at 4:00 P.M. under double-blind, random-assignment conditions on separate days as previously described (Lesch et al., 1991). For measurement of plasma ACTH and cortisol, blood was collected at −30, 0, 15, 30, 45, 60, 75, 90, 105, 120, 150, and 180 minutes, and sublingual body temperature was recorded at −60, −30, 0, 30, 60, 90, 120, 150, and 180 minutes with a high-resolution thermistor probe. The hypothermic, ACTH, and cortisol responses to IPS were calculated as the net (IPS–placebo difference) area under the curve (AUC$_{0-180}$) via trapezoidal integration. *HTR1A-1019* and *5-HTTLPR* genotypes were determined as previously reported (Lesch et al., 1996; Strobel et al., 2003). The effect of the *HTR1A-1019* and *5-HTTLPR* genotypes on IPS-induced hypthermia and on ACTH and cortisol concentrations was tested by analysis of variance (ANOVA).

subserve. Examples of endophenotypes may be cognitive functions such as attentional processes (Fossella et al., 2002), or brain activations captured via functional neuroimaging techniques (Furmark et al., 2004; Hariri et al., 2002, 2005; Heinz et al., 2005).

In a recent study (Canli, Amin, Constable, & Lesch, 2005), we employed this endophenotype approach to assess whether there is any evidence for an effect of the *HTR1A-1019* polymorphism on emotional attention. We used the emotional word Stroop task, in which word stimuli are printed in different ink colors and participants are asked to identify, as quickly and accurately as possible, the color of the ink for each word. Although word meaning is irrelevant in this task, emotional words may be more distracting than neutral words and thus result in slower reaction times (RTs). The first part of our study, using a sample of healthy volunteers (*n* = 65), was a behavioral evaluation of the impact that the *HTR1A-1019* polymorphism may have on RTs in the emotional word Stroop task. In the second part of the study, we used fMRI in a sample of 30 healthy volunteers to identify brain regions in which activation during performance of the emotional word Stroop task varied as a function of the *HTR1A-1019* polymorphism.

Our prior experience with this task (Canli, Amin, Haas, Omura, & Constable, 2004) and work by other investigators (Compton et al., 2003; Isenberg et al., 1999; Shin et al., 2001; Whalen et al., 1998) identified a priori regions of interest where genetic variation may affect neural function. Furthermore, by using emotional stimuli that could be either positive or negative in valence, we would be able to assess whether genetic variation in the *HTR1A-1019* would be specific to negative stimuli—as one might expect, given its association with anxiety- and depression-related traits as well as PD (Rothe et al., 2004; Strobel et al., 2003). Finally, to address the question whether any effect of the *HTR1A-1019* would generalize to other serotonergic polymorphisms (i.e., to obtain discriminant validity), participants were also genotyped for the *5-HTTLPR* polymorphism, which has similarly been associated with anxiety and depression (Caspi et al., 2003; Lesch et al., 1996).

Our behavioral study revealed that RTs for negative, relative to neutral, words were significantly slower for *HTR1A-1019* SNP heterozygous individuals (C/G) than for homozygous subjects (C/C and G/G, respectively), whereas RTs did not differ significantly between the two homozygous groups (see Figure 13.4). Importantly, this effect was specific to negatively valenced words and the *HTR1A-1019* polymorphism (no effect of genotype was seen for the *5-HTTLPR*). Additional analyses revealed that the effect size was 2.4 times greater for a *HTR1A-1019* genotype effect on RT, compared to a genotype effect on self-reported neuroticism. This is empirical support for the view that endophenotype measures are more sensitive to genetic variation than self-report measures are.

The analysis of the fMRI data was focused on two a priori regions of interest, the anterior cingulate cortex and the inferior parietal lobule, based on our prior work (Canli, Amin, Haas, et al., 2004). Although there were no significant activation differences in the anterior cingulate as a function of *HTR1A*-1019 genotype, heterozygous subjects showed significantly greater activation than homozygous subjects did in response to negative, relative to neutral, words in the right inferior parietal lobule (Figure 13.4). The cluster that represented this activation difference was localized within an a priori region of interest, remained significant after corrections for multiple comparisons, and was very large in size (comprising several hundred voxels). Peak activation within this cluster represented an effect size of *HTR1A* genotype that was 6.6 times greater than the effect size of *HTR1A* on self-reported neuroticism. Thus there is a progressive amplification of the effect size that genetic variation has on self-reported personality traits, on RT measures of cognition, and on fMRI-based measures of brain activation, consistent with the endophenotype approach. Further analyses confirmed that the observed effects of *HTR1A* on Stroop processing of negative words were valence- and gene-specific.

The greater reactivity in heterozygous than in homozygous individuals is consistent with the concept of "molecular heterosis," according to which a phenotype associated with a polymorphic gene is more strongly expressed in heterozygous than in homozygous individuals (Comings & MacMurray, 2000). Furthermore, the specificity of the effect for negatively valenced stimuli is consistent with the role of *HTR1A* variation in anxiety- and depression-related traits (Strobel et al., 2003). However, the association with self-reported neuroticism and harm avoidance has been found with both heterozygous and homozygous carriers of the G allele. This suggests that the expression of molecular heterosis may depend on which measure of phenotype is selected (Comings & MacMurray, 2000).

LOOKING FORWARD

Taken together, we find converging evidence from behavioral and functional imaging data that heterozygous carriers of a functional *HTR1A-1019* polymorphism, which has previously been associated with anxiety- and depression-related traits, show greater attention to negative emotional stimuli. This provides evidence for molecular heterosis in cognition and its associated neural substrate. Functionally, this suggests that the degree of genetic transcriptional activity is not always linearly related to phenotype expression and may therefore indicate an interaction with additional variables that have not yet been identified. Therefore, although we have provided evidence for molecular heterosis in a specific cognitive paradigm and a specific neural locus, future work will need to identify the mechanism by which these nonlinear processes operate. It remains to be shown in future studies whether molecular heterosis is more likely to be the rule or the exception in characterizing gene–brain–cognition correlations.

ACKNOWLEDGMENTS

We would like to thank G. Ortega and N. Steigerwald for excellent technical a-ssistance. The work reported here was supported by grants from the Deutsche Forschungsgemeinschaft (No. SFB 581, No. KFO 125/1-1) and the European Commission (No. NEWMOOD LSHM-CT-2003-503474) to Klaus-Peter Lesch, and by grants from Stony Brook University, the National Science Foundation (No. BCS-0224221), and the National Institute of Mental Health (No. 1R13MH06783501A1) to Turhan Canli.

REFERENCES

Arias, B., Arranz, M. J., Gasto, C., Catalan, R., Pintor, L., Gutierrez, B., et al. (2002). Analysis of structural polymorphisms and C-1018G promoter variant of the 5-HT(1A) receptor gene as putative risk factors in major depression. *Molecular Psychiatry, 7*, 930–932.

Bengel, D., Murphy, D. L., Andrews, A. M., Wichems, C. H., Feltner, D., Heils, A., et al. (1998). Altered brain serotonin homeostasis and locomotor insensitivity to 3, 4-methylenedioxymethamphetamine ("Ecstasy") in serotonin transporter-deficient mice. *Molecular Pharmacology, 53*, 649–655.

Bhagwagar, Z., Rabiner, E. A., Sargent, P. A., Grasby, P. M., & Cowen, P. J. (2004). Persistent reduction in brain serotonin1A receptor binding in recovered depressed men measured by positron emission tomography with [11C]WAY-100635. *Molecular Psychiatry, 9*, 386–392.

Blier, P., & Ward, N. M. (2003). Is there a role for 5-HT1A agonists in the treatment of depression? *Biological Psychiatry, 53*, 193–203.

Canli, T., Amin, Z., Constable, R. T., & Lesch, K. P. (2005). *Evidence for molecular heterosis in cognition.* Manuscript submitted for publication.

Canli, T., Amin, Z., Haas, B., Omura, K., & Constable, R. T. (2004). A double dissociation between mood states and personality traits in the anterior cingulate. *Behavioral Neuroscience, 118*, 897–904.

Caspi, A., Sugden, K., Moffitt, T. E., Taylor, A., Craig, I. W., Harrington, H., et al. (2003). Influence of life stress on depression: Moderation by a polymorphism in the 5-HTT gene. *Science, 301*, 386–389.

Chalmers, D. T., Kwak, S. P., Mansour, A., Akil, H., & Watson, S. J. (1993). Corticosteroids regulate brain hippocampal 5-HT1A receptor mRNA expression. *Journal of Neuroscience, 13*, 914–923.

Cheetham, S. C., Crompton, M. R., Katona, C. L., & Horton, R. W. (1990). Brain 5-HT1 binding sites in depressed suicides. *Psychopharmacology (Berlin), 102*, 544–548.

Cloninger, C. R., Svrakic, D. M., & Przybeck, T. R. (1993) A psychobiological model of temperament and character. *Archives of General Psychiatry, 30*, 975–990.

Comings, D. E., & MacMurray, J. P. (2000). Molecular heterosis: A review. *Molecular Genetics and Metabolism, 71*, 19–31.

Compton, R. J., Banich, M. T., Mohanty, A., Milham, M. P., Herrington, J., Miller, G. A., et al. (2003). Paying attention to emotion: An fMRI investigation of cognitive and emotional Stroop tasks. *Cognitive, Affective, and Behavioral Neuroscience, 3*, 81–96.

Costa, P., Jr., & McCrae, R. R. (1992). *Revised NEO Personality Inventory (NEO PI-R) and NEO Five-Factor Inventory (NEO FFI).* Odessa, FL: Psychological Assessment Resources.

Crowe, R. R., Goedken, R., Samuelson, S., Wilson, R., Nelson, J., & Noyes, R., Jr. (2001). Genomewide survey of panic disorder. *American Journal of Medical Genetics, 105*, 105-109.

David, S. P., Murthy, N. V., Rabiner, E. A., Munafo, M. R., Johnstone, E. C., Jacob, R., et al. (2005). A functional genetic variation of the serotonin (5-HT) transporter affects 5-HT1A receptor binding in humans. *Journal of Neuroscience, 25*, 2586-2590.

De Vry, J. (1995). 5-HT1A receptor agonists: recent developments and controversial issues. *Psychopharmacology (Berlin), 121*, 1–26.

Di Pino, G., Mössner, R., Lesch, K. P., Lauder, J. M., & Persico, A. M. (2004). Serotonin roles in neurodevelopment: More than just neural transmission. *Current Neuropharmacology, 2*, 403–417.

Drevets, W. C., Frank, E., Price, J. C., Kupfer, D. J., Holt, D., Greer, P. J., et al. (1999). PET imaging of serotonin 1A receptor binding in depression. *Biological Psychiatry, 46*, 1375-1387.

Fabre, V., Rioux, A., Lesch, K. P., Murphy, D. L., Lanfumey, L., Hamon, M., et al. (2000). Altered expression and coupling of the serotonin 5-HT1A and 5-HT1B receptors in knock-out mice lacking the 5-HT transporter. *European Journal of Neuroscience, 12*, 2299–2310.

Flügge, G. (1995). Dynamics of central nervous 5-HT1A-receptors under psychosocial stress. *Journal of Neuroscience, 15*, 7132–7140.

Fossella, J., Sommer, T., Fan, J., Wu, Y., Swanson, J. M., Pfaff, D. W., et al. (2002). Assessing the molecular genetics of attention networks. *BMC Neuroscience, 3*, 14.

Furmark, T., Tillfors, M., Garpenstrand, H., Marteinsdottir, I., Langstrom, B., Oreland, L., et al. (2004). Serotonin transporter polymorphism related to amygdala excitability and symptom severity in patients with social phobia. *Neuroscience Letters, 362*, 189–192.

Griebel, G. (1995). 5-Hydroxytryptamine-interacting drugs in animal models of anxiety disorders: More than 30 years of research. *Pharmacology and Therapeutics, 65*, 319–395.

Groenink, L., Pattij, T., De Jongh, R., Van der Gugten, J., Oosting, R. S., Dirks, A., et al. (2003). 5-HT(1A) receptor knockout mice and mice overexpressing corticotropin-releasing hormone in models of anxiety. *European Journal of Pharmacology, 463*, 185–197.

Gross, C., & Hen, R. (2004). *The developmental origins of anxiety. Nature Reviews Neuroscience, 5*, 545–552.

Gross, C., Zhuang, X., Stark, K., Ramboz, S., Oosting, R., Kirby, L., et al. (2002). Serotonin1A receptor acts during development to establish normal anxiety-like behaviour in the adult. *Nature, 416*, 396–400.

Hamer, D. (2002). Genetics: Rethinking behavior genetics. *Science, 298*, 71–72.

Hamon, M., Gozlan, H., El Mestikawy, S., Emerit, M. B., Boanos, F., & Schlechter, L. (1990) The central 5-HT1A receptors: pharmacological, biochemical, functional and regulatory properties. *Annals of the New York Academy of Sciences, 600,* 114–131.

Hariri, A. R., Drabant, E. M., Munoz, K. E., Kolachana, B. S., Mattay, V. S., Egan, M. F., et al. (2005). A susceptibility gene for affective disorders and the response of the human amygdala. *Archives of General Psychiatry, 62,* 146–152.

Hariri, A. R., Mattay, V. S., Tessitore, A., Kolachana, B., Fera, F., Goldman, D., et al. (2002). Serotonin transporter genetic variation and the response of the human amygdala. *Science, 297,* 400–403.

Heinz, A., Braus, D. F., Smolka, M. N., Wrase, J., Puls, I., Hermann, D., et al. (2005). Amygdala–prefrontal coupling depends on a genetic variation of the serotonin transporter [Electronic version]. *Nature Neuroscience, 8,* 20–21.

Heisler, L. K., Chu, H. M., Brennan, T. J., Danao, J. A., Bajwa, P., Parsons, L. H., et al. (1998). Elevated anxiety and antidepressant-like responses in serotonin 5-HT1A receptor mutant mice. *Proceedings of the National Academy of Sciences USA, 95,* 15049–15054.

Hensler, J. G. (2003). Regulation of 5-HT1A receptor function in brain following agonist or antidepressant administration. *Life Sciences, 72,* 1665–1682.

Hjorth, S., Bengtsson, H. J., Kullberg, A., Carlzon, D., Peilot, H., & Auerbach, S. B. (2000). Serotonin autoreceptor function and antidepressant drug action. *Journal of Psychopharmacology, 14,* 177–185.

Holmes, A., Yang, R. J., Lesch, K. P., Crawley, J. N., & Murphy, D. L. (2003). Mice lacking the serotonin transporter exhibit 5-HT1A receptor-mediated abnormalities in tests for anxiety-like behavior. *Neuropsychopharmacology, 28,* 2077–2088.

Huang, Y. Y., Battistuzzi, C., Oquendo, M. A., Harkavy-Friedman, J., Greenhill, L., Brodsky, B., et al. (2004). Human 5-HT1A receptor C-1019G polymorphism and psychopathology. *International Journal of Neuropsychopharmacology, 7,* 441–451.

Isenberg, N., Silbersweig, D., Engelien, A., Emmerich, S., Malavade, K., Beattie, B., et al. (1999). Linguistic threat activates the human amygdala. *Proceedings of the National Academy of Sciences USA, 96,* 10456–10459.

Kendler, K. S., Neale, M. C., Kessler, R. C., Heath, A. C., & Eaves, L. J. (1993). Major depression and phobias: the genetic and environmental sources of comorbidity. *Psychological Medicine, 23,* 361–371.

Knowles, J. A., Fyer, A. J., Vieland, V. J., Weissman, M. M., Hodge, S. E., Heiman, G. A., et al. (1998). Results of a genome-wide genetic screen for panic disorder. *American Journal of Medical Genetics, 81,* 139–147.

Lemonde, S., Du, L., Bakish, D., Hrdina, P., & Albert, P. R. (2004). Association of the C(-1019)G 5-HT1A functional promoter polymorphism with antidepressant response. *International Journal of Neuropsychopharmacology, 7,* 501–506.

Lemonde, S., Turecki, G., Bakish, D., Du, L., Hrdina, P. D., Bown, C. D., et al. (2003). Impaired repression at a 5-hydroxytryptamine 1A receptor gene polymorphism associated with major depression and suicide. *Journal of Neuroscience, 23,* 8788–8799.

Lerer, B., Gelfin, Y., Gorfine, M., Allolio, B., Lesch, K. P., & Newman, M. E. (1999). 5-HT1A receptor function in normal subjects on clinical doses of fluoxetine: Blunted temperature and hormone responses to ipsapirone challenge. *Neuropsychopharmacology, 20,* 628–639.

Lesch, K. P. (2001). Variation of serotonergic gene expression: Neurodevelopment and the complexity of response to psychopharmacologic drugs. *European Neuropsychopharmacology, 11,* 457–474.

Lesch, K. P. (2003). Genetic dissection of anxiety and related disorders. In D. Nutt & T. Ballenger (Eds.), *Anxiety disorders* (pp. 229–250). Oxford: Blackwell.

Lesch, K. P. (2005). Genetic alterations of the murine serotonergic gene pathway: the neurodevelopmental basis of anxiety. In F. Holsboer & A. Ströhle (Eds.), *Handbook of experimental pharmacology: Vol. 169. Anxiety and anxiolytic drugs* (pp. 71–112). New York: Springer.

Lesch, K. P., Bengel, D., Heils, A., Sabol, S. Z., Greenberg, B. D., Petri, S., et al. (1996). Association of anxiety-related traits with a polymorphism in the serotonin transporter gene regulatory region. *Science, 274,* 1527–1531.

Lesch, K. P., Disselkamp-Tietze, J., & Schmidtke, A. (1990). 5-HT1A receptor function in depression: Effect of chronic amitriptyline treatment. *Journal of Neural Transmission (General Section), 80,* 157–161.

Lesch, K. P., Hoh, A., Schulte, H. M., Osterheider, M., & Muller, T. (1991). Long-term fluoxetine treatment decreases 5-HT1A receptor responsivity in obsessive–compulsive disorder. *Psychopharmacology (Berlin), 105,* 415–420.

Lesch, K. P., Mayer, S., Disselkamp-Tietze, J., Hoh, A., Wiesmann, M., Osterheider, M., et al. (1990). 5-HT1A receptor responsivity in unipolar depression: Evaluation of ipsapirone-induced ACTH and cortisol secretion in patients and controls. *Biological Psychiatry, 28,* 620–628.

Lesch, K. P., & Mössner, R. (1999). 5-HT1A receptor inactivation: Anxiety or depression as a murine experience. *International Journal of Neuropsychopharmacology, 2,* 327–331.

Lesch, K. P., Wiesmann, M., Hoh, A., Muller, T., Disselkamp-Tietze, J., Osterheider, M., et al. (1992). 5-HT1A receptor–effector system responsivity in panic disorder. *Psychopharmacology (Berlin), 106,* 111–117.

Lesch, K. P., Zeng, Y., Reif, A., & Gutknecht, L. (2003). Anxiety-related traits in mice with modified genes of the serotonergic pathway. *European Journal of Pharmacology, 480,* 185–204.

Li, Q., Wichems, C., Heils, A., Lesch, K. P., & Murphy, D. L. (2000). Reduction in the density and expression, but not G-protein coupling, of serotonin receptors (5-HT1A) in 5-HT transporter knock-out mice: Gender and brain region differences. *Journal of Neuroscience, 20,* 7888–7895.

Lopez, J. F., Chalmers, D. T., Little, K. Y., & Watson, S. J. (1998). A. E. Bennett Research Award. Regulation of serotonin1A, glucocorticoid, and mineralocorticoid receptor in rat and human hippocampus: implications for the neurobiology of depression. *Biological Psychiatry, 43,* 547–573.

Mayorga, A. J., Dalvi, A., Page, M. E., Zimov-Levinson, S., Hen, R., & Lucki, I. (2001). Antidepressant-like behavioral effects in 5-hydroxytryptamine(1A) and 5-hydroxytryptamine(1B) receptor mutant mice. *Journal of Pharmacology and Experimental Therapeutics, 298,* 1101–1107.

Neumeister, A., Bain, E., Nugent, A. C., Carson, R. E., Bonne, O., Luckenbaugh, D. A., et al. (2004). Reduced serotonin type 1A receptor binding in panic disorder. *Journal of Neuroscience, 24,* 589–591.

Nishiguchi, N., Shirakawa, O., Ono, H., Nishimura, A., Nushida, H., Ueno, Y., et al. (2002). Lack of an association between 5-HT1A receptor gene structural polymorphisms and suicide victims. *American Journal of Medical Genetics, 114,* 423–425.

Olivier, B., Pattij, T., Wood, S. J., Oosting, R., Sarnyai, Z., & Toth, M. (2001). The 5-HT(1A) receptor knockout mouse and anxiety. *Behavioral Pharmacology, 12,* 439–450.

Olivier, B., Soudijn, W., & van Wijngaarden, I. (1999). The 5-HT1A receptor and its ligands: Structure and function. *Progress in Drug Research, 52,* 103–165.

Parks, C. L., Robinson, P. S., Sibille, E., Shenk, T., & Toth, M. (1998). Increased anxiety of mice lacking the serotonin1A receptor. *Proceedings of the National Academy of Sciences USA, 95,* 10734–10739.

Parsons, L. H., Kerr, T. M., & Tecott, L. H. (2001). 5-HT(1A) receptor mutant mice exhibit enhanced tonic, stress-induced and fluoxetine-induced serotonergic neurotransmission. *Journal of Neurochemistry, 77,* 607–617.

Ramboz, S., Oosting, R., Amara, D. A., Kung, H. F., Blier, P., Mendelsohn, M., et al. (1998). Serotonin receptor 1A knockout: An animal model of anxiety-related disorder. *Proceedings of the National Academy of Sciences USA, 95,* 14476–14481.

Richer, M., Hen, R., & Blier, P. (2002). Modification of serotonin neuron properties in mice lacking 5-HT1A receptors. *European Journal of Pharmacology, 435,* 195–203.

Rothe, C., Gutknecht, L., Freitag, C. M., Tauber, R., Franke, P., Fritze, J., et al. (2004). Association of a functional -1019CG 5-HT1A receptor gene polymorphism with panic disorder with agoraphobia. *International Journal of Neuropsychopharmacology, 7,* 189–192.

Santarelli, L., Saxe, M., Gross, C., Surget, A., Battaglia, F., Dulawa, S., et al. (2003). Requirement of hippocampal neurogenesis for the behavioral effects of antidepressants. *Science, 301,* 805–809.

Sargent, P. A., Kjaer, K. H., Bench, C. J., Rabiner, E. A., Messa, C., Meyer, J., et al. (2000). Brain serotonin1A receptor binding measured by positron emission tomography with [11C]WAY-100635: effects of depression and antidepressant treatment. *Archives of General Psychiatry, 57,* 174–180.

Serretti, A., Artioli, P., Lorenzi, C., Pirovano, A., Tubazio, V., & Zanardi, R. (2004). The C(-1019)G polymorphism of the 5-HT1A gene promoter and antidepressant response in mood disorders: Preliminary findings. *International Journal of Neuropsychopharmacology, 7,* 453–460.

Shen, H. W., Hagino, Y., Kobayashi, H., Shinohara-Tanaka, K., Ikeda, K., Yamamoto, H., et al. (2004). Regional differences in extracellular dopamine and serotonin assessed by *in vivo* microdialysis in mice lacking dopamine and/or serotonin transporters. *Neuropsychopharmacology, 29,* 1790–1799.

Shin, L. M., Whalen, P. J., Pitman, R. K., Bush, G., Macklin, M. L., Lasko, N. B., et al. (2001). An fMRI study of anterior cingulate function in posttraumatic stress disorder. *Biological Psychiatry, 50,* 932–942.

Sibille, E., Pavlides, C., Benke, D., & Toth, M. (2000). Genetic inactivation of the serotonin(1A) receptor in mice results in downregulation of major GABA(A) receptor alpha subunits, reduction of GABA(A) receptor binding, and benzodiazepine-resistant anxiety. *Journal of Neuroscience, 20,* 2758–2765.

Strobel, A., Gutknecht, L., Zheng, Y., Reif, A., Brocke, B., & Lesch, K. P. (2003). Allelic variation of serotonin receptor 1A function is associated with anxiety- and depression-related traits. *Journal of Neural Transmission, 110,* 1445–1453.

Toth, M. (2003). 5-HT(1A) receptor knockout mouse as a genetic model of anxiety. *European Journal of Pharmacology, 463,* 177–184.

Whalen, P. J., Bush, G., McNally, R. J., Wilhelm, S., McInerney, S. C., Jenike, M. A., et al. (1998). The emotional counting Stroop paradigm: A functional magnetic resonance imaging probe of the anterior cingulate affective division. *Biological Psychiatry, 44,* 1219–1228.

Wissink, S., Meijer, O., Pearce, D., van der Burg, B., & van der Saag, P. T. (2000). Regulation of the rat serotonin-1A receptor gene by corticosteroids. *Journal of Biological Chemistry, 275,* 1321–1326.

14

Genetically Driven Variation in Serotonin Function

IMPACT ON AMYGDALA REACTIVITY AND INDIVIDUAL DIFFERENCES IN FEARFUL AND ANXIOUS PERSONALITY

Ahmad R. Hariri

The 20th century bore witness to an explosion of inquiry regarding both the biological and social nature of individual differences in human behavior, including such complex emergent phenomena as character, temperament, and personality. Early attempts to characterize human behavior within both Darwinian and Mendelian frameworks were, at best, overly simplistic and poorly informed. For example, the complex nature of most genotype–phenotype links (e.g., pleitropic and polygenic traits), as well as of familial transmission of behavioral traits, was largely unknown. At worst, these early forays into the heritability of behaviors were politically and socially destructive (e.g., the eugenics movement). In the mid-20th century, however, the triumph of empirically based population and quantitative genetics ushered in the modern era of behavioral genomics (Weinberger & Goldman, in press). Since that time, research has increasingly focused on identifying specific biological pathways that contribute to complex cognitive and emotional behaviors—an endeavor paramount to our understanding of how individual differences in these behaviors emerge and how such differences may confer vulnerability to psychiatric disease.

Recent advances in both molecular genetics and noninvasive functional neuroimaging have begun to provide the tools necessary to explore these as well as other behaviorally relevant biological mechanisms. With completion of a rough draft of the reference human genome sequence (Lander et al., 2001;

295

Venter et al., 2001), a major effort is underway to identify common variations in this sequence that affect gene function (i.e., functional polymorphisms), and subsequently to understand how such functional variations alter human biology. Since approximately 70% of all genes are expressed in the brain, many of these functional polymorphisms will influence how the brain processes information. Functional neuroimaging (e.g., positron emission tomography [PET], functional magnetic responance imaging [fMRI], electroencephalography [EEG], and magnetoencephalography [MEG]), because of its capacity to assay information processing in discrete brain circuits within individuals, has unique potential as a tool for characterizing functional genomics in the brain. The goals of this chapter are to (1) describe the conceptual basis for and potential of this synthetic approach, referred to as "imaging genomics"; (2) highlight recent studies of the relationship between genetic variation in serotonergic neurotransmission and brain function that exemplify this approach; and (3) discuss the relevance of genetically driven variation in amygdala reactivity for individual differences in the personality trait of harm avoidance.

WHY STUDY GENES?

Genes have unparalleled potential impact on all levels of biology. In the context of disease states, particularly behavioral disorders, genes not only transcend phenomenological diagnosis; they represent mechanisms of disease. Moreover, genes offer the potential to identify at-risk individuals and biological pathways for the development of new treatments. Although most human behaviors cannot be explained by genes alone, and certainly much variance in aspects of brain information processing will not be genetically determined, variations in genetic sequence that affect gene function will contribute some variance to these more complex phenomena. This conclusion is implicit in the results of studies of twins, which have revealed heritabilities ranging from 40% to 70% for various aspects of cognition, temperament, and personality (Plomin, Owen, & McGuffin, 1994). In the case of psychiatric illness, genes appear to be the only consistent risk factors that have been identified across populations, and the lion's share of susceptibility to major psychiatric disorders is accounted for by inheritance (Moldin & Gottesman, 1997).

Although the strategy for finding susceptibility genes for complex disorders by traditional linkage and association methods may seem relatively straightforward (albeit not easily achieved), developing a useful and comprehensive understanding of the mechanisms by which such genes increase biological risk is a much more daunting challenge. The "candidate gene association approach" has been a particularly popular strategy for attempting to meet this challenge (Vink & Boomsma, 2002). "Genetic association" is a test of a relationship between a particular phenotype and a specific allele of a gene. This approach usually begins with selecting a biological aspect of a particular condition or disease, then identifying variants in genes thought to affect the candidate biological process, and next searching for evidence that the frequency of a particular variant ("allele") is increased in populations having the disease or condition. A significant increase in allele frequency in the selected population is evidence of association. When a particular allele is significantly associated (i.e., is in linkage) with a particular phenotype, it is potentially a causative factor in determining that phenotype.

THE ROLE OF FUNCTIONAL NEUROIMAGING

Traditionally, the impact of genetic polymorphisms on human behavior has been examined by using assays such as clinical evaluations, personality questionnaires, and neuropsychological batteries. Although a few such studies have reported significant associations between specific genetic polymorphisms and behaviors, their collective results have been weak and inconsistent (Malhotra & Goldman, 1999). This is not surprising, given the considerable individual variability and subjectivity of such behavioral measures. Because such behavioral assays are vague and imprecise, it has been necessary to use very large samples, often exceeding several hundred subjects, to identify even small gene effects (Glatt & Freimer, 2002). In addition, behavioral probes and neuropsychological tests allow for the use of alternative task strategies by different individuals, which may obscure potential gene effects on the underlying neural substrates meant to be engaged by the tests.

Because the response of brain regions subserving specific cognitive and emotional processes may be more objectively measurable than the subjective experience of these same processes, functional genetic polymorphisms may have a more robust impact at the level of brain than at the level of behavior. Thus functional polymorphisms in genes that are only weakly related to behaviors and, in an extended fashion, to psychiatric syndromes may be strongly related to the function of specific neural systems involved in processing cognitive and emotional information in brain and, in turn, mediating and moderating behavior. This is the underlying assumption of what we have called "imaging genomics" (Hariri & Weinberger, 2003b). The potential for marked differences at the neurobiological level, in the absence of significant differences in behavioral measures, underscores the need for a direct assay of brain function. Accordingly, imaging genomics within the context of a "candidate gene association approach" provides an ideal opportunity to further our understanding of biological mechanisms contributing to individual differences in behavior and personality. Moreover, imaging genomics provides a unique tool with which to explore and evaluate the functional impact of brain-relevant genetic polymorphisms potentially more incisively and with greater sensitivity than directly examining behavior.

Functional neuroimaging techniques—especially those that are noninvasive, such as fMRI and EEG/MEG—typically require no more than a few minutes of subject participation to acquire substantial data sets, reflecting the acquisition of many hundreds of repeated measures of brain function within a single subject. Thus these techniques, in contrast to their behavioral counterparts, may require considerably fewer subjects (tens vs. hundreds) to identify significant gene effects on the response characteristics of the brain. Moreover, the efficiency of these techniques allows for the ability to investigate the specificity of gene effects by examining their influence on multiple functional systems (e.g., prefrontal, striatal, limbic) in a single subject in one experimental session. This capacity to rapidly assay differences in the brain responses of different information-processing systems, with enhanced power and sensitivity, places functional neuroimaging at the forefront of available tools for the *in vivo* study of functional genetic variation.

Of course, the protocol for imaging genomics involves first identifying a meaningful variation in the DNA sequence within a candidate gene. For the variant to be meaningful, it should have an impact at the molecular and cellular level in gene or protein function (i.e., should be a functional variant), and the distribution of such effects at the level of brain systems involved in specific forms of information processing should be predictable. For example, a genetic variation in the gene for the serotonin transporter (5-HT) that affects the availability of synaptic 5-HT would be expected to affect amygdala function, because 5-HT is important in amygdala physiology (see below). Finally, the contributions of abnormalities in these systems to complex behaviors and emergent phenomena, possibly including psychiatric syndromes, can then be understood from a more biological perspective.

5-HT AND EMOTIONAL BEHAVIOR

Converging evidence from animal and human studies using a myriad of experimental approaches has revealed that 5-HT is a critical neurotransmitter in the generation and regulation of emotional behavior (Lucki, 1998). Serotonergic neurotransmission has also been an efficacious target for the pharmacological treatment of mood and anxiety disorders, including depression, obsessive–compulsive disorder, and panic disorder (Blier & de Montigny, 1999). Moreover, genetic variation in several key 5-HT subsystems (presumably resulting in altered central serotonergic tone and neurotransmission) has been associated with various aspects of personality and temperament, as well as with susceptibility to affective illness (Murphy et al., 1998; Reif & Lesch, 2003). Although many of these findings have led to novel insights about the neurobiology of complex behaviors and psychiatric disease, the enthusiasm for their collective results has been tempered by weak, inconsistent, and failed attempts at replication.

The inability to substantiate these relationships through consistent replication in independent cohorts may simply reflect methodological issues, such as inadequate controls for nongenetic factors (e.g., age, gender, and population stratification), insufficient power, and/or inconsistency in the methods applied. Alternatively, and perhaps more importantly, such inconsistency may

The path from here to there...

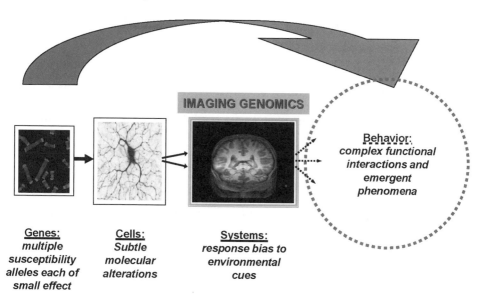

FIGURE 14.1. The increasingly divergent path from genes to behavior. Imaging genomics allows for the estimation of genetic effects at the level of brain information processing, which represents a more proximate biological link to genes as well as an obligatory intermediate of behavior. Adapted from Hariri and Weinberger (2003a).

reflect the underlying biological nature of the relationship between allelic variants in 5-HT genes (each with presumably small effect) and observable behaviors in the domain of mood and emotion (which typically reflect complex functional interactions and emergent phenomena). Given that the biological impact of a variation in a gene traverses an increasingly divergent path from cells to neural systems to behavior (see Figure 14.1), the response of brain regions subserving emotional processes in humans (e.g., amygdala, hippocampus, prefrontal cortex, anterior cingulate gyrus) may be more objectively measurable than the subjective experience of these same processes. Thus functional polymorphisms in 5-HT genes that are only weakly related to behaviors or psychiatric syndromes may be more strongly related to the integrity of these underlying neural systems (Hariri & Weinberger, 2003a).

5-HT, THE AMYGDALA, AND EMOTIONAL BEHAVIOR

The amygdala is a central brain structure in the generation of both typical and pathological emotional behavior, especially fear (LeDoux, 2000). Furthermore, the amygdala is densely innervated by serotonergic neurons, and 5-HT receptors are abundant throughout amygdala subnuclei (Azmitia & Gannon, 1986). Thus the activity of this subcortical region may be uniquely sensitive to alterations in serotonergic neurotransmission, and any resulting variability in amygdala excitability is likely to contribute to individual differences in emergent phenomena such as mood and temperament.

A substantial number of functional neuroimaging studies have revealed that human facial expressions, especially those depicting fear and anger, are robust and consistent provocateurs of amygdala activation (Davis & Whalen, 2001; Zald, 2003). The consistency of amygdala engagement in response to fearful or threatening facial expressions probably reflects the intrinsic survival value of such stimuli (Darwin, 1872/1998), as conspecifics represent both the greatest threat to our safety (signaled by angry facial expressions) and the most valuable source of information about danger in our environment (signaled by fearful facial expressions). Functional neuroimaging studies of genetic variation in serotonergic neurotransmission, as highlighted below, can capitalize on this inherent sensitivity by utilizing angry and fearful facial expressions as primary stimuli; they can thus maximize the ability to detect robust amygdala activation in all subjects, and can ensure that substantial variance in this response exists across subjects.

Furthermore, functional neuroimaging has provided important advances in our understanding of how different brain regions interact to regulate emotional behavior. Specifically, several landmark imaging studies have revealed that engagement of the prefrontal cortex, through a variety of cognitive tasks, results in the modulation and possibly the inhibition of the amygdala (Beauregard, Levesque, & Bourgouin, 2001; Hariri, Bookheimer, & Mazziotta, 2000; Keightley et al., 2003; Lange et al., 2003; Nakamura et al., 1998; Narumoto et al., 2000). Collectively, these results suggest that the dynamic interactions of the amygdala and prefrontal cortex may be critical in regulating emotional behavior (Hariri, Mattay, Tessitore, Fera, & Weinberger, 2003). Although fMRI, especially when it utilizes event-related strategies, allows for a rough estimation of how these and other brain regions interact during the processing of emotional material, imaging techniques that offer far superior temporal resolution, such as EEG and MEG, will be needed to more carefully explore the dynamic interplay of these neural circuits and the effects that variations in 5-HT subsystem genes have on this functional connectivity.

GENETIC VARIATION IN THE 5-HT TRANSPORTER

The 5-HT transporter (5-HTT) plays an important role in serotonergic neurotransmission by facilitating reuptake of 5-HT from the synaptic cleft. In 1996, a relatively common polymorphism was identified in the human 5-HTT gene (*SLC6A4*), located on chromosome 17q11.1–17q12 (Heils et al., 1996). The polymorphism is a variable repeat sequence in the promoter region (*5-HTTLPR*), resulting in two common alleles: the short (S) variant, comprising

14 copies of a 20- to 23-base-pair repeat unit; and the long (L) variant, comprising 16 copies. In populations of European ancestry, the frequency of the S allele is approximately .40, and the genotype frequencies are in Hardy–Weinberg equilibrium (L/L = .36, L/S = .48, S/S = .16). These relative allele frequencies, however, can vary substantially across populations (Gelernter, Kranzler, & Cubells, 1997).

Following the identification of this polymorphism, Lesch and colleagues (1996) demonstrated *in vitro* that the *5-HTTLPR* alters both *SLC6A4* transcription and level of 5-HTT function. Cultured human lymphoblast cell lines homozygous for the L allele have higher concentrations of 5-HTT messenger RNA (mRNA) and express nearly twofold greater 5-HT reuptake than do cells possessing either one or two copies of the S allele. Subsequently, both *in vivo* imaging measures of radioligand binding to 5-HTT (Heinz et al., 2000) and postmortem calculation of 5-HTT density (Little et al., 1998) in humans reported nearly identical reductions in 5-HTT binding levels associated with the S allele as observed *in vitro* (but see Patkar et al., 2004; Shioe et al., 2003; van Dyck et al., 2004). These data are consistent with ß-CIT single-photon emission computed tomography studies in humans and nonhuman primates reporting an inverse relationship between 5-TT availability and cerebrospinal fluid concentrations of 5-hydroxyindoleacetic acid, a 5-HT metabolite (Heinz et al., 1998, 2002); they indicate that the *5-HTTLPR* is functional and has an impact on serotonergic neurotransmission.

In their initial study, Lesch and colleagues (1996) also demonstrated that individuals carrying the S allele are slightly more likely to display abnormal levels of anxiety than are L/L homozygotes. Since their original report, others have confirmed the association between the *5-HTTLPR* S allele and heightened anxiety (Du, Bakish, & Hrdina, 2000; Katsuragi et al., 1999; Mazzanti et al., 1998; Melke et al., 2001), and have also demonstrated that individuals possessing the S allele more readily acquire conditioned fear responses (Garpenstrand, Annas, Ekblom, Oreland, & Fredrikson, 2001) and develop affective illness (Lesch & Mössner, 1998) than do those homozygous for the L allele. Recent studies utilizing pharmacological challenge paradigms of the 5-HT system suggest that these differences in affect, mood, and temperament may reflect *5-HTTLPR*-driven variation in 5-HTT expression and subsequent changes in synaptic concentrations of 5-HT (Moreno et al., 2002; Neumeister et al., 2002; Whale, Clifford, & Cowen, 2000). Furthermore, reduced 5-HTT availability, which presumably exists in *5-HTTLPR* S-allele carriers, has been associated with mood disturbances including major depression (Caspi et al., 2003; Malison et al., 1998), as well as with the severity of depression and anxiety in various psychiatric disorders (Eggers et al., 2003; Heinz et al., 2002; Willeit et al., 2000).

Not surprisingly, however, several additional studies have failed to identify a relationship between *5-HTTLPR* genotype and subjective measures of emotion and personality (Bail et al., 1997; Deary et al., 1999; Flory et al., 1999; Glatt & Freimer, 2002; Katsuragi et al., 1999). These failures probably reflect the vagueness and subjectivity of the behavioral measurements, but they also raise some concern that the relationship may be spurious (Ohara, Nagai, Tsukamoto, Tani, & Suzuki, 1998). In addition, such replication failures may reflect inadequate control for nongenotype factors such as gender and ethnicity (Williams et al., 2003), as well as chronic alcohol use (Heinz et al., 2000; Little et al., 1998) and exposure to environmental stress (Caspi et al., 2003)—all of which have been shown to influence the effect of the *5-HTTLPR* on both brain and behavior (see also Reif & Lesch, 2003).

Although the potential influence of genetic variation in 5-HTT function on human mood and temperament was bolstered by subsequent studies demonstrating increased anxiety-like behavior and abnormal fear conditioning in 5-HTT knockout mice (Holmes, Lit, Murphy, Gold, & Crawley, 2003), the underlying neurobiological correlates of this functional relationship remain unknown. Because the physiological response of the amygdala during the processing of fearful or threatening stimuli may be more objectively measurable than the subjective experience of emotionality, the *5-HTTLPR* may have a more obvious impact at the level of amygdala biology than at the level of individual responses to questionnaires or ratings of emotional symptoms.

IMAGING GENOMICS OF THE *5-HTTLPR* AND AMYGDALA REACTIVITY

In 2002, our research group at the National Institute of Mental Health utilized an imaging genomics strategy with fMRI to directly explore the neural basis of the apparent relationship between the *5-HTTLPR* and emotional behavior (Hariri, Mattay, Tessitore, Kolachana, et al., 2002). Specifically, we hypothesized that *5-HTTLPR* S-allele carriers, who presumably have relatively lower 5-HTT function and higher synaptic concentrations of 5-HT (analogous to the 5-HTT knockout mice) and have been reported to be more anxious and fearful, would exhibit greater amygdala activity in response to fearful or threatening stimuli than those homozygous for the L allele, who presumably have lower levels of synaptic 5-HT and have been reported to be less anxious and fearful (analogous to the contrasting wild-type mice).

In our initial study, subjects from two independent cohorts ($n = 14$ in each) were divided into equal groups based on their *5-HTTLPR* genotype, with the groups matched for age, gender, IQ, and task performance. During scanning, the subjects performed a simple perceptual processing task involving the matching of fearful and angry human facial expressions. Importantly, this task has been effective at consistently engaging the amygdala across multiple subject populations and experimental paradigms (Hariri et al., 2000; Hariri, Mattay, Tessitore, Fera, et al., 2002; Hariri, Tessitore, et al., 2002; Tessitore et al., 2002). Consistent with our hypothesis, we found that subjects carrying the less efficient *5-HTTLPR* S allele exhibited significantly increased amygdala activity in comparison with subjects homozygous for the L allele (Hariri, Mattay, Tessitore, Kolachana, et al., 2002). In fact, the difference in amygdala activity between *5-HTTLPR* genotype groups in this study was nearly fivefold, accounting for 20% of the total variance in the amygdala response during this experience—an effect size greater than any previously reported behavioral associations. This initial finding suggested that the increased anxiety and fearfulness associated with individuals possessing the *5-HTTLPR* S allele may reflect the hyperresponsiveness of their amygdalas to relevant environmental stimuli.

Recently, three independent functional imaging studies have reported identical *5-HTTLPR* S-allele-driven amygdala hyperreactivity in cohorts of healthy German (Heinz et al., 2005) and Italian (Bertolino et al., in press) volunteers, as well as in Dutch patients with social phobia (Furmark et al., 2004). Moreover, we have also replicated our initial finding of *5-HTTLPR* S effects on amygdala reactivity in a large, independent cohort of volunteers (*n* = 92). This large sample also allowed for the exploration of both sex-specific and S-allele load effects on amygdala function, and, in turn, dimensions of temperament associated with depression and anxiety (see below).

Specifically, we again observed that *5-HTTLPR* S-allele carriers exhibit significantly increased right amygdala activation in response to our fMRI challenge paradigm (Hariri et al., 2005; see Figure 14.2). In addition, our latest data reveal that *5-HTTLPR* S-allele-driven amygdala hyperresponsivity is equally pronounced in both sexes and independent of S-allele load. The equivalent effect of one or two S alleles on amygdala function is consistent with the original observations of Lesch and colleagues (1996) on the influence of the *5-HTTLPR* on *in vitro* gene transcription efficiency and subsequent 5-HT availability. The absence of sex differences suggests that the increased prevalence of mood disorders in females may be related to factors other than the direct risk effect of the *5-HTTLPR* S allele.

The collective results of these imaging genomics studies reveal that the *5-HTTLPR* S allele has a robust effect on human amygdala function. Importantly, the absence of group differences in age, gender, IQ, and ethnicity in each of these studies indicates that the observed effects are not likely to reflect systematic variation in such nongenotype factors. Rather, the data suggest that heritable variation in 5-HT signaling associated with the *5-HTTLPR* results in relatively heightened amygdala responsivity to salient environmental cues. That these results primarily emerged in samples of ethnically matched, healthy volunteers who were carefully screened to exclude any lifetime history of psychiatric illness or treatment argues that they represent genetically determined biological traits not related to manifest psychiatric illness.

5-HTTLPR, AMYGDALA REACTIVITY, AND HARM AVOIDANCE

In contrast to these striking imaging genomics findings of *5-HTTLPR* S-allele-driven amygdala hyperreactivity, attempts to link these effects on brain function with measures of emergent behavioral phenomena—namely, the person-

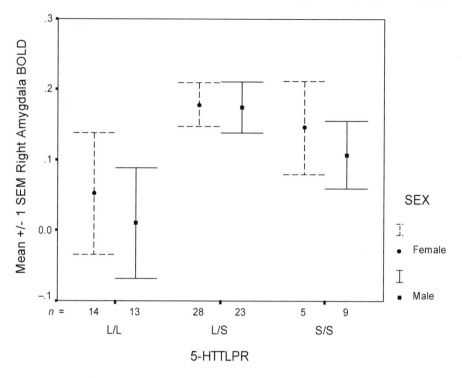

FIGURE 14.2. *5-HTTLPR* effects on amygdala reactivity. Line graphs represent the mean (± *SEM*) blood-oxygen-level-dependent (BOLD) signal change in the right amygdala. There was a main effect of *5-HTTLPR* genotype on right amygdala activation, with S-allele carriers having significantly greater activity than L-allele homozygotes, $F(1, 33) = 4.72$, $p = .04$. Adapted from Hariri et al. (2005).

ality trait of harm avoidance—have failed to detect any significant relationships. Specifically, in both our initial and replication studies, we did not detect any significant *5-HTTLPR* genotype effects on subjective behavioral measures of anxiety-like or fear-related traits as indexed by the Harm Avoidance (HA) subscale of the Tridimensional Personality Questionnaire (TPQ)—a personality measure putatively related to trait anxiety and 5-HT function (Cloninger, 1986; Cloninger et al., 1993). Although the sample sizes and thus power in both of our imaging cohorts were small relative to those of traditional behavioral association studies, the absence of an effect of the *5-HTTLPR* on HA is consistent with several published reports in larger samples (Schinka, Busch, & Robichaux-Keene, 2004). Thus our results and those of previous studies suggest that the *5-HTTLPR* does not have a robust and consistent effect on the dimensions of anxious and fearful personality measured by the HA subscale of the TPQ. Moreover, we failed to find any relationship, independent of *5-HTTLPR* genotype or other factors (e.g., age, gender, IQ), between amygdala reactivity and HA scores in a subsample of 83 subjects with overlapping fMRI and behavioral data sets (Hariri et al., 2005; see Figure 14.3).

These findings provide compelling evidence that genetically driven differences in the response of brain regions underlying emotional behavior may be readily investigated in relatively small sample populations, in the absence of significant differences in behavioral measures. They also raise the intriguing possibility that *5-HTTLPR* S-allele-driven variation in phasic amygdala function creates a bias toward a heightened brain response to environmental threat, but that this relative hyperresponsivity alone does not predict individual differences in harm avoidance. Although it is likely that constitutive variation in 5-HT signaling affects the biology of distributed brain systems beyond the amygdala, we and others have focused on the effects of the *5-HTTLPR* on amygdala function because this region plays a central role in the generation of behavioral arousal and orientation, as well as in specific emotional states such as fear.

TOWARD A SYNTHESIS

It is important to emphasize that the *5-HTTLPR* S allele's effect on amygdala reactivity in our studies, as well as those by Heinz and colleagues (2005) and Bertolino and colleagues (in press), exist in samples of healthy volunteers with no history of mood or other psychiatric disorders. This is consistent with a recent fMRI study reporting that although amygdala hyperexcitability reflects a stable, heritable trait associated with inhibited behavior, it does not by itself predict the development of mood disorders (Schwartz, Wright, Shin, Kagan, & Rauch, 2003). The study of Caspi and colleagues (2003) suggests that the existence of significant stressors in the environment of individuals carrying the *5-HTTLPR* S allele is necessary to tip the balance further toward the development of pathology and illness. Similarly, abnormal social behavior (Champoux et al., 2002) and 5-HT metabolism (Bennett et al., 2002) have been reported in rhesus macaques with the *5-HTTLPR* S-allele homologue, but only in peer-reared (and thus environmentally stressed) individuals.

This shift toward pathology may reflect the effects of environmental stress on brain regions, most notably the prefrontal cortex, that are critical in the regulation of amygdala activity (Hariri et al., 2003; Keightley et al., 2003; Rosenkranz, Moore, & Grace, 2003). For example, the experience of environmental insult before the maturation of relatively late-developing prefrontal regulatory circuits (Lewis, 1997) may result in further biased amygdala drive in S-allele carriers. Such relative amygdala hyperactivity and prefrontal hypoactivity have been documented in mood disorders (Phillips, Drevets, Rauch, & Lane, 2003; Siegle, Steinhauer, Thase, Stenger, & Carter, 2002), and thus may reflect critical predictive biological markers.

The importance, and perhaps even necessity, of such environmental stressors' acting on an extended neural circuitry in facilitating *5-HTTLPR* S-

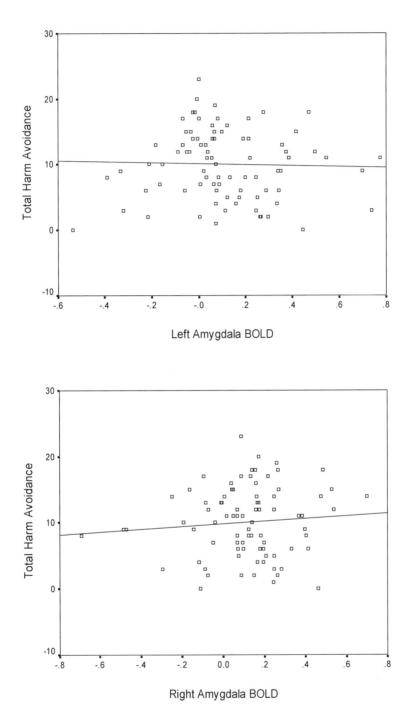

FIGURE 14.3. Amygdala reactivity and harm avoidance. Plots illustrate the absence of significant correlations between either left (r = –0.032, p = .77) or right (r = .086, p = .44) amygdala activity and total Harm Avoidance scores in a sample of 83 subjects. Adapted from Hariri et al. (2005).

allele influences on behavior is underscored by the absence of significant genotype or genotype × sex effects on HA, as well as correlations between
amygdala reactivity and HA, in our replication study in healthy subjects
(Hariri et al., 2005). This suggests that *5-HTTLPR*-driven variation in the
responsivity of the amygdala, though robust and consistent, does not necessarily result in altered mood and temperament per se. Rather, our current
results suggest that individual differences in complex, emergent phenomena,
such as harm avoidance, probably reflect the effects of genetic variation on a
distributed brain system involved in not only mediating physiological and
behavioral arousal (e.g., amygdala), but also regulating and integrating this
arousal in the service of adaptive responses to environmental challenges (e.g.,
prefrontal cortex).

Along these lines, two recent imaging genomics studies have reported
increased prefrontal responsivity during the monitoring of performance errors
(Fallgatter et al., 2004), and increased functional coupling of the amygdala
and prefrontal cortex during affect processing (Heinz, Smolka, & Braus,
2004), in healthy S-allele carriers. Thus intact dynamic interactions of the
amygdala and prefrontal cortex may be critical for typical behavioral responses in individuals possessing the *5-HTTLPR* S allele. As the impact of
genetically driven variation in dopamine availability (e.g., the catechol-*O*-
methyltransferase gene, or *COMT*) on prefrontal function has been well documented (Egan et al., 2001; Mattay & Goldberg, 2004), it will be of increasing
importance to model heritable variation in both amygdala and prefrontal
activity in exploring the influence of genes on behavior. We have begun to
examine the direct and interactive effects of several functional polymorphisms
(e.g., *5-HTTLPR* and *COMT*) on the dynamics of the amygdala and prefrontal cortex during the generation, integration, and regulation of affect. Furthermore, we are now exploring the impact of early environmental stress on
such genetically driven variation in brain function, and are examining how
this combination of effects contributes to the etiology of mood and other
affectively laden disorders in large longitudinal studies of children and adolescents.

LOOKING FORWARD

A focus on brain phenotypes allows for a more incisive assessment of genetic
effects—as evidenced by multiple replications of our initial report of 5-HTT
effects on amygdala reactivity—by examining biological systems more proximate to underlying molecular and cellular effects of specific genetic variants.
This increased power and sensitivity is reflected in the dramatically reduced
sample sizes (tens rather than hundreds) required to demonstrate robust
genetic effects on brain function. Moreover, understanding genetic effects on
distinct brain circuitry (e.g., amygdala and medial prefrontal cortex) has the
potential to inform many different behavioral phenotypes (e.g., fear, anxiety,

impulsivity, aggression) dependent on and supported by the underlying circuitry. Although "imaging genomics" provides a powerful new approach to the study of genes, brain, and behavior, its true potential will only be realized by aggressively expanding the scope and scale of the experimental protocols. Although single-gene effects on brain function can be readily documented in samples as small as 14 subjects, examining the contributions of multiple genes acting in response to variable environmental pressures is ultimately necessary for the development of truly predictive markers that account for the majority of variance in any given phenotype, such as stress resiliency. Ultimately, we anticipate that such a mechanistic understanding will allow for the early identification of individuals at greater risk for emotional regulatory problems that can have long-term health-related implications.

ACKNOWLEDGMENTS

I would like to thank Daniel R. Weinberger, MD, for his inspirational and pioneering work in imaging genomics, as well as his continued support and tutelage. Our research reported in this chapter was supported by the National Alliance for Research on Schizophrenia and Affective Disorders, and by the Intramural Research Program of the National Institute of Mental Health.

REFERENCES

Azmitia, E. C., & Gannon, P. J. (1986). The primate serotonergic system: A review of human and animal studies and a report on *Macaca fascicularis*. *Advances in Neurology, 43*, 407–468.

Ball, D., Hill, L., Freeman, B., Eley, T. C., Strelau, J., Riemann, R., et al. (1997). The serotonin transporter gene and peer-rated neuroticism. *NeuroReport, 8*, 1301–1304.

Beauregard, M., Levesque, J., & Bourgouin, P. (2001). Neural correlates of conscious self-regulation of emotion. *Journal of Neuroscience, 21*, 1–6.

Bennett, A. J., Lesch, K. P., Heils, A., Long, J. C., Lorenz, J. G., Shoaf, S. E., et al. (2002). Early experience and serotonin transporter gene variation interact to influence primate CNS function. *Molecular Psychiatry, 7*, 118–122.

Bertolino, A., Arciero, G., Rubino, V., Latorre, V., De Candia, M., Mazzola, V., et al. (in press). Variation of human amygdala response during threatening stimuli as a function of 5–HTTLPR genotype and personality style. *Biological Psychiatry*.

Blier, P., & de Montigny, C. (1999). Serotonin and drug-induced therapeutic responses in major depression, obsessive–compulsive and panic disorders. *Neuropsychopharmacology, 21*, 91S–98S.

Caspi, A., Sugden, K., Moffitt, T. E., Taylor, A., Craig, I. W., Harrington, H., et al. (2003). Influence of life stress on depression: Moderation by a polymorphism in the 5–HTT gene. *Science, 301*, 386–389.

Champoux, M., Bennett, A., Shannon, C., Higley, J. D., Lesch, K. P., & Suomi, S. J.

(2002). Serotonin transporter gene polymorphism, differential early rearing, and behavior in rhesus monkey neonates. *Molecular Psychiatry, 7,* 1058–1063.

Cloninger, C. R. (1986). A unified biosocial theory of personality and its role in the development of anxiety states. *Psychiatric Development, 4,* 167–226.

Cloninger, C. R., Svrakic, D. M., & Przybeck, T. R. (1993). A psychobiological model of temperament and character. *Archives of General Psychiatry, 50,* 975–990.

Darwin, C. (1998). *The expression of the emotions in man and animals* (3rd ed.). New York: Oxford University Press. (Original work published 1872)

Davis, M., & Whalen, P. J. (2001). The amygdala: Vigilance and emotion. *Molecular Psychiatry, 6,* 13–34.

Deary, I. J., Battersby, S., Whiteman, M. C., Connor, J. M., Fowkes, F. G., & Harmar, A. (1999). Neuroticism and polymorphisms in the serotonin transporter gene. *Psychological Medicine, 29,* 735–739.

Du, L., Bakish, D., & Hrdina, P. D. (2000). Gender differences in association between serotonin transporter gene polymorphism and personality traits. *Psychiatric Genetics, 10,* 159–164.

Egan, M. F., Goldberg, T. E., Kolachana, B. S., Callicott, J. H., Mazzanti, C. M., Straub, R. E., et al. (2001). Effect of COMT Val108/158 Met genotype on frontal lobe function and risk for schizophrenia. *Proceedings of the National Academy of Sciences USA, 98,* 6917–6922.

Eggers, B., Hermann, W., Barthel, H., Sabri, O., Wagner, A., & Hesse, S. (2003). The degree of depression in Hamilton Rating Scale is correlated with the density of presynaptic serotonin transporters in 23 patients with Wilson's disease. *Journal of Neurology, 250,* 576–580.

Fallgatter, A. J., Herrmann, M. J., Roemmler, J., Ehlis, A. C., Wagener, A., Heidrich, A., et al. (2004). Allelic variation of serotonin transporter function modulates the brain electrical response for error processing. *Neuropsychopharmacology, 29,* 1506–1511.

Flory, J. D., Manuck, S. B., Ferrell, R. E., Dent, K. M., Peters, D. G., & Muldoon, M. F. (1999). Neuroticism is not associated with the serotonin transporter (5–HTTLPR) polymorphism. *Molecular Psychiatry, 4,* 93–96.

Furmark, T., Tillfors, M., Garpenstrand, H., Marteinsdottir, I., Langstrom, B., Oreland, L., & Fredrikson, M. (2004). Serotonin transporter polymorphism linked to amygdala excitability and symptom severity in patients with social phobia. *Neuroscience Letters, 362,* 1–4.

Garpenstrand, H., Annas, P., Ekblom, J., Oreland, L., & Fredrikson, M. (2001). Human fear conditioning is related to dopaminergic and serotonergic biological markers. *Behavioral Neuroscience, 115,* 358–364.

Gelernter, J., Kranzler, H., & Cubells, J. F. (1997). Serotonin transporter protein (SLC6A4) allele and haplotype frequencies and linkage disequilibria in African- and European-American and Japanese populations and in alcohol-dependent subjects. *Human Genetics, 101,* 243–246.

Glatt, C. E., & Freimer, N. B. (2002). Association analysis of candidate genes for neuropsychiatric disease: The perpetual campaign. *Trends in Genetics, 18,* 307–312.

Hariri, A. R., Bookheimer, S. Y., & Mazziotta, J. C. (2000). Modulating emotional responses: Effects of a neocortical network on the limbic system. *NeuroReport, 11,* 43–48.

Hariri, A. R., Drabant, E. M., Munoz, K. E., Kolachana, B., Mattay, V. S., Egan, M.

F., et al. (2005). A susceptibility gene for affective disorders and the response of the human amygdala. *Archives of General Psychiatry, 62,* 146–152.

Hariri, A. R., Mattay, V. S., Tessitore, A., Fera, F., Smith, W. G., & Weinberger, D. R. (2002). Dextroamphetamine modulates the response of the human amygdala. *Neuropsychopharmacology, 27,* 1036–1040.

Hariri, A. R., Mattay, V. S., Tessitore, A., Fera, F., & Weinberger, D. R. (2003). Neocortical modulation of the amygdala response to fearful stimuli. *Biological Psychiatry, 53,* 494–501.

Hariri, A. R., Mattay, V. S., Tessitore, A., Kolachana, B., Fera, F., Goldman, D., et al. (2002). Serotonin transporter genetic variation and the response of the human amygdala. *Science, 297,* 400–403.

Hariri, A. R., Tessitore, A., Mattay, V. S., Fera, F., & Weinberger, D. R. (2002). The amygdala response to emotional stimuli: A comparison of faces and scenes. *NeuroImage, 17,* 317–323.

Hariri, A. R., & Weinberger, D. R. (2003a). Functional neuroimaging of genetic variation in serotonergic neurotransmission. *Genes, Brain, and Behavior, 2,* 314–349.

Hariri, A. R., & Weinberger, D. R. (2003b). Imaging genomics. *British Medical Bulletin, 65,* 259–270.

Heils, A., Teufel, A., Petri, S., Stober, G., Riederer, P., Bengel, D., & Lesch, K. P. (1996). Allelic variation of human serotonin transporter gene expression. *Journal of Neurochemistry, 66,* 2621–2624.

Heinz, A., Braus, D. F., Smolka, M. N., Wrase, J., Puls, I., Hermann, D., et al. (2005). Amygdala–prefrontal coupling depends on a genetic variation of the serotonin transporter. *Nature Neuroscience, 8,* 20–21.

Heinz, A., Higley, J. D., Gorey, J. G., Saunders, R. C., Jones, D. W., Hommer, D., et al. (1998). *In vivo* association between alcohol intoxication, aggression, and serotonin transporter availability in nonhuman primates. *American Journal of Psychiatry, 155,* 1023–1028.

Heinz, A., Jones, D. W., Bissette, G., Hommer, D., Ragan, P., Knable, M., et al. (2002). Relationship between cortisol and serotonin metabolites and transporters in alcoholism. *Pharmacopsychiatry, 35,* 127–134.

Heinz, A., Jones, D. W., Mazzanti, C., Goldman, D., Ragan, P., Hommer, D., et al (2000). A relationship between serotonin transporter genotype and in vivo protein expression and alcohol neurotoxicity. *Biological Psychiatry, 47,* 643–649.

Heinz, A., Smolka, M., & Braus, D. (2004). Amygdala activation, prefrontal metabolism and the serotonin transporter. *Biological Psychiatry, 55,* 43.

Holmes, A., Lit, Q., Murphy, D. L., Gold, E., & Crawley, J. N. (2003). Abnormal anxiety-related behavior in serotonin transporter null mutant mice: The influence of genetic background. *Genes, Brain, and Behavior, 2,* 365–380.

Katsuragi, S., Kunugi, H., Sano, A., Tsutsumi, T., Isogawa, K., Nanko, S., et al. (1999). Association between serotonin transporter gene polymorphism and anxiety-related traits. *Biological Psychiatry, 45,* 368–370.

Keightley, M. L., Winocur, G., Graham, S. J., Mayberg, H. S., Hevenor, S. J., & Grady, C. L. (2003). An fMRI study investigating cognitive modulation of brain regions associated with emotional processing of visual stimuli. *Neuropsychologia, 41,* 585–596.

Lander, E. S., Linton, L. M., Birren, B., Nusbaum, C., Zody, M. C., Baldwin, J., et al. (2001). Initial sequencing and analysis of the human genome. *Nature, 409,* 860–921.

Lange, K., Williams, L. M., Young, A. W., Bullmore, E. T., Brammer, M. J., Williams, S. C., et al. (2003). Task instructions modulate neural responses to fearful facial expressions. *Biological Psychiatry, 53*, 226–232.

LeDoux, J. E. (2000). Emotion circuits in the brain. *Annual Review of Neuroscience, 23*, 155–184.

Lesch, K. P., Bengel, D., Heils, A., Sabol, S. Z., Greenberg, B. D., Petri, S., et al. (1996). Association of anxiety-related traits with a polymorphism in the serotonin transporter gene regulatory region. *Science, 274*, 1527–1531.

Lesch, K. P., & Mossner, R. (1998). Genetically driven variation in serotonin uptake: Is there a link to affective spectrum, neurodevelopmental, and neurodegenerative disorders? *Biological Psychiatry, 44*, 179–192.

Lewis, D. A. (1997). Development of the prefrontal cortex during adolescence: Insights into vulnerable neural circuits in schizophrenia. *Neuropsychopharmacology, 16*, 385–398.

Little, K. Y., McLaughlin, D. P., Zhang, L., Livermore, C. S., Dalack, G. W., McFinton, P. R., et al. (1998). Cocaine, ethanol, and genotype effects on human midbrain serotonin transporter binding sites and mRNA levels. *American Journal of Psychiatry, 155*, 207–213.

Lucki, I. (1998). The spectrum of behaviors influenced by serotonin. *Biological Psychiatry, 44*, 151–162.

Malhotra, A. K., & Goldman, D. (1999). Benefits and pitfalls encountered in psychiatric genetic association studies. *Biological Psychiatry, 45*, 544–550.

Malison, R. T., Price, L. H., Berman, R., van Dyck, C. H., Pelton, G. H., Carpenter, L., et al. (1998). Reduced brain serotonin transporter availability in major depression as measured by [123I]-2 beta-carbomethoxy-3 beta-(4–iodophenyl)tropane and single photon emission computed tomography. *Biological Psychiatry, 44*, 1090–1098.

Mattay, V. S., & Goldberg, T. E. (2004). Imaging genetic influences in human brain function. *Current Opinion in Neurobiology, 14*, 239–247.

Mazzanti, C. M., Lappalainen, J., Long, J. C., Bengel, D., Naukkarinen, H., Eggert, M., et al. (1998). Role of the serotonin transporter promoter polymorphism in anxiety-related traits. *Archives of General Psychiatry, 55*, 936–940.

Melke, J., Landen, M., Baghei, F., Rosmond, R., Holm, G., Bjorntorp, P., et al. (2001). Serotonin transporter gene polymorphisms are associated with anxiety-related personality traits in women. *American Journal of Medical Genetics, 105*, 458–463.

Moldin, S. O., & Gottesman, I. I. (1997). At issue: Genes, experience, and chance in schizophrenia—positioning for the 21st century. *Schizophrenia Bulletin, 23*, 547–561.

Moreno, F. A., Rowe, D. C., Kaiser, B., Chase, D., Michaels, T., Gelernter, J., et al. (2002). Association between a serotonin transporter promoter region polymorphism and mood response during tryptophan depletion. *Molecular Psychiatry, 7*, 213–216.

Murphy, D. L., Andrews, A. M., Wichems, C. H., Li, Q., Tohda, M., & Greenberg, B. (1998). Brain serotonin neurotransmission: An overview and update with an emphasis on serotonin subsystem heterogeneity, multiple receptors, interactions with other neurotransmitter systems, and consequent implications for understanding the actions of serotonergic drugs. *Journal of Clinical Psychiatry, 59*(Suppl. 15), 4–12.

Nakamura, K., Kawashima, R., Nagumo, S., Ito, K., Sugiura, M., Kato, T., et al. (1998). Neuroanatomical correlates of the assessment of facial attractiveness. *NeuroReport, 9,* 753–757.

Narumoto, J., Yamada, H., Iidaka, T., Sadato, N., Fukui, K., Itoh, H., et al. (2000). Brain regions involved in verbal or non-verbal aspects of facial emotion recognition. *NeuroReport, 11,* 2571–2576.

Neumeister, A., Konstantinidis, A., Stastny, J., Schwarz, M. J., Vitouch, O., Willeit, M., et al. (2002). Association between serotonin transporter gene promoter polymorphism (5HTTLPR) and behavioral responses to tryptophan depletion in healthy women with and without family history of depression. *Archives of General Psychiatry, 59,* 613–620.

Ohara, K., Nagai, M., Tsukamoto, T., Tani, K., & Suzuki, Y. (1998). Functional polymorphism in the serotonin transporter promoter at the SLC6A4 locus and mood disorders. *Biological Psychiatry, 44,* 550–554.

Patkar, A. A., Berrettini, W. H., Mannelli, P., Gopalakrishnan, R., Hoehe, M. R., Bilal, L., et al. (2004). Relationship between serotonin transporter gene polymorphisms and platelet serotonin transporter sites among African-American cocaine-dependent individuals and healthy volunteers. *Psychiatric Genetics, 14,* 25–32.

Phillips, M. L., Drevets, W. C., Rauch, S. L., & Lane, R. (2003). Neurobiology of emotion perception: II. Implications for major psychiatric disorders. *Biological Psychiatry, 54,* 515–528.

Plomin, R., Owen, M. J., & McGuffin, P. (1994). The genetic basis of complex human behaviors. *Science, 264,* 1733–1739.

Reif, A., & Lesch, K. P. (2003). Toward a molecular architecture of personality. *Behavioral Brain Research, 139,* 1–20.

Rosenkranz, J. A., Moore, H., & Grace, A. A. (2003). The prefrontal cortex regulates lateral amygdala neuronal plasticity and responses to previously conditioned stimuli. *Journal of Neuroscience, 23,* 11054–11064.

Schinka, J. A., Busch, R. M., & Robichaux-Keene, N. (2004). A meta-analysis of the association between the serotonin transporter gene polymorphism (5-HTTLPR) and trait anxiety. *Molecular Psychiatry, 9,* 197–202.

Schwartz, C. E., Wright, C. I., Shin, L. M., Kagan, J., & Rauch, S. L. (2003). Inhibited and uninhibited infants "grown up": Adult amygdalar response to novelty. *Science, 300,* 1952–1953.

Shioe, K., Ichimiya, T., Suhara, T., Takano, A., Sudo, Y., Yasuno, F., et al. (2003). No association between genotype of the promoter region of serotonin transporter gene and serotonin transporter binding in human brain measured by PET. *Synapse, 48,* 184–188.

Siegle, G. J., Steinhauer, S. R., Thase, M. E., Stenger, V. A., & Carter, C. S. (2002). Can't shake that feeling: Event-related fMRI assessment of sustained amygdala activity in response to emotional information in depressed individuals. *Biological Psychiatry, 51,* 693–707.

Tessitore, A., Hariri, A. R., Fera, F., Smith, W. G., Chase, T. N., Hyde, T. M., et al. (2002). Dopamine modulates the response of the human amygdala: A study in Parkinson's disease. *Journal of Neuroscience, 22,* 9099–9103.

van Dyck, C. H., Malison, R. T., Staley, J. K., Jacobsen, L. K., Seibyl, J. P., Laruelle, M., et al. (2004). Central serotonin transporter availability measured with [^{123}I]beta-CIT SPECT in relation to serotonin transporter genotype. *American Journal of Psychiatry, 161,* 525–531.

Venter, J. C., Adams, M. D., Myers, E. W., Li, P. W., Mural, R. J., Sutton, G. G., et al. (2001). The sequence of the human genome. *Science, 291*, 1304–1351.

Vink, J. M., & Boomsma, D. I. (2002). Gene finding strategies. *Biological Psychology, 61*, 53–71.

Weinberger, D. R., & Goldman, D. (in press). Psychiatric disorders. In J. D. Watson, J. A. Witkowski, & J. R. Inglis (Eds.),*Rereading heredity in relation to eugenics: Contemporary reflections on the promise of human genetics.* Cold Spring Harbor, NY: Cold Spring Harbor Laboratory.

Whale, R., Clifford, E. M., & Cowen, P. J. (2000). Does mirtazapine enhance serotonergic neurotransmission in depressed patients? *Psychopharmacology (Berlin), 148*, 325–326.

Willeit, M., Praschak-Rieder, N., Neumeister, A., Pirker, W., Asenbaum, S., Vitouch, O., et al. (2000). [123I]-beta-CIT SPECT imaging shows reduced brain serotonin transporter availability in drug-free depressed patients with seasonal affective disorder. *Biological Psychiatry, 47*, 482–489.

Williams, R. B., Marchuk, D. A., Gadde, K. M., Barefoot, J. C., Grichnik, K., Helms, M. J., et al. (2003). Serotonin-related gene polymorphisms and central nervous system serotonin function. *Neuropsychopharmacology, 28*, 533–541.

Zald, D. H. (2003). The human amygdala and the emotional evaluation of sensory stimuli. *Brain Research Reviews, 41*, 88–123.

V

Individual Differences
in Children

15

Etiology of Psychopathic Tendencies in Children

DISTINGUISHING A GENETICALLY VULNERABLE SUBGROUP OF CHILDREN WITH ANTISOCIAL BEHAVIOR

Essi Viding and Robert Plomin

Psychopathy is an adult diagnosis that includes both affective–interpersonal impairment (callous–unemotional [CU] traits—e.g., lack of empathy, lack of guilt, shallow emotions) and overt antisocial behavior (Hart & Hare, 1997). One can also find children who exhibit CU traits and conduct problems (CP), and who thus could be said to have psychopathic tendencies (Frick, 1998; Viding, 2004). As such, individuals with psychopathy (adults) or CP + CU traits (children) represent a subset of those who would meet diagnostic criteria for antisocial personality disorder (APD) in adulthood or conduct disorder (CD) in childhood (Blair, 2001; Frick, 1998; Hart & Hare, 1997). In the fourth edition of the *Diagnostic and Statistical Manual of Mental Disorders* (DSM-IV) and its text revision (DSM-IV-TR; American Psychiatric Association, 1994, 2000), diagnostic criteria for these childhood and adulthood manifestations of antisocial behavior (i.e., APD and CD) include overt antisocial acts (such as violence toward other people or stealing), but do not distinguish subgroups of antisocial individuals on the basis of their CU profile (Hart & Hare, 1997). Most adults diagnosed with APD do not fulfill the diagnostic criteria for psychopathy, as defined by Hare and colleagues, given that they lack the concomitant CU features (Hart & Hare, 1997). In the same vein, not all children who have CD display CU traits.[1]

Children who show antisocial behavior from early childhood are at great risk for showing antisocial and criminal behavior in adulthood—a pattern known as "life-course-persistent antisocial behavior" (Moffitt, 2003). Such

317

individuals are likely to be 10 times more costly to the society than the average citizen (Scott, Knapp, Henderson, & Maughan, 2001); the interpersonal cost of these individuals to those who cross their paths is impossible to estimate. The early onset of these behaviors and their costliness make it important to understand the early origins of these behaviors, in order to intervene to prevent their onset. One theme of this chapter is that CU traits may be a risk factor that makes children vulnerable for life-course-persistent antisocial behavior of a particularly serious nature (Frick, 1998; Frick & Hare, 2001). Indeed, antisocial individuals who present with CU traits (individuals with psychopathy) start offending at a young age and continue across the lifespan with acts that are often predatory in nature (Hart & Hare, 1997). The predatory nature of their crimes reflects these individuals' lack of empathy (CU personality core). A recent study found that psychopathic murderers were highly likely to have committed premeditated murder, whereas this was not the case for nonpsychopathic murderers, whose offense was often a result of a heated dispute or a "crime of passion" (Woodworth & Porter, 2002). Even when residing in a correctional institution, individuals with psychopathy are six times more likely to offend than their convicted peers (Wong, 1985). The distinct pattern of offending (e.g., more premeditated crime and recidivism) seen in those with psychopathy defined by the personality-based approach (Hart & Hare, 1997), as well as the growing body of evidence for a characteristic neurocognitive profile (e.g., dysfunction in processing others' distress and punishment to self, linked to possible amygdala damage; Blair, 2003), attests to the importance of the CU traits in defining psychopathic personality disorder.

Mirroring the findings on adults, children with CU + CP have a greater number and variety of CP, and are also more likely to come into contact with the police than children with CP who do not have elevated CU trait scores (Christian, Frick, Hill, Taylor, & Frazer, 1997). Children with CU + CP are also less distressed about their behavioral problems than other children with extreme externalizing pathology; this suggests that CU traits moderate the level of distress experienced by the perpetrators (Barry et al., 2000), presumably facilitating the persistent antisocial conduct seen in these individuals. Children with CU + CP show a neurocognitive profile that is similar to the profile found in adults with psychopathy. This finding raises the possibility that psychopathy may be a developmental disorder with CU personality markers that can be delineated successfully in children. Research also suggests that these personality traits may go hand in hand with neurocognitive impairment in affective processing (Blair, 2001).

MEASUREMENT OF PSYCHOPATHY AND CU + CP

Cleckley (1941) first proposed the classic definition of psychopathy as a constellation of deviant personality traits, such as lack of empathy, lack of guilt, shallow affect, and manipulation of others. Building on this tradition, Hare developed the Psychopathy Checklist—Revised (PCL-R; Hare, 1991), a diagnostic instrument that indexes not just the extreme antisocial behavior seen in psychopathy, but also the CU markers at the core of the disorder (i.e., two aspects of psychopathy). The PCL-R is by far the most commonly used instrument to assess psychopathy in prison settings and has both good reliability and validity. Youth and screening versions of the PCL-R have additionally been developed for use in incarcerated populations (Forth, Kosson, & Hare, 2004; Hart, Cox, & Hare, 1995). Instruments also exist for self-report of psychopathic traits in both prison and wider populations; these include the Levenson's Self-Report Psychopathy Scale (Levenson, Kiehl, & Fitzpatrick, 1995), the Psychopathic Personality Inventory (PPI; Lilienfield & Andrews, 1996), and the Youth Psychopathic Traits Inventory (Andershed, Gustafson, Kerr, & Stattin, 2002). Finally, the Antisocial Process Screening Device (APSD; Frick & Hare, 2001) was designed to provide an age-appropriate measure of CU traits alongside measurement of impulsivity and narcissism. Frick (1998) conceptualized CU traits as risk factors for life-course-persistent antisocial behavior. Both teachers and parents can complete the APSD (Frick & Hare, 2001).

GENETIC STUDIES ON ANTISOCIAL BEHAVIOR AND PSYCHOPATHIC TRAITS

Given the early emergence of antisocial behavior in individuals with psychopathy and its long-term impact—even as compared with other antisocial individuals—it is important to gain information about the heritable and environmental origins of the CU traits, as well as about their function as risk factors for early-emerging antisocial behavior (which is itself a risk marker for life-course-persistent antisocial behavior). Broadening this understanding will inform future research, as well as the design of prevention and treatment programs. Genetic study designs are crucial for mapping the etiology of CU traits. This section briefly describes what is known about the genetic and environmental origins of antisocial behavior and psychopathic traits. This short review highlights the twin method, the most commonly used behavioral genetic study design, in answering a number of interesting questions that go beyond demonstrating heritability.

Rhee and Waldman (2002) recently conducted a meta-analysis of behavioral genetic studies on antisocial behavior and estimated that on average, about 41% of the variance on antisocial behavior was due to genetic factors, about 16% to shared environmental factors, and about 43% to nonshared environmental factors (these terms are defined in detail below). These estimates were based on findings from 51 studies that varied in sample size from very small (fewer than 100 participants) to large (thousands of participants); used different methods to infer estimates of heritability and environmental influence (twin, adoption, and sibling study designs); collected data on different age groups (children, juveniles, and adults); applied different definitions of antisocial behavior; and used different informants. However, the basic finding is that antisocial behavior is moderately heritable.

The Twin Method

Before we briefly review the small existing literature on the etiology of psychopathic personality traits, it is pertinent to provide a short description of the twin method and its use in antisocial behavior research. The twin study design can be used to estimate the proportion of variance on a trait that can be attributed to genetic, shared environmental, and nonshared environmental factors (Plomin, DeFries, McClearn, & McGuffin, 2001). It exploits the fact that monozygotic (MZ) twins are 100% similar genetically, while dizygotic (DZ) twins are on average 50% similar. If MZ twins resemble each other more closely than DZ twins do, genetic influences on a trait are inferred. The "heritability" statistic refers to the extent of genetic influences on individual differences on a trait. It is a population statistic and does not denote the amount of genetic influence on a particular trait within an individual. A rough heritability estimate can be calculated as twice the difference of MZ and DZ correlations, because MZ twins are twice as similar genetically as DZ twins. To the extent that MZ resemblance is not twice as great as DZ resemblance, "shared environmental" influences on a trait are inferred as residual twin resemblance not explained by genetic factors. These are environmental influences that act to make the twins similar to each other, such as prenatal events and life experiences affecting both twins in the same way. "Nonshared environmental" influences—environmental influences that act to make twins dissimilar to each other—are indicated to the extent that MZ resemblance is less than unity. The nonshared environmental estimate encompasses environmental factors that serve to make twins different from each other plus measurement error; of course, measurement error can be considered separately if an index of reliability is available. The major premise of the twin method is the "equal-environments" assumption (i.e., the assumption that MZ and DZ twins experience equal environments). This assumption has been shown to be reasonable in general (Plomin et al., 2001) and specifically in relation to behavior problems, including CD (Cronk et al., 2002).

Although simple MZ and DZ twin correlations provide a rough picture of the genetic and environmental influences on a trait, in practice twin analyses are conducted via maximum-likelihood model fitting. This approach tests the fit of the model and alternative models to the data, makes assumptions explicit, provides powerful estimates of genetic and environmental parameters using all of the data simultaneously, and gives standard error of estimates (Neale & Cardon, 1992).

Use of sufficiently large twin samples permits questions that go beyond demonstrating that antisocial behavior is heritable. It is possible to investigate genetic and environmental influences on comorbidity between antisocial behavior and other behavioral problems by analyzing twin 1's antisocial behavior and twin 2's score on another behavior. For example, there is suggestive evidence of overlapping genetic influences for conduct disturbance and hyperactivity (Silberg et al., 1996). It is also possible to ask developmental questions by assessing antisocial behavior over time and investigating whether genetic or environmental variables contribute to its continuity or change by measuring twin 1's phenotypic score at age 1 and twin 2's phenotypic score at age 2. As an example, a recent study suggested that continuity of aggressive antisocial behavior is genetically mediated (Eley, Lichtenstein, & Moffitt, 2003). The twin design can also be used to study heterogeneity within a behavioral phenotype. Groups of antisocial individuals can be divided on some distinct behavioral or personality marker to see whether etiological influences differ for different subtypes. For instance, early-onset antisocial behavior appears to be more heritable than adolescence-limited antisocial behavior—a finding that has been argued to reflect the transient, almost normative nature of adolescent antisocial behavior (Moffitt, 2003). The higher heritability estimate for antisocial behavior in young children may reflect a genetic predisposition to such behavior, particularly when antisocial behavior is pervasive over different settings (Arseneault et al., 2003).

Twin Studies of Psychopathic Personality Traits

Only two published twin studies to date have explicitly addressed psychopathic personality traits in adults. Blonigen, Carlson, Krueger, and Patrick (2003) collected data from 353 adult male twins; their study used the PPI (Lilienfeld & Andrews, 1996), a self-report measure designed to assess the personality domain of psychopathy. This instrument shows substantial positive correlations with several indices of Cleckley's (1941) classic clinical description of psychopathy, but it is not divided into two scales like the PCL-R, as it was developed to assess psychopathic traits in the general population rather than the syndrome of psychopathy in antisocial individuals. The PPI includes 163 items and forms a global index of psychopathic personality and eight subscales: Machiavellian Egocentricity, Social Potency, Fearlessness, Cold-Heartedness, Impulsive Nonconformity, Blame Externalization, Carefree Nonplanfulness, and Stress Immunity. Most of the individual subscales showed modest to moderately high heritabilities (h^2 = .29–.56), moderate nonshared environmental estimates, and negligible shared environmental influence. The heritability estimates were similar to or slightly higher than those typically found for self-report personality questionnaires (Loehlin, 1992).

Taylor, Loney, Bobadilla, Iacono, and McGue (2003) conducted a study with a sample of 398 young adult twin pairs. They created two scales to correspond to the personality and antisocial behavior aspects of the PCL-R, using items from the Minnesota Temperament Inventory. The scales were labeled Detachment (e.g., "I am insincere," "I have shallow feelings") and Antisocial (e.g., "I engage in misbehavior," "I do not learn from punishment"). Taylor and colleagues reported findings similar to those of Bloningen and colleagues for the heritability of the psychopathic personality dimension (h^2 = .42 for Detachment). The heritability estimate for the Antisocial scale was also in line with previous findings (h^2 = .39). Both scales also showed substantial influence of nonshared environment (with the measurement error incorporated in this term) and no influence of shared environment. In addition to these univariate analyses, Taylor and colleagues conducted a bivariate analysis to explore the etiological relationship between Detachment and Antisocial ratings. In their sample, genetic influences on these two trait measures overlapped substantially. There were also some common nonshared environmental influences (or common measurement error) that contributed to individual differences in both traits.

Because the sample sizes of the two studies described above were relatively small by standards of twin studies of self-report personality questionnaires (Loehlin, 1992), replication is needed in other twin samples. Furthermore, the samples were unselected, and the size of the samples prevented meaningful comparisons of heritabilities for the extremes of psychopathic personality traits. Finally, one of these studies was conducted on adults and the other on young adults, whereas for people interested in prevention and treatment efforts, data from childhood on similar (CU) personality traits and their etiological relationship with antisocial behavior is needed.

With this in mind, we have recently conducted the first twin studies of CU traits in preadolescent children. As mentioned above, none of the previous studies have reported on the etiology of extreme CU traits, or on whether the etiology of extreme CP/antisocial behavior differs for those individuals with CU (CU + CP) and those without CU (CP only). It is the combination of extreme CU traits and extreme antisocial behavior that characterizes individuals with psychopathy (or CU + CP, in the case of children), and it is therefore crucial to focus genetically informative research on the extremes of the sample distribution, in addition to studying the etiology of individual differences. In order to focus future molecular genetic investigations, we have also studied the etiological origins of the relationship between CU traits and antisocial behavior in 7-year-old twins.

ETIOLOGY OF CU TRAITS, CP, AND THEIR CO-OCCURRENCE IN CHILDREN

Sample and Measures

The sampling frame for our study consisted of 7,374 twins from the 1994 and 1995 birth cohorts of the Twins Early Development Study (TEDS). The average age of the participants at the time of assessment was 7.1 years (SD = 0.23 years). The sample and its history are described in detail elsewhere (Trouton, Spinath, & Plomin, 2002). Teachers provided ratings of CU and antisocial behavior (i.e., CP). We created a novel CU scale by using seven items available in the TEDS: three items from the APSD (Frick & Hare, 2001), as well as four items from the Strengths and Difficulties Questionnaire (SDQ; Goodman, 1997). These items either were original CU items ("Does not show feelings or emotions," "Feels bad or guilty when he/she does something wrong" [reverse-scored], "Is concerned about how well he/she does at school" [reverse-scored]) or were selected to reflect CU (e.g., "Considerate of other people's feelings" [reverse-scored]). None of the items overlapped with any of the CP items.

Teacher ratings on the CU scale showed good internal consistency ($\alpha =$ .74). Our CP scale was the SDQ 5-item scale used to assess conduct problems (e.g., "Often fights with other children or bullies them," "Often has temper tantrums or hot tempers"). The SDQ scales have good reliability and validity (Goodman, 1997), and the teacher ratings on the CP scale showed good internal consistency in the TEDS sample ($\alpha = .71$). The CU and CP scale scores correlated .49, indicating that although there was overlapping variance, the scales were not measuring the same construct.

Heritability of Extreme CU Traits and Extreme CP

We found that elevated levels of CU traits (top 10%) were under strong genetic influence (heritability of .67; Viding et al., 2005). This finding was broadly in line with the findings on the etiology of the individual differences in psychopathic personality traits reported in the adult studies (Bloningen et al., 2003; Taylor et al., 2003). It also corresponded closely to the findings on the etiology of individual differences in CU traits in our own twin sample (see the next section of this chapter). A small shared environmental influence on CU traits was also detected at the extreme (see Figure 15.1). After establishing that elevated levels of the CU traits were substantially heritable in children, we conducted further research on children with elevated levels of CP (top 10%) who either had or did not have elevated levels of CU traits. When we separated children with elevated levels of CP into these two groups, the most interesting result emerged (see Figure 15.1): We found CP in children with elevated levels of CU traits to be under extremely high genetic influence (group heritability of .81) and no influence of shared environment. In contrast, CP in children without elevated levels of CU traits showed modest genetic influence (group heritability of .30) and moderate environmental influence (group shared environmental influence = .34, group nonshared environmental influence = .26). This is a novel finding and represents an etiologically based refinement for theories of antisocial behavior. It indicates that there is heterogeneity within the early-onset group that warrants further investigation. CU traits appear to be an interesting marker for this heterogeneity. It is worth noting that our finding was replicated when 5%, 10%, and 15% cutoffs were used to select extreme groups for both CU traits and CP. It is also worth noting that our method did not mean that we merely measured heritability for more severe antisocial behavior in children

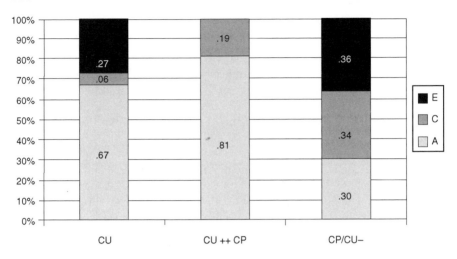

FIGURE 15.1. Callous–unemotional (CU) traits were strongly heritable at the extreme ($h^2g = .67$). Furthermore, conduct problems (CP) were strongly heritable in children with elevated levels of CU traits (CU + CP; $h^2g[\text{CP}] = .81$), but only moderately heritable in children without elevated levels of CU traits (CP/CU–; $h^2g[\text{CP}] = .31$).

with CU + CP. If we took varying severity cutoffs for antisocial behavior without any regard for the level of CU traits, the heritability of antisocial behavior at different cutoffs did not change.

These findings of etiological heterogeneity have implications for future research on development of antisocial behavior. We are currently following up the twins at 9 years of age and will be able to assess whether the two subgroups of children with early-onset antisocial behavior (i.e., those with and without CU traits) show different patterns of stability for their antisocial behavior, or differ in their environmental risk factors. Because we are using a twin design, we can also address whether genetic or environmental effects are primarily responsible for any change or continuity in antisocial behavior in the two subgroups. The finding of high heritability in the subgroup of children with early-onset antisocial behavior and CU traits also suggests that molecular genetic research may be particularly fruitful in this group. In contrast, children with early-onset antisocial behavior, but without elevated levels of CU traits, had a strong shared environmental influence on their antisocial behavior. Using theoretically defined environmental measures to identify specific shared environmental factors (Caspi et al., 2004; Jaffee, Caspi, Moffitt, & Taylor, 2001), assessing DNA polymorphisms to identify specific genes (Plomin, DeFries, Craig, & McGuffin, 2003), and assessing their interaction (Caspi et al., 2002) and correlation (Plomin, 1994) will be particularly important for future research efforts. These issues are discussed in more detail later in this chapter.

Bivariate Analysis of CP and CU Traits

The finding that heritability is high for early-onset CP in children with both CU traits and CP provides strong support for the use of CU traits to designate children with early-onset CP who may have distinct causal processes leading to their antisocial behavior. However, this finding does not provide data on the reason for the correlation between CU and CP. That is, this pattern of findings could occur because individual differences in CU and CP are both highly heritable, but the co-occurrence could be due to environmental factors. Alternatively, both CU and CP could have strong genetic components, and the covariation among these domains could also show strong genetic mediation. In addition to studying the genetic contribution to the phenotypic covariance between CU and CP, it is also possible to investigate the extent to which CU and CP are genetically correlated (i.e., the extent to which overlapping genetic influences act on both traits, independent of their contribution to the phenotypic covariance). If CU and CP are genetically correlated, molecular genetic analyses should focus on finding the common genes that mediate the risk for CU + CP. If CU and CP are not genetically correlated, then it would not be useful to study groups with CU + CP, because it would make it more difficult to identify genes if the CU + CP combination is actually a mix of two genetically distinct disorders.

We used bivariate model-fitting analysis to investigate these questions (Viding, Frick, & Plomin, 2005). Univariate estimates derived from the bivariate model-fitting analysis indicated that individual differences in both CU and CP were substantially heritable at the age of 7 (Table 15.1). Environmental influences on both CU and CP were mainly of the nonshared kind (Table 15.1). Our analyses indicated that about 75% of the phenotypic correlation of .49 between CP and CU was genetically mediated (Table 15.1). Bivariate model-fitting analysis also allows the estimation of the genetic correlation (r_g), which denotes the extent to which genes influencing phenotype 1 also influence phenotype 2. CU traits shared substantial amount of overlapping genetic influences with CP (r_g = .58; Table 15.1). Nonshared environmental influences showed moderate overlap (Table 15.1).

These findings provide novel insights into CU traits in children and their relationship with CP. First of all, these CU traits show strong heritability in children—perhaps even higher than what has been observed in adult twin studies of psychopathic personality traits. Furthermore, genes appear to drive the phenotypic relationship observed between CU and CP, and there is substantial overlap in the genes important for CU traits and CP. The shared genetic influences between CU and CP suggest that molecular genetic research should concentrate on the group with CU + CP. If the genetic overlap between CU and CP had proven to be minimal, it would have suggested that the genetic risk for the two dimensions is distinct. This would have implied that the hunt for CU + CP polymorphisms should be conducted separately for the CU and CP dimensions. Instead, our findings suggest that the combination of

TABLE 15.1. Estimates Derived from the Bivariate
Model-Fitting Analysis

	CU	CP
Total variance due to:		
A	.64 (.55–.71)	.59 (.51–.67)
C	.06 (.00–.14)	.06 (.00–.14)
E	.30 (.28–.33)	.35 (.32–.37)
Phenotypic relationship mediated by:		
biv h^2		.75 (.60–.88)
biv c^2		.05 (.05–.18)
biv e^2		.20 (.17–.20)
Correlations:		
r_g		.58 (.50–.66)
r_c		.41 (.00–1.0)
r_e		.30 (.30–.34)

Note. Standardized Additive Genetic (A), shared environmental (C), and
nonshared environmental (E) components; bivariate heritability (biv h^2),
bivariate shared environmental (biv c^2), and bivariate nonshared environmental (biv e^2) estimates; and genetic (r_g), shared environment (r_c),
and nonshared environment (r_e) correlations between CU and CP. Findings are from the full ACE correlated-factors model (with 95% confidence intervals).

CU and CP should guide selection criteria in future molecular genetic studies.
Polymorphisms associated with CU + CP can eventually be used to enrich longitudinal study designs to investigate gene–environment interactions.

Environmental influences for CU and CP appear to operate in a child-
and trait-specific manner (Viding et al., 2005). As an example, parental treatment may differ for twins, and this differential treatment may cause differences in levels of CU and CP. It is also good to remember that the genetic
parameter in quantitative genetic analyses also includes effects of gene–
environment correlation. For example, children with a particular genotype
may evoke a certain reaction from their environment or may actively seek out
certain kinds of activities, all of which would reinforce the measured trait. If
genes that mediate the association between CU and CP can be identified, theoretically meaningful environmental measures can be used to test such hypotheses.

It should be pointed out that not all genetic influences on the individual
differences in CU and CP were overlapping in our study (Viding et al., 2005).
The nonoverlapping genetic variance has been proposed to imply some independence in the biological substrates underlying CU and CP (Taylor et al.,
2003). However, both Taylor and colleagues' (2003) study and our own
individual-differences analysis addressed the entire continuum of scores. Such
individual-differences analyses do not necessarily translate to results for the
more clinically relevant issue of extreme groups. We would not rule out the
possibility that CP-unique and CU-unique genetic influences may be impor-

tant for the development of CU + CP. One could, for example, envisage epistatic interaction between genes for CP and CU, in that CP-unique genes might have particularly risk-predisposing effects in the presence of CU-unique genes, and vice versa. Many such issues will only be solved as we find genes associated with CU + CP. Nonetheless, based on our recent findings that there is substantial genetic overlap between CU and CP, and that the phenotypic relationship is strongly mediated by overlapping genetic influences, we have suggested that the common genes may be the easiest to find (Viding et al., 2005). They are also likely to be the genes that are most important for determining CU + CP group membership.

LOOKING FORWARD

The findings presented in this chapter form a starting point for a program of research that hopes to capitalize on interdisciplinary research approaches. First, longitudinal work including measured environmental variables in a genetically informative study design that can disentangle gene–environment interactions and correlations will provide important information about the development of persistent antisocial behavior. Second, the strong heritability of CU traits, as well as CP in individuals who also have CU traits, encourages the molecular genetic investigation on antisocial behavior to concentrate on the group with CU. Third, studying brain and cognitive correlates of CU + CP in a genetically informative framework will provide crucial insights into genes–brain–behavior pathways to antisocial behavior.

The Developmental Angle

Behavioral genetic methods are powerful in informing the causal theory of the development of antisocial behavior. Longitudinal measurement of both antisocial behavior and CU traits will enable us to explore the genetic and environmental influences on the persistence of antisocial behavior and associated moderating factors, such as CU traits. It will be particularly interesting to incorporate measured environmental variables in a longitudinal genetic design. The finding of substantial shared environmental influence for antisocial behavior in children without elevated levels of CU traits indicates that family-wide environmental influences that are not acting on a child's genotype are important for the development of antisocial behavior in this subgroup (Viding et al., 2005). In contrast, environmental influences acting in tandem with the genotype, as well as environmental influences unique to a child, appear more important for the development of antisocial behavior in children with elevated levels of CU traits. We are in the process of charting common and unique environmental risk factors for antisocial behavior in these two etiologically distinct subtypes. Recent advances in the study of environmental risk factors within genetically informative samples have provided clues about such risk factors (e.g., maltreatment and maternal negative emotionality) that have a truly environmentally mediated effect on antisocial behavior (e.g., Caspi et al., 2004; Jaffee et al., 2004).

Gene Hunting

Common behavioral disorders, such as antisocial behavior disorders, are currently proposed to be the quantitative extremes of the same genetic effects that operate throughout the distribution (Plomin, Owen, & McGuffin, 1994). In this model of quantitative trait loci (QTLs), many genes of varying but modest effect size are hypothesized to be involved in the development of any complex quantitative trait, and these genes are thought to act in a probabilistic manner. There has been slow progress in identifying QTLs, as they are neither sufficient nor necessary to cause extreme behavioral outcome, and thus require very large sample sizes to detect their small effects. They can be said to act together with other risk or protective genes to increase or reduce the risk of disorder. Furthermore, a risk gene may have to be combined with environmental risk before a clinically significant outcome is produced. It is thus important to understand that genes are not blueprints determining outcome.

There is now suggestive evidence that a number of serotonin pathway genes may be associated with impulsive antisocial, aggressive, and violent behavior (Lesch, 2003). Not all of these findings have been replicated; however, this may not be so surprising, given the heterogeneous nature of the samples under study, the different levels of environmental risk between samples, and the fact that the genes are QTLs of small effect size. The molecular genetic research on antisocial behavior so far has primarily concentrated on impulsive antisocial and violent behavior. We are currently trying to find genes associated with CU traits (postulated to be associated with instrumental aggression), using our twin sample and a novel DNA-pooling strategy comparing composite DNA from large samples of groups of individuals high versus low on the quantitative trait (Butcher et al., 2004). Pooled DNA will be genotyped on microarrays (gene chips) that can genotype more than 500,000 DNA markers.

If we find genes associated with CU + CP, these genes can then be used to answer questions about comorbidity, development, and effects of environment with much greater precision. For example, we can assess the extent to which the same genes associated with CU + CP are also associated with some other phenotypes, such as hyperactivity. We can also see whether these genes are associated with persistent risk for antisocial behavior. Perhaps the most exciting possibilities lie in the realm of using measured genes to study gene–environment interaction. The study of gene–environment interaction is possibly the most exciting follow-up for finding genes associated with behavior. As an example, a recent study by Caspi and colleagues (2002) demonstrated the involvement of a risk monoamine oxidase A allele in antisocial behavior, but only if the carrier of the vulnerable genotype had also experienced childhood maltreatment.

Genes–Brain–Behavior Pathways

Substantial amount is already known about neurocognitive correlates of adult psychopathy, as well as of CU + CP. Current research implicates emotion-related dysfunction in the amygdala and orbito-frontal cortex (both important for emotion processing) as possible brain correlates of adult psychopathy (Blair, 2001, 2003; Kiehl et al., 2001). Preliminary neuropsychological evidence suggests that similar brain dysfunction is found in children with CU + CP (Blair, 2001; Viding, 2004). Furthermore, both adults with psychopathy and children with CU + CP perform poorly in cognitive tasks assessing ability to make a distinction between moral and conventional transgressions, as well as cognitive tasks assessing ability to attribute guilt and sympathy (Blair, 2001; Viding, 2004). Both the brain and cognitive dysfunction found in adults with psychopathy and in children with CU + CP might be related to genetic vulnerability. An ongoing study of ours within the TEDS is investigating these issues, using cognitive tasks. The cognitive tasks within a twin study approach will allow us to estimate the overlap of genetic influences between a trait (CU) and associated cognitions (e.g., ability to attribute guilt and sympathy).

Brain imaging studies in genetically informative samples should also be at the forefront of our future research agenda. For example, if we select phenotypically discordant DZ twins who differ on crucial allelic variants and set them to perform a theoretically meaningful task in the scanner, we could find out about contributions of specific genes to functional brain differences associated with antisocial behavior. As there is ever-increasing knowledge about developmental vulnerability periods of particular brain areas, best timing for the environmental modulation of genetic risk could be cued with such study designs. Use of MZ twins discordant for the disorder in a similar scanning experiment would yield information about nonshared environmental influences on brain/cognitive function crucial for the development of antisocial behavior. Aside from the obvious target of preventing environmental risk, knowledge of the nature of environmental risk that predisposes to cognitive differences in genetically identical individuals could direct efforts at cognitive restructuring in therapy. That is, this knowledge could cue the provision of environments that would counter the risk. Lastly, individuals with identical risk genes but different levels of environmental risk could be scanned at different developmental stages, to document developmental processes associated with maladaptive cognitions and antisocial outcome.

Practical Relevance

Do the findings from behavioral genetic studies (both quantitative genetic studies and those including measured genes and measured environments) on CU traits/antisocial behavior actually yield results that have any practically relevant bearing? In other words, do the genetic investigations provide information that goes beyond basic science? We would argue that they do. Genetic research is important for studying the causality and "mode of operation" of environmental risk factors in affecting antisocial behavior outcome (Caspi et al., 2002).

Behavioral genetic research to date also cautions against entertaining ideas of gene therapy for antisocial behavior. Genes with variants that are common in the population are more than likely to have multiple functions—some of which are desirable, others not. Hence a risk gene may have many functions over and above increasing risk for disorder. When this information is combined with the fact that genes interact in complex systems, as well as with environmental risk factors, it seems pertinent to conclude that removing the effects of one gene via gene therapy is unlikely to be effective (National Committee on Bioethics, 2002).

This does not mean that genotype information will be irrelevant for possible future therapeutic intervention. For example, demonstration of genetically heterogeneous subtypes of early-onset antisocial behavior suggests the possibility of subtype-specific risk gene variants (Viding et al., 2005). Early knowledge of such risk genes may come to guide prevention efforts prior to the emergence of clear, overt behavioral/personality markers for the disorder. Because cognitive-behavioral approaches are likely to feature strongly in the antisocial behavior intervention, developing better understanding of the genes–brain–cognition–behavior pathways for particular subtypes (with or without CU traits)—especially within a longitudinal, developmental framework—could provide crucial insights for intervention.

As a final argument, we would suggest that increased knowledge about genetic influences on different variants of antisocial behavior will eventually lead to etiology-based diagnosis in antisocial behavior disorders. Current diagnostic systems rely on overt behaviors, thus yielding diagnostic categories consisting of etiologically heterogeneous groups of individuals, who (unsurprisingly) do not respond in a similar manner to prevention and treatment efforts (Uhl & Grow, 2004).

CONCLUSIONS

This chapter has provided an outline on the research to the etiology of CU traits and their relationship with antisocial behavior. Current research suggests that CU traits mark a subgroup of individuals genetically vulnerable to antisocial behavior. Future longitudinal, developmental research combining genetic, neurocognitive, and epidemiological methods will help to develop a better understanding of various pathways to antisocial behavior. Such research should be focused on the development of more precise environmental and cognitive-behavioral interventions. However, achieving this precision will not be possible without concurrent study of genetic factors and their contribution to the development of antisocial behavior.

ACKNOWLEDGMENTS

For our own research reported here, we are indebted to the parents of the twins in the Twins Early Development Study (TEDS). TEDS is supported by a programme grant (No. G9424799) from the U.K. Medical Research Council. The research on CU traits also receives support from the U.K. National Forensic Mental Health R&D Programme and the Economic and Social Research Council (Grant Nos. MRD 12-37 and PTA-026-27-0076).

NOTE

1. Note that the terms "psychopathic personality traits" and "callous–unemotional (CU) traits" are used to refer to broadly similar concepts in this chapter. We have tried to take care not to imply that children are psychopathic; hence our preference for using the term "CU traits" to refer to the personality variables in children. The term "conduct problems (CP)" is used interchangeably with "antisocial behavior" when we are talking about children. The acronym "CU + CP" (CU traits coupled with CP) is used to define a syndrome covering both CU traits and overt antisocial behavior in children. It remains to be seen how many children with CU + CP will go on to develop psychopathy in adulthood. Paul Frick and colleagues (e.g., Frick et al., 2003) and our own research group (e.g., Viding, Blair, Moffitt, & Plomin, 2005) are currently conducting longitudinal research to answer this question.

REFERENCES

American Psychiatric Association. (1994). *Diagnostic and statistical manual of mental disorders* (4th ed.). Washington, DC: Author.

American Psychiatric Association. (2000). *Diagnostic and statistical manual of mental disorders* (4th ed., text rev.). Washington, DC: Author.

Andershed, H. A., Gustafson, S. B., Kerr, M., & Stattin, H. (2002). The usefulness of self-reported psychopathy-like traits in the study of antisocial behaviour among non-referred adolescents. *European Journal of Personality, 16,* 383–402.

Arseneault, L., Moffitt, T. E., Caspi, A., Taylor, A., Rijsdijk, F. V., Jaffee, S. R., et al. (2003). Strong genetic effects on cross-situational antisocial behaviour among 5–year-old children according to mothers, teachers, examiner–observers, and twins' self-reports. *Journal of Child Psychology and Psychiatry, 44*(6), 832–848.

Barry, C. T., Frick, P. J., DeShazo, T. M., McCoy, M. G., Ellis, M., & Loney, B. R. (2000). The importance of callous–unemotional traits for extending the concept of psychopathy to children. *Journal of Abnormal Psychology, 109,* 335–340.

Blair, R. J. R. (2001). Neurocognitive models of aggression, the antisocial personality disorders, and psychopathy. *Journal of Neurology, Neurosurgery and Psychiatry, 71,* 727–731.

Blair, R. J. R. (2003). Neurobiological basis of psychopathy. *British Journal of Psychiatry, 182,* 5–7.

Blonigen, D. M., Carlson, R. F., Krueger, R. F., & Patrick, C. J. (2003). A twin study of self-reported psychopathic personality traits. *Personality and Individual Differences, 35,* 179–197.

Butcher, L. M., Meaburn, E., Liu, L., Fernandes, C., Hill, L., Al-Chalabi, A., et al. (2004). Genotyping pooled DNA on microarrays: A systematic genome screen of thousands of SNPs in large samples to detect QTLs for complex traits. *Behavior Genetics, 34,* 549–555.

Caspi, A., McClay, J., Moffitt, T. E., Mill, J., Martin, J., Craig, I. W., et al. (2002). Role of genotype in the cycle of violence in maltreated children. *Science, 297,* 851–854.

Caspi, A., Moffitt, T. E., Morgan, J., Rutter, M., Taylor, A., Arseneault, L., et al. (2004). Maternal expressed emotion predicts children's antisocial behavior problems: Using monozygotic-twin differences to identify environmental effects on behavioral development. *Developmental Psychology, 40,* 149–161.

Christian, R., Frick, P. J., Hill, N., Tyler, L. A., & Frazer, D. (1997). Psychopathy and conduct problems in children: II. Subtyping children with conduct problems based on their interpersonal and affective style. *Journal of the American Academy of Child and Adolescent Psychiatry, 36,* 233–241.

Cleckley, H. C. (1941). *The mask of sanity: An attempt to reinterpret the so-called psychopathic personality.* St Louis, MO: Mosby.

Cloninger, C. R., & Gottesman, I. I. (1987). Genetic and environmental factors in antisocial behavior disorders. In S. A. Mednick, T. E. Moffitt, & S. A. Stack (Eds.), *The causes of crime: New biological approaches* (pp. 92–109). Cambridge, UK: Cambridge University Press.

Cronk, N. J., Slutske, W. S., Madden, P. A., Bucholz, K. K., Reich, W., & Heath, A. C. (2002). Emotional and behavioral problems among female twins: An evaluation of the equal environments assumption. *Journal of the American Academy of Child and Adolescent Psychiatry, 41,* 829–837.

Eley, T. C., Lichtenstein, P., & Moffitt, T. E. (2003). A longitudinal behavioral genetic analysis of the etiology of aggressive and nonaggressive antisocial behavior. *Development and Psychopathology, 15*(2), 383–402.

Forth, A. E., Kosson, D. S., & Hare, R. D. (2004). *The Psychopathy Checklist: Youth Version.* Toronto: Multi-Health Systems.

Frick, P. J. (1998). *Conduct disorders and severe antisocial behavior.* New York: Plenum Press.

Frick, P. J., Cornell, A. H., Bodin, S. D., Dane, H. E., Barry, C. T., & Loney, B. R. (2003). Callous–unemotional traits and developmental pathways to severe conduct problems. *Developmental Psychology, 39,* 372–378.

Frick, P. J., & Hare, R. D. (2001). *The Antisocial Process Screening Device (ASPD).* Toronto: Multi-Health Systems.

Goodman, R. (1997). The Strengths and Difficulties Questionnaire: A research note. *Journal of Child Psychology and Psychiatry, 38,* 581–586.

Hare, R. D. (1991). *The Hare Psychopathy Checklist—Revised.* Toronto: Multi-Health Systems.

Hart, S. D., Cox, D. N., & Hare, R. D. (1995). *The Hare Psychopathy Checklist: Screening Version.* Toronto: Multi-Health Systems.

Hart, S. D., & Hare, R. D. (1997). Psychopathy: Assessment and association with criminal conduct. In D. M. Stoff & J. Breiling (Eds.), *Handbook of antisocial behavior* (pp. 22–35). New York: Wiley.

Jaffee, S. R., Caspi, A., Moffitt, T. E., & Taylor, A. (2004). Physical maltreatment victim to antisocial child: Evidence of an environmentally mediated process. *Journal of Abnormal Psychology, 113,* 44–55.

Kiehl, K. A., Smith, A. M., Hare, R. D., Mendrek, A., Forster, B. B., Brink, J., et al. (2001). Limbic abnormalities in affective processing by criminal psychopaths as revealed by functional magnetic resonance imaging. *Biological Psychiatry, 50*(9), 677–684.

Lesch, K. P. (2003). The serotonergic dimension of aggression and violence. In M. P. Mattson (Ed.), *Neurobiology of aggression* (pp. 33–63). Totowa, NJ: Humana Press.

Levenson, M. R., Kiehl, K. A., & Fitzpatrick, C. M. (1995). Assessing psychopathic attributes in a noninstitutionalized population. *Journal of Personality and Social Psychology, 68,* 151–158.

Lilienfeld, S. O., & Andrews, B. P. (1996). Development and preliminary validation of a self-report measure of psychopathic personality traits in noncriminal populations. *Journal of Personality Assessment, 66,* 488–524.

Loehlin, J. C. (1992). *Genes and environment in personality development.* Newbury Park, CA: Sage.

Moffitt, T. E. (2003). Life-course-persistent and adolescence antisocial behavior. In B. B. Lahey, T. E. Moffitt, & A. Caspi (Eds.), *Causes of conduct disorder and juvenile delinquency* (pp. 49–75). New York: Guilford Press.

National Committee on Bioethics. (2002). *Genetics and human behavior: The ethical context.* Chicago: American Academy of Pediatrics.

Neale, M. C., & Cardon, L. R. (1992). *Methodology for genetic studies of twins and families.* Dordrecht, The Netherlands: Kluwer Academic.

Plomin, R. (1994). Genetics and experience. *Current Opinion in Psychiatry, 7,* 297–299.

Plomin, R., DeFries, J. C., Craig, I. W., & McGuffin, P. (2003). *Behavioral genetics in the postgenomic era.* Washington, DC: American Psychological Association.

Plomin, R., DeFries, J. C., McClearn, G. E., & McGuffin, P. (2001). *Behavioral genetics* (4th ed.). New York: Worth.

Plomin, R., Owen, M. J., & McGuffin, P. (1994). The genetic basis of complex human behaviors. *Science, 264,* 1733–1739.

Rhee, S. H., & Waldman, I. D. (2002). Genetic and environmental influences on antisocial behavior: A meta-analysis of twin and adoption studies. *Psychological Bulletin, 128*(3), 490–529.

Rushton, J. P. (1996). Self-report delinquency and violence in adult twins. *Psychiatric Genetics, 6,* 87–89.

Scott, S., Knapp, M., Henderson, J., & Maughan, B. (2001). Financial cost of social exclusion: Follow up study of antisocial children into adulthood. *British Medical Journal, 323,* 191.

Silberg, J., Rutter, M., Meyer, J., Maes, H., Hewitt, J., Simonoff, E., et al. (1996). Genetic and environmental influences on the covariation between hyperactivity and conduct disturbance in juvenile twins. *Journal of Child Psychology and Psychiatry, 37*(7), 803–816.

Taylor, J., Loney, B. R., Bobadilla, L., Iacono, W. G., & McGue, M. (2003). Genetic and environmental influences on psychopathy trait dimensions in a community sample of male twins. *Journal of Abnormal Child Psychology, 31,* 633–641.

Trouton, A., Spinath, F. M., & Plomin, R. (2002). Twins Early Development Study (TEDS): A multivariate, longitudinal genetic investigation of language, cognition and behaviour problems in childhood. *Twin Research, 5,* 444–448.

Uhl, G. R., & Grow, R. W. (2004). The burden of complex genetics in brain disorders. *Archives of General Psychiatry, 61,* 223–229.

Viding, E. (2004). Annotation: Understanding the development of psychopathy. *Journal of Child Psychology and Psychiatry, 45*(8), 1329–1337.

Viding, E., Blair, R. J. R., Moffitt, T. E., & Plomin, R. (2005). Strong genetic risk for psychopathic syndrome in children. *Journal of Child Psychology and Psychiatry, 46,* 592–597.

Viding, E., Frick, P. J., & Plomin, R. (2005). *Genetic influences on the relationship between callous–unemotional traits and conduct problems in 7–year-old twins.* Manuscript submitted for publication.

Wong, S. (1985). *Criminal and institutional behaviors of psychopaths.* Ottawa: Programs Branch Users Report, Ministry of the Solicitor General of Canada.

Woodworth, M., & Porter, S. (2002). In cold blood: Characteristics of criminal homicides as a function of psychopathy. *Journal of Abnormal Psychology, 111,* 436–445.

16

A Cognitive-Behavioral Genetic Approach to Emotional Development in Childhood and Adolescence

Jennifer Y. F. Lau and Thalia C. Eley

According to a recent nationwide survey carried out in the United Kingdom, "emotional disorders," including anxiety and depressive conditions, constitute one of the main categories of psychiatric problems diagnosed in children and adolescents in the community (Meltzer, Gatward, Goodman, & Ford, 2000). While this study revealed a point prevalence estimate of 4% for categorically defined disorders, subclinical symptoms have also been found to be common, and show similar degrees of psychosocial impairment and service utilization (Angold, Costello, Farmer, Burns, & Erkanli, 1999). Among the longer-term detrimental effects of these conditions is a strong persistence of symptoms into adulthood, where they continue to have negative effects on social adjustment and functioning (Fombonne, Wostear, Cooper, Harrington, & Rutter, 2001). Given these negative outcomes, an improved understanding of the different risk factors involved in anxiety and depression, and of how these are expressed during childhood and adolescence, is essential to the planning of preventive interventions.

Behavioral genetic research has provided an abundance of information on the genetic and environmental origins of anxiety and depression in children and adolescents. This chapter begins by providing a brief outline of the key principles governing behavioral genetic methodology and describing how these have been applied in developmental research on anxiety and depression phenotypes. It then moves on to more recent and exciting research in the field that is examining genetic (and environmental) risk mechanisms on anxiety and depression, thus posing the question of *how* these risks are expressed. In particular, two new approaches are discussed that address the interplay between genetic and environmental factors in these phenotypes, and the role of traditionally defined cognitive variables in accounting for some genetic (and environmental) risk factors in anxiety and depression.

BEHAVIORAL GENETIC STUDIES OF ANXIETY AND DEPRESSION

Behavioral genetic studies seek to understand the causes of variation in behavioral outcomes (for an introduction to the study of behavioral genetics, the reader is referred to Plomin, DeFries, McClearn, & McGuffin, 2001). These causes can be divided into those that are genetic and those that can be attributed to the environment. Indexing and quantifying these different sources of influence form the basis of most behavioral genetic designs (see Table 16.1). Through such twin and family studies, the importance of genetic factors in the etiology of anxiety and depression in childhood and adolescence has now been well accepted. Estimates of heritability typically account for about a third of the variance in anxiety symptoms, with the remainder of the risk being attributable to moderate shared environmental influences and substantial nonshared environmental influences (Eley & Gregory, 2004). For depression, a similar profile of effects is obtained, but with a somewhat lesser contribution from the shared environment (Eley, 1999; Rice, Harold, & Thapar, 2002b). Studies comparing the magnitude of genetic and environmental effects obtained at different developmental stages (e.g., childhood and adolescence) have revealed, however, that the relative estimates of these types of effects may change across time (Rice, Harold, & Thapar, 2002a; Scourfield et al., 2003). Specifically, with both phenotypes, genes may have an increased effect in adolescence, whereas in childhood shared environmental effects play a larger role. Whether this is due to newer "developmental" genes emerging in adolescence, as suggested by recent evidence (Scourfield et al., 2003), has not been fully clarified, although conflicting evidence that genes are responsible for continuity and stability of symptoms across time rather than change also exists (O'Connor, Neiderhiser, Reiss, Hetherington, & Plomin, 1998; Silberg et al., 1999).

Whereas univariate analyses partition variance in a single measure into genetic and environmental constituents, twin analyses of the covariance between *two* measures can address the extent to which genetic and environmental factors influencing one measure also influence the other. Studies applying these bivariate analyses to measures of anxiety and depression have shown that the co-occurrence of these two types of symptoms is mostly due to overlapping genes, but that environmental contributions are largely specific (Eley & Stevenson, 1999; Thapar & McGuffin, 1997). In other words, anxiety and depression appear to have common genetic risk mechanisms, but to be influ-

TABLE 16.1. Behavioral Genetic Methodology

The basic aim of behavioral genetic designs is to determine how much of variation in a measured phenotype is due to genetic (and/or environmental) effects. The simplest way in which this can be done is to compare the extent to which different family members resemble one another on behavioral characteristics. Given that different members differ in their genetic relatedness to one another—for instance, siblings share on average half of their segregating genes with one another, while only sharing one-quarter of their genes with their first cousins—it is plausible to attribute any greater similarity among sibling pairs than among first cousins to shared genetic effects. However, such a conclusion is limited by the fact that siblings are also much more likely to share a family environment than they are to share such an environment with their cousins, and thus the family design is not equipped to adequately distinguish shared genetic from shared environmental influences.

By far the most useful and widely available design with respect to decomposing and quantifying genetic and environmental effects is the twin design, which to date has contributed the majority of findings on the genetic underpinnings of anxiety and depression. In brief, twin data allow the comparison of phenotypic similarity among monozygotic (MZ) or identical twins and dizygotic (DZ) or fraternal twins. Whereas MZ twins share all of their genetic material (A), DZ twins, like ordinary sibling pairs, share on average only half of their segregating genes (½A). In contrast, both types of twins share their family environment (C) to the same degree. As aspects of this environment contribute to the similarity among all family members (including twins), this is known as the "shared environment." Finally, as family members (and twins) also differ from one another in certain respects, these differences are accounted for by individual-specific or "nonshared environmental" effects (E).

As investigators can define each of these three sources of influence (termed A, C, and E) that contribute to variation on a phenotype, MZ and DZ resemblances can be re-expressed in such terms. Specifically, correlations between MZ twins (rMZ) are equal to A + C, while correlations between DZ twins (rDZ) are due to ½A + C. Thus any difference in twin correlations between MZ and DZ pairs can provide a rough estimate of genetic effects (A). Any resemblance in MZ twins that is not due to genetic effects is accounted for by aspects of the family environment shared between family members (shared environment, or C). Finally, differences between MZ twins (calculated as $1 - r$MZ) are explained as unique or individual-specific factors (nonshared environment, or E) in the phenotype. Although such comparisons offer a simple method of signposting the effect of genes relative to the environment on different phenotypic measures, conclusions drawn from twin analyses are not without their limitations; these include the equal-environments assumption, chorionicity, assortative mating, and generalizability.

The "equal-environments assumption" is the assumption that MZ and DZ twins experience shared environment to the same degree, and this proposition has been questioned by some investigators. For instance, because of their closer physical resemblance, MZ twins may be treated more alike by others than DZ twins may be; this treatment may inflate the MZ twins' experience of the shared environment and overall resemblance, leading to artificial increases in heritability.

(continued)

TABLE 16.1. *(continued)*

However, detailed observational studies indicate that the increased similarity of treatment of MZ twins relative to DZ twins is entirely due to the increased similarity of their behavior, which elicits more similar responses from others. This is therefore fundamentally a genetic effect and is correctly interpreted as such. "Chorionicity" refers to the number of chorions (the "chorion" is the sac within which, in a singleton, the fetus develops). For all DZ twins there are two chorions, but for two-thirds of MZ twins there is just one chorion, leading to the possibility that increased MZ resemblance may be due to chorion sharing rather than to shared genes. "Assortative mating" refers to the tendency of individuals to seek mates who are similar to themselves. This phenomenon, which has been well documented, may then lead to increased genetic variance within families that results in increased genetic effects. The final question regarding the validity of twin designs is the extent to which twins are representative of the general (nontwin) population. However, existing studies addressing this issue indicate that with the exception of a slight initial delay in language development, twins are largely indistinguishable from nontwins. These limitations imply that any derived estimates of heritability should not be taken as absolutes, but rather as indications of the role of genes in different phenotypes, and should not diminish the overall importance of the genetic contribution. In fact, as will be seen later in this chapter, the principles of the twin design can be applied in more complex model-fitting approaches to test hypotheses relating to genetic and environmental risk mechanisms in anxiety and depression.

---

enced by different sets of social factors. Although studies confirming this genetic relationship have mainly used concurrent anxiety and depression symptoms (i.e., symptoms co-occurring in the same time frame), a more recent study showed that earlier symptoms of anxiety (including overanxious disorder and simple phobias between ages 8 and 13) reflected the same genetic risk as pubertal depression (ages 14–17) (Silberg, Rutter, & Eaves, 2001). Surprisingly, no shared genetic links between concurrent measures of prepubertal anxiety and depression were found, suggesting that this shared liability is expressed across development.

In summary, these earlier twin and family studies of anxiety and depression have proved useful in highlighting the roles of genetics and the environment in these emotional phenotypes. In addition, they have explored various aspects of these risk factors, including their differential roles during development, as well as how they account for the co-occurrence of these symptoms phenotypically. However, little is still known about *how* genetic and environmental risk effects are expressed, or about the mechanisms that are involved in creating vulnerability to these disorders. In order to bridge the gap between identifying risk factors and developing treatments and therapies, it is essential to understand the "intermediate" processes by which liabilities are translated in the brain into cognition and behavior. In the next two sections, we discuss two novel approaches that provide some insight into these "intermediate" processes, using data from several large twin studies in the United Kingdom.

GENE–ENVIRONMENT INTERACTIONS AND CORRELATIONS

Accumulating evidence suggests that the genetic and environmental effects on anxiety and depression are not independent risk factors, but instead interact and correlate with one another to increase vulnerability to these phenotypes. Specifically, genetic risks are known to influence environmental risk exposure ("gene–environment correlation") and to increase susceptibility to negative environmental stressors ("gene–environment interaction") (Lau & Eley, 2004b). Examining these two processes of interplay between genetic and environmental influences on anxiety and depression is one approach to learning about the risk mechanisms leading to emotional disorders.

Gene–Environment Correlations

Evidence that gene–environment correlations are important to anxiety and depression comes from a range of twin and family designs. Because such correlations essentially refer to the co-occurrence of genetic and environmental effects on phenotypic variation, support for these correlations primarily involves demonstrating that an environmental risk variable also shows genetic influence. Many environmental predictors of anxiety and depression, such as negative life events and aspects of the parent–child relationship, have been found to show genetic effects (Lau, Rijsdijk, & Eley, in press; Pike, McGuire, Hetherington, Reiss, & Plomin, 1996; Saudino, Pedersen, Lichtenstein, McClearn, & Plomin, 1997). Moreover, such genetic effects also overlap with genes that are implicated in outcome measures of emotional symptoms. This indicates that genetic risks for these phenotypes may in part be expressed through an exposure to environmental risk, and this exposure has been suggested to arise in three ways: "passive," "evocative," or "active" processes (Scarr & McCartney, 1983).

Passive gene–environment correlation arises when the parental genetic makeup influences both the child's genotype and the rearing environment provided for the child. For example, a child may inherit his or her mother's depressogenic genes, together with being exposed to a repertoire of negative parenting styles. Evocative processes apply when a child's genetic propensities elicit, through cognitive variables or temperamental traits, certain reactions from other people. Thus infants who are frequently crying and irritable may evoke more negative responses from their parents than cheerful, smiling babies may. Finally, active types of gene–environment correlation occur when individuals select, modify, or construct their experiences based on genetically mediated dispositions, such as personality traits. Sociable youngsters may choose to spend more of their time with other children, thus increasing the levels of social contact in their environment, while inhibited children may spend more time in isolation and thus may experience increased feelings of loneliness.

As yet, it is fairly difficult to distinguish among these three types of gene–environment correlations at an analytical level, and often only an overall effect can be demonstrated. However, it has been suggested that such correlation processes may be expressed at different points in development: Passive forms may be more salient during infancy and early childhood, whereas evocative and active processes may become more important as children begin to experience environments outside the family and play a more active role in shaping their own experiences. One study that has explored these developmental trends included a comparison of the relative contribution of genetic and environmental factors to the relationship between negative life events and depression in two different age groups (8–11 and 12–17 years) (Rice, Harold, & Thapar, 2003). Their results showed that genes did play a larger role in this association in the older adolescent sample compared to the child sample, thus suggesting that active gene–environment correlation becomes a stronger influence on depression symptoms across development. These increased effects could also potentially account for the larger genetic effects found during adolescence by previous studies.

Gene–Environment Interactions

Given that genes may be expressed through the creation of environmental risks, genetic influences are also hypothesized to influence an individual's susceptibility to such risks (gene–environment interaction). An alternative way of conceptualizing these interaction effects is that the occurrence of the environmental risk factor elicits or activates the genetic predisposition to the phenotype. In either scenario, an interaction arises when one variable (e.g., a genetic risk factor) has differential effects at varying levels of the other (e.g., an environmental risk factor). We can better illustrate this point by means of a figure. Figure 16.1 presents the results of a family-based design, which utilized data from 1818 adolescent offspring and 1294 parents from the G1219 study (a large community U.K.-based study investigating familial resemblance for emotional and behavioral problems) to examine the effects of parental education and genetic vulnerability on adolescent depressive symptoms (Eley, Liang, et al., 2004). The index of genetic vulnerability here had previously been created by using quantitative genetic modeling techniques to estimate maximum familial liability to anxiety, depression, and neuroticism, as indicated by scores from the parent sample and from the adolescents' siblings (Sham et al., 2000). Such an index is thought to reflect the effects of shared genes among family members. Although both this measure of genetic relatedness and a dichotomous variable of parental education (no vs. some qualifications) predicted high depression scores in adolescent offspring, what was most striking about these results was the significant interaction between these variables. Specifically, adolescents whose parents reported no educational qualifications, *and* who were in the highest third of scorers on the genetic risk index, were

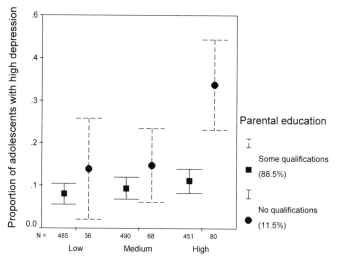

FIGURE 16.1. Effects of parental education and genetic risk on severe depression. From Eley et al. (2004). Copyright 2004 by the American Academy of Child and Adolescent Psychiatry. Reprinted by permission.

three times more likely to be grouped among the high depression scorers. In other words, the effects of genetic vulnerability varied greatly at different levels of the environmental risk moderator.

Although these findings can illustrate the effects of interactions, they are limited in their capacity to disentangle the effects of shared genes from those of shared environmental factors in the familial vulnerability composite index (see Table 16.1). These confounding influences can be distinguished in twin studies, where the examination of monozygotic (MZ) and dizygotic (DZ) twin correlations allows the variance due to genetic, shared environmental, and nonshared environmental factors to be partitioned. One method of investigating interaction effects in twin studies, featured in many earlier studies of gene–environment interactions, involves the comparison of estimated genetic effects in different environmental strata. Thus a significant difference between heritability estimated in one environmental condition and that estimated in another signifies an interaction. For instance, in one adult sample of female twins, heritability for depression symptoms was significantly decreased in the presence of a marital relationship (Heath, Eaves, & Martin, 1998). Presumably, being in a stable relationship is indicative to some degree of higher levels of social support received by this subset of adult females than by their unmarried counterparts, and the effect of having this social buffer attenuated the genetic risk for depression.

Although many of these studies appear supportive of gene–environment interactions, many investigators fail to recognize that such results may reflect correlations between genes and environments, rather than interactions (Lau & Eley, 2004a). To use the study described above as an example, Heath and colleagues' (1998) results are also consistent with the interpretation that genetic risk for depression, perhaps mediated through personality traits, may influence individuals' social relationships (including their marital status). In other words, gene–environment correlations may be responsible for the observed interaction effect. True interactions are premised on the assumption that genotypes are randomly distributed over the range of environmental conditions, but a violation of this assumption can arise when allelic frequencies are higher in individuals exposed to a certain environmental condition (i.e., gene–environment correlation) (Eaves, Silberg, & Erkanli, 2003). Thus any genetic influences on an environmental measure also involved in the phenotype must be taken into account by studies testing for interactions.

One approach to resolving this issue has been to examine environmental stressors that reflect negligible or minimal genetic influence. A study utilizing this method (Silberg, Rutter, Neale, & Eaves, 2001) demonstrated a significant interaction between genetic risk and a composite index of three life events in their effects on anxiety and depression symptoms in adolescent female twins. Although the choice of three life events minimizes confounding the effects of gene–environment correlation with those of gene–environment interaction, a drawback is that the occurrences of "dependent" life events (i.e., those that may be influenced through personality traits by genes) are ignored, leading to a rather restricted use of available data on environmental risk factors. A more recent and sophisticated approach is to model gene–environment correlations alongside gene–environment interactions (Purcell, 2002). In one study, several distinct pathways to depression symptoms in adolescence were supported (Eaves et al., 2003). In the first pathway, prepubertal anxiety symptoms were found to act as an early influence on later depression through shared genetic effects. These common effects, apart from having main effects on depression outcome, also influenced exposure to negative life events (gene–environment correlation). Life events either influenced depression directly or were found to moderate the effects of the common genetic factor, shared with anxiety, on depression. Finally, genetic factors that were not shared with anxiety (i.e., those that were specific to depression) were also moderated by the occurrence of life events.

Our own data on a subsample of the G1219 study also provide support for the combined effects of gene–environment interaction and gene–environment correlation on adolescent depression symptoms; we examined both negative life events and maternal punitive disciplinary style (Lau & Eley, 2004a). Both measures of environmental risk were found to be moderately heritable, and to share common genetic effects with depression symptoms. Moreover, genetic effects on depression symptoms were found to be moderated by each environmental risk variable. In other words, we demonstrated gene–environment interactions in the presence of a genetic correlation between the environmental risk measure and the phenotypic outcome. These findings both increase the validity of interaction effects and support their co-occurence in influencing emotional symptoms. Genetic influences were found to increase across levels of environmental risk.

Although gene–environment interactions and correlations are now widely established as important risk mechanisms, with more recent evidence highlighting their combined effects on emotional phenotypes (particularly depression), the evidence has mainly relied on quantitative genetic findings. This approach, though useful in exploring the nature of genetic effects, uses an indirect measure of genetic influence, as inferred from genetic relationships among family members. A more direct and precise method of measuring genetic effects is to use DNA variants, or "polymorphisms." In molecular genetic studies, specific sections of DNA called "markers," usually within genes but sometimes just close to them, are examined. Markers vary across the population, leading to different variants called "alleles" in different individuals. These markers are also called "polymorphisms," reflecting the different versions identified within and across populations. The most useful markers are those where the different alleles have an effect on the function of the gene; these are known as "functional polymorphisms," because they provide direct information about the action of the gene. However, it is also common to use more anonymous markers, in the hope that these may be closely linked to (and therefore always inherited with) the gene of interest. Several different sampling approaches can be taken in molecular genetic studies, but for the studies described here, the method chosen is that of case–control comparison, in which genetic polymorphism frequencies are compared between the two groups, much as any other type of risk factor would be.

One of the first and most exciting studies with regard to an emotional phenotype in this field reported a significant interaction between a functional polymorphism in the serotonin (5-HT) transporter gene-linked promoter region (*5-HTTLPR*) and the effect of life events on depression symptoms in an adult sample (Caspi et al., 2003). The *5-HTTLPR*, which is involved in regulatory processes during stress (Hariri et al., 2002), is an excellent candidate for interaction with environmental stress; it exists in two forms, a long and a short allele. The latter has been associated with lower transcriptional efficiency (Lesch et al., 1996). Individuals carrying this short allele of the *5-HTTLPR* reported higher levels and more severe symptoms of depression in response to life events that had occurred over the last 5 years. Furthermore, this allele also moderated the longitudinal prediction from child maltreatment to adult depression, indicating that the effects of this genetic factor may have been expressed earlier in development.

We found data consistent with the hypothesis that this gene–environment interaction is operational during earlier stages of life (Eley, Sugden, et al., 2004). Using family-based measures of environmental risk, including social adversity, family life events, and parental employment level, we found a significant interaction between this composite risk variable and the *5-HTTLPR* in female adolescents. Specifically, the effects of this environmental risk moderator were stronger among those carrying the short allele. Together, these findings suggest that this genetic variant is likely to express itself by influencing susceptibility to environmental risks across development.

INTERMEDIATE PHENOTYPES AND GENETIC RISK

The second approach to understanding genetic and environmental risk mechanisms in anxiety and depression is to search for intermediate phenotypes that may reflect or even mediate the risks associated with these influences. As described in the previous section, genes may express themselves through processes of interplay with the environment, such as the creation of environmental risks, or by increasing susceptibility to these risks. Thus it is plausible that these effects act primarily on core processes associated with stress reactivity. "Stress reactivity," however, is a broad term encompassing several different levels of analysis, including physiological, cognitive, and behavioral reactivity. The approach chosen here is based on a top-down approach (behavior–cognitions–brain–genes) rather than a bottom-up approach (genes–protein–function–behavior), although the latter is just as valid a perspective to take, and in fact a combination of the two approaches would be most beneficial. Our starting point therefore has been to examine cognitive factors and personality traits that have traditionally been implicated in the development of these emotional behaviors, and that have the potential to act as markers of genetic and environmental risks. In particular, three sets of processes are discussed: attributional style and depression; anxiety sensitivity and anxiety; and state and trait anxiety.

Attributional Style and Depression

Attributional style is a well-known risk factor for depression (Seligman, 1974; Seligman et al., 1984). Specifically, the "learned helplessness" theory (Abramson, Seligman, & Teasdale, 1978), later reformulated as the "hopelessness" theory (Alloy, Abramson, Metalsky, & Hartlage, 1988), identifies individuals who attribute negative events to internal (directed to the self), stable (likely to persist across time), and global (likely to affect many aspects of life) causes as having an increased vulnerability to depression. Such individuals may exhibit the opposite pattern of attributions for positive events, interpreting these as occurring for external, unstable, and specific reasons (Gladstone & Kaslow, 1995). This differential style of responding to events in the environment—an example of cognitive reactivity—is thought to be fully expressed in the presence of life events.

Given the strong and more recently prospective associations that have been demonstrated between attributional style and depression symptoms (e.g.,

Hankin, Abramson, & Siler, 2001), and that have largely been used as support for the role of attributional style as a vulnerability factor for the phenotype, we set out to unravel its genetic and environmental etiology. Previous psychosocial studies have focused entirely on "social" correlates of attributional style, including learning and modeling from parental patterns of attribution and negative parenting styles (Alloy et al., 1999; Garber & Flynn, 2001). However, the possibility that it also reflects a heritable component has not been fully addressed. Similarly, its association with depression has generally been depicted as a diathesis–stress relationship, such that environmental factors are crucial to the expression of this relationship. It has not been considered that perhaps attributional style reflects a genetic vulnerability to depression, which is elicited by environmental stressors. In other words, attributional style may be directly involved in gene–environment interaction processes as described previously.

Using self-reported data on attributional style and depression symptoms in over 1300 adolescent twin and sibling pairs from the G1219 twin study, we examined the genetic and environmental structure of attributional style, as well as its association with depression (Lau, Rijsdijk, & Eley, in press). Support for attributional style as a heritable rather than just a learned trait was obtained through findings of a moderate genetic influence, small (and nonsignificant) shared environmental contributions, and considerable nonshared environmental influences. Second, in terms of its association with depression, we demonstrated that genes were as important as the environment to this relationship, accounting for just under half of the covariance between the two measures. Thus these results support the idea that, as an aspect of cognitive reactivity, attributional style is heritable. Furthermore, some of this genetic liability is also involved, in addition to environmental factors, in the relationship of attributional style with depression. Whether this suggests that a negative attributional style is directly implicated in gene–environment interaction processes is unresolved and requires more research.

Although these findings fit in with our hypothesis that attributional style acts as a marker of genetic risk for depression, preliminary results from a younger twin sample suggests that this marker is only expressed during adolescence. Specifically, using similar twin analyses on the same measures collected in children age 8, we found very small and nonsignificant genetic effects on both attributional style and its association with depression, despite the fact that their phenotypic correlation was comparable to that in the adolescent sample. In contrast, shared environmental effects were proportionately larger in the younger children. This suggests that despite attributional style co-occurring with depression early in childhood, its genetic effects do not become apparent until adolescence. These findings are compatible to some degree with findings from cognitive studies that attributional style only becomes fully operational in adolescence, where it interacts with negative life stress to precipitate symptoms.

Anxiety Sensitivity and Anxiety

Within the field of cognitive risk factors for anxiety, one that has been attract-ing increasing attention is "anxiety sensitivity." This is defined as "the fear of anxiety sensations which arises from beliefs that these sensations have harm-ful somatic, social or psychological consequences" (Taylor, 1999). Originally, anxiety sensitivity was proposed as a unitary construct that increases risk for anxiety in general and panic in particular. However, subsequent analyses of relevant data indicated the presence of subfactors within the construct. These two approaches were brought together by the proposal of a hierarchical factor structure, with one first-order factor and several (usually three) second-order factors (Zinbarg & Barlow, 1997). These second-order factors reflect con-cerns about physical phenomena (e.g., worry about fast heart rate), concerns about mental illness (e.g., worry about loss of cognitive control), and social concerns that apply to visible symptoms of anxiety (e.g., worry about blush-ing). This factor structure has been widely replicated in both adults and chil-dren (Muris, Schmidt, Merckelbach, & Schouten, 2001; Silverman, Ginsburg, & Goedhart, 1999; Zinbarg & Barlow, 1997). Given the potential impor-tance of anxiety sensitivity in precipitating vulnerability to anxiety, our aims were to explore this phenotypic structure further, in terms of its etiological structure. We therefore set out, first, to replicate this structure in our own data; second, to examine the genetic and environmental influences on the three second-order factors; and third, to examine the genetic and environmen-tal structure of these three factors.

Using data from over 1600 pairs of twins and siblings from the G1219 study, we first tested (in group 1—one random member of each pair), and then replicated (in group 2), the three-factor hierarchical structure (Eley & Brown, 2004). We found that this structure did indeed provide good fit in both groups. We therefore created three scales as the sum of the items loading onto the three second-order factors. The next stage was to examine the genetic and environmental influences on our three scales. To date, theories of anxiety sensitivity have had little to say about its origins, and much more to say about its role in the etiology of anxiety. Thus we were interested in examining the possible effects of genetic factors on the variation in each of the three anxiety sensitivity scales, and on the covariation between them. We found moderate heritability for all three scales (18% to 31%). Multivariate genetic models revealed that a higher-order factor structure provided the best description of the data at the genetic and environmental level—as it does at the phenotypic level. Of note, the latent phenotype (higher-order factor) influencing all three subscales was highly heritable (60%), indicating that much of the genetic influence on these three scales is shared. In contrast, the environmental influ-ences were largely specific to each variable. Preliminary examination of the genetic and environmental links between these three scales on the one hand and anxiety and depression symptoms on the other indicates a moderate level of genetic sharing, but also shared environmental influences. These data thus indicate that although it is possible to identify subscales of anxiety sensitivity, these are all related to one another via a higher-order factor, through which much of the genetic influence on each is mediated. Only some of these shared genetic effects are also involved in anxiety and depression symptoms.

State and Trait Anxiety

It has been recognized for some time that anxiety is not a unitary construct, but instead may be composed of various dimensions underlying different aspects of vulnerability to the phenotype (Smoller & Tsuang, 1998). One common distinction that has been made is between "state anxiety" and "trait anxiety" (Spielberger, 1966). State anxiety is the transitory pattern of emotions elicited by environmental stressors, including physiological arousal and symptoms of apprehension, worry, and tension. It therefore represents the environmentally reactive component of anxiety. Trait anxiety, however, refers to individual differences in the predisposition to respond to threatening situations, and is often characterized as a personality disposition toward anxiety. Although both of these independently define anxiety, it is the association between the two—the expression of trait anxiety as state anxiety—that may be suggestive of how vulnerability to anxiety symptoms is expressed. Specifically, individuals with high levels of trait anxiety may be predisposed to exhibit intense and prolonged symptoms of state anxiety in the face of threat (Spielberger, 1966). Extrapolating from this, we suggest that trait anxiety reflects a biological—in particular, a genetic—disposition to anxiety mediated through an individual's personality. In comparison, state anxiety may represent the product of an interaction between this disposition and a stressor. In other words, the association between state and trait anxiety may reflect a process of gene–environment interaction in creating anxiety symptoms.

There is some evidence both from an earlier and from our own behavioral genetic designs examining the genetic and environmental influences on state and trait anxiety, which supports their purported roles in manifesting the anxiety phenotype (Lau, Eley, & Stevenson, 2004; Legrand, McGue, & Iacono, 1999). In both studies, which used twins in the age ranges 8–16 (Lau, Eley, & Stevenson, 2004) and 10–12 or 16–18 (Legrand et al., 1999), state anxiety was largely environmentally influenced, with contributions from both shared and nonshared environmental factors. Trait anxiety, by contrast, showed moderate genetic influences and substantial nonshared environmental contributions. In terms of the association between the two measures of anxiety, which was only examined in our analyses, we found that nonshared environmental factors were an important source of influence, but that there was also a modest but significant effect of genes. Thus there is some support for the idea that state and trait anxiety are vulnerability mechanisms reflecting a genetic interplay with the environment in creating anxiety symptoms.

CONCLUSIONS

In summary, much has been learned about the mechanisms by which genetic and environmental factors may influence behavior. Notably, genetic effects may be expressed through either correlations or interactions with the environment, thus influencing exposure to environmental risks or susceptibility to these risks. Molecular genetic analyses, which seek to identify specific DNA variants that underlie genetic risks in behavioral phenotypes, must take these findings seriously. First, the need to take into account the moderating effect of environmental factors is crucial. Neglecting to do so may result in heterogeneity between samples, and may be the reason for many negative findings regarding genetic associations in the literature. For example, there may be individuals within the sample who have incomplete penetration, such that they possess the risk allele but do not expressed the associated behavioral manifestations, due to a lack of exposure to the adverse environment. If these individuals are then included in the sample as "controls," this may well result in nonsignificant comparisons in genotypic frequencies between the cases and controls. Accordingly, investigators must control for environmental exposure. Second, given that the genes involved in emotional behaviors may also be expressed through environmental risk exposure, this suggests that "exposure to risks" may be considered as an additional endophenotype for study in conjunction with phenotypic measures.

More recent evidence from our own data highlights the importance of considering gene–environment interactions together with potential gene–environment correlations in quantitative designs, so that one set of processes does not lead to contaminated and biased estimates of the other. Understanding these processes in more detail has also influenced how we can incorporate findings from other disciplines of the behavioral sciences to improve our knowledge of genetic risk mechanisms. By identifying variables that have received adequate support as vulnerability factors in the development of anxiety and depression, we can speculate on whether these reflect the genetic and environmental risks also demonstrated in these phenotypes. Attributional style, which has traditionally been conceptualized as a cognitive diathesis for stress in depression, has been shown by our data to be moderately heritable, with genetic influences involved in its association with depression. Interestingly, the finding that the genetic effects are only apparent in adolescent samples also suggests these effects' potential in explaining age-related increases in depression symptoms, increased heritability of symptoms, and possibly "new" developmental genetic influences that have been characterized in earlier phenotypic and genetic studies of this age range.

Our examination of the structure of anxiety sensitivity suggests that a higher-order factor mediates genetic influences on all three aspects of this vulnerability construct. This indicates that although it may be useful for clinical reasons to distinguish among physical, mental, and social concerns, from a molecular genetic point of view it is probably therefore not worth examining anxiety sensitivity scales independently. The distinction between state and trait anxiety also further highlights how we can separate the more genetically influenced components of anxiety from the environmentally mediated ones. Yet examining their association is just as beneficial in understanding the wider picture of how these different components may interact in creating vulnerability to anxiety.

LOOKING FORWARD

In summary, the application of behavioral genetics to childhood emotional disorders such as anxiety and depression has moved the field beyond examining the *extent* of genetic and environmental influences, to asking questions about the *nature* of these effects and how they may be expressed. As such, we have aimed to highlight not just the level of impact of genetic and environmental influences, but also their interplay in the development of symptoms, as well as more exciting areas involving the integration of cognitive and personality measures within genetic designs. These have included the examination of intermediate processes by which genetic and environmental risks may influence behavioral outcomes. These top-down approaches should occur in parallel with investigation of bottom-up processes, including the use of molecular genetics to examine the role of specific genes. Eventually, dialogue between these two perspectives should meet at the level of the brain, highlighting potentially different avenues for prevention and intervention of these often lifelong and debilitating conditions.

ACKNOWLEDGMENTS

Our studies described in this chapter were supported by the W. T. Grant Foundation and by a Medical Research Council training fellowship to Thalia C. Eley. Jennifer Y. F. Lau was supported by a Medical Research Council doctoral studentship. We would like to thank the families who took part, and would also like to thank Robert Plomin, Abram Sterne, Richard Williamson, Pak Sham, Maria Napolitano, Alessandra Iervolino, Richard Rowe, Barbara Maughan, Fruhling Rijsdijk, Georgina Hosang, Alice Gregory, Fiona McCleod, and Jasmine Singh for support and help with different aspects of these projects.

REFERENCES

Abramson, L. Y., Seligman, M. E. P., & Teasdale, J. D. (1978). Learned helplessness in humans: Critique and reformulation. *Journal of Abnormal Psychology, 87,* 49–74.

Alloy, L. B., Abramson, L. Y., Metalsky, G. I., & Hartlage, S. (1988). The hopelessness theory of depression: Attributional aspects. *British Journal of Clinical Psychology, 27,* 5–21.

Alloy, L. B., Abramson, L. Y., Whitehouse, W. G., Hogan, M. E., Tashman, N. A., Steinberg, D. L., et al. (1999). Depressogenic cognitive styles: Predictive validity, information processing and personality characteristics, and developmental origins. *Behaviour Research and Therapy, 37,* 503–531.

Angold, A., Costello, E. J., Farmer, E. M., Burns, B. J., & Erkanli, A. (1999). Impaired but undiagnosed. *Journal of the American Academy of Child and Adolescent Psychiatry, 38,* 129–137.

Caspi, A., Sugden, K., Moffitt, T. E., Taylor, A., Craig, I. W., Harrington, H., et al. (2003). Influence of life stress on depression: Moderation by a polymorphism in the 5-HTT gene. *Science, 301,* 386–389.

Eaves, L., Silberg, J., & Erkanli, A. (2003). Resolving multiple epigenetic pathways to adolescent depression. *Journal of Child Psychology and Psychiatry, 44,* 1006–1014.

Eley, T. C. (1999). Behavioral genetics as a tool for developmental psychology: Anxiety and depression in children and adolescents. *Clinical Child and Family Psychology Review, 2,* 21–36.

Eley, T. C., & Brown, T. A. (2004). Phenotypic and genetic/environmental structure of anxiety sensitivity in adolescents. *Behavior Genetics, 34*(6), 637.

Eley, T. C., & Gregory, A. M. (2004). Behavioral genetics. In T. L. Morris & J. S. March (Eds.), *Anxiety disorders in children and adolescents* (2nd ed., pp. 71–97). New York: Guilford Press.

Eley, T. C., Liang, H., Plomin, R., Sham, P., Sterne, A., Williamson, R., et al. (2004). Parental vulnerability, family environment and their interactions as predictors of depressive symptoms in adolescents. *Journal of the American Academy of Child and Adolescent Psychiatry, 43,* 298–306.

Eley, T. C., & Stevenson, J. (1999). Exploring the covariation between anxiety and depression symptoms: A genetic analysis of the effects of age and sex. *Journal of Child Psychology and Psychiatry, 40,* 1273–1284.

Eley, T. C., Sugden, K., Gregory, A. M., Sterne, A., Plomin, R., & Craig, I. W. (2004). Gene–environment interaction analysis of serotonin system markers with adolescent depression. *Molecular Psychiatry, 9,* 908–918.

Fombonne, E., Wostear, G., Cooper, V., Harrington, R., & Rutter, M. (2001). The Maudsley long-term follow-up of child and adolescent depression: 2. Suicidality, criminality and social dysfunction in adulthood. *British Journal of Psychiatry, 179,* 218–223.

Garber, J., & Flynn, C. (2001). Predictors of depressive cognitions in young adolescents. *Cognitive Therapy and Research, 25*(4), 353–376.

Hankin, B. L., Abramson, L. Y., & Siler, M. (2001). A prospective test of the hopelessness theory of depression in adolescence. *Cognitive Therapy and Research, 25*(5), 607–632.

Hariri, A. R., Mattay, V. S., Tessitore, A., Kolachana, B., Fera, F., Goldman, D., et al. (2002). Serotonin transporter genetic variation and the response of the human amygdala. *Science, 297,* 400–403.

Heath, A. C., Eaves, L. J., & Martin, N. G. (1998). Interaction of marital status and genetic risk for symptoms of depression. *Twin Research,* 119–122.

Lau, J. Y. F., & Eley, T. C. (2004a). *Gene–environment interactions and correlations on adolescent depression.* Manuscript submitted for publication.

Lau, J. Y. F., & Eley, T. C. (2004b). Gene–environment interactions and correlations in psychiatric disorders. *Current Psychiatry Reports, 6*(2), 119–124.

Lau, J. Y. F., Eley, T. C., & Stevenson, J. (in press). Examining the state–trait relationship: A behavioral genetic approach. *Journal of Abnormal Child Psychology.*

Lau, J. Y. F., Rijsdijk, F. V., & Eley, T. C. (in press). I think, therefore I am: A twin study of attributional style in adolescents. *Journal of Child Psychology and Psychiatry.*

Legrand, L. N., McGue, M., & Iacono, W. G. (1999). A twin study of state and trait anxiety in childhood and adolescence. *Journal of Child Psychology and Psychiatry, 40,* 953–958.

Lesch, K. P., Bengel, D., Heils, A., Zhang Sabol, S., Greenburg, B. D., Petri, S., et al. (1996). Association of anxiety-related traits with a polymorphism in the serotonin transporter gene regulatory region. *Science, 274,* 1527–1531.

Meltzer, H., Gatward, R., Goodman, R., & Ford, T. (2000). *Mental health of children and adolescents in Great Britain.* London: Her Majesty's Stationery Office.

Muris, P., Schmidt, H., Merckelbach, H., & Schouten, E. (2001). Anxiety sensitivity in adolescents: Factor structure and relationships to trait anxiety and symptoms of anxiety disorders and depression. *Behaviour Research and Therapy, 39,* 89–100.

O'Connor, T. G., Neiderhiser, J. M., Reiss, D., Hetherington, E. M., & Plomin, R. (1998). Genetic contributions to continuity, change, and co-occurrence of antisocial and depressive symptoms in Adolescence. *Journal of Child Psychology and Psychiatry, 39,* 323–336.

Pike, A., McGuire, S., Hetherington, E. M., Reiss, D., & Plomin, R. (1996). Family environment and adolescent depressive symptoms and antisocial behavior: A multivariate genetic analysis. *Developmental Psychology, 32,* 590–603.

Plomin, R., DeFries, J. C., McClearn, G. E., & McGuffin, P. (2001). *Behavioral genetics* (4th ed.). New York: Worth.

Purcell, S. (2002). Variance components models for gene–environment interaction in twin analysis. *Twin Research, 5,* 554–571.

Rice, F., Harold, G. T., & Thapar, A. (2002a). Assessing the effects of age, sex and shared environment on the genetic aetiology of depression in childhood and adolescence. *Journal of Child Psychology and Psychiatry, 43,* 1039–1051.

Rice, F., Harold, G. T., & Thapar, A. (2002b). The genetic aetiology of childhood depression: A review. *Journal of Child Psychology and Psychiatry, 43,* 65–80.

Rice, F., Harold, G. T., & Thapar, A. (2003). Negative life events as an account of age-related differences in the genetic aetiology of depression in childhood and adolescence. *Journal of Child Psychology and Psychiatry, 44,* 977–987.

Saudino, K. J., Pedersen, N. L., Lichtenstein, P., McClearn, G. E., & Plomin, R. (1997). Can personality explain genetic influences on life events? *Journal of Personality and Social Psychology, 72,* 196–206.

Scarr, S., & McCartney, K. (1983). How people make their own environments: A theory of genotype–environmental effects. *Child Development, 54,* 424–435.

Scourfield, J., Rice, F., Thapar, A., Harold, G. T., Martin, N., & McGuffin, P. (2003). Depressive symptoms in children and adolescents: Changing aetiological influences with development. *Journal of Child Psychology and Psychiatry, 44,* 968–976.

Seligman, M. E. P. (1974). Depression and learned helplessness. In R. J. Friedman & M. M. Katz (Eds.), *The psychology of depression: Contemporary theory and research* (pp. 83–113). Washington, DC: Winston.

Seligman, M. E. P., Peterson, C., Kaslow, N. J., Tanenbaum, R. L., Alloy, L. B., &

Abramson, L. Y. (1984). Attributional style and depressive symptoms among children. *Journal of Abnormal Psychology, 93,* 235–238.

Sham, P. C., Sterne, A., Purcell, S., Cherny, S. S., Webster, M., Rijsdijk, F. V., et al. (2000). GENESiS: Creating a composite index of the vulnerability to anxiety and depression in a community-based sample of siblings. *Twin Research, 3,* 316–322.

Silberg, J., Pickles, A., Rutter, M., Hewitt, J., Simonoff, E., Maes, H., et al. (1999). The influence of genetic factors and life stress on depression among adolescent girls. *Archives of General Psychiatry, 56,* 225–232.

Silberg, J. L., Rutter, M., & Eaves, L. (2001). Genetic and environmental influences on the temporal association between earlier anxiety and later depression in girls. *Biological Psychiatry, 49,* 1040–1049.

Silberg, J., Rutter, M., Neale, M., & Eaves, L. (2001). Genetic moderation of environmental risk for depression and anxiety in adolescent girls. *British Journal of Psychiatry, 179,* 116–121.

Silverman, W. K., Ginsburg, G. S., & Goedhart, A. W. (1999). Factor structure of the childhood anxiety sensitivity index. *Behaviour Research and Therapy, 37,* 903–917.

Smoller, J. W., & Tsuang, M. T. (1998). Panic and phobic anxiety: Defining phenotypes for genetic studies. *American Journal of Psychiatry, 155,* 1152–1162.

Spielberger, C. D. (1966). *Anxiety and behavior.* New York: Academic Press.

Taylor, S. (1999). *Anxiety sensitivity.* Mahwah, NJ: Erlbaum.

Thapar, A., & McGuffin, P. (1997). Anxiety and depressive symptoms in childhood: A genetic study of comorbidity. *Journal of Child Psychology and Psychiatry, 38,* 651–656.

Zinbarg, R. E., & Barlow, D. (1997). Hierarchical structure and general factor saturation of the Anxiety Sensitivity Index: Evidence and implications. *Psychological Assessment, 9,* 277–284.

17

Cognitive and Biological Functioning in Children at Risk for Depression

Ian H. Gotlib, Jutta Joormann, Kelly L. Minor, and Rebecca E. Cooney

Major depressive disorder (MDD) is a devastating, sometimes fatal psychological disorder that afflicts nearly one-fifth of the population, making it one of the most prevalent of all psychiatric disorders. MDD is characterized by at least a 2-week period of persistent sad mood or loss of interest or pleasure in daily activities, as well as a number of associated symptoms, such as weight loss or gain, appetite loss, sleep disturbance, psychomotor retardation, fatigue, feelings of worthlessness, and concentration difficulties (American Psychiatric Association, 2000). Clinically significant depression is a pressing societal problem, placing a burden of almost $50 billion per year on the American economy and accounting for over 20% of costs for all mental illness (Stewart, Ricci, Chee, Hahn, & Morganstein, 2003). Moreover, depressive disorders are associated with both an elevated risk of suicide (Hirschfeld & Goodwin, 1988) and an increased risk of mortality from other causes (Murphy, Monson, Olivier, Sobol, & Leighton, 1987).

MDD is a recurrent disorder. It is estimated that 24% of women and 15% of men will experience at least one episode of clinically significant depression (Kessler et al., 2003). Importantly, approximately 80% of these individuals will experience more than one major depressive episode over the course of their lives (Boland & Keller, 2002). At least 50% of depressed patients have been found to relapse within 2 years of recovery (e.g., Keller & Shapiro, 1981); individuals with three or more previous episodes of depression may have a relapse rate as high as 40% within only 12–15 weeks after recovery (Keller et al., 1992; Mueller et al., 1996). Indeed, the risk for experiencing a new episode of depression has been found to increase by 16% with every episode (Solomon et al., 2000). This high rate of recurrence almost certainly reflects the presence of stable factors that place certain individuals at increased risk for developing MDD, and for experiencing depressive episodes repeatedly over the course of their lives. Given the high prevalence and the personal and societal costs of this disorder, efforts to identify vulnerability factors for both the onset and the recurrence of depression are particularly pressing.

In this context, in addition to examining characteristics of individuals who are already experiencing MDD, investigators have been focusing increasingly on factors associated with *risk* for MDD. Because first episodes of depression are occurring at increasingly younger ages (Kessler et al., 2003), and because early-onset depression has been found to have particularly pernicious effects, predicting both poorer course and more adverse outcomes (e.g., Lewinsohn, Rohde, Seeley, Klein, & Gotlib, 2000), researchers have underscored the importance of assessing the functioning of children and adolescents in helping to understand risk for this disorder. In fact, two populations have been of particular interest to researchers. First, based on the rationale that factors that serve to increase individuals' vulnerability for depression should be detectable before the first onset of a depressive episode, investigators have begun to examine children of depressed parents, who are known to be at high risk for developing a depressive disorder. In fact, having parents who suffer from depression is associated with a threefold increase in the risk to the offspring for developing a depressive episode. Second, children and young adolescents who have already had a diagnosable depressive episode are at elevated risk for developing recurrent episodes. Epidemiological studies have found that depression during adolescence predicts a two- to threefold increase in the risk for adult depression. Given these figures, it is clear that a high priority for current research is to identify the factors and mechanisms that place offspring of depressed parents at elevated risk for depression, and that contribute to the recurrence of depressive episodes. Thus investigators have begun to examine the functioning of offspring of depressed parents, and in particular of depressed mothers, in an attempt to understand the processes that operate to place people at elevated risk for the onset of this disorder. In addition, investigators have begun to focus on children and adolescents who have been diagnosed with depression, to understand processes that are implicated in the recurrence of depressive episodes.

In attempting to identify potential risk factors and mechanisms of risk for depression, it is helpful to turn to the formulation that what characterizes depressed individuals is not so much an abnormal initial response to a stressor, such as a stressful life event, but rather the maintenance of the ensuing affective state. Thus it may be that prolonged or incomplete recovery from affective states, and accompanying cognitive, physiological, and neural changes following exposure to a stressor, are important risk factors for depression. In this context, investigators have examined a number of psychological and biological factors both in offspring of depressed parents and in children and adolescents who have been diagnosed with a depressive disorder. Whereas some studies have attempted to delineate individual differences in the processing of emotional information in these children, other investigations have focused on individual differences in neuroendocrine responses, and still other research has investigated neural activation in response to stressors. These studies have significantly advanced our understanding of childhood depression and have helped to refine our hypotheses about risk factors. Nevertheless, it is important to note that these literatures are developing independently of each other. We believe that in order to gain a more comprehensive understanding of risk factors and mechanisms of risk for depression, it is critical that we begin to integrate research on cognitive and affective aspects of depression with investigations of biological factors. The purposes of this chapter are to briefly review these literatures, and to present preliminary results from a study designed to integrate psychological and biological functioning in children at elevated risk for the development of MDD. We turn first to a discussion of risk for depression among children of depressed parents, and then discuss briefly the constructs of emotion regulation and stress reactivity as they interact with risk.

CHILDREN AT RISK FOR DEPRESSION

Research examining depression during childhood and adolescence clearly demonstrates that children can become depressed. Although depressive disorders are less common in early childhood, prevalence rates of depression become comparable to rates in adults by middle adolescence. Consequently, investigators have postulated that mood disorders usually have their first manifestation in middle to late adolescence, making this a particularly vulnerable period for the development of depression (Hankin et al., 1998). Importantly, follow-up studies have shown that depression in childhood and adolescence tends to recur (Kovacs & Paulaukas, 1984), and that continuity exists between childhood and adult mood disorders. Indeed, longitudinal studies have found that children and adolescents with depression tend to have recurrent depressive episodes as adults (e.g., Harrington, Fudge, Rutter, Pickles, & Hill, 1990). Moreover, Pine, Cohen, Gurley, Brook, and Ma (1998) found that depressive disorders in young adulthood are often preceded by depression during adolescence. Thus studying children and adolescents diagnosed with MDD has the possibility of significantly advancing our understanding of risk factors for the recurrence of MDD.

Much has been written about the adverse effects of mothers' depression on their children. In fact, negative effects of maternal depression have been found in children ranging in age from infancy through adolescence (e.g., Rahman, Lovel, Bunn, Igbal, & Harrington, 2004; Whiffen & Gotlib, 1989).

Beardslee, Versage, and Gladstone (1998), Hammen (1997), and Williamson, Birmaher, Axelson, Ryan, and Dahl (2004) recently reported that having parents who suffer from depression is associated with a three- to fivefold increase in the risk to the offspring for developing a depressive episode during early adolescence. Maternal depression has been found to be associated with an earlier onset and more severe course of depression in the offspring (Lieb, Isensee, Hofler, Pfister, & Wittchen, 2002), and with an increased risk in the children for substance abuse and anxiety disorders (for reviews of these literatures, see Cummings & Davies, 1994; Gotlib & Goodman, 1999).

In addition to these adverse diagnostic outcomes, maternal depression has been found to be consistently associated with increased rates of behavior problems, socioemotional maladjustment, and deficits in cognitive/intellectual functioning. Moreover, these difficulties have been observed in offspring ranging in age from infancy through adolescence (see Gotlib & Goodman, 1999, for a detailed review of this literature). Importantly, the results of longitudinal investigations indicate that a parent's recovery from the depressive episode during which a child was assessed is not associated with improved functioning in the child, regardless of the developmental period during which the parent's episode of depression occurred—a finding that underscores the importance of prevention of depression to maximize the emotional health of the offspring of depressed mothers.

Given these figures and the ultimate goal of preventing depression among young children of depressed parents, it is critical that we identify the factors and mechanisms placing these offspring at elevated risk for this disorder. Although investigators have provided important data regarding the magnitude of this risk, we know little about the specific factors that are implicated in the development of depression in these offspring, or about the mechanisms involved in the intergenerational transmission of risk. While there is a genetic component that contributes to these children's risk for depression (Wallace, Schneider, & McGuffin, 2002), it is almost certain that the effects of parental depression on offspring are transmitted through multiple mechanisms— including the heritability of depression; innate dysfunctional neuroregulatory mechanisms; exposure to, and modeling of, negative maternal cognitions, behaviors, and affect; the stressful context of the children's lives; and an inability to deal effectively with stress and to regulate negative emotions (Goodman & Gotlib, 1999). Thus, although the children of depressed parents are genetically at risk for depression, the stress of living with their depressed parents and inadequate skills for coping with this stress significantly increase the risk for depression in these children (Hammen, 1997). Understanding the operation of these factors and mechanisms is crucial if we are to develop effective programs to prevent the onset of this debilitating disorder.

Although there have been a small number of investigations examining different aspects of depression and of risk for depression in children, each study has typically focused on one relatively narrow domain of risk, such as cognitive (e.g., Taylor & Ingram, 1999), neuroendocrine (e.g., Goodyer, Herbert, Tamplin, & Altham, 2000a), or neurobiological functioning (Thomas et al., 2001). It is clear, however, that progress in understanding the mechanisms underlying the transmission of risk for depression from parent to child will be made most rapidly by adopting an integrative approach in research in this area (cf. Goodman & Gotlib, 1999). In this chapter, therefore, we review the results of studies examining psychological and biological factors that have been implicated in increasing risk for depression, and we present initial findings from an integrative study of the offspring of depressed mothers. We begin by outlining the theoretical framework and by reviewing the literatures assessing cognitive, neuroendocrine, and neural aspects of depression; we indicate for each domain how these factors may be implicated in risk for this disorder. We then describe preliminary results of a study currently being conducted in our laboratory, in which we are assessing the psychological and biological functioning of 11- to 14-year-old daughters of mothers with a history of recurrent depression. As we describe in greater detail later, in conducting this study we are utilizing an integrative framework in which we are focusing explicitly on the constructs of emotion regulation and stress reactivity in understanding the mechanisms underlying risk for depression.

EMOTION REGULATION, STRESS REACTIVITY, AND RISK FOR DEPRESSION

Contemporary models of adult depression are explicitly diathesis–stress formulations, positing that events perceived as stressful will trigger, or interact with, an "endogenous" vulnerability that contributes to the onset of the disorder (cf. Monroe & Simons, 1991). From this perspective, therefore, a comprehensive understanding of risk for depression involves not only identifying the processes related to vulnerability to this disorder, but determining how these processes and factors are triggered by stressful or aversive experiences to lead to depression. To date, research examining diathesis–stress models of depression has focused primarily on identifying cognitive factors that might underlie increased risk for the onset and recurrence of depression. Indeed, a large body of empirical research suggests that individual differences in the processing of emotional information support and sustain depressive states. Despite the promise of these findings, however, it is becoming increasingly apparent that cognitive theories of depression have significant limitations. For example, no real connections have been made between cognitive theories of depression and other aspects of depressive functioning. Investigators examining information processing in depression have focused narrowly on immediate attention to and memory for discrete valenced stimuli. There is a growing consensus, however, that depression involves a dysregulation not only of cognitions, but also of emotions (Barlow, 1991), of temperament (e.g., Watson & Clark, 1995), of motivated responses to emotionally valenced information (e.g., Henriques & Davidson, 2000), and of biological functioning (Posener, DeBattista, Williams, & Schatzberg, 2001). Indeed, developing literatures now highlight the importance of biological aspects of emotion regulation and responsivity to emotional stimuli (Davidson, Pizzagalli, & Nitschke, 2002; Rottenberg, Wilhelm, Gross, & Gotlib, 2002). It is clear, therefore, that the study of cognitive aspects of depression must be expanded by adopting a broader, more integrative perspective on the processing of emotional stimuli by depressed individuals.

In this context, recent research attempting to understand the development of negative outcomes in depression has focused on the constructs of stress exposure; stress reactivity and recovery; and, in particular, emotion regulation and other self-regulatory processes that are engaged in response to stress. Overall, three factors are of particular importance in understanding the heightened vulnerability of children of depressed parents: (1) the amount of stress present in the children's environment; (2) the perception and evaluation of this stress and/or stressors by the children, which determine their immediate response to the stressors (stress reactivity); and (3) the children's regulatory skills in response to the stressors, which determine the long-term consequences of exposure to the stressors (emotion regulation). The construct of "emotion regulation," which evolved from the broader concept of "coping," involves the utilization of behavioral and cognitive strategies in efforts to modulate affective intensity and duration (Thompson, 1994). This construct is becoming increasingly important in understanding the onset and maintenance of depression. Theorists have suggested that what characterizes individuals who are vulnerable to depression is not so much an abnormal initial response to a stressor, such as a stressful life event, but rather an inability to regulate the duration and intensity of the ensuing negative affect (e.g., Teasdale, 1988). In understanding risk for depression from this perspective, therefore, it is important to examine prolonged or incomplete recovery from negative affective states, and the accompanying physiological and neural changes that follow exposure to a stressor.

Unfortunately, the little research that has examined emotion regulation in depression has been conducted primarily with self-report measures. These measures are susceptible to demand characteristics and do not permit the assessment of automatic regulation processes. Perhaps more importantly, as we have noted earlier, there is a pressing need to broaden the range of methodologies that are used to study vulnerability to depression. For example, baseline hypothalamic–pituitary–adrenal (HPA) axis functioning and HPA reactivity and recovery, which probably reflect reactions to stress and the ability to regulate negative emotions, have recently been found to be aberrant in samples of depressed adults (Reus, Wolkowitz, & Frederick, 1997) and children (Goodyer, Park, Netherton, & Herbert, 2001). Similarly, investigators examining brain activation have begun to delineate neural correlates of emotion regulation (Ochsner, Bunge, Gross, & Gabrieli, 2002). Finally, an important aspect of emotion regulation and stress reactivity is response to rewarding experiences. Depressed persons have been found to report feeling both higher levels of negative affect and lower levels of positive affect than do nondepressed controls (Watson, Clark, & Carey, 1988). In addition, recent studies have shown that the lack of responsiveness to reward is what predicts recovery from depression (Joormann & Siemer, 2004; Kasch, Rottenberg, Arnow, & Gotlib, 2002).

Only recently have researchers begun to integrate these areas of research. Young and Nolen-Hoeksema (2001), for example, have demonstrated that the use of maladaptive emotion regulation strategies, such as rumination, is associated with heightened cortisol levels in healthy adults. In this chapter, we present an integrative assessment of emotion regulation and of stress reactivity and recovery in a group of young girls at risk for depression. We use a range of methodologies, including self-report measures, information-processing performance, HPA axis functioning and reactivity, and neural responses to emotional stimuli following exposure to stressful experiences. In the following sections, we briefly describe the assessment of emotion regulation and stress reactivity and recovery in depression from the perspectives of information processing, neuroendocrine functioning, and patterns of neural activation, and we provide an overview of the relevant literature summarizing studies on adults with depression, children with depression, and children at risk for the onset of depression.

INFORMATION PROCESSING IN DEPRESSION

One of the major approaches over the past two decades to understanding the etiology of MDD, the functioning of depressed individuals, and vulnerability to this disorder is information-processing theory, which is driven in large part by cognitive models of depression. In general, these models emphasize the importance of cognitive constructs, such as schemas, in placing individuals at elevated risk for experiencing episodes of depression and in hindering the recovery process (Beck, 1967; Bower, 1981; Teasdale, 1988). Thus cognitive theories posit that vulnerable and depressed individuals selectively attend to negative stimuli, filter out positive stimuli, and perceive negative or neutral information as being more negative than is actually the case. Moreover, cognitive theories posit further that because of these negative schemas, depressed individuals are characterized by a negative bias in recall, demonstrating better recall for negative than for neutral or positive material. Negative schemas, developed through adverse early experiences, are posited to be latent until they are activated when individuals experience a stressful life event. Depressive affect innervates the negative schemas (which operate at an automatic, as opposed to strategic, level of functioning) and reinforces their activity.

Depressed Adults

Empirical studies of depressed adults have generally provided support for cognitive formulations of depression. Early studies of the cognitive functioning of depressed individuals relied on self-report methodologies, which were cor-

rectly criticized both for being susceptible to response bias and for not adequately assessing automatic processing (see Gotlib & McCabe, 1992). These
self-report methodologies have been largely replaced by more sophisticated
procedures, many derived from research in experimental cognitive psychology, to examine the cognitive functioning of depressed individuals (Gotlib &
MacLeod, 1997). For example, over the past 20+ years in our laboratory, we
have used information-processing paradigms to examine attentional interference, selective attention, and memory biases in depressed individuals.
We developed the emotion Stroop task (Gotlib & Cane, 1987; Gotlib &
McCann, 1984), as well as other information-processing tasks—such as the
deployment-of-attention task (Gotlib, McLachlan, & Katz, 1988; McCabe &
Gotlib, 1995; McCabe, Gotlib, & Martin, 2000), the emotion dichotic listening task (McCabe & Gotlib, 1993), and, more recently, the emotion faces
dot probe attentional task (Gotlib, Krasnoperova, Neubauer, & Joormann,
2004)—to assess cognitive biases in depressed persons. Using these tasks, we
have documented biases in attention in both subclinically depressed college
students (e.g., Gotlib et al., 1988) and patients diagnosed with MDD (e.g.,
Gotlib & Cane, 1987; Gotlib, Krasnoperova, et al., 2004). Compared to
matched nondepressed control participants, we have found depressed adults
to be characterized by greater attention to negative than to neutral or positive stimuli. In another series of studies, we have also found evidence of
depression-associated biases in memory (e.g., Gilboa & Gotlib, 1997; Gilboa,
Roberts, & Gotlib, 1997; Gotlib, Kasch, et al., 2004), such that depressed
individuals exhibit better memory for negative than for neutral or positive
information.

Depressed Children

Critical to a developmental approach to understanding cognitive biases in
depressed adults is the question of whether depressed children resemble their
adult counterparts with respect to their cognitive functioning. Unfortunately,
research on information-processing biases in depressed children clearly lags
behind investigations of depressed adults. As in the adult literature, studies
relying on self-report measures indicate that depressed children endorse more
cognitive errors and more negative attributions than do nondepressed children
(e.g., Tems, Stewart, Skinner, Hughes, & Emslie, 1993). Again, however,
investigators have moved to information-processing methodologies to assess
cognitive dysfunction in depressed children. The few studies conducted in this
area to date have focused primarily on depressed children's memory for positive and negative information. In an early investigation, Whitman and
Leitenberg (1990) asked children to recall their performance on a verbal task
on which feedback was provided. Whitman and Leitenberg found that
depressed children recalled fewer of the words they had previously gotten correct than did nondepressed children. More recently, Bishop, Dalgleish, and
Yule (2004) presented positive and negative emotional stories to children who

scored low and high on a measure of depressive symptoms, and found that children with high levels of depressive symptoms showed enhanced recall of the negative emotional stories. Finally, two studies have examined memory for emotional stimuli in children diagnosed with depression. Neshat-Doost, Taghavi, Moradi, Yule, and Dalgleish (1998) presented nondepressed and depressed children with a series of positive, negative, and neutral words; they found that, in contrast to the nondepressed children, depressed children recalled more negative than positive words. Similarly, Timbremont and Braet (2004) administered a self-referent encoding task to depressed children, and reported that they endorsed more negative words on the task and recalled fewer positive words than did nondepressed controls.

Children at Risk for Depression

It is clear from the results of these studies that depressed adults and depressed children alike are characterized by biases in their processing of emotional information. Cognitive theorists posit that such schema-driven biases precede the onset of depressive episodes, and therefore should be evident in individuals at risk for depression before they have experienced an episode of depression. However, few studies have been conducted examining the role of cognitive factors in the onset of depression in adults, and even fewer have been reported with children. In adults, biases in information processing have been found to predict increases in depressive symptoms (as opposed to the onset of diagnosable depression) in women after they tested positive for cervical cancer (MacLeod & Hagan, 1992), in pregnant women following birth (Bellew & Hill, 1991), and in undergraduate students (Rude, Wenzlaff, Gibbs, Vane, & Whitney, 2002). Four studies have reported results that mirror these findings in samples of children. Hammen and Zupan (1984) demonstrated the potential utility of information-processing tasks in identifying children at risk for developing depression, demonstrating that compared with children of nondepressed mothers, offspring of depressed mothers tended to recall more negative than positive words that they had judged as self-relevant. Jaenicke and colleagues (1987) examined memory for self-encoded positive and negative adjectives in the school-age children of mothers with unipolar depression, a medical illness, or no disorders. Jaenicke and colleagues found that the children of depressed mothers remembered proportionally fewer positive words that they had endorsed than did the children of medically ill mothers or the offspring of mothers with no disorders; there were no differences among the three groups of children in the proportion of negative adjectives they recalled.

Recent work examining cognitive factors associated with increased vulnerability to depression has suggested that negative schemas must be "primed," or "activated," by inducing a negative mood in individuals who are at risk for this disorder (e.g., Ingram & Siegle, 2002). In this context, Taylor and Ingram (1999) found that under an induced negative mood, children of depressed mothers endorsed fewer positive words than did children of parents with no history of psychiatric disorder. Finally, in a study conducted recently in our laboratory, we induced a negative mood state in children of parents with bipolar disorder and children of never-disordered parents, and then administered an emotion Stroop task and a self-referent encoding task to the children (Gotlib, Traill, Montoya, Joormann, & Chang, 2005). In contrast to the control offspring, we found the children of bipolar parents to exhibit an attentional bias for social-threat and irritable-manic words on the emotion Stroop task, and better recall of negative words that they had endorsed on the self-referent encoding task.

Taken together, the results of these studies indicate that depressed children and adults are characterized by biases in attention to, and memory for, negative emotional material. There is also growing evidence of the operation of negative cognitive schemas in children at elevated risk for depression, particularly as these children experience negative mood states—a finding that supports the possibility that the cognitive biases apparent in depressed adults may have their origins in childhood. It is critical to note, however, that little evidence currently indicates that negative cognitive schemas play a causal role in the onset of diagnosable depressive episodes, either in children or in adults. In adults, investigators examining the role of information-processing biases in depression have found cognitive dysfunction to predict subsequent increases in depressive symptomatology. In samples of children and adolescents, researchers have demonstrated that offspring of depressed parents exhibit biases in their processing of emotional information; there is no evidence to date in children, however, that these biases play a role in either the exacerbation of depressive symptoms or the development of a depressive episode. This is an important consideration, and one that we discuss in greater detail later in this chapter.

NEUROENDOCRINE ASPECTS OF EMOTION REGULATION/COPING IN DEPRESSION

Recent research on coping and emotion regulation has focused on neuroendocrine and neural functioning as an alternative to self-report methodologies—a shift that has helped to elucidate the biological foundations of emotion dysregulation. The HPA system and the resultant production of cortisol are conceptualized as the psychophysiological substrates for the regulation and coping systems. The HPA system represents the core of human stress response, secreting cortisol when under stress as a means of mobilizing the resources necessary for sustaining the physical and psychological activity needed for action (Stansbury & Gunnar, 1994). Indeed, investigators have argued that levels of cortisol produced under stress reflect individuals' ability to regulate and cope (Gunnar, Marvinney, Isensee, & Fisch, 1989). Moreover, tonic HPA functioning is also of interest because basal cortisol varies across the day, promotes various adaptive functions, and may reflect individuals' baseline physiological and emotional arousal. Given that the functioning of the HPA system is so integrally related to the human stress response, it is not surprising that atypical patterns of both basal HPA functioning and HPA reactivity have been documented in various psychiatric disorders, including depression (cf. Gunnar & Cheatham, 2003).

Depressed Adults

The major cognitive and biological theories of depression implicate stress, often in the form of stressful life events, in the onset of this disorder. In a diathesis–stress formulation, for example, Beck (1967) postulated that in individuals who are vulnerable to depression, negative cognitive schemas are activated by personally relevant stressors; from a more biological perspective, Post (1992) presented a "kindling" formulation of the relation between stress and depression, arguing that less stress is required to precipitate each successive episode of depression (see also Kendler, Kessler, Neale, Heath, & Eaves, 1993; Young & Nolen-Hoeksema, 2001). Given this emphasis on the association between stress and depression, it is not surprising that the potential role of cortisol irregularity in adult depression has been the focus of research for over four decades (Michael & Gibbons, 1963). Dinan (1996) has hypothesized that stressful life events lead to the production of elevated levels of cortisol, which in turn reduce brain serotonin function, resulting in the onset of depression. Consistent with this hypothesis and with theoretical postulates emphasizing the elevated levels of stress in depression, the results of empirical studies generally indicate that MDD is associated with HPA axis overactivity, as reflected in both tonic cortisol hypersecretion and cortisol hypersecretion following an acute stressor (Parker, Schatzberg, & Lyons, 2003).

It is important to note that there is some variability in this general pattern of cortisol hypersecretion as a function of the specific depressive samples studied, the ways cortisol levels have been measured (e.g., quantification of rhythm amplitude, timing of secretion bursts, mean levels over the course of a 24-hour period), and the media in which the cortisol has been assessed (e.g., urine, plasma, cerebrospinal fluid, saliva) (e.g., Galard, Catalan, Castellanos, & Gallart, 2002; Maes, Calabrese, & Meltzer, 1994; Yehuda, Boisoneau, Mason, & Giller, 1993). Nevertheless, there is ample evidence that MDD is associated with HPA axis dysfunction. Moreover, results of studies examining the suppression of dexamethasone, a synthetic glucocorticoid that suppresses cortisol, indicate that HPA axis dysregulation may play a role in the recurrence of depression (Targum, 1984). Considered collectively, therefore, depressed adults appear to be characterized by dysregulation of HPA axis functioning, presumably reflecting difficulties in emotion regulation and coping with the effects of stress. Indeed, consistent with a diathesis–stress perspective, HPA axis dysfunction may represent a trait-like vulnerability factor for depression, interacting with environmental stress to precipitate recurrences of depressive episodes. In part to examine the veracity of this formulation, investigators have begun to assess HPA axis functioning in sample of depressed children and, more recently, in samples of children who are at elevated risk for depression.

Depressed Children

In contrast to the relatively consistent findings of hypercortisolemia in depressed adults, results of studies examining HPA axis functioning in depressed children and adolescents are equivocal. For example, a number of researchers have reported that, unlike depressed adults, depressed youth are not characterized by general cortisol hypersecretion over the course of the diurnal cycle (e.g., Birmaher et al., 1992; Dahl et al., 1991). Instead, depressed adolescents have been found to exhibit high cortisol levels during the evening, when the HPA axis is typically quiescent (De Bellis et al., 1996; Goodyer, Park, & Herbert, 2001). Interestingly, Goodyer, Herbert, Moor, and Altham (1991) found that elevated levels of evening cortisol secretion among depressed youth normalize following recovery from a depressive episode, suggesting that cortisol hypersecretion might be a state characteristic of depression.

Countering this position, however, there are data indicating that levels of cortisol secretion among depressed youth during a depressive episode have predictive utility. For example, although Rao and colleagues (1996) did not find differences between depressed and nondepressed adolescents in levels of evening cortisol secretion, they reported that within their sample of depressed adolescents, elevations in evening cortisol levels predicted a recurrent course of the disorder at a 7-year follow-up assessment. Similarly, Mathew and colleagues (2003) found that elevations of daytime cortisol in depressed adolescents predicted subsequent suicide attempts over a 10-year follow-up period. Thus, although depression-associated dysfunction of the HPA axis has not consistently been found in children and adolescents in cross-sectional investigations, there is evidence to suggest that basal levels of diurnal cortisol secretion predict recurrence of depression and suicide attempts.

These longitudinal findings may reflect the relation between HPA axis functioning and coping under stress, indicating that depressed adolescents are less capable than are their nondepressed counterparts of coping effectively with stressors in their environment. Consistent with this formulation, several investigators have reported heightened levels of HPA axis reactivity to stress in children and adolescents with clinically significant internalizing symptoms (e.g., Granger, Weisz, McCracken, Ikeda, & Douglas, 1996; Watamura, Donzella, Alwin, & Gunnar, 2003). For example, Ashman, Dawson, Panagiotides, Yamada, and Wilkinson (2002) found that although children with clinically significant internalizing symptoms and control children without psychiatric disorders did not differ with respect to levels of basal cortisol, the internalizing children exhibited a greater cortisol response to a laboratory stressor. From a different perspective, Granger and colleagues (1996) found that increased cortisol reactivity to a laboratory stressor predicted internalizing symptoms and the presence of anxiety disorders among clinic-referred children at a 6-month follow-up assessment. Finally, in samples of depressed children, Luby and colleagues (2003) found depressed preschoolers to exhibit HPA axis reactivity in response to a discrete stressor, and Coplan and colleagues (2002) found elevated levels of cortisol in anticipation of a laboratory stressor (carbon dioxide inhalation) among those children and adolescents diagnosed with depression and/or anxiety who were sensitive to the anxiogenic effects of the challenge. Interestingly, depressed/anxious children in that study who did not respond to the respiratory procedure did not differ from healthy controls in their cortisol response. These findings indicate that depressed youth are characterized by relatively high levels of cortisol reactivity in response to relevant stressors, and that elevated cortisol reactivity may be a significant predictor of increases in depressive symptoms.

Children at Risk for Depression

The results of the studies described above suggest that the pattern of HPA functioning and reactivity in depressed children and adolescents is similar to that found in depressed adults. Moreover, there is some evidence that levels of cortisol activity among depressed children may predict the course of the disorder. Little research, however, has examined whether HPA dysregulation functions as a risk factor for the onset of a depressive episode in youth. Ashman and colleagues (2002) found abnormal HPA reactivity in response to a laboratory stressor in children whose mothers were depressed but who themselves were not depressed. More recently, Halligan, Herbert, Goodyer, and Murray (2004) reported that having depressed mothers was associated with higher and more variable morning cortisol levels in their children. In a prospective study, Essex, Klein, Cho, and Kalin (2002) found that preschool-age children of depressed mothers exhibited elevated cortisol levels, and that these were associated with subsequent higher levels of mental health symptoms in first grade. Finally, in a 3-year longitudinal study, Goodyer, Herbert, Tamplin, and Altham (2000b) demonstrated that peak levels of morning cortisol and late afternoon levels of dehydroepiandrosterone (DHEA, another hormone that indexes HPA activity) among adolescents predicted the subsequent onset of MDD. In fact, DHEA hypersecretion was found in this sample to precede the onset of the depressive episode.

In sum, although few studies have been reported, the limited findings from investigations of children and adolescents at risk for depression indicate that these children differ from their low-risk counterparts with respect to their HPA functioning. Compared to children at low risk for depression, high-risk children have been found to be characterized by elevated and/or more variable levels of cortisol secretion. It appears, therefore, that dysregulated HPA axis functioning, both tonic and in response to a stressor, may serve as a risk factor for the development of a major depressive episode in children. Indeed, these data are consistent with Goodman and Gotlib's (1999) formulation that a critical consequence of maternal depression for a child is chronic activation of the HPA axis as a result of the stress of living with a depressed parent, and thus that such a child has an impaired ability to cope effectively with stress. In testing this formulation more explicitly, these data underscore the importance of assessing both exposure to stress and neuroendocrine functioning in children at elevated risk for depression. And in this context of broadening the scope of investigations in this area, it is important to note that chronic activation of the HPA axis, resulting in high levels of cortisol, can also disrupt functioning in regions of the brain that are responsible for the regulation of emotion (e.g., the prefrontal cortex, the anterior cingulate cortex [ACC], and the amygdala), thereby probably interfering with individuals' ability to cope with stress (Goodman & Gotlib, 1999). No studies, however, have examined cortisol secretion in response to stress in school-age or adolescent offspring of depressed parents. Later in this chapter, we present data from such an investigation—but we turn first to a brief examination of neural functioning in depressed adults and children, and in children at risk for depression.

NEURAL BASES OF EMOTION REGULATION AND REWARD RESPONSIVITY IN DEPRESSION

Although investigators have long speculated about deficits in neural functioning in depression, only relatively recently have advances in neuroimaging allowed researchers to examine neural aspects of depressive disorders. Indeed, depression has now been found to be associated with abnormalities of several cortical and subcortical regions, including the hippocampus, prefrontal cortex, ACC, and amygdala (e.g., Davidson et al., 2002; Mayberg, 2002). Initial research in this area focused largely on differences between currently depressed and nondepressed adults in the volume of these anatomical structures. Drawing on recent findings concerning the involvement of specific structures in emotion regulation, more recent investigations have examined depression-associated differences in patterns of neural activation in response to the processing of emotional stimuli.

Depressed Adults

A number of morphometric studies using magnetic resonance imaging (MRI) have reported atrophy in the hippocampus (Bremner et al., 2000), subgenual ACC (Drevets, Price, & Simpson, 1997), and amygdala (e.g., Sheline, Sanghavi, Mintun, & Gado, 1999) in patients diagnosed with MDD. Interestingly, the decrease in the volume of the amygdala appears to be found more consistently in patients with relatively long histories of depressive episodes; in individuals in their first episode of depression, amygdalar volume has been found to be abnormally increased (e.g., Frodl et al., 2003).

Researchers have also documented depression-associated abnormalities in the function of these structures. For example, investigators using positron emission tomography (PET) imaging to examine serotonin agonist binding in the hippocampus have found reduced serotonin receptor binding/density in depressed patients (e.g., Sheline, Mittler, & Mintun, 2002). Similarly, Saxena and colleagues (2001) reported evidence of depression-associated decreased glucose metabolism in the hippocampus. These results have led researchers to posit that neuronal loss in hippocampus in depression is due to stress-induced hypercortisolemia (Pariante & Miller, 2001)—a position consistent with findings that degree of hippocampal loss is positively correlated with lifetime duration of depression (Sheline et al., 1999). In contrast, abnormal elevations in cerebral blood flow, blood oxygenation, and glucose metabolism have been found in the amygdala and the subgenual ACC in depressed individuals (Drevets, 2000; Siegle, Steinhauer, Thase, Stenger, & Carter, 2002). Interestingly, these results are consistent with the finding that effective response to antidepressants is associated with a decrease in metabolic activity in the subgenual ACC (Mayberg et al., 1999). Finally, a number of investigators have reported depression-associated amygdala responsivity in response to fearful or negative faces (e.g., Breiter et al., 1996)—a pattern that also appears to diminish with pharmacotherapy (Sheline et al., 2001; see Davidson et al., 2002, for an extended discussion of this literature).

Siegle and colleagues (2002) have provided what may be the first demonstration of how the amygdala in depression may be involved in sustained processing of negative emotional material that interferes with responsivity to neutral material. Interestingly, self-reported levels of rumination were significantly correlated with left amygdala activity (Siegle et al., 2002). Work done by Elliott, Rubinsztein, Sahakian, and Dolan (2000, 2002) has identified medial and orbital prefrontal regions as critical to mood-congruent processing biases. During an emotional go/no-go task, Elliott and colleagues (2002) detected attenuated engagement of the posterior orbito-frontal cortex (OFC) in depressed participants for emotionally valenced trials in contrast to neutral trials. The supposition that orbito-frontal areas may be distinctly involved in mediation of emotional processing is buttressed by neuroanatomical data. The OFC is highly interconnected with both the hippocampus and amygdala and is thought to inhibit posterior structures, particularly structures putatively involved in inappropriate emotional responses (Dias, Robbins, & Roberts, 1996). The Siegle and colleagues study, which detected increased processing of negative words in the amygdala and related decreased dorsolateral prefrontal cortex (DLPFC) activity, is consistent with a model of inverse functionality between limbic and prefrontal activity. Davidson and colleagues (2002) have posited that the DLPFC may modulate activity in the amygdala; disinhibition or decreased activity of the DLPFC may be related to patterns of hyperresponsivity in limbic regions such as the amygdala. Moreover, the DLPFC is considered a key component in executive control, working memory, and attention (Kane & Engle, 2002). Pochon and colleagues (2002) have further suggested that limbic inhibition of the DLPFC may serve to override top-down emotional control processes by selecting which representations to maintain.

Depressed and At-Risk Children

In contrast to this growing literature in adults, neuroimaging studies of depressed children are rare, and imaging studies of children at risk for depression are virtually nonexistent. MacMillan and colleagues (2003) reported marginally significant elevations in amygdala volume among depressed adolescents. In a study investigating the neural response to sadness-eliciting film clips in nondisordered children, Levesque and colleagues (2003) found increased left amygdala activation. Using a clinical sample, Thomas and colleagues (2001) examined patterns of neural activation in depressed and anxious children, relative to healthy controls, as they viewed fearful and neutral faces. Thomas et al. found that whereas the anxious children exhibited an exaggerated amygdala response to the fearful faces, the five depressed girls in this study demonstrated a blunted amygdala response to the fearful faces. This blunted neural response is intriguing, because it mirrors findings of blunted psychophysiological reactivity to emotional stimuli among depressed adults (e.g., Rottenberg, Gross, Wilhelm, Najmi, & Gotlib, 2002; Rottenberg, Kasch, Gross, & Gotlib, 2002).

It is impossible to determine from these investigations, of course, whether abnormalities in neural functioning represent symptoms or consequences of depression, or whether they might be predictors of depression. Unfortunately, researchers have not assessed the neural functioning of high-risk individuals before the onset of MDD, in order to examine whether dysfunctional patterns of neural response to emotional stimuli might constitute a risk factor for this disorder. In the following section, we describe preliminary results of an ongoing study of young daughters of mothers with recurrent depression in which we are examining biases in information processing, levels of cortisol secretion, and patterns of neural activation as possible risk factors for depression.

PSYCHOBIOLOGICAL FUNCTIONING OF GIRLS AT RISK FOR DEPRESSION

The research that we have reviewed thus far indicates that, with few exceptions, depressed adults are characterized by negative biases in attention and memory functioning; by dysregulated HPA axis functioning, as reflected by elevated levels of cortisol secretion; and by abnormalities in both the structure and function of the hippocampus, ACC, and amygdala. There is also a smaller (and less consistent) literature indicating that depressed children may share a subset of these same characteristics. Given that these indices of emotion dysregulation and dysfunction appear to characterize children and adults while they are depressed, an important question concerns the role that these difficulties and deficits may play in the onset of this disorder. Unfortunately, as we described above, there is little research addressing this question. To begin to fill this gap, we have initiated a study examining the psychobiological functioning of a group of participants at elevated risk for the onset of depression. If dysfunction in the processing of emotional information, dysregulation of the HPA axis in response to stress, or abnormalities in patterns of neural activation contribute to the onset of a depressive episode, we would expect these characteristics to be observable in individuals who have not experienced an episode of depression, but who are at increased risk for the development of this disorder.

To test this formulation, we have begun a study in which we are examining biases in the processing of emotional material, abnormalities in HPA axis functioning, and dysfunctional patterns of neural activation in response to mood and valenced stimuli in young girls of mothers with recurrent depression. As we have noted in detail earlier in this chapter, offspring of depressed parents are at elevated risk for developing depression themselves. And given the higher prevalence of MDD among women than among men, daughters of depressed parents are at particularly high risk for the development of depression.

Participants in this ongoing study are 11- to 14-year-old daughters and their biological mothers. All of the daughters are being interviewed with the Washington University Kiddie Schedule for Affective Disorders and Schizophrenia (K-SADS; Geller et al., 2001); their mothers complete the K-SADS with reference to their daughters. Regardless of the diagnostic status of the mothers, all daughters in this study must have never had a diagnosable Axis I disorder. Mothers are interviewed with the Structured Clinical Interview for DSM (SCID-I; First, Spitzer, Gibbon, & Williams, 1996), to establish whether they meet diagnostic criteria for having had two discrete episodes of MDD within their daughters' lifetime ("recurrent depressed" mothers) or for never having had an Axis I disorder ("never-disordered" mothers). At the time of testing, recurrent depressed mothers must not be experiencing an episode. Thus no mother or daughter meets criteria for a current diagnosis of MDD at the time of her first participation in the study.

We are collecting data from both mothers and daughters that assess psychobiological aspects of depression, emotion regulation, and stress reactivity. Mothers and daughters participate in emotion information-processing tasks with a negative-mood-inducing component; converse with each other about a stressful topic, during (and following) which salivary cortisol is collected; undergo a stressful interview, during (and following) which salivary cortisol is collected (daughters only); and, if they are able, participate in a functional MRI (fMRI) scanning session in which neural aspects of emotion regulation are assessed. Below we outline briefly the assessments we conduct in these areas and the initial results of these assessments.

Biases in the Processing
of Emotional Information

Mothers and daughters complete the self-referent encoding task (SRET) and the emotion faces dot probe task after participating in a negative-mood-inducing procedure. In the SRET, participants indicate whether positive and negative adjectives are self-referent, and are then given an incidental recall task. In the emotion faces dot probe task, participants are required to detect a dot probe in the spatial location of either a neutral or an emotional (sad or happy) face. Faster response latencies to detect the probe in the location of the sad faces reflect selective attention to those faces.

We obtained the expected results in the two groups of mothers: Compared to the 14 control mothers, the 14 recurrent depressed mothers (all of whom were in remission at the time of testing) both endorsed and recalled more negative words as self-descriptive on the SRET, and selectively attended to sad faces on the emotion faces dot probe task. More important, however, was the performance of the two groups of daughters. Despite equivalent self-reports concerning the effects of the negative-mood-inducing procedure, compared with the 14 control daughters, the 14 at-risk daughters endorsed more negative words on the SRET, recalled both fewer positive and more negative words on the SRET, and exhibited a strong selective attention to sad faces on the emotion faces dot probe task (Figures 17.1, 17.2, and 17.3). These data replicate results presented earlier, indicating that both depressed adults and depressed children exhibit preferential processing of negative stimuli. Moreover, these results extend these findings, and strongly suggest that information-processing biases play an important role in increasing vulnerability to depression.

Salivary Cortisol Secretion in Response to Stress

To assess HPA axis functioning in response to stress, all daughters undergo a 15-minute stress session. They complete a 3-minute serial subtraction task followed by a 12-minute social competence interview, developed to induce emotional arousal by discussing stressful life situations. Four saliva samples are collected over the course of 50 minutes: one sample immediately before task instructions, and three samples at 15, 30, and 45 minutes after the onset of the stressor. Following the laboratory stressor (i.e., during collection of the final two samples), participants watch a neutral videotape. As can be seen in Figure 17.4, the high-risk daughters exhibited both an elevated immediate response to the stressor and a slowed cortisol recovery. These data indicate that stress activates the HPA axis in individuals at heightened risk for depression to a greater extent than is the case for nonvulnerable individuals, and suggest a mechanism by which stress may play a role in the onset of depression in people vulnerable to the development of this disorder.

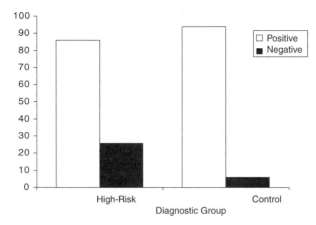

FIGURE 17.1. Endorsement on the SRET.

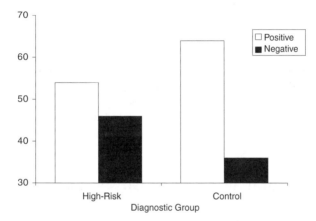
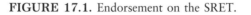

FIGURE 17.2. Recall on the SRET.

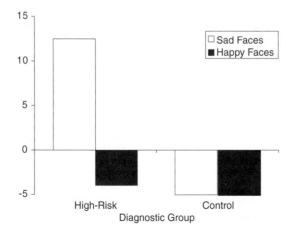

FIGURE 17.3. Bias scores on the dot probe task.

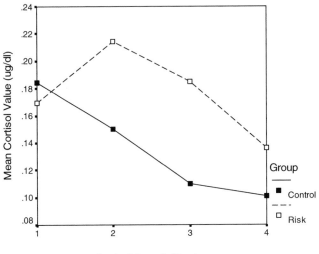

FIGURE 17.4. Cortisol response to laboratory stressor in 10 at-risk and 10 control girls. Note: Sample 1 was taken before the stressor; Sample 2 was taken directly after 15 minutes of stress induction; Sample 3 was taken 15 minutes after the stressor ended; Sample 4 was taken 30 minutes after the stressor ended.

Patterns of Neural Activation in Girls at Risk for Depression

Daughters who are eligible to be scanned participate in two tasks in the scanner: a mood repair task and a reward responsivity task. In the mood repair task, we are examining neural markers of a potentially compromised ability to use happy autobiographical memories to "repair" a sad mood. In this task, daughters undergo a negative-mood-inducing procedure in the scanner and are then asked to remember positive events that made them feel good. In the reward responsivity task, designed to examine reward processing, daughters perform a task in which, on each trial, they can anticipate gaining (reward) or losing (punishment) points that they can redeem for preselected prizes.

Whole-brain imaging data consisting of 24 contiguous slices (4 mm each) were acquired with a General Electric 1.5-tesla Signa scanner, using a spiral in–out sequence (Glover & Law, 2001). All images were preprocessed and analyzed with Analysis of Functional Neural Images software (Cox, 1996). Individual maps were thresholded at an exploratory omnibus threshold of $p <$ .001, overlaid on T1-weighted structural scans, and examined for significant activations. Preliminary results from four at-risk and four control girls indicate that, despite comparable mood ratings, the mood repair procedure induced activation in the amygdala only in the at-risk girls (Figure 17.5). Group differences between the two groups of daughters were also found for the reward responsivity task. As expected, both control and at-risk daughters exhibited activation of the ventral striatum while anticipating reward. Most importantly, however, only the high-risk girls also exhibited increased ACC activation in response to obtaining reward; in contrast, the controls girls showed activated ACC during the punishment condition (Figure 17.6). These data suggest that instantiation of a sad mood state in high-risk girls entails a broader recruitment of areas involved in emotional processing than is the case in control girls, and that the process of positive autobiographical memory retrieval to repair a negative mood is more challenging or aversive for girls at risk for depression. Moreover, the finding of ACC activation in the high-risk girls in response to reward is intriguing in light of the role of the ACC in conflict monitoring; it suggests that the possibility of receiving reward is not entirely a positive experience for girls at risk for depression. Interestingly, in previous studies the ACC has been related to anhedonia in depressed adults (Mitterschiffthaler et al., 2003), again suggesting another link between this structure and risk for depression.

Finally, we should note that although the data we have presented from this project are important in underscoring the significance of emotion regulation and stress reactivity in girls at risk for depression, much work remains to be done to integrate findings across the various domains of investigation. We have examined girls at risk for depression, using information-processing, neuroendocrine, and fMRI methodologies. We are now beginning to examine coherence across these domains, in order to gain a more comprehensive understanding of the interplay of risk factors for depression. For example, we are finding that within the group of at-risk daughters of mothers with recur-

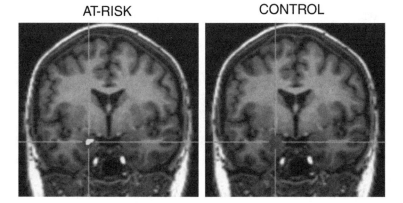

FIGURE 17.5. Amygdala activation during mood repair.

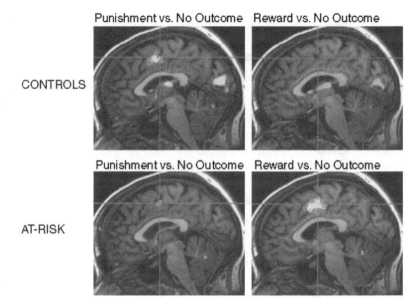

FIGURE 17.6. ACC activation during anticipation of reward.

rent depression, less reactivity in cortisol and mood is related to a stronger bias toward negative stimuli on the dot probe task. Similarly, recall of negative words is associated with more reactivity in cortisol and mood ratings. These are promising, if limited, data, but they do indicate how cross-domain assessment can increase our understanding of factors and mechanisms involved in elevated risk for depression.

LOOKING FORWARD

There are now substantial literatures delineating psychological and biological aspects of depression in adults and children. In addition, there is a small but growing literature elucidating factors involved in increasing risk for depression. In this chapter, we have briefly reviewed these literatures, and have also presented preliminary results from a study designed to examine psychobiological aspects of risk for depression. Understanding the interrelationships among these various domains of functioning as they affect risk for depression is a critical direction for future research. Indeed, it is only through such an integration that we can generate cogent and promising new experimental questions and methodologies in this area. Findings from future work following these lines should contribute to the development of an integrative psychobiological theory of risk for depression, and should help us to gain a better understanding of factors involved in the onset and recurrence of this disorder. In the longer term, of course, such results will facilitate our understanding of the psychological and biological bases of depression, and will permit the development of early identification and prevention programs for this debilitating disorder.

REFERENCES

American Psychiatric Association. (2000). *Diagnostic and statistical manual of mental disorders* (4th ed., text rev.). Washington, DC: Author.

Ashman, S. B., Dawson, G., Panagiotides, H., Yamada, E., & Wilkinson, C. W. (2002). Stress hormone levels of children of depressed mothers. *Development and Psychopathology, 14*(2), 333–349.

Barlow, D. H. (1991). Disorders of emotions: Clarification, elaboration, and future directions. *Psychological Inquiry, 2,* 97–105.

Beardslee, W., Versage, E., & Gladstone, T. (1998). Children of affectively ill parents: A review of the past 10 years. *Journal of the American Academy of Child and Adolescent Psychiatry, 37*(11), 1134–1141.

Beck, A. T. (1967). *Depression: Clinical, experimental, and theoretical aspects.* New York: Harper & Row.

Bellew, M., & Hill, A. B. (1991). Schematic processing and the prediction of depression following childbirth. *Personality and Individual Differences, 12*(9), 943–949.

Birmaher, B., Ryan, N. D., Dahl, R., Rabinovich, H., Ambrosini, P., Williamson, D. E., et al. (1992). Dexamethasone suppression test in children with major depressive disorder. *Journal of the American Academy of Child and Adolescent Psychiatry, 31*(2), 291–297.

Bishop, S. J., Dalgleish, T., & Yule, W. (2004). Memory for emotional stories in high and low depressed children. *Memory, 12*(2), 214–230.

Boland, R. J., & Keller, M. B. (2002). Course and outcome of depression. In I. H. Gotlib & C. L. Hammen (Eds.), *Handbook of depression* (pp. 43–60). New York: Guilford Press.

Bower, G. H. (1981). Mood and memory. *American Psychologist, 36,* 129–148.

Breiter, H. C., Etcoff, N. L., Whalen, P. J., Kennedy, W. A., Rauch, S. L., Buckner, R. L., et al. (1996). Response and habituation of the human amygdala during visual processing of facial expression. *Neuron, 17,* 875–887.

Bremner, J. D., Narayan, M., Anderson, E. R., Staib, L. H., Miller, H. L., & Charney, D. S. (2000). Hippocampal volume reduction in major depression. *American Journal of Psychiatry, 157*(1), 115–118.

Coplan, J. D., Moreau, D., Chaput, F., Martinez, J. M., Hoven, C. W., Mandell, D. J., et al. (2002). Salivary cortisol concentrations before and after carbon-dioxide inhalations in children. *Biological Psychiatry, 51*(4), 326–333.

Cox, R. W. (1996). AFNI: Software for analysis and visualization of functional magnetic resonance neuroimages; *Computers and Biomedical Research, 29,* 162–173.

Cummings, E. M., & Davies, P. T. (1994). Maternal depression and child development. *Journal of Child Psychology and Psychiatry, 35*(1), 73–112.

Dahl, R. E., Ryan, N. D., Puig-Antich, J., Nguyen, N. A., al-Shabbout, M., Meyer, V. A., et al. (1991). 24-hour cortisol measures in adolescents with major depression: A controlled study. *Biological Psychiatry, 30*(1), 25–36.

Davidson, R. J., Pizzagalli, D., & Nitschke, J. B. (2002). The representation and regulation of emotion in depression: Perspectives from affective neuroscience. In I. H. Gotlib & C. L Hammen (Eds.), *Handbook of depression* (pp. 219–244). New York: Guilford Press.

De Bellis, M. D., Dahl, R. E., Perel, J. M., Birmaher, B., al-Shabbout, M., Williamson, D. E., et al. (1996). Nocturnal ACTH, cortisol, growth hormone, and prolactin secretion in prepubertal depression. *Journal of the American Academy of Child and Adolescent Psychiatry, 35*(9), 1130–1138.

Dias, R., Robbins, T. W., & Roberts, A. C. (1996). Dissociation in prefrontal cortex of affective and attentional shifts. *Nature, 380,* 69–72.

Dinan, T. (1996). Serotonin and the regulation of hypothalamic–pituitary–adrenal axis function. *Life Sciences, 58*(20), 1683–1694.

Drevets, W. C. (2000). Neuroimaging studies of mood disorders. *Biological Psychiatry, 48,* 813–829.

Drevets, W. C., Price, J. L., & Simpson, J. R. (1997). Subgenual prefrontal cortex abnormalities in mood disorders. *Nature, 386,* 824–827.

Elliott, R., Rubinsztein, J. S., Sahakian, B. J., & Dolan, R. J. (2000). Selective attention to emotional stimuli in a verbal go/no-go task: An fMRI study. *NeuroReport, 11*(8), 1739–1744.

Elliott, R., Rubinsztein, J. S., Sahakian, B. J., & Dolan, R. J. (2002). The neural basis of mood-congruent processing biases in depression. *Archives of General Psychiatry, 59*(7), 597–604.

Essex, M. J., Klein, M. H., Cho, E., & Kalin, N. H. (2002). Maternal stress beginning in infancy may sensitize children to later stress exposure: Effects on cortisol and behavior. *Biological Psychiatry, 52*(8), 776–784.

First, M. B., Spitzer, R. L., Gibbon, M., & Williams, J. B. (1996). *Structured Clinical Interview for DSM-IV.* Washington, DC: American Psychiatric Association.

Frodl, T., Meisenzahl, E. M., Zetzsche, T., Born, C., Jäger, M., Groll, C., et al. (2003). Larger amygdala volumes in first depressive episode as compared to recurrent major depression and healthy control subjects. *Biological Psychiatry, 53,* 338–344.

Galard, R., Catalan, R., Castellanos, J. M., & Gallart, J. M. (2002). Plasma corticotropin-releasing factor in depressed patients before and after the dexamethasone suppression test. *Biological Psychiatry, 51*(6), 463–468.

Geller, B., Zimerman, B., Williams, M., Bolhofner, K., Craney, J. L., DelBello, M. P., et al. (2001). Reliability of the Washington University in St. Louis Kiddie Schedule for Affective Disorders and Schizophrenia (WASH-U-KSADS) mania and rapid cycling sections. *Journal of the American Academy of Child and Adolescent Psychiatry, 40,* 450–455.

Gilboa, E., & Gotlib, I. H. (1997). Cognitive biases and affect persistence in previously dysphoric and neverdysphoric individuals. *Cognition and Emotion, 11,* 517–538.

Gilboa, E., Roberts, J. E., & Gotlib, I. H. (1997). The effects of induced and naturally occurring dysphoric mood on biases in selfevaluation and memory. *Cognition and Emotion, 11,* 65–82.

Glover, G. H., & Law, C. S. (2001). Spiral-in/out BOLD fMRI for increased SNR and reduced susceptibility artifacts. *Magnetic Resonance Medicine, 46,* 515–522.

Goodman, S. H., & Gotlib, I. H. (1999). Risk for psychopathology in the children of depressed mothers: A developmental model for understanding mechanisms of transmission. *Psychological Review, 106,* 458–490.

Goodyer, I., Herbert, J., Moor, S., & Altham, P. (1991). Cortisol hypersecretion in depressed school-age children and adolescents. *Psychiatry Research, 37,* 237–244.

Goodyer, I. M., Herbert, J., Tamplin, A., & Altham, P. M. E. (2000a). First-episode major depression in adolescents: Affective, cognitive and endocrine characteristics of risk status and predictors of onset. *British Journal of Psychiatry, 176*(2), 142–149.

Goodyer, I. M., Herbert, J., Tamplin, A., & Altham, P. M. E. (2000b). Recent life events, cortisol, dehydroepiandrosterone and the onset of major depression in high-risk adolescents. *British Journal of Psychiatry, 177,* 499–504.

Goodyer, I. M., Park, R. J., & Herbert, J. (2001). Psychosocial and endocrine features of chronic first-episode major depression in 8–16 year olds. *Biological Psychiatry, 50*(5), 351–357.

Goodyer, I. M., Park, R. J., Netherton, C. M., & Herbert, J. (2001). Possible role of cortisol and dehydroepiandrosterone in human development and psychopathology. *British Journal of Psychiatry, 179*(3), 243–249.

Gotlib, I. H., & Cane, D. B. (1987). Construct accessibility and clinical depression: A longitudinal investigation. *Journal of Abnormal Psychology, 96,* 199–204.

Gotlib, I. H., & Goodman, S. H. (1999). Children of parents with depression. In W. K. Silverman & T. H. Ollendick (Eds.), *Developmental issues in the clinical treatment of children* (pp. 415–432). Needham Heights, MA: Allyn & Bacon.

Gotlib, I. H., Kasch, K. L., Traill, S., Joormann, J., Arnow, B., & Johnson, S. L. (2004). Coherence and specificity of information-processing biases in depression and social phobia. *Journal of Abnormal Psychology, 113,* 386–398.

Gotlib, I. H., Krasnoperova, E., Neubauer, D. L., & Joormann, J. (2004). Attentional biases for negative interpersonal stimuli in clinical depression. *Journal of Abnormal Psychology, 113,* 127–135.

Gotlib, I. H., & MacLeod, C. (1997). Information processing in anxiety and depression: A cognitive developmental perspective. In J. Burack & J. Enns (Eds.), *Attention, development, and psychopathology* (pp. 350–378). New York: Guilford Press.

Gotlib, I. H., & McCabe, S. B. (1992). An information-processing approach to the study of cognitive functioning in depression. In E. F. Walker, B. A. Cornblatt, & R. H. Dworkin (Eds.), *Progress in experimental personality and psychopathology research* (Vol. 15, pp. 131–161). New York: Springer.

Gotlib, I. H., & McCann, C. D. (1984). Construct accessibility and depression: An examination of cognitive and affective factors. *Journal of Personality and Social Psychology, 47,* 427–439.

Gotlib, I. H., McLachlan, A. L., & Katz, A. N. (1988). Biases in visual attention in depressed and nondepressed individuals. *Cognition and Emotion, 2,* 185–200.

Gotlib, I. H., Traill, S. K., Montoya, R. L., Joormann, J., & Chang, K. (2005). Attention and memory biases in the offspring of parents with bipolar disorder: Indications from a pilot study. *Journal of Child Psychology and Psychiatry, 46,* 84–93.

Granger, D. A., Weisz, J. R., McCracken, J. T., Ikeda, S. C., & Douglas, P. (1996). Reciprocal influences among adrenocortical activation, psychosocial processes, and the behavioral adjustment of clinic-referred children. *Child Development, 67*(6), 3250–3262.

Gunnar, M. R., & Cheatham, C. L. (2003). Brain and behavior interfaces: Stress and the developing brain. *Infant Mental Health Journal, 24(3)*, 195–211.

Gunnar, M. R., Marvinney, D., Isensee, J., & Fisch, R. O. (1989). Coping with uncertainty: New models of the relations between hormonal, behavioral, and cognitive processes. In D. S. Palermo (Ed.), *Coping with uncertainty: Behavioral and developmental perspectives* (pp. 101–129). Hillsdale, NJ: Erlbaum.

Halligan, S. L., Herbert, J., Goodyer, I. M., & Murray, L. (2004). Exposure to postnatal depression predicts elevated cortisol in adolescent offspring. *Biological Psychiatry, 55*(4), 376–381.

Hammen, C. (1997). Children of depressed parents: The stress context. In S. A. Wolchik & I. N. Sandler (Eds.), *Handbook of children's coping: Linking theory and intervention* (pp. 131–157). New York: Plenum Press.

Hammen, C., & Zupan, B. A. (1984). Self-schemas, depression, and the processing of personal information in children. *Journal of Experimental Child Psychology, 37,* 598–608.

Hankin, B. L., Abramson, L. Y., Moffitt, T. E., Silva, P. A., McGee, R., & Angell, K. E. (1998). Development of depression from preadolescence to young adulthood: Emerging gender differences in a 10–year longitudinal study. *Journal of Abnormal Psychology, 107,* 128–140.

Harrington, R., Fudge, H., Rutter, M., Pickles, A., & Hill, J. (1990). Adult outcomes of childhood and adolescent depression: I. Psychiatric status. *Archives of General Psychiatry, 47,* 465–473.

Henriques, J. B., & Davidson, R. J. (2000). Decreased responsiveness to reward in depression. *Cognition and Emotion, 14,* 711–724.

Hirschfeld, R. M. A., & Goodwin, F. K. (1988). Mood disorders. In J. A. Talbott, R. E. Hales, & S. C. Yudofsky (Eds.), *Textbook of psychiatry* (pp. 403–441). Washington, DC: American Psychiatric Press.

Ingram, R. E., & Siegle, G. J. (2002). Contemporary methodological issues in the study of depression: Not your father's Oldsmobile. In I. H. Gotlib & C. L. Hammen (Eds.), *Handbook of depression* (pp. 86–114). New York: Guilford Press.

Jaenicke, C., Hammen, C., Zupan, B., Hiroto, D., Gordon, D., Adrian, C., et al. (1987). Cognitive vulnerability in children at risk for depression. *Journal of Abnormal Child Psychology, 15,* 559–572.

Joormann, J., & Siemer, M. (2004). Memory accessibility, mood regulation, and dysphoria: Difficulties in repairing sad mood with happy memories? *Journal of Abnormal Psychology, 113*(2), 179–188.

Kane, M. J., & Engle, R. W. (2002). The role of prefrontal cortex in working-memory capacity, executive attention, and general fluid intelligence: An individual-differences perspective. *Psychonomic Bulletin and Review, 9*(4), 637–671.

Kasch, K. L., Rottenberg, J., Arnow, B., & Gotlib, I. H. (2002). Behavioral activation and inhibition systems and the severity and course of depression. *Journal of Abnormal Psychology, 111,* 589–597.

Keller, M. B., Lavori, P. W., Mueller, T. I., Endicott, J., Coryell, W., Hirschfeld, R. M. A., et al. (1992). Time to recovery, chronicity, and levels of psychopathology in major depression: A 5year prospective followup of 431 subjects. *Archives of General Psychiatry, 49,* 809–816.

Keller, M. B., & Shapiro, R. W. (1981). Major depressive disorder: Initial results from a oneyear prospective naturalistic followup study. *Journal of Nervous and Mental Disease, 169,* 761–768.

Kendler, K. S., Kessler, R. C., Neale, M. C., Heath, A. C., & Eaves, L. J. (1993). The prediction of major depression in women: Toward an integrated etiologic model. *American Journal of Psychiatry, 150,* 1139–1148.

Kessler, R. C., Berglund, P., Demler, O., Jin, R., Koretz, D., Merikangas, K. R., et al. (2003). The epidemiology of major depressive disorder: Results from the National Comorbidity Survey Replication (NCS-R). *Journal of the American Medical Association, 289,* 3095–3105.

Kovacs, M., & Paulaukas, S. L. (1984). Developmental stage and the expression of depressive disorders in children: An empirical analysis. *New Directions for Child Development, 26,* 59–80.

Levesque, J., Joanette, Y., Mensour, B., Beaudoin, G., Leroux, J. M., Bourgouin, P., et al. (2003). Neural correlates of sad feelings in healthy girls. *Neuroscience, 121*(3), 545–551.

Lewinsohn, P. M., Rohde, P., Seeley, J. R., Klein, D. N., & Gotlib, I. H. (2000). Natural course of adolescent major depressive disorder in a community sample: Predictors of recurrence in young adults. *American Journal of Psychiatry, 157,* 1584–1591.

Lieb, R., Isensee, B., Hofler, M., Pfister, H., & Wittchen, H. U. (2002). Parental major depression and the risk of depression and other mental disorders in offspring: A prospective–longitudinal community study. *Archives of General Psychiatry, 59,* 365–374.

Luby, J. L., Heffelfinger, A., Mrakotsky, C., Brown, K., Hessler, M., & Spitznagel, E. (2003). Alteration in stress cortisol reactivity in depressed preschoolers relative to psychiatric and no-disorder comparison groups. *Archives of General Psychiatry, 60*(12), 1248–1255.

MacLeod, C., & Hagan, R. (1992). Individual differences in the selective processing of threatening information, and emotional responses to a stressful life event. *Behaviour Research and Therapy, 30*(2), 151–161.

MacMillan, S., Szeszko, P. R., Moore, G. J., Madden, R., Lorch, E., Ivey, J., et al. (2003). Increased amygdala: Hippocampal volume ratios associated with severity of anxiety in pediatric major depression. *Journal of Child and Adolescent Psychopharmacology, 13,* 65–73.

Maes, M., Calabrese, J. R., & Meltzer, H. Y. (1994). The relevance of the in- versus outpatient status for studies on HPA-axis in depression: Spontaneous hypercortisolism is a feature of major depressed inpatients and not of major depression per se. *Progress in Neuro-Psychopharmacology and Biological Psychiatry, 18*(3), 503–517.

Mathew, S. J., Coplan, J. D., Goetz, R. R., Feder, A., Greenwald, S., Dahl, R. E., et al. (2003). Differentiating depressed adolescent 24h cortisol secretion in light of their adult clinical outcome. *Neuropsychopharmacology, 28*(7), 1336–1343.

Mayberg, H. S. (2002). Mapping mood: An evolving emphasis on frontal–limbic interactions. In D. T. Stuss & R. T. Knight (Eds.), *Principles of frontal lobe function* (pp. 376–391). Oxford: Oxford University Press.

Mayberg, H. S., Liotti, M., Brannan, S. K., McGinnis, S., Mahurin, R. K., & Jerabek, P. A. (1999). Reciprocal limbic–cortical function and negative mood: Converging PET findings in depression and normal sadness. *American Journal of Psychiatry, 156*(5), 675–682.

McCabe, S. B., & Gotlib, I. H. (1993). Attentional processing in clinically depressed subjects: A longitudinal investigation. *Cognitive Therapy and Research, 17,* 359–377.

McCabe, S. B., & Gotlib, I. H. (1995). Selective attention and clinical depression: Performance on a deployment-of-attention task. *Journal of Abnormal Psychology, 104,* 359–377.

McCabe, S. B., Gotlib, I. H., & Martin, R. A. (2000). Cognitive vulnerability for depression: Deployment of attention as a function of history of depression and current mood state. *Cognitive Therapy and Research, 24,* 427–444.

Michael, R. P., & Gibbons, J. L. (1963). Interrelationships between the endocrine system and neuropsychiatry. *International Review of Neurobiology, 11,* 243–302.

Mitterschiffthaler, M. T., Kumari, V., Malhi, G. S., Brown, R. G., Giampietro, V. P., Brammer, M. J., et al. (2003). Neural response to pleasant stimuli in anhedonia: An fMRI study. *NeuroReport, 14,* 177–182.

Monroe, S. M., & Simons, A. D. (1991). Diathesis–stress theories in the context of life-stress research: Implications for depressive disorders. *Psychological Bulletin, 110,* 406–425

Mueller, T. I., Keller, M. B., Leon, A. C., Solomon, D. A., Shea, M. T., Coryell, W., & Endicott, J. (1996). Recovery after 5 years of unremitting major depressive disorder. *Archives of General Psychiatry, 53,* 794–799.

Mueller, T. I., & Leon, A. C. (1996). Recovery, chronicity, and levels of psychopathology in major depression. *Psychiatric Clinics of North America, 19*(1), 85–102.

Murphy, J. M., Monson, R. R., Olivier, D. C., Sobol, A. M., & Leighton, A. H. (1987). Affective disorders and mortality: A general population study. *Archives of General Psychiatry, 44,* 473–480.

Neshat-Doost, H. T., Taghavi, M. R., Moradi, A. R., Yule, W., & Dalgleish, T. (1998). Memory for emotional trait adjectives in clinically depressed youth. *Journal of Abnormal Psychology, 107,* 642–650.

Ochsner, K. N., Bunge, S. A., Gross, J. J., & Gabrieli, J. D. E. (2002). Rethinking feelings: An fMRI study of the cognitive regulation of emotion. *Journal of Cognitive Neuroscience, 14*(8), 1215–1229.

Pariante, C. M., & Miller, A. H. (2001). Glucocorticoid receptors in major depression: Relevance to pathophysiology and treatment. *Biological Psychiatry, 49,* 391–404.

Parker, K. J., Schatzberg, A. F., & Lyons, D. M. (2003). Neuroendocrine aspects of hypercortisolism in major depression. *Hormones and Behavior, 43*(1), 60–66.

Pine, D., Cohen, P., Gurley, D., Brook, J., & Ma, Y. (1998). The risk for early-adulthood anxiety and depressive disorders in adolescents with anxiety and depressive disorders. *Archives of General Psychiatry, 55*(1), 56–64.

Pochon, J. B., Levy, R., Poline, J. B., Crozier, S., Lehericy, S., Pillon, B., et al. (2001). The role of dorsolateral prefrontal cortex in the preparation of forthcoming actions: An fMRI study. *Cerebral Cortex, 11,* 260–266.

Posener, J. A., DeBattista, C., Williams, G. H., & Schatzberg, A. F. (2001). Cortisol feedback during the HPA quiescent period in patients with major depression. *American Journal of Psychiatry, 158,* 2083–2085.

Post, R. M. (1992). Transduction of psychosocial stress into the neurobiology of recurrent affective disorder. *American Journal of Psychiatry, 149,* 999–1010.

Rahman, A., Lovel, H., Bunn, J., Iqbal, Z., & Harrington, R. (2004). Mothers' mental health and infant growth: A case–control study from Rawalpindi, Pakistan. *Child: Care, Health and Development, 30*(1), 21–27.

Rao, U., Dahl, R. E., Ryan, N. D., Birmaher, B., Williamson, D. E., Giles, D. E., et al. (1996). The relationship between longitudinal clinical course and sleep and cortisol changes in adolescent depression. *Biological Psychiatry, 40*(6), 474–484.

Reus, V., Wolkowitz, O., & Frederick, S. (1997). Antiglucocorticoid treatments in psychiatry. *Psychoneuroendocrinology, 22*(Suppl. 1), S121–S124.

Rottenberg, J., Gross, J. J., Wilhelm, F. H., Najmi, S., & Gotlib, I. H. (2002). Crying threshold and intensity in major depressive disorder. *Journal of Abnormal Psychology, 111*, 302–312.

Rottenberg, J., Kasch, K. L., Gross, J. J., & Gotlib, I. H. (2002). Sadness and amusement reactivity differentially predict concurrent and prospective functioning in major depressive disorder. *Emotion, 2*, 135–146.

Rottenberg, J., Wilhelm, F. H., Gross, J. J., & Gotlib, I. H. (2002). Respiratory sinus arrhythmia as a predictor of outcome in major depressive disorder. *Journal of Affective Disorders, 71*, 265–272.

Rude, S. S., Wenzlaff, R. M., Gibbs, B., Vane, J., & Whitney, T. (2002). Negative processing biases predict subsequent depressive symptoms. *Cognition and Emotion, 16*(3), 423–440.

Saxena, S., Brody, A. L, Ho, M. L., Alborzian, S., Ho, M. K., Maidment, K. M., et al. (2001). Cerebral metabolism in major depression and obsessive–compulsive disorder occurring separately and concurrently. *Biological Psychiatry, 50*, 159–170.

Sheline, Y. I., Barch, D. M., Donnelly, J. M., Ollinger, J. M., Snyder, A. Z., & Mintun, M. A. (2001). Increased amygdala response to masked emotional faces in depressed subjects resolves with antidepressant treatment: An fMRI study. *Biological Psychiatry, 50*(9), 651–658.

Sheline, Y. I., Mittler, B. L., & Mintun, M. A. (2002). The hippocampus and depression. *European Psychiatry, 17*, 300–305.

Sheline, Y. I., Sanghavi, M., Mintun, M. A., & Gado, M. H. (1999). Depression duration but not age predicts hippocampal volume loss in medically healthy women with recurrent major depression. *Journal of Neuroscience, 19*(12), 5034–5043.

Siegle, G. J., Steinhauer, S. R., Thase, M. E., Stenger, V. A., & Carter, C. S. (2002). Can't shake that feeling: Event-related fMRI assessment of sustained amygdala activity in response to emotional information in depressed individuals. *Biological Psychiatry, 51*(9), 693–707.

Solomon, D., Keller M., Leon, A., Mueller, T., Lavori, P., Shea, M., et al. (2000). Multiple recurrences of major depressive disorder. *American Journal of Psychiatry, 157*(2), 229–233.

Stansbury, K., & Gunnar, M. R. (1994). Adrenocortical activity and emotion regulation. In N. A. Fox (Ed), The development of emotion regulation: Biological and behavioral considerations. *Monographs of the Society for Research in Child Development, 59*(2–3, Serial No. 240), 108–134, 250–283.

Stewart, W., Ricci, J., Chee, E., Hahn, S., & Morganstein, D. (2003). Cost of lost productive work time among U.S. workers with depression. *Journal of the American Medical Association, 289*, 3135–3144.

Targum, S. D. (1984). Persistent neuroendocrine dysregulation in major depressive disorder: A marker for early relapse. *Biological Psychiatry, 19*(3), 305–318.

Taylor, L., & Ingram, R. E. (1999). Cognitive reactivity and depressotypic information processing in children of depressed mothers. *Journal of Abnormal Psychology,* *108,* 202–208.

Teasdale, J. D. (1988). Cognitive vulnerability to persistent depression. *Cognition and Emotion, 2,* 247–274.

Tems, C. L., Stewart, S. M., Skinner, J. R., Hughes, C. W., & Emslie, G. (1993). Cognitive distortions in depressed children and adolescents: Are they state dependent or traitlike? *Journal of Clinical Child Psychology, 22,* 316–326.

Thomas, K. M., Drevets, W. C., Dahl, R. E., Ryan, N. D., Birmaher, B., Eccard, C. H., et al. (2001). Amygdala response to fearful faces in anxious and depressed children. *Archives of General Psychiatry, 58*(11), 1057–1063.

Thompson, R. A. (1994). Emotion regulation: A theme in search of definition. In N. A. Fox (Ed.), The development of emotion regulation: Biological and behavioral considerations. *Monographs of the Society for Research in Child Development, 59*(2–3, Serial No. 240), 25–52, 250–283.

Timbremont, B., & Braet, C. (2004). Cognitive vulnerability in remitted depressed children and adolescents. *Behaviour Research and Therapy, 42(4),* 423–437.

Wallace, J., Schneider, T., & McGuffin, P. (2002). Genetics of depression. In I. H. Gotlib & C. L. Hammen (Eds.), *Handbook of depression* (pp. 169–191). New York: Guilford Press.

Watamura, S. E., Donzella, B., Alwin, J., & Gunnar, M. R. (2003). Morning to afternoon increases in cortisol concentrations for infants and toddlers at child care: Age differences and behavioral correlates. *Child Development, 74,* 1006–1020.

Watson, D., & Clark, L. A. (1995). Depression and the melancholic temperament. *European Journal of Personality, 9,* 351–366.

Watson, D., Clark, L. A., & Carey, G. (1988). Positive and negative affectivity and their relation to anxiety and depressive disorders. *Journal of Abnormal Psychology, 97,* 346–353.

Whiffen, V. E., & Gotlib, I. H. (1989). Infants of postpartum depressed mothers: Temperament and cognitive status. *Journal of Abnormal Psychology, 98,* 274–279.

Whitman, P. B., & Leitenberg, H. (1990). Negatively biased recall in children with self-reported symptoms of depression. *Journal of Abnormal Child Psychology, 18,* 15–27.

Williamson, D., Birmaher, B., Axelson, D., Ryan, N., & Dahl, R. (2004). First episode of depression in children at low and high familial risk for depression. *Journal of the American Academy of Child Psychiatry, 43*(3), 291–297.

Yehuda, R., Boisoneau, D., Mason, J. W., & Giller, E. L. (1993). Glucocorticoid receptor number and cortisol excretion in mood, anxiety, and psychotic disorders. *Biological Psychiatry, 34*(1–2), 18–25.

Young, E. A., & Nolen-Hoeksema, S. (2001). Effects of ruminations on the saliva cortisol response to a social stressor. *Psychoneuroendocrinology, 26*(3), 319–329.

VI

Personality in Animals

18

Using Mouse Models to Unravel Aggressive Behavior

Silvana Chiavegatto

The prevalence of violence in our society has stimulated both social and biological scientists to search for the predictors and causes of this destructive human behavior. The striking individual aggression differences among humans, as well as among other mammals, may reflect physiological factors, experiential history, or the interaction of both. "Aggression" is defined here as any behavior directed at causing physical or mental injury, although the classification of an act as "aggressive" depends on subjective judgments of intention and causality. In both humans and animals, the term "aggression" comprises a variety of heterogeneous engaged behaviors. In nature, conflicts are most likely to occur over limited resources, such as territories, food, and mates; consequently, the social interaction resolves which subject gains access to the disputed resource. In many cases, a submissive attitude on the part of one animal forestalls the need for any actual contest over a resource. Animals may also participate in psychological intimidation by engaging in threat displays or ritualized combat, in which dominance is determined, but no physical damage is inflicted. Accordingly, aggression and submission may represent the endpoints of a single behavioral continuum, or, alternatively, two independent but interacting dimensions of the behaving individual. Mouse models have played an important role in the elucidation of biological and molecular pathways underlying human disease. This approach is progressively becoming an accepted way to study the genetic foundation of psychiatric disorders. The present chapter focuses on the contributions of mouse models to the biological and molecular understanding of aggression.

AGGRESSIVE BEHAVIOR IN MICE:
IS IT A GOOD MODEL?

Because aggression is a primitive yet highly conserved vertebrate behavior, it is reasonable to expect that the molecular mechanisms underlying aggression are comparable among vertebrates. Species-specific features of aggression are probably the results of adjustment of novel molecules as modulators superimposed on the primary neural circuits. There are several advantages of using rodent models, such as the desirable ability to control the environment (raising, housing, testing), and the attractive possibility of manipulating the animal model in a hormonal, pharmacological, and genetic manner (Sluyter et al., 2003). Laboratory mice are the species most often used in aggression studies. The genetic concordance between humans and mice is over 90%, thus strengthening the likelihood that similar behavioral traits will share similar genetic candidates.

Researchers devoted to the ethological analysis of patterns of aggression in mice have tentatively classified these behaviors into several types (reviewed in Nelson & Chiavegatto, 2000, 2001), with the different types of aggression appearing to have different neuroendocrine bases (reviewed in Maxson, 1999). No simple extrapolation of animal aggression subtypes to aggression in humans is possible, mainly because of the impact of complex cultural variables on behavior. Therefore, research into subtypes of human aggression has been rather limited.

Laboratory mice are fairly docile, and their expression of aggressive behavior is usually induced by artificial or environmental situations. Predatory aggression is presumably motivated by hunger, and thus differs from other types of aggression motivated by social factors (e.g., isolation-induced aggression). Maternal aggression, which serves to protect the offspring from intruders, requires hormonal changes associated with the production of offspring to be expressed (Gammie & Nelson, 1999). Territorial and intermale aggressions are aimed to obtain access to resources through territoriality or dominance hierarchies, respectively. In general, there is a potentially close correspondence between the situations and/or stimuli that elicit hostility in mice and humans. Moreover, there is no evidence that emotions and motivations associated with aggression differ significantly between humans and other mammals, although the cognitive representations of these are undoubtedly more elaborate and differentiated in humans (Adams, 1980; Blanchard & Blanchard, 2003).

Importantly, studies using aggressive mice have revealed and confirmed underlying mechanisms from neuroendocrine and other physiological systems relevant to aspects of human violent behavior, such as the involvement of serotonin (5-HT). In this sense, the use of mice has demonstrated reliability and validity in modeling aggressive behavior, and it can be considered a valuable method or process to identify novel mechanisms related to aggression.

MEASURING AGGRESSION IN MICE

Rodents can exhibit a large pattern of responses when confronted with an unknown conspecific. The responses vary from investigative to aggressive behaviors, depending on various factors such as social status (dominant or not), type of rearing (isolated or group-housed), place of confrontation (new or familiar), experimental design (naive or experienced), and gender.

Mouse models of aggression in a laboratory rely on the offensive components of social interactions in mice. "Offensive" behavior, in this context, is characterized by initiation on the part of the aggressive animal that often leads to damage to the opponents (Krsiak, 1974). It follows a defined temporal course and occurs in episodic fashion, with epochs of intense aggressive behavior alternating with relative quiescence (Miczek, 1983). In male mice, isolation for several weeks induces an extensive repertoire of natural agonistic behaviors—namely, aggressive behavior and reactions to aggression (Miczek & Krsiak, 1979). A singly housed mouse is then allowed to interact with a nonaggressive group-housed male mouse in an unfamiliar or neutral arena (isolation-induced aggression paradigm) or in his own home cage (resident–intruder paradigm; see Figure 18.1). The basic sequence of acts and postures during offensive attack is simple and stereotyped. The isolated mouse approaches the opponent, assumes an offensive sideways posture and/or offensive upright posture, and finally engages in a bite-and-kick attack. The sideways intimidation is a lateral rotation of the body directed toward an opponent, accompanied by piloerection. The most evident element of aggressive behavior in mice is the attack bite, which is aimed preferentially at the back or flanks of the adversary, and is associated with kicking movements of the rear legs. During or immediately before this rapid sequence, the aggressive mouse displays several tail rattles (vigorous and quick shakings of the tail), which may reflect a state of high arousal (Miczek, Maxson, Fish, & Faccidomo, 2001). Following the burst of attack, there may be a refractory period of several minutes during which no further attack occurs; instead, several nonagonistic activities, such as grooming, rearing, walking, or anogenital sniffing, may take place. The entire sequence may last from several seconds to several minutes, depending upon the strength of offensive motivation in the attacking animal and the defensive/submissive tactics of the contestant. Each occurrence of these behavioral elements can be measured in terms of frequency, as well as the duration of specific behaviors in a fixed interval. The latency to the first attack bite and percentage of animals fighting are also determined. More detailed analysis can usually be obtained from video-recorded encounters, and produces information on the patterns of aggressive behavior, such as the sequential structure of the behavior and its burst-like character (Miczek et al., 1989).

Conspecific confrontations in the laboratory need to be very well done in order to obtain consistent results. The environmental situations regarding the encounter should be carefully controlled, because the experience of the aggres-

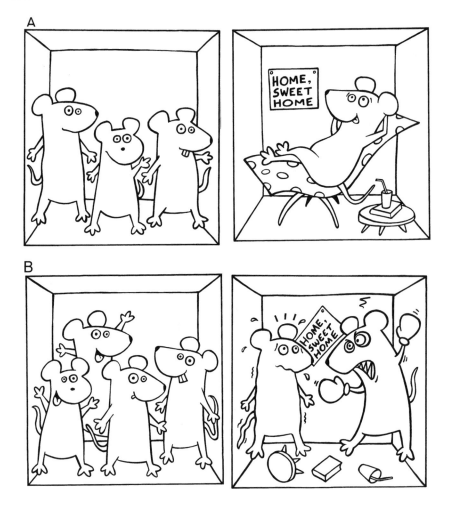

FIGURE 18.1. Resident–intruder model of aggression in male mice. (A) Left cage showing group-housed male adult mice (docile); in the right cage is an isolated male mouse (resident). (B) One group-housed mouse is introduced into the resident's cage. The isolated mouse displays aggressive behaviors against the intruder.

sive experimental mouse (naive to the paradigm or not), as well as variation in the behavior of the opponent (changes in social investigation or activity, previous experience with the paradigm, etc.), can mislead data analysis (Roubertoux, Le Roy, Mortaud, Perez-Diaz, & Tordjman, 1999). A previously defeated or naive opponent can elicit different reactions from the tested mouse. This potential problem can be reduced, however, when group-housed opponents are determined before the onset of the study to be nonaggressive, and an appropriate number of them are employed.

Although aggressive behavior in female mice can also occur toward other females in a territorial-like fashion, it is much more evident during the postpartum period (Gandelman, 1972). This so-called "maternal aggression" is highest during the first 2 weeks of lactation and is absent after the pups are weaned, suggesting an important control by suckling stimulation (Garland & Svare, 1988). Lactating mice, in contrast to the passivity exhibited by nonparturient animals, display immediate and intense aggressive behavior toward both male and female mouse intruders, and are believed to be motivated by protection of the litter (for a review, see Lonstein & Gammie, 2002). Maternal aggression in females is characterized by short-latency attacks of high intensity, mostly directed toward the head/neck region of the opponent and usually without the introductory threatening behaviors typically displayed by male animals confronted with an intruder. Because male and female mice express aggressive behavior in different patterns (continuously vs. temporarily, respectively), it seems that gender-specialized mechanisms were developed for the control of aggression (Gammie, Huang, & Nelson, 2000). The extent to which maternal aggression and male aggression in mice share a common neural basis remains to be investigated.

GENETIC AND MOLECULAR APPROACHES

Neurobehavioral studies have advanced substantially through the use of mouse genetics. Behavior genetic studies of aggressive behavior in mice have successfully demonstrated its inheritance. The first genetic studies on mouse aggression reported inbred strain differences in fighting, indicating an effect of genetic variants on individual differences in offensive behaviors (Ginsburg & Allee, 1942; Scott, 1942). Subsequent support of this view came from breeding studies that selected specific levels of fighting as behavioral phenotypes (Cairns, MacCombie, & Hood, 1983; Lagerspetz, Tirri, & Lagerspetz, 1968; Southwick & Clark, 1968). In the 1990s, with the significant technological advances in molecular biology, many genes were related to aggressive behavior (for reviews, see Maxson & Canastar, 2003; Nelson & Chiavegatto, 2001). The availability of genetic engineering techniques, and the consequent possibility of generating animal mutants carrying specific alterations in their genomes, represented a turning point in behavior genetics. By the use of these techniques, genes can be multiplied (in transgenic animals) or deleted (in gene knockout animals) at will, facilitating the understanding of the physiological significance of their protein products (Koller & Smithies, 1992).

There are two approaches to behavioral analysis using genetic techniques: the direct approach, in which behavioral differences are tracked down to the controlling genes; and the reverse approach, in which interesting genes are manipulated and their behavioral consequences are then studied. As any complex behavior does, aggression probably depends on many genetic points, perturbations in any of which may lead to dysfunctional outcomes. Using the reverse approach to behavioral analysis proved to be very important to the aggression studies, because it not only confirmed the pharmacologically derived knowledge in the underlying mechanisms, but also brought many new candidates into focus. Nevertheless, as with all behavioral techniques, there are some potential caveats (reviewed in Gerlai, 1996; Nelson, 1997; Nelson & Young, 1998). In the generation of null mice, there is a possibility that proteins exerting an important role in the control of particular behavior may also be indispensable for the correct development of specific brain circuits, and that their absence may promote fatal errors in neural tissue development. Alternatively, other genes or proteins may substitute for the function of the deleted gene product in a compensatory way, and thus may abolish the impact of gene ablation on the phenotype (false-negative result), or even lead to secondary phenotypical alterations that are not directly related to the function of the gene of interest (false-positive result). An additional confounding issue is the effect of background genes linked to the targeted locus. Ignoring the genetic background may lead to misinterpretation of results (see discussion by Gerlai, 1999). These shortcomings can be partially circumvented by the use of conditional mutants, in which the transgene is expressed only under specific circumstances (pharmacological treatment, cell-specific expression, etc.) or deleted only upon pharmacological intervention (e.g., LoxP) (Golic, 1994; Kilby, Snaith, & Murray, 1993).

In summary, because aggression is a complex and often variable trait, it is probably influenced by a large number of genes as well as by environmental factors. In order to understand this complex network of interactions, it is necessary to collect converging evidence by using a variety of techniques; these include ablation studies, as well as pharmacological, genetic, and molecular manipulations.

IMPLICATION OF 5-HT IN AGGRESSION

Typical and hyperaggressive individuals share some focal motives for aggression, implying deficiencies in mechanisms that act to control aggression. Accordingly, findings of unusual physiological parameters—such as reduced 5-HT metabolites in cerebrospinal fluid (Brown et al., 1982; Linnoila et al., 1983; Virkkunen, Goldman, Nielsen, & Linnoila, 1995), reduced prefrontal cortex size or activity (Raine et al., 1998), and a blunted response of prolactin to a 5-HT agonist (fenfluramine challenge) (Coccaro, 1992; Manuck et al., 1998)—have been found in impulsively violent humans. Reduced 5-HT levels or turnover in the brains of laboratory animals have also been extensively reported (see review by Lesch & Merschdorf, 2000). Several neurotransmitters have also been implicated in aggression, but the data on 5-HT are most compelling (Miczek, Fish, De Bold, & De Almeida, 2002). The 5-HT system generally depresses aggression in animals and violent behavior in humans. Drugs that inhibit 5-HT synthesis, such as parachlorophenylalanine (pCPA); a tryptophan-free diet; and lesions of 5-HT neurons all decrease 5-HT levels and elevate aggression in nonhuman animals (Chiavegatto et al., 2001; Gibbons, Barr, Bridger, & Leibowitz, 1978, 1979; Hole, Johnson, & Berge, 1977; Valzelli, Bernasconi, & Garattini, 1981). On the other hand, reduction in aggression has been obtained by treatment with 5-HT precursors, 5-HT reuptake inhibitors, and 5-HT releasing agents, in addition to 5-HT$_{1A}$ and 5-HT$_{1B}$ agonists (Chiavegatto et al., 2001; de Almeida, Nikulina, Faccidomo, Fish, & Miczek, 2001; Gibbons, Barr, Bridger, & Leibowitz, 1981; Gibbons et al., 1978; Miczek et al., 2001; Nelson & Chiavegatto, 2001; Olivier, Mos, van Oorschot, & Hen, 1995; Rolinski & Herbut, 1981).

Additional evidence for the participation of 5-HT in aggression comes from gene-targeting strategies. Mutant mice in which functional integrity of the 5-HT system was affected showed an altered aggressive phenotype (for reviews, see in Miczek et al., 2001; Nelson & Chiavegatto, 2001).

In this context, the 5-HT$_{1B}$ receptor knockout mice have attracted much attention. 5-HT$_{1B}$ receptors are expressed in a variety of brain regions, such as the raphe nuclei, periaqueductal grey, lateral septum, basal ganglia, and hippocampus; they either presynaptically inhibit 5-HT release or act as heteroreceptors modulating the release of other neurotransmitters. Both male and female 5-HT$_{1B}$$^{-/-}$ mice are more aggressive (Bouwknecht et al., 2001; Saudou et al., 1994)—a finding consistent with the antiaggressive effect of several 5-HT$_{1B}$ agonists, including eltoprazine (Olivier, Mos, & Rasmussen, 1990), CP-94,253 (Chiavegatto et al., 2001; Fish, Faccidomo, & Miczek, 1999), zolmitriptan (de Almeida et al., 2001), and anpirtoline (de Almeida & Miczek, 2002; Miczek et al., 2001; Rilke, Will, Jahkel, & Oehler, 2001) when administered in rodents.

Interestingly, the highly aggressive behavior of 5-HT$_{1B}$ null mice can be reduced by administration of the nonselective 5HT$_{1B}$ agonist eltoprazine (one of the so-called "serenics") in much the same way as in wild-type (WT) mice (Ramboz et al., 1996). Because eltoprazine additionally activates 5-HT$_{1A}$ receptors, these results suggest that the 1B subtype is not the only type of 5-HT receptors modulating aggression; the 1A receptors may also have a role.

Although agonists of 5-HT$_{1A}$ receptors also decrease aggression in rodents (Miczek, Hussain, & Faccidomo, 1998; Olivier et al., 1995), mice lacking 5-HT$_{1A}$ receptors are more anxious, less reactive, and possibly less aggressive (Zhuang et al., 1999). The absence of 5-HT$_{1A}$ receptors and the docile phenotype of these mice are in accordance with the increased postsynaptic 5-HT$_{1A}$ receptor availability in limbic and cortical regions reported in highly aggressive mice (Korte et al., 1996). However, the lack of both presynaptic autoreceptors and postsynaptic receptors in the 5-HT$_{1A}$$^{-/-}$ mice makes the interpretation of data complex and difficult. Recently, mice expressing 5-HT$_{1A}$ receptors exclusively in forebrain regions and in a time-controlled manner were developed (Gross et al., 2002). This study implicates the postsynaptic type of 5-HT_{1A} receptors in anxiety-like behaviors associated with their critical expression during the early postnatal period, but unfortunately the authors did not investigate aggression in these animals.

Whereas both 5HT_{1A} and 5-HT_{1B} receptors control 5-HT release, regional brain metabolic alterations in both 5HT_{1A} and 5-HT_{1B} receptor knockout mice do not show clear correlations with the changes in monoamine level/turnover in each distinct area (Ase, Reader, Hen, Riad, & Descarries, 2000). Taken together, these data suggest singular contributions of these two receptors at diverse postsynaptic sites promoting the known 5-HT inhibitory effects on aggression.

The participation of other 5-HT receptor subtypes in aggression is presently not clear. The lack of selective and specific agonists and antagonists makes the pharmacological data confusing. It is expected that in the near future, genetic manipulation of these receptors, coupled with behavior analysis, can provide new evidence regarding the contribution of each type of 5-HT receptor to aggressive behavior.

The 5-HT transporter (5-HTT) significantly modulates 5-HT levels by controlling its reuptake at the synapse. The absence of the 5-HTT gene in 5-$\text{HTT}^{-/-}$ mice leads to increased basal levels of extracellular 5-HT and several compensatory alterations in 5-HT homeostasis (see overview by Murphy et al., 2001). Consistent with reduced aggression after administration of 5-HTT inhibitors, male 5-$\text{HTT}^{-/-}$ mice are less aggressive than WT animals (Holmes, Murphy, & Crawley, 2002).

It is clear from the reported evidence that individual differences in aggressiveness are associated with perturbed homeostasis of the 5-HT system. The investigation of the molecular mechanisms underlying compromised 5-HT neurotransmission is an important subject for exploration in the research on aggressive behavior.

ADDITIONAL CANDIDATES EMERGING FROM GENETIC MANIPULATIONS

Studies that have applied selective targeting and mutation of specific genes have identified several new candidates putatively involved in aggression (Table 18.1). These genes have been implicated through either increases or decreases in aggression after behavioral phenotyping of mutant animals.

A behavioral role in aggression for the gaseous neurotransmitter nitric oxide (NO) was first reported in the mid-1990s (Nelson et al., 1995) and has recently been reviewed (Chiavegatto, Demas, & Nelson, 2005). The neuronal isoform of its synthetic enzyme (nNOS) was deleted by homologous recombination, and the aggressiveness of the males against their conspecifics became salient across a battery of behavioral phenotypes of these null mutants. Interestingly, as soon as these animals arrived at the lab, students and caretakers informally observed high levels of aggression among male cage-mates when

TABLE 18.1. Gene Candidates Putatively Involved in Male Aggression, According to Genetic and Molecular Research

Proteins, and genes involved in their expression	Type of mutation	Effects on aggressive behavior	References
Neurotransmitters, neuropeptides			
Acetylcholine (ACh)			
—	Genetically hypercholinergic rats[a]	Increase	Pucilowski et al. (1990)
Ache	AChE[-/-] mice	Decrease[b]	Duysen et al. (2002)
Adenosine			
Adora1	A$_1$[-/-] mice	Increase	Gimenez-Lort et al. (2002)
Adora2a	A$_{2A}$[-/-] mice	Increase	Ledent et al. (1997)
Arginine vasopressin (AVP)			
Avpr1b	V1bR[-/-] mice	Decrease	Wersinger et al. (2002)
Cannabinoid (CB)			
Cnr1	CB1[-/-] mice	Increase	Martin et al. (2002)
Dopamine			
Drd2	D$_{2L}$[-/-] mice	Decrease	Vukhac et al. (2001)
Slc6a3	DAT[-/-] mice	Increase[c]	Rodriguiz et al. (2004)
Gamma-aminobutyric acid (GABA)			
Gad2	GAD65[-/-] and GAD65[+/-] mice	Decrease	Stork, Ji, et al. (2000)
Histamine			
Hrh1	H$_1$[-/-] mice	Decrease	Yanai et al. (1998)
Melanocortin (α-MSH)			
Mc5r	MC5R[-/-] mice	Decrease	Morgan et al. (2004)
Nitric oxide (NO)			
Nos1	nNOS[-/-] mice	Increase	Nelson et al. (1995), Chiavegatto et al. (2001)
Nos2	Endothelial NOS[-/-] mice	Decrease	Demas et al. (1999)
Norepinephrine			
Adra2c	α$_{2C}$[-/-] mice	Increase	Sallinen et al. (1998)
	α$_{2C}$ overexpressed mice	Decrease	Sallinen et al. (1998)
Slc6a2	NET[-/-] mice	Increase[d]	Haller et al. (2002)
Opioid peptides			
Penk1	enk[-/-] mice	Increase	Konig et al. (1996)
Pnoc	N/OFQ[-/-] mice	Increase[e]	Ouagazzal et al. (2003)
Pomc1	C57BL/6-Pomc[tm1Low] mice	Increase[f]	Vaanholt et al. (2003)
Oxytocin (OT)			
Oxt	OT[-/-] mice	Decrease/ increase	De Vries et al. (1997), Winslow et al. (2000)
Serotonin (5-HT)			
Htr1b	5-HT$_{1B}$[-/-] mice	Increase	Saudou et al. (1994)
Htr1a	5-HT$_{1A}$[-/-] mice	Decrease	Zhuang et al. (1999)
Slc6a4	5-HTT[-/-] mice	Decrease	Holmes et al. (2002)
Substance P (SP)			
Tacr1	NK-1[-/-] mice	Decrease	De Felipe et al. (1998)

(continued)

TABLE 18.1. *(continued)*

Proteins, and genes involved in their expression	Type of mutation	Effects on aggressive behavior	References
Steroid hormones			
Ar	Androgen receptor null mice	Decrease	Sato et al. (2004)
Cyp19a1	Aromatase P450$^{-/-}$ mice	Decrease	Toda et al. (2001), Matsumoto et al. (2003a, 2003b)
Esr1	Estrogen receptor $\alpha^{-/-}$ mice	Decrease	Ogawa et al. (1997, 2000)
Esr2	Estrogen receptor $\beta^{-/-}$ mice	Increase	Ogawa et al. (1999), Nomura et al. (2002)
Esr1 + Esr2	Estrogen receptor $\alpha\beta^{-/-}$ mice	Decrease	Ogawa et al. (2000)
Pgr	Progression receptor$^{-/-}$ male mice	Decrease[g]	Schneider et al. (2003)
Metabolic enzymes			
Monoamine oxidase A (MAO-A)			
Maoa	MAO-A$^{-/-}$	Increase	Cases et al. (1995), Popova et al. (2001)
MAOA	MAO-A point mutation in humans	Increase	Brunner et al. (1993)
Catechol-O-methyltransferase (COMT)			
Comt	COMT $^{-/-}$ mice	No difference	Gogos et al. (1998)
	COMT $^{+/-}$ mice	Increase	Gogos et al. (1998)
Neutral endopeptidase (NEP)			
Mme	NEP$^{-/-}$ mice	Increase	Fischer et al. (2000)
Cytokines/growth factors (neurotrophins)			
Interleukin-6 (IL-6)			
Il6	IL-6$^{-/-}$ mice	Increase	Alleva et al. (1998)
	IL-6 overexpression in mice	Decrease	Alleva et al. (1998)
Transforming growth factor α (TGFα)			
Tgfa	TGFα overexpression in mice	Increase	Hilakivi-Clarke et al. (1992)
Brain-derived neurotrophic factor (BDNF)			
Bdnf	BDNF$^{+/-}$ mice	Increase	Lyons et al. (1999)
Signaling molecules			
α-Ca^{2+}-calmodulin-dependent kinase II (α-CaMKII)			
Camk2a	α-CaMKII$^{-/-}$ mice	Decrease	Chen et al. (1994)
	α-CaMKII$^{+/-}$ mice	Increase	Chen et al. (1994)
Neural cell adhesion molecule (NCAM)			
Ncam	NCAM$^{-/-}$ and NCAM$^{+/-}$ mice	Increase	Stork et al. (1997), Stork, Welzl, et al. (2000)
	NCAM180 expression in NCAM$^{-/-}$ mice	Normal	Stork, Welzl, et al. (2000)
Regulator of G protein signaling-2 (RGS2)			
Rgs2	Rgs2$^{-/-}$ mice	Decrease	Oliveira-Dos-Santos et al. (2000)

(continued)

TABLE 18.1. *(continued)*

Proteins, and genes involved in their expression	Type of mutation	Effects on aggressive behavior	References
Signaling molecules *(cont.)*			
Breakpoint cluster region (BCR)			
Bcr	Bcr⁻/⁻ mice	Increase	Voncken et al. (1998)
VGF polypeptide			
Vgf	VGF⁻/⁻ mice	Decrease	Hahm et al. (1999)
β2-microglobulin			
B2m	ß2m⁻/⁻ mice	Decrease	Loconto et al. (2003)
Fyn tyrosine kinase			
Fyn	Fyn⁻/⁻ mice	Decrease	Miyakawa et al. (2001)
Guanosine diphosphate (GDP) dissociation inhibitor 1			
Gdi1	Gdi1⁻/⁻ mice	Decrease	D'Adamo et al. (2002)
Cell adhesion molecule with homology to L1CAM			
Chl1	Chl1⁻/⁻ mice	Decrease	Frints et al. (2003)
Cation channel			
Trpc2	Trp2⁻/⁻ mice	Decrease	Leypold et al. (2002), Stowers et al. (2002)
Transcription factors			
Nr2e1	Tailless⁻/⁻ mice	Increase[b]	Monaghan et al. (1997)
Nr2e1	Frc mice (spontaneous mutation)	Increase[b]	Young et al. (2002)
Fev	Pet-1⁻/⁻ mice	Increase	Hendricks et al. (2003)
Function unknown			
Gene trap ROSA b-geo 22			
Gtrgeo22	Rosa22⁻/⁻ mice	Decrease	Campbell et al. (2002)

[a]Selectively bred for their divergent physiological responses to cholinergic drug challenges.
[b]The mutants have several other impairments.
[c]In dyadic testing condition.
[d]As intruder in the first encounter.
[e]Only when group-housed.
[f]ß-Endorphin-deficient mice counterattack as intruder.
[g]Only toward infants.

these males were moved from individual shipping containers to group-housing conditions. When aggression was systematically analyzed, male nNOS⁻/⁻ residents engaged in three to four times more aggressive encounters than WT mice in the resident–intruder test of aggression. Confrontations staged in novel environments (in dyadic or group encounters) showed that approximately 90% of the aggressive attacks were initiated by the mutants (Nelson et al., 1995).

Subsequently, another piece of evidence strengthened the involvement of nNOS-derived NO in aggression. WT male mice treated with 7-nitroindazole, a relatively specific drug that blocks nNOS activity *in vivo*, showed substantially increased aggressive behavior associated with a marked reduction of NOS activity in brain homogenates (Demas et al., 1997). These pharmacological data confirm the behavioral results obtained in nNOS$^{-/-}$ mice, ruling out a possible contribution of compensatory mechanisms or strain differences to the aggressive behavioral phenotype of nNOS null mice.

Several additional investigations were conducted in these mutant animals, in order to understand the mechanisms underlying NO in male mice aggression. There were no evident sensorimotor deficits or differences in blood testosterone concentrations between genotypes, either before or after agonistic encounters. Data on castrated nNOS$^{-/-}$ males suggest that although testosterone is required, it is not sufficient to elevate aggression in the knockouts (Kriegsfeld, Dawson, Dawson, Nelson, & Snyder, 1997). Monoamines and their metabolites were quantified by high-performance liquid chromatography in different brain areas of male mice from both genotypes. Although dopamine and norepinephrine concentrations were unchanged, the 5-HT metabolism (5-hydroxyindoleacetic acid [5-HIAA]/5-HT) was significantly reduced in several brain regions, including the cortex, hypothalamus, midbrain, and cerebellum, of male nNOS$^{-/-}$ mice in comparison to the WT mice (Chiavegatto et al., 2001). Unexpectedly, the alterations in 5-HT turnover were due to increased concentration of 5-HT, with no changes in 5-HIAA in most brain regions studied. This disturbed 5-HT neurochemical profile was not accompanied by alterations in the density or distribution of 5-HT axon terminals detectable by 5-HT immunocytochemistry in either sagittal or coronal male nNOS$^{-/-}$ mouse brain slices (Chiavegatto et al., 2001).

The elevated aggressive phenotype in the nNOS male knockout mice could be ameliorated by pharmacological increase of 5-HT metabolism, using its precursor 5-hydroxytryptophan. Conversely, the same increased level of aggressive behavior was induced in WT mice after a regimen of pCPA injections (a 5-HT synthesis inhibitor) that dramatically reduced 5-HT turnover in the brains of WT mice (Chiavegatto et al., 2001). These data demonstrated that, among other downstream effects, the absence of nNOS disturbs 5-HT metabolism associated with increased male aggressive behavior.

Because alterations in 5-HT metabolism could reveal disturbed 5-HT receptor function or even induce regulation of 5-HT receptor levels, the auto- as well as heteroreceptors 5-HT$_{1A}$ and 5-HT$_{1B}$ were investigated in male nNOS$^{-/-}$ and WT mice. Although the 5-HT$_{1A}$ agonist 8-OH-DPAT and the 5-HT$_{1B}$ agonist CP-94,253 dose-dependently decreased aggression in both genotypes, significantly higher concentrations of both agonists were necessary to reduce aggressive behavior of the nNOS knockouts (Chiavegatto et al., 2001). Although the effects of pharmacological inhibition of nNOS on 5-HT neurotransmission remain to be determined, our results suggest hypofunction of the 5HT$_{1A}$ and 5-HT$_{1B}$ receptors in the brains of male nNOS$^{-/-}$ mice, thus revealing a requirement of the neuronal isoform of NOS for the integrity of the brain 5-HT system.

Another gene candidate, which at decreased levels is implicated in aggression, is the gene controlling the production of brain-derived neurotrophic factor (BDNF). The BDNF null mice show early postnatal lethality, but the heterozygous mice (with one functional BDNF gene) have forebrain BDNF messenger RNA and protein levels that are 50% of those of WT mice, and they have a typical life span. These animals develop enhanced intermale aggressiveness that can be ameliorated by the selective 5-HT reuptake inhibitor fluoxetine. In addition, young adult $BDNF^{+/-}$ mice show blunted c-fos induction by the specific 5-HT releaser–uptake inhibitor dexfenfluramine, as well as alterations in the expression of several 5-HT receptors in the cortex, hippocampus, and hypothalamus. Forebrain 5-HT levels and fiber density in $BDNF^{+/-}$ mice are typical at an early age but undergo premature age-associated decrements (Lyons et al., 1999). Indeed, the 5-HT_{1A} receptor function—specifically, the capacity of the 5-HT_{1A} receptor to activate G proteins—is attenuated in $BDNF^{+/-}$ mice (Hensler, Ladenheim, & Lyons, 2003).

The neural cell adhesion molecule (NCAM) was first found to be involved in aggressive behavior after genetic manipulations in which its gene was disrupted. Both the null mutant and the heterozygous male mice exhibited high anxiety and aggression. Plasma testosterone concentrations did not differ between genotypes, either before or after behavioral testing (Stork, Welzl, Cremer, & Schachner, 1997). The reduction of the atypical emotional phenotype was obtained with 5-HT_{1A} agonists, but lower doses were required to mutants in comparison to the WT mice (Stork et al., 1999). Such increased response to 5-HT_{1A} receptor stimulation suggests a functional change in the 5-HT system of $NCAM^{-/-}$ mice. The typical behavioral phenotype of these male mutants could be rescued by the transgene expression of one NCAM isoform, the NCAM 180. The regularization of aggressive behavior was accompanied by regularization of 5-HT_{1A} function (Stork, Welzl, et al., 2000).

These studies, together with the various candidates listed in Table 18.1, demonstrate the power of using genetically modified mice to probe the neurobiological mechanisms underlying aggression.

COMMON MECHANISM?

It has become evident from pharmacological, genetic, and molecular approaches that homeostasis of the 5-HT system has an impact on aggression. Most molecules/systems discussed so far that interfere with aggressive behavior also influence the signaling properties of 5-HT. It seems that changes in 5-HT concentration, turnover, or metabolism in particular brain areas, and/or modifications in the expression, activity, or function of 5-HT receptors affect aggression in converging ways. It is tempting to speculate that the integrity of the complex interacting pathways modulated by the 5-HT system is a common downstream influence on the expression of aggressive behavior.

LOOKING FORWARD

Aggressive behavior as a complex behavioral personality trait seems to be under the influence of many genes in an intricate network of processes that is gradually being untangled by new genetic and molecular techniques associated with mouse models. Thus genetically transmitted variation in this system might be expected to contribute to individual differences in heritable behavioral traits related to aggression. It is my belief that the use of mouse models for the study of mechanisms underlying individual variation in the susceptibility to display aggressive acts can make a contribution toward understanding of the human spectrum of aggression. In this sense, we can envisage in the near future the possibility of diagnosing, and of using pharmacological tools to treat, this behavioral disorder.

ACKNOWLEDGMENTS

I am grateful to Randy J. Nelson for introducing me to this field, and to FAPESP-Brazil (01/09079-1 and 01/01637-5) for financial support.

REFERENCES

Adams, D. B. (1980). Motivational systems of agonistic behavior in muroid rodents: A comparative review and neural model. *Aggressive Behavior, 6*, 295–346.

Alleva, E., Cirulli, F., Bianchi, M., Bondiolotti, G. P., Chiarotti, F., De Acetis, L., et al. (1998). Behavioural characterization of interleukin-6 overexpressing or deficient mice during agonistic encounters. *European Journal of Neuroscience, 10*(12), 3664–3672.

Ase, A. R., Reader, T. A., Hen, R., Riad, M., & Descarries, L. (2000). Altered serotonin and dopamine metabolism in the CNS of serotonin 5-HT(1A) or 5-HT(1B) receptor knockout mice. *Journal of Neurochemistry, 75*(6), 2415–2426.

Blanchard, D. C., & Blanchard, R. J. (2003). What can animal aggression research tell us about human aggression? *Hormones and Behavior, 44*(3), 171–177.

Bouwknecht, J. A., Hijzen, T. H., van der Gugten, J., Maes, R. A., Hen, R., & Olivier, B. (2001). Absence of 5-HT(1B) receptors is associated with impaired impulse control in male 5-HT(1B) knockout mice. *Biological Psychiatry, 49*(7), 557–568.

Brown, G. L., Ebert, M. H., Goyer, P. F., Jimerson, D. C., Klein, W. J., Bunney, W. E., et al. (1982). Aggression, suicide, and serotonin: Relationships to CSF amine metabolites. *American Journal of Psychiatry, 139*(6), 741–746.

Brunner, H. G., Nelen, M., Breakefield, X. O., Ropers, H. H., & van Oost, B. A. (1993). Abnormal behavior associated with a point mutation in the structural gene for monoamine oxidase A. *Science, 262*, 578–580.

Cairns, R. B., MacCombie, D. J., & Hood, K. E. (1983). A developmental–genetic analysis of aggressive behavior in mice: I. Behavioral outcomes. *Journal of Comparative Psychology, 97*(1), 69–89.

Campbell, P. K., Waymire, K. G., Heier, R. L., Sharer, C., Day, D. E., Reimann, H., et al. (2002). Mutation of a novel gene results in abnormal development of spermatid flagella, loss of intermale aggression and reduced body fat in mice. *Genetics, 162*(1), 307–320.

Cases, O., Seif, I., Grimsby, J., Gaspar, P., Chen, K., Pournin, S., et al. (1995). Aggressive behavior and altered amounts of brain serotonin and norepinephrine in mice lacking MAOA. *Science, 268,* 1763–1766.

Chen, C., Rainnie, D. G., Greene, R. W., & Tonegawa, S. (1994). Abnormal fear response and aggressive behavior in mutant mice deficient for alpha-calcium-calmodulin kinase II. *Science, 266,* 291–294.

Chiavegatto, S., Dawson, V. L., Mamounas, L. A., Koliatsos, V. E., Dawson, T. M., & Nelson, R. J. (2001). Brain serotonin dysfunction accounts for aggression in male mice lacking neuronal nitric oxide synthase. *Proceedings of the National Academy of Sciences USA, 98*(3), 1277–1281.

Chiavegatto, S., Demas, G. E., & Nelson, R. J. (2005). Nitric oxide and aggression. In R. J. Nelson (Ed.), *Biology of aggression.* New York: Oxford University.

Coccaro, E. F. (1992). Impulsive aggression and central serotonergic system function in humans: An example of a dimensional brain–behavior relationship. *International Clinical Psychopharmacology, 7*(1), 3–12.

D'Adamo, P., Welzl, H., Papadimitriou, S., Raffaele di Barletta, M., Tiveron, C., Tatangelo, L., et al. (2002). Deletion of the mental retardation gene Gdi1 impairs associative memory and alters social behavior in mice. *Human Molecular Genetics, 11,* 2567–2580.

de Almeida, R. M., & Miczek, K. A. (2002). Aggression escalated by social instigation or by discontinuation of reinforcement ("frustration") in mice: Inhibition by Anpirtoline, a 5-HT(1B) receptor agonist. *Neuropsychopharmacology, 27*(2), 171–181.

de Almeida, R. M., Nikulina, E. M., Faccidomo, S., Fish, E. W., & Miczek, K. A. (2001). Zolmitriptan—a 5-HT1B/D agonist, alcohol, and aggression in mice. *Psychopharmacology (Berlin), 157*(2), 131–141.

De Felipe, C., Herrero, J. F., O'Brien, J. A., Palmer, J. A., Doyle, C. A., Smith, A. J., et al. (1998). Altered nociception, analgesia and aggression in mice lacking the receptor for substance P. *Nature, 392,* 394–397.

Demas, G. E., Eliasson, M. J., Dawson, T. M., Dawson, V. L., Kriegsfeld, L. J., Nelson, R. J., & Snyder, S. H. et al. (1997). Inhibition of neuronal nitric oxide synthase increases aggressive behavior in mice. *Molecular Medicine, 3*(9), 610–616.

Demas, G. E., Kriegsfeld, L. J., Blackshaw, S., Huang, P., Gammie, S. C., Nelson, R. J., et al. (1999). Elimination of aggressive behavior in male mice lacking endothelial nitric oxide synthase. *Journal of Neuroscience, 19,* RC30.

DeVries, A. C., Young, W. S., III, & Nelson, R. J. (1997). Reduced aggressive behaviour in mice with targeted disruption of the oxytocin gene. *Journal of Neuroendocrinology, 9*(5), 363–368.

Duysen, E. G., Stribley, J. A., Fry, D. L., Hinrichs, S. H., & Lockridge, O. (2002). Rescue of the acetylcholinesterase knockout mouse by feeding a liquid diet: Phenotype of the adult acetylcholinesterase deficient mouse. *Brain Research: Developmental Brain Research, 137*(1), 43–54.

Fischer, H. S., Zernig, G., Schuligoi, R., Miczek, K. A., Hauser, K. F., Gerard, C., et al. (2000). Alterations within the endogenous opioid system in mice with targeted deletion of the neutral endopeptidase ('enkephalinase') gene. *Regulatory Peptides, 96*(1–2), 53–58.

Fish, E. W., Faccidomo, S., & Miczek, K. A. (1999). Aggression heightened by alcohol or social instigation in mice: Reduction by the 5-HT(1B) receptor agonist CP-94,253. *Psychopharmacology (Berlin), 146*(4), 391–399.

Frints, S. G., Marynen, P., Hartmann, D., Fryns, J. P., Steyaert, J., Schachner, M., et al. (2003). CALL interrupted in a patient with non-specific mental retardation: gene dosage-dependent alteration of murine brain development and behavior. *Human Molecular Genetics, 12*, 1463–1474.

Gammie, S. C., Huang, P. L., & Nelson, R. J. (2000). Maternal aggression in endothelial nitric oxide synthase-deficient mice. *Hormones and Behavior, 38*(1), 13–20.

Gammie, S. C., & Nelson, R. J. (1999). Maternal aggression is reduced in neuronal nitric oxide synthase-deficient mice. *Journal of Neuroscience, 19*, 8027–8035.

Gandelman, R. (1972). Mice: Postpartum aggression elicited by the presence of an intruder. *Hormones and Behavior, 3*(1), 23–28.

Garland, M., & Svare, B. (1988). Suckling stimulation modulates the maintenance of postpartum aggression in mice. *Physiology and Behavior, 44*(3), 301–305.

Gerlai, R. (1996). Gene-targeting studies of mammalian behavior: Is it the mutation or the background genotype? *Trends in Neurosciences, 19*(5), 177–181.

Gerlai, R. (1999). Targeting genes associated with mammalian behavior: Past mistakes and future solutions. In W. E. Crusio & R. Gerlai (Eds.), *Handbook of molecular-genetic techniques for brain and behavior research* (Vol. 13, pp. 364–375). Amsterdam: Elsevier.

Gibbons, J. L., Barr, G. A., Bridger, W. H., & Leibowitz, S. F. (1978). Effects of para-chlorophenylalanine and 5-hydroxytryptophan on mouse killing behavior in killer rats. *Pharmacology, Biochemistry and Behavior, 9*(1), 91–98.

Gibbons, J. L., Barr, G. A., Bridger, W. H., & Leibowitz, S. F. (1979). Manipulations of dietary tryptophan: Effects on mouse killing and brain serotonin in the rat. *Brain Research, 169*(1), 139–153.

Gibbons, J. L., Barr, G. A., Bridger, W. H., & Leibowitz, S. F. (1981). L-Tryptophan's effects on mouse killing, feeding, drinking, locomotion, and brain serotonin. *Pharmacology, Biochemistry and Behavior, 15*(2), 201–206.

Gimenez-Llort, L., Fernandez-Teruel, A., Escorihuela, R. M., Fredholm, B. B., Tobena, A., Pekny, M., et al. (2002). Mice lacking the adenosine A1 receptor are anxious and aggressive, but are normal learners with reduced muscle strength and survival rate. *European Journal of Neuroscience, 16*(3), 547–550.

Ginsburg, B., & Allee, W. C. (1942). Some effects of conditioning on social dominance and subordination in inbred strains of mice. *Physiological Zoology, 15*, 485–506.

Gogos, J. A., Morgan, M., Luine, V., Santha, M., Ogawa, S., Pfaff, D., et al. (1998). Catechol-O-methyltransferase-deficient mice exhibit sexually dimorphic changes in catecholamine levels and behavior. *Proceedings of the National Academy of Sciences USA, 95*(17), 9991–9996.

Golic, K. G. (1994). Local transposition of P elements in *Drosophila melanogaster* and recombination between duplicated elements using a site-specific recombinase. *Genetics, 137*(2), 551–563.

Gross, C., Zhuang, X., Stark, K., Ramboz, S., Oosting, R., Kirby, L., et al. (2002).

Serotonin1A receptor acts during development to establish normal anxiety-like behaviour in the adult. *Nature, 416,* 396–400.

Hahm, S., Mizuno, T. M., Wu, T. J., Wisor, J. P., Priest, C. A., Kozak, C. A., et al. (1999). Targeted deletion of the Vgf gene indicates that the encoded secretory peptide precursor plays a novel role in the regulation of energy balance. *Neuron, 23*(3), 537–548.

Haller, J., Bakos, N., Rodriguiz, R. M., Caron, M. G., Wetsel, W. C., & Liposits, Z. (2002). Behavioral responses to social stress in noradrenaline transporter knockout mice: Effects on social behavior and depression. *Brain Research Bulletin, 58*(3), 279–284.

Hendricks, T. J., Fyodorov, D. V., Wegman, L. J., Lelutiu, N. B., Pehek, E. A., Yamamoto, B., et al. (2003). Pet-1 ETS gene plays a critical role in 5-HT neuron development and is required for normal anxiety-like and aggressive behavior. *Neuron, 37*(2), 233–247.

Hensler, J. G., Ladenheim, E. E., & Lyons, W. E. (2003). Ethanol consumption and serotonin-1A (5–HT1A) receptor function in heterozygous BDNF (+/-) mice. *Journal of Neurochemistry, 85*(5), 1139–1147.

Hilakivi-Clarke, L. A., Arora, P. K., Sabol, M. B., Clarke, R., Dickson, R. B., & Lippman, M. E. (1992). Alterations in behavior, steroid hormones and natural killer cell activity in male transgenic TGF alpha mice. *Brain Research, 588*(1), 97–103.

Hole, K., Johnson, G. E., & Berge, O. G. (1977). 5,7–Dihydroxytryptamine lesions of the ascending 5-hydroxytryptamine pathways: habituation, motor activity and agonistic behavior. *Pharmacology, Biochemistry and Behavior, 7*(3), 205–210.

Holmes, A., Murphy, D. L., & Crawley, J. N. (2002). Reduced aggression in mice lacking the serotonin transporter. *Psychopharmacology (Berlin), 161*(2), 160–167.

Kilby, N. J., Snaith, M. R., & Murray, J. A. (1993). Site-specific recombinases: Tools for genome engineering. *Trends in Genetics, 9*(12), 413–421.

Koller, B. H., & Smithies, O. (1992). Altering genes in animals by gene targeting. *Annual Review of Immunology, 10,* 705–730.

Konig, M., Zimmer, A. M., Steiner, H., Holmes, P. V., Crawley, J. N., Brownstein, M. J., et al. (1996). Pain responses, anxiety and aggression in mice deficient in pre-proenkephalin. *Nature, 383,* 535–538.

Korte, S. M., Meijer, O. C., de Kloet, E. R., Buwalda, B., Keijser, J., Sluyter, F., et al. (1996). Enhanced 5-HT1A receptor expression in forebrain regions of aggressive house mice. *Brain Research, 736*(1–2), 338–343.

Kriegsfeld, L. J., Dawson, T. M., Dawson, V. L., Nelson, R. J., & Snyder, S. H. (1997). Aggressive behavior in male mice lacking the gene for neuronal nitric oxide synthase requires testosterone. *Brain Research, 769*(1), 66–70.

Krsiak, M. (1974). Behavioral changes and aggressivity evoked by drugs in mice. *Research Communications in Chemical Pathology and Pharmacology, 7*(2), 237–257.

Lagerspetz, K. Y., Tirri, R., & Lagerspetz, K. M. (1968). Neurochemical and endocrinological studies of mice selectively bred for aggressiveness. *Scandinavian Journal of Psychology, 9*(3), 157–160.

Ledent, C., Vaugeois, J. M., Schiffmann, S. N., Pedrazzini, T., El Yacoubi, M.,

Vanderhaeghen, J. J., et al. (1997). Aggressiveness, hypoalgesia and high blood pressure in mice lacking the adenosine A2a receptor. *Nature, 388,* 674–678.

Lesch, K. P., & Merschdorf, U. (2000). Impulsivity, aggression, and serotonin: A molecular psychobiological perspective. *Behavioral Sciences and the Law, 18*(5), 581–604.

Leypold, B. G., Yu, C. R., Leinders-Zufall, T., Kim, M. M., Zufall, F., & Axel, R. (2002). Altered sexual and social behaviors in trp2 mutant mice. *Proceedings of the National Academy of Sciences USA, 99*(9), 6376–6381.

Linnoila, M., Virkkunen, M., Scheinin, M., Nuutila, A., Rimon, R., & Goodwin, F. K. (1983). Low cerebrospinal fluid 5-hydroxyindoleacetic acid concentration differentiates impulsive from nonimpulsive violent behavior. *Life Sciences, 33*(26), 2609–2614.

Loconto, J., Papes, F., Chang, E., Stowers, L., Jones, E. P., Takada, T., et al. (2003). Functional expression of murine V2R pheromone receptors involves selective association with the M10 and M1 families of MHC class Ib molecules. *Cell, 112*(5), 607–618.

Lonstein, J. S., & Gammie, S. C. (2002). Sensory, hormonal, and neural control of maternal aggression in laboratory rodents. *Neuroscience and Biobehavioral Reviews, 26*(8), 869–888.

Lyons, W. E., Mamounas, L. A., Ricaurte, G. A., Coppola, V., Reid, S. W., Bora, S. H., et al. (1999). Brain-derived neurotrophic factor-deficient mice develop aggressiveness and hyperphagia in conjunction with brain serotonergic abnormalities. *Proceedings of the National Academy of Sciences USA, 96,* 15239–15244.

Manuck, S. B., Flory, J. D., McCaffery, J. M., Matthews, K. A., Mann, J. J., & Muldoon, M. F. (1998). Aggression, impulsivity, and central nervous system serotonergic responsivity in a nonpatient sample. *Neuropsychopharmacology, 19*(4), 287–299.

Martin, M., Ledent, C., Parmentier, M., Maldonado, R., & Valverde, O. (2002). Involvement of CB1 cannabinoid receptors in emotional behaviour. *Psychopharmacology (Berlin), 159*(4), 379–387.

Matsumoto, T., Honda, S., & Harada, N. (2003a). Alteration in sex-specific behaviors in male mice lacking the aromatase gene. *Neuroendocrinology, 77*(6), 416–24.

Matsumoto, T., Honda, S., & Harada, N. (2003b). Neurological effects of aromatase deficiency in the mouse. *Journal of Steroid Biochemistry and Molecular Biology, 86*(3–5), 357–365.

Maxson, S. C. (1999). Genetic influences on aggressive behaviors. In D. W. Pfaff, W. Berrettini, T. H. Joh, & S. C. Maxson (Eds.), *Genetic influences on neural and behavioral functions* (pp. 405–416). Boca Raton, FL: CRC Press.

Maxson, S. C., & Canastar, A. (2003). Conceptual and methodological issues in the genetics of mouse agonistic behavior. *Hormones and Behavior, 44*(3), 258–262.

Miczek, K. A. (1983). Ethological analysis of drug action on aggression and defense. *Progress in Neuropsychopharmacology and Biological Psychiatry, 7*(4–6), 519–524.

Miczek, K. A., Fish, E. W., De Bold, J. F., & De Almeida, R. M. (2002). Social and neural determinants of aggressive behavior: Pharmacotherapeutic targets at serotonin, dopamine and gamma-aminobutyric acid systems. *Psychopharmacology (Berlin), 163*(3–4), 434–458.

Miczek, K. A., Haney, M., Tidey, J., Vatne, T., Weerts, E., & DeBold, J. F. (1989). Temporal and sequential patterns of agonistic behavior: Effects of alcohol, anxiolytics and psychomotor stimulants. *Psychopharmacology (Berlin)*, 97(2), 149–151.

Miczek, K. A., Hussain, S., & Faccidomo, S. (1998). Alcohol-heightened aggression in mice: Attenuation by 5-HT1A receptor agonists. *Psychopharmacology (Berlin)*, 139(1–2), 160–168.

Miczek, K. A., & Krsiak, M. (1979). Drug effects on agonistic behavior. In T. Thompson & P. B. Dews (Eds.), *Advances in behavioral pharmacology* (Vol. 2, pp. 87–162). New York: Academic Press.

Miczek, K. A., Maxson, S. C., Fish, E. W., & Faccidomo, S. (2001). Aggressive behavioral phenotypes in mice. *Behavioural Brain Research*, 125(1–2), 167–181.

Miyakawa, T., Yagi, T., Takao, K., & Niki, H. (2001). Differential effect of Fyn tyrosine kinase deletion on offensive and defensive aggression. *Behavioural Brain Research*, 122(1), 51–56.

Monaghan, A. P., Bock, D., Gass, P., Schwager, A., Wolfer, D. P., Lipp, H. P., et al. (1997). Defective limbic system in mice lacking the tailless gene. *Nature*, 390, 515–517.

Morgan, C., Thomas, R. E., & Cone, R. D. (2004). Melanocortin-5 receptor deficiency promotes defensive behavior in male mice. *Hormones and Behavior*, 45(1), 58–63.

Murphy, D. L., Li, Q., Engel, S., Wichems, C., Andrews, A., Lesch, K. P., et al. (2001). Genetic perspectives on the serotonin transporter. *Brain Research Bulletin*, 56(5), 487–494.

Nelson, R. J. (1997). The use of genetic "knockout" mice in behavioral endocrinology research. *Hormones and Behavior*, 31(3), 188–196.

Nelson, R. J., & Chiavegatto, S. (2000). Aggression in knockout mice. *ILAR Journal*, 41(3), 153–162.

Nelson, R. J., & Chiavegatto, S. (2001). Molecular basis of aggression. *Trends in Neurosciences*, 24(12), 713–719.

Nelson, R. J., Demas, G. E., Huang, P. L., Fishman, M. C., Dawson, V. L., Dawson, T. M., et al. (1995). Behavioural abnormalities in male mice lacking neuronal nitric oxide synthase. *Nature*, 378, 383–386.

Nelson, R. J., & Young, K. A. (1998). Behavior in mice with targeted disruption of single genes. *Neuroscience and Biobehavioral Reviews*, 22(3), 453–462.

Nomura, M., Durbak, L., Chan, J., Smithies, O., Gustafsson, J. A., Korach, K. S., et al. (2002). Genotype/age interactions on aggressive behavior in gonadally intact estrogen receptor beta knockout (betaERKO) male mice. *Hormones and Behavior*, 41(3), 288–296.

Ogawa, S., Chan, J., Chester, A. E., Gustafsson, J. A., Korach, K. S., & Pfaff, D. W. (1999). Survival of reproductive behaviors in estrogen receptor beta gene-deficient (betaERKO) male and female mice. *Proceedings of the National Academy of Sciences USA*, 96(22), 12887–12892.

Ogawa, S., Chester, A. E., Hewitt, S. C., Walker, V. R., Gustafsson, J. A., Smithies, O., et al. (2000). Abolition of male sexual behaviors in mice lacking estrogen receptors alpha and beta (alpha beta ERKO). *Proceedings of the National Academy of Sciences USA*, 97, 14737–14741.

Ogawa, S., Lubahn, D. B., Korach, K. S., & Pfaff, D. W. (1997). Behavioral effects of estrogen receptor gene disruption in male mice. *Proceedings of the National Academy of Sciences USA*, 94(4), 1476–1481.

Oliveira-Dos-Santos, A. J., Matsumoto, G., Snow, B. E., Bai, D., Houston, F. P.,

Whishaw, I. Q., et al. (2000). Regulation of T cell activation, anxiety, and male aggression by RGS2. *Proceedings of the National Academy of Sciences USA, 97,* 12272–12277.

Olivier, B., Mos, J., & Rasmussen, D. (1990). Behavioural pharmacology of the serenic, eltoprazine. *Drug Metabolism and Drug Interactions, 8*(1–2), 31–83.

Olivier, B., Mos, J., van Oorschot, R., & Hen, R. (1995). Serotonin receptors and animal models of aggressive behavior. *Pharmacopsychiatry, 28*(Suppl. 2), 80–90.

Ouagazzal, A. M., Moreau, J. L., Pauly-Evers, M., & Jenck, F. (2003). Impact of environmental housing conditions on the emotional responses of mice deficient for nociceptin/orphanin FQ peptide precursor gene. *Behavioural Brain Research, 144*(1–2), 111–117.

Popova, N. K., Skrinskaya, Y. A., Amstislavskaya, T. G., Vishnivetskaya, G. B., Seif, I., & de Meier, E. (2001). Behavioral characteristics of mice with genetic knockout of monoamine oxidase type A. *Neuroscience and Behavioral Physiology, 31*(6), 597–602.

Pucilowski, O., Eichelman, B., Overstreet, D. H., Rezvani, A. H., & Janowsky, D. S. (1990). Enhanced affective aggression in genetically bred hypercholinergic rats. *Neuropsychobiology, 24*(1), 37–41.

Raine, A., Meloy, J. R., Bihrle, S., Stoddard, J., LaCasse, L., & Buchsbaum, M. S. (1998). Reduced prefrontal and increased subcortical brain functioning assessed using positron emission tomography in predatory and affective murderers. *Behavioral Sciences and the Law, 16*(3), 319–332.

Ramboz, S., Saudou, F., Amara, D. A., Belzung, C., Segu, L., Misslin, R., et al. (1996). 5-HT1B receptor knock out—behavioral consequences. *Behavioural Brain Research, 73*(1–2), 305–312.

Rilke, O., Will, K., Jahkel, M., & Oehler, J. (2001). Behavioral and neurochemical effects of anpirtoline and citalopram in isolated and group housed mice. *Progress in Neuro-Psychopharmacology and Biological Psychiatry, 25*(5), 1125–1144.

Rodriguiz, R. M., Chu, R., Caron, M. G., & Wetsel, W. C. (2004). Aberrant responses in social interaction of dopamine transporter knockout mice. *Behavioural Brain Research, 148*(1–2), 185–198.

Rolinski, Z., & Herbut, M. (1981). The role of the serotonergic system in foot shock-induced behavior in mice. *Psychopharmacology (Berlin), 73*(3), 246–251.

Roubertoux, P. L., Le Roy, I., Mortaud, S., Perez-Diaz, F., & Tordjman, S. (1999). Measuring aggression in the mouse. In W. E. Crusio & R. T. Gerlai (Eds.), *Handbook of molecular-genetic techniques for brain and behavior research* (Vol. 13, pp. 696–709). Amsterdam: Elsevier.

Sallinen, J., Haapalinna, A., Viitamaa, T., Kobilka, B. K., & Scheinin, M. (1998). Adrenergic alpha2C-receptors modulate the acoustic startle reflex, prepulse inhibition, and aggression in mice. *Journal of Neuroscience, 18*(8), 3035–3042.

Sato, T., Matsumoto, T., Kawano, H., Watanabe, T., Uematsu, Y., Sekine, K., et al. (2004). Brain masculinization requires androgen receptor function. *Proceedings of the National Academy of Sciences USA, 101*(6), 1673–1678.

Saudou, F., Amara, D. A., Dierich, A., LeMeur, M., Ramboz, S., Segu, L., et al. (1994). Enhanced aggressive behavior in mice lacking 5-HT1B receptor. *Science, 265,* 1875–1878.

Schneider, J. S., Stone, M. K., Wynne-Edwards, K. E., Horton, T. H., Lydon, J., O'Malley, B., et al. (2003). Progesterone receptors mediate male aggression toward infants. *Proceedings of the National Academy of Sciences USA, 100*(5), 2951–2956.

Scott, J. P. (1942). Genetic difference in the social behavior of inbred strains of mice. *Journal of Heredity, 33*, 11–15.

Sluyter, F., Arseneault, L., Moffitt, T. E., Veenema, A. H., de Boer, S., & Koolhaas, J. M. (2003). Toward an animal model for antisocial behavior: Parallels between mice and humans. *Behavioral Genetics, 33*(5), 563–574.

Southwick, C. H., & Clark, L. H. (1968). Interstrain differences in aggressive behavior and exploratory activity of inbred mice. *Communications in Behavioral Biology, 1*, 49–59.

Stork, O., Ji, F. Y., Kaneko, K., Stork, S., Yoshinobu, Y., Moriya, T., et al. (2000). Postnatal development of a GABA deficit and disturbance of neural functions in mice lacking GAD65. *Brain Research, 865*(1), 45–58.

Stork, O., Welzl, H., Cremer, H., & Schachner, M. (1997). Increased intermale aggression and neuroendocrine response in mice deficient for the neural cell adhesion molecule (NCAM). *European Journal of Neuroscience, 9*(6), 1117–1125.

Stork, O., Welzl, H., Wolfer, D., Schuster, T., Mantei, N., Stork, S., et al. (2000). Recovery of emotional behaviour in neural cell adhesion molecule (NCAM) null mutant mice through transgenic expression of NCAM180. *European Journal of Neuroscience, 12*(9), 3291–3306.

Stork, O., Welzl, H., Wotjak, C. T., Hoyer, D., Delling, M., Cremer, H., et al. (1999). Anxiety and increased 5-HT1A receptor response in NCAM null mutant mice. *Journal of Neurobiology, 40*(3), 343–355.

Stowers, L., Holy, T. E., Meister, M., Dulac, C., & Koentges, G. (2002). Loss of sex discrimination and male–male aggression in mice deficient for TRP2. *Science, 295*, 1493–1500.

Toda, K., Saibara, T., Okada, T., Onishi, S., & Shizuta, Y. (2001). A loss of aggressive behaviour and its reinstatement by oestrogen in mice lacking the aromatase gene (Cyp19). *Journal of Endocrinology, 168*(2), 217–220.

Vaanholt, L. M., Turek, F. W., & Meerlo, P. (2003). Beta-endorphin modulates the acute response to a social conflict in male mice but does not play a role in stress-induced changes in sleep. *Brain Research, 978*(1–2), 169–176.

Valzelli, L., Bernasconi, S., & Garattini, S. (1981). p-Chlorophenylalanine-induced muricidal aggression in male and female laboratory rats. *Neuropsychobiology, 7*(6), 315–320.

Virkkunen, M., Goldman, D., Nielsen, D. A., & Linnoila, M. (1995). Low brain serotonin turnover rate (low CSF 5-HIAA) and impulsive violence. *Journal of Psychiatry and Neuroscience, 20*(4), 271–275.

Voncken, J. W., Baram, T. Z., Gonzales-Gomez, I. I., van Schaick, H., Shih, J. C., Chen, K., et al. (1998). Abnormal stress response and increased fighting behavior in mice lacking the bcr gene product. *International Journal of Molecular Medicine, 2*(5), 577–583.

Vukhac, K. L., Sankoorikal, E. B., & Wang, Y. (2001). Dopamine D2L receptor- and age-related reduction in offensive aggression. *NeuroReport, 12*(5), 1035–1038.

Wersinger, S. R., Ginns, E. I., O'Carroll, A. M., Lolait, S. J., & Young, W. S., III. (2002). Vasopressin V1b receptor knockout reduces aggressive behavior in male mice. *Molecular Psychiatry, 7*(9), 975–984.

Winslow, J. T., Hearn, E. F., Ferguson, J., Young, L. J., Matzuk, M. M., & Insel, T. R.

(2000). Infant vocalization, adult aggression, and fear behavior of an oxytocin null mutant mouse. *Hormones and Behavior, 37*(2), 145–155.

Yanai, K., Son, L. Z., Endou, M., Sakurai, E., Nakagawasai, O., Tadano, T., et al. (1998). Behavioural characterization and amounts of brain monoamines and their metabolites in mice lacking histamine H1 receptors. *Neuroscience, 87*(2), 479–487.

Young, K. A., Berry, M. L., Mahaffey, C. L., Saionz, J. R., Hawes, N. L., Chang, B., et al. (2002). Fierce: A new mouse deletion of Nr2e1; violent behaviour and ocular abnormalities are background-dependent. *Behavioural Brain Research, 132*(2), 145–158.

Zhuang, X., Gross, C., Santarelli, L., Compan, V., Trillat, A. C., & Hen, R. (1999). Altered emotional states in knockout mice lacking 5-HT1A or 5-HT1B receptors. *Neuropsychopharmacology, 21*(2, Suppl.), 52S–60S.

19

Searching for Genetic and Environmental Contributions to Personality and Happiness in Chimpanzees (*Pan troglodytes*)

Alexander Weiss and James E. King

CHIMPANZEE NATURAL HISTORY

Chimpanzees are our closest living nonhuman relatives—cousins with whom we shared a common African ancestor some 5–6 million years ago (Purvis, 1995; Sarich & Wilson, 1967; Wilson & Sarich, 1969). Consequently, approximately 98% of our genetic material is shared with chimpanzees. Chimpanzees display evidence of several behavioral abilities and characteristics, including language ability and a theory of mind, that were previously assumed to be unique to the human animal (de Waal, 1996; Hare, Call, & Tomasello, 2001; Rumbaugh & Savage-Rumbaugh, 1994; Whiten, 1997; Whiten et al., 1999).

Almost all wild nonhuman primates form year-round troops or populations, in which the same individuals come into mutual contact over extended time. However, chimpanzees (as well as a few monkey species) display a more sophisticated organization in the form of "fission–fusion" sociality, in which members of one population are constantly forming, splitting, and reforming new smaller subgroups (Chapmin, White, & Wrangham, 1993).

One dramatic feature of wild chimpanzee groups is the practice of lethal territorial defense (Pusey, 2001; Wrangham & Peterson, 1996); small groups of males patrol the boundaries of their group's territory, and savagely attack and often kill individual males from adjoining territories. Successful attacks may result in expanded territory size. Pusey (2001) showed that there is a positive relationship between female weight and territory size, thus suggesting that successful territorial defense contributes to evolutionary fitness.

Another important aspect of the social structure of chimpanzees and other primates is the existence of dominance hierarchies. The dominant male chimpanzees typically have first access to valued resources, such as food and females in estrus (de Waal, 2000). Dominant females also live a charmed life, with more and heavier infants (Pusey, Williams, & Goodall, 1999), and they often intervene positively in disputes (de Waal, 2000). In his descriptions of the life of chimpanzees in the chimpanzee colony at the Arnhem Zoo, de Waal (2000) emphasized several behavioral characteristics present in chimpanzees that ascended to the highest levels of the dominance hierarchy. Among others, they included the ability to form alliances, fearlessness, assertiveness, and aggressiveness. Dominance status of wild male chimpanzees is closely related to reciprocal activities with other males, including cooperation against a third individual and grooming (Arnold & Whiten, 2003; Watts, 2002). This is also likely to be the case in humans: Former Speaker of the House of Representatives Newt Gingrich, who read de Waal's *Chimpanzee Politics* (2000), noted that similar reciprocal behaviors helped him ascend to his position as Speaker (N. Gingrich, personal communication, June 28, 2004).

These characteristics that promote high dominance can be classified in terms of the five-factor model (FFM) of personality (McCrae & Costa, 2003)—namely, high extraversion (the ability to form alliances and assertiveness), low neuroticism (fearlessness), and low agreeableness (aggressiveness).

The belief that chimpanzees or other apes have personality traits like those in humans is not new. Darwin (1872/1998) was an early advocate of the view that other animals, especially apes, share basic behavioral and emotional tendencies with humans. Later, Wolfgang Köhler (1924/1925) and Robert Yerkes (1925, 1929, 1939, 1943) included frequent personality-descriptive adjectives in describing the individual chimpanzees whose behavior and learning were the subjects of these classic works. The adjectives applied to chimpanzees in these publications encompass all five factors of the FFM. However, the chimpanzee personality descriptions were probably intended to provide only some interesting background to the authors' main purpose—a description of behaviors and learning capabilities of apes. The view that animal personality and temperament is a peripheral issue, not a component part of the serious scientific questions addressed by animal behavior researchers, has persisted until the present time (Gosling, 2001).

One primary reason for this state of affairs was probably the reluctance of comparative psychologists and ethologists to engage in "anthropomorphism"—a force so strong that Jane Goodall was even frowned upon at first for giving chimpanzees names (Goodall, 1986). Fortunately, there is currently a revival of interest in animal personality research and, with this, an increased interest in the personality of chimpanzees and other great apes. Detailed descriptions of individual chimpanzees in their natural habitat, including personality-relevant attributes, were pioneered by Goodall (1968, 1986) and may have been partly responsible for this change.

ANIMAL PERSONALITY RESEARCH

An important development that probably led to an increased interest in animal personality research was the development of the FFM (McCrae & Costa, 2003). The FFM posits that five personality domains—"neuroticism," "extraversion," "openness to experience," "agreeableness," and "conscientiousness"—are biologically based emotional and behavioral dispositions. Evidence that these personality domains are heritable (Bouchard & Loehlin, 2001), show mostly stability in adulthood (McCrae & Costa, 2003), and are found across different cultures (McCrae, 2001) and species (Gosling, 2001; Gosling & John, 1999) supports this basic tenet of the FFM.

Modern research on ape personality can be traced back to Buirski and Plutchik (1991), who used a modified version of the Emotions Profile Index to rate chimpanzees at the Gombe Stream Reserve in Tanzania. One chimpanzee, Passion, had a profile indicating that she was unusually aggressive, distrustful, and depressed. In addition, she was far less timid, controlled, and gregarious than the other chimpanzees. Approximately a year after the ratings were made, she and her daughter, Pom, began to kidnap, murder, and eat the infants of other chimpanzees—a behavior that was never previously observed in any chimpanzees.

Gold and Maple (1994) later obtained adjectival ratings of gorillas in zoological parks. Factor analysis revealed analogues of neuroticism, extraversion, and agreeableness, as well as a distinct factor related to dominance. Their questionnaire did not include items that would have measured openness to experience or conscientiousness.

A later study (King & Figueredo, 1997) used a 43-item adjectival rating form that included items representing all five human factors. Interrater reliabilities of ratings were comparable to those in ratings of humans. In addition, upon factor-analyzing these adjectives, they found five factors that were analogous to those found in humans and a sixth, chimpanzee-specific factor that they designated as "dominance." Later research on chimpanzee personality indicated that this factor structure and both age and sex differences generalized from the zoo chimpanzees they were derived from to a sample of chimpanzees in an African sanctuary (King, Weiss, & Farmer, 2005).

The correlation between personality ratings and overt behavior is a fundamental part of the construct validity of personality constructs. Pederson, King, and Landau (in press) demonstrated a pattern of correlations between personality factors and behaviors in zoo-housed chimpanzees. For example, aggressive behaviors were positively correlated with Dominance and negatively associated with agreeableness and dependability—a result consistent with the defining items in each factor.

CHIMPANZEE HAPPINESS

Interestingly, the history of research on animal happiness or subjective well-being has paralleled the history of research on happiness in humans. In both the human and animal cases, the approach to the study of happiness ignored philosophical traditions (e.g., Schopenauer, 1859/1969).

However, until recently psychologists ignored the philosophical wisdom about human happiness, and instead defined happiness primarily by the absence of psychopathology (Seligman, 2002). Similarly, in nonhuman animals, subjective well-being is commonly inferred by the absence of aberrant behaviors such as motor stereotypies and self-injurious behavior (Baker & Aureli, 1997) or problems in breeding (Johnson, Petto, & Sehgal, 1991), or by the presence of species-specific behaviors (Rosenblum, 1991).

Recent researchers of human happiness argue that happiness or subjective well-being is more than the absence of psychopathology, and they focus more on the positive contributions to happiness (Seligman, 2002). This line of research has led to a number of surprising findings, including that one's level of happiness is heritable (Lykken & Tellegen, 1996); is mostly stable over the life span, and only temporarily affected by positive and negative life events (Eid & Diener, 2004); and is predicted largely by personality, especially extraversion and neuroticism (Diener, 1998).

A similar new positive approach to animal happiness is emerging. King and Landau (2003) created a rating scale for zoo-housed chimpanzees comparable to those used to assess human happiness (see Table 19.1). It included items designed to measure the balance of positive versus negative moods, ability to achieve goals, and the amount of pleasure derived from social interactions; it also included a global item asking the rater how happy he or she would be if the rater were the rated chimpanzee. Although on the surface these items may seem subjective, the interrater reliabilities were high (see Table 2 in King & Landau, 2003). In addition, ratings of chimpanzee subjective well-being were stable over time and were strongly correlated with personality dimensions—namely, dominance, extraversion, and dependability (King & Landau, 2003).

HERITABILITY OF CHIMPANZEE PERSONALITY

The heritability of personality and subjective well-being in zoo-housed chimpanzees is an important avenue for better understanding of the evolutionary as well as the proximal origins of these phenotypes. The availability of detailed pedigrees across zoos allows estimation of the proportion of phenotypic variance due to genetic and environmental effects. However, use of

TABLE 19.1 Items Used to Assess Chimpanzee Subjective Well-Being

Item	Construct assessed
"Estimate the amount of time each of the chimpanzees in your zoo is happy, contented, enjoying itself, or otherwise in a positive mood. Assume that at other times the chimpanzees are unhappy, bored, frightened, or otherwise in a negative mood."	Balance of positive and negative moods
"Estimate, for each chimpanzee in your zoo, the extent to which social interactions with other chimpanzees are satisfying, enjoyable experiences as opposed to being sources of fright, distress, frustration, or some other negative experience. It is not the number of social interactions that should be estimated, but the extent to which social interactions that do occur are a positive experience."	Pleasure derived from social interations
"Estimate, for each chimpanzee in your zoo, the extent to which it is effective or successful in achieving its goals or wishes. Examples of goals would be achieving desired social interactions, achieving a desired dominance status, and having access to desirable locations, devices, or materials in the enclosure."	Perceived personal control
"Imagine how happy you would be if you were that chimpanzee for a week. You would be exactly like that chimpanzee. You would behave the same way as that chimpanzee, would perceive the world the same way as that chimpanzee, and would feel things the same way as that chimpanzee."	Global satisfaction

detailed pedigrees also permits assessment of different types of shared environmental influences; this capability is lacking in traditional twin studies.

Among chimpanzees, most shared environmental effects are likely to come from differences in the maternal environment (see, e.g., Goodall, 1986). The maternal environment can influence the offspring in two possible ways. The first is through "heritable maternal effects"—often called "indirect genetic effects"—in which some heritable phenotype of the mother affects the maternal environment afforded her infant, which in turn directly affects the infant's phenotype (personality or happiness, in our case) (Willham, 1972). A hypothetical example of a heritable maternal effect would be if a heritable disposition toward aggression in a mother caused her to behave in a way that influenced her offspring's subjective well-being. Of course, these heritable rearing environments do not necessarily have to manifest themselves as behavioral traits of the mother; they may include physical characteristics such as the quality of her milk and a myriad of other possibilities. If heritable maternal effects are present, individuals raised by genetically related mothers will be more similar to each other than would be expected only from their genetic relatedness to each other.

The second potential maternal influence consists of "nonheritable maternal effects," in which some aspect of the maternal environment that is unrelated to a heritable characteristic of the mother may have an effect on the phenotype of her offspring. Unlike heritable maternal effects, individuals with related mothers should be no more similar to one another than would be predicted from how genetically related they are to one another. Thus nonheritable maternal effects are similar to the shared environmental effects described by behavior geneticists (Rowe, 1994).

One commonly overlooked advantage of using animals in zoos for genetic studies is that the zoo environment may permit a more thorough investigation into environmental sources of variance. One problem with trying to locate nonshared environmental influences in humans is that humans, and probably other animals in their natural environment, pick and create niches (Gosling, Ko, Mannarelli, & Morris, 2002; Scarr & McCartney, 1983) that are compatible with their personalities. Consequently, a high correlation will emerge between the individual's heritable personality traits and the environment. This gene × environment correlation will reduce the measured size of shared environmental effects (see Zuckerman, Chapter 3, this volume, for a detailed discussion of the effect of the shared environment on heritability estimates).

Captive chimpanzees, on the other hand, are more limited than humans with respect to the available environmental and social niches. They have no control over their enclosure size, the amount of crowding, the degree of enrichment, and other possible shared environmental influences that may influence their personality or subjective well-being. Also, to prevent inbreeding and promote outbreeding, zoos exchange chimpanzees. These exchanges increase the genetic diversity among chimpanzees within an enclosure. Furthermore, to the extent that personality traits are heritable, the exchanges will increase the variability of personality within the enclosure. These facts suggest that because the self-selection of environments is reduced in zoos, a more accurate and nonattenuated assessment of the shared and nonshared environmental influences, particularly the chimpanzee–environment fit, is possible as well.

GOALS

Our goals are twofold. First, we review our previous findings regarding genetic influences on chimpanzee personality, subjective well-being, and the covariance between these two phenotypes. Second, we describe and present the results of a series of new analyses that test for a variety of possible shared and nonshared environmental influences on chimpanzee personality or subjective well-being.

REVIEW OF PREVIOUS STUDIES

In an earlier study (Weiss, King, & Figueredo, 2000), we estimated the influence of genes, shared zoo environments, and nonshared environments in a sample of 145 chimpanzees that were housed in zoos around the United States and Australia. Since the chimpanzees were not organized into neat, self-contained nuclear family groups, the pedigrees were complex, and the number of independent pairs of related individuals was low.

Therefore, we took advantage of quantitative genetic approaches commonly used to assess the genetic and environmental sources of variance in herds of agriculturally important animals such as cattle. Large cattle herds have the same type of complex genetic relationships as populations of zoo chimpanzees. Our initial approach used the "symmetric differences squared" (SDS) technique; SDS is based on multiple-regression analysis. We regressed squared differences of all possible chimpanzee pairs onto two variables, one reflecting genetic effects and the other the shared zoo effects. The genetic variable was 1 minus the degree of relatedness of each pair; the shared zoo effect was whether the pair shared a common zoo enclosure (variable = 0) or was in different enclosures (variable = 1) (Grimes & Harvey, 1980). The unstandardized regression weights attached to each of these two predictor variables were equal to twice the amount of variance contributed by genes and zoo environments. The intercept was equal to twice the amount of variance due to the nonshared environment plus error. Thus dividing one of these weights by the sum of all the weights gave the proportions of variance for heritability (h^2), shared zoo effects (z^2), and nonshared environmental effects plus error (e^2) (Grimes & Harvey, 1980).

We found that approximately 66% of the variance in the dominance factor was the result of genetic differences among individuals. In addition, there was evidence that dependability was moderately heritable, but this effect was not significant. Shared zoo effects accounted for almost none of the variance in any of the six factors; nonshared environmental effects and error accounted for the remaining variance (see Table 19.2).

TABLE 19.2. Proportions of Variance in Chimpanzee Personality Factors Attributable to Genetic and Environmental Sources of Variance

Factor	Full model			Restricted model		
	h^2	z^2	e^2	h^2	z^2	e^2]
Dominance	0.80[*]	−0.10	0.31	0.63[*]	n.e.	0.37
Extraversion	−0.39	0.02	1.36	−0.35	n.e.	1.35
Dependability	0.22	−0.01	0.79	0.21	n.e.	0.79
Agreeableness	0.06	−0.02	0.96	0.03	n.e.	0.97
Emotional stability	0.05	0.01	0.93	0.08	n.e.	0.92
Openness	−0.16	0.03	1.12	−0.11	n.e.	1.11

Note. SDS analyses sometimes yield negative estimates; these estimates should be treated as being equal to zero (Grimes & Harvey, 1980). From Weiss, King, & Figueredo (2000). Copyright 2000 by Kluwer Academic Publishers. Adapted by permission.
[*]$p < .001$.

The lack of any significant heritability for the chimpanzee analogues of the human FFM is inconsistent with research on the behavior genetics of human personality dimensions (Bouchard & Loehlin, 2001), which typically indicates heritabilities of approximately .50. This may have been a result of the relatively small sample of chimpanzees, or of the fact that dominance was a large factor that accounted for most of the variance among personality descriptors. However, as the dominance factor was a blend of adjectival descriptors for all five human factors, this suggests some consistency between the human and chimpanzee heritability findings. In addition, the negligible shared environmental effect of zoos on personality variance is entirely consistent with findings from behavior genetic studies of human personality (Bouchard & Loehlin, 2001).

A follow-up study, using 128 chimpanzees from the original study, sought to extend the findings with respect to dominance by (1) assessing the possible contribution of heritable and nonheritable maternal effects, (2) assessing the contribution of genetic and environmental effects on subjective well-being, and (3) determining whether the covariance between dominance and subjective well-being was a result of shared genetic or environmental effects.

Because of the increased complexity of the analyses, we used another quantitative genetic analysis commonly used by agricultural researchers. This approach incorporates a restricted maximum-likelihood approach (MTDFREML; Boldman, Kriese, Van Vleck, Van Tassell, & Kachman, 1995) to find the genetic and environmental variance coefficients that are best able to reproduce the properties of a sample. These properties are expressed in matrices reflecting the proportion of genes shared among subjects, the genetic relatedness of the subjects' mothers, whether paired subjects have the same mother, and the subjects' phenotype scores. Specific information about the algorithms used in the analysis is available elsewhere (Weiss, 2002; Weiss, King, & Enns, 2002).

We tested several models, and the model with the best fit, as assessed by Akaike's information criterion (1987), included largely correlated genetic and largely uncorrelated nonshared environmental effects contributing to individual differences in dominance and subjective well-being. It did not include any nonheritable maternal effects for dominance or subjective well-being. Shared zoo effects were small. There were also moderate heritable maternal effects on subjective well-being (see Figure 19.1). As eliminating the heritable maternal effects did not significantly reduce the degree of model fit, or change the other parameter estimates (Weiss et al., 2002), this was deemed an alternative model.

As in the prior study, dominance was significantly heritable (Weiss et al., 2000). Subjective well-being was also significantly heritable—a result entirely consistent with the human literature (Lykken & Tellegen, 1996).

In addition, two novel findings emerged. First, there was some evidence for the possible presence of heritable maternal effects on subjective well-being. Two previous papers, one on humans (Furnham & Cheng, 2000) and one on

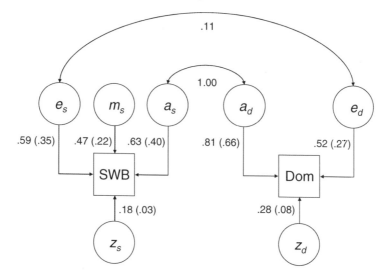

FIGURE 19.1. The best fitting model. The sizes for additive genetic (a), heritable maternal (m), nonheritable maternal (c), zoo (z), and nonshared environmental (e) effects are indicated by the path coefficients. The proportions of variance accounted for by these effects are next to these path coefficients in parentheses. SWB and s both represent subjective well-being; Dom and d both represent dominance. From Weiss, King, and Enns (2002). Copyright 2002 by the American Psychological Association. Adapted by permission.

chimpanzees (Bard & Gardner, 1996), suggested a possible maternal link to subjective well-being.

The most important finding in this study was the high genetic correlation between dominance and subjective well-being. Unrotated factor analysis of the items making up dominance and subjective well-being suggested that these results did not arise because these items were markers of a single latent variable (Weiss et al., 2002). It was important to verify the factorial independence of dominance and subjective well-being, because a genetic correlation between two indices of the same latent variable would be a somewhat trivial finding.

ENVIRONMENTAL EFFECTS ON CHIMPANZEE PERSONALITY

Since there are several possible environmental influences on dominance and subjective well-being in zoo habitats, we sought out the most likely candidates. The first, physical characteristics of an enclosure, was focused on the effects of habitat size and chimpanzee density. It has been noted that higher population densities within enclosures lead to increased stress, because within these enclosures chimpanzees are not able to avoid contact with others as easily (de Waal, 2000). However, Nieuwenhuijsen and de Waal (1982) found that increased crowding in a zoo population of chimpanzees resulted in more grooming, but no increase in aggression. Apparently a behavioral homeostasis in chimpanzees serves to regulate aggression under the increased stress of crowding. An interesting question is then whether there are constant personality differences between zoos with different degrees of crowding.

The second environmental effect that we examined was potential for social support from relatives. In humans, subjective well-being is higher in individuals who are married or who regularly attend church (Myers, 2000). In addition, support from kin, friends, or the community may be protective against circumstances that can reduce happiness (Buss, 2000; Hamilton, 1964; Trivers, 1971). There is considerable evidence that social support is important to chimpanzees. First, it is a major factor in attaining dominance. Frans de Waal (2000) noted that to become a dominant male, not only must the male align himself with other chimpanzees, but he must also cut off his opponent from his allies (see also Arnold & Whiten, 2003; Watts, 2002). It should also not be surprising that in chimpanzees, social support, especially from more dominant animals, can protect individuals from coming to harm or experiencing other adverse consequences, and that dominant females typically have healthier offspring (Pusey, 2001).

Another possible factor that may contribute to chimpanzee dominance or subjective well-being is how well an individual chimpanzee fits in its social environment. One interpretation of this would be the similarity of an individual's personality to those of others in the immediate vicinity. In humans, this is one component of what is known as the "person–environment fit." There is some evidence that higher congruence between an individual and the environment leads the individual to be happier (Moskowitz & Cotes, 1995). These findings are also consistent with findings showing that happier individuals tend to have more friends (Myers, 2000).

Among chimpanzees, the fit between a chimpanzee and the social environment may very well contribute to dominance and subjective well-being. With respect to the former, it may be easier for a chimpanzee to form coalitions with other chimpanzees that have similar personality traits; hence the animal would be more likely to be bold, to act aggressively, and to behave in other ways that would lead it to be rated higher on those adjectives constituting the dominance factor. Although there are no ethological observations bearing on this hypothesis, it would not be surprising if chimpanzee happiness is also influenced by whether individual chimpanzees can find compatible social niches.

ENVIRONMENTAL CORRELATES OF DOMINANCE AND SUBJECTIVE WELL-BEING

We tested these hypotheses on possible environmental predictors of dominance and subjective well-being, using data from 128 chimpanzees residing in

13 zoos. Twelve of the zoos were located in the United States, and one was located in Australia (see Table 19.3). Of these chimpanzees, there were 49 males and 79 females with mean ages of 16.8 and 20.0, respectively. Ages ranged from 3 to 55 years, indicating that the sample included juveniles and old adults (see Weiss et al., 2002, for more information about this sample).

The degree of relatedness of all 8,128 pairs of chimpanzees was computed with the Animal Breeder's Toolkit software package (Golden, Snelling, & Mallinckrodt, 1992). Table 19.4 displays the number of chimpanzee pairs of different degrees of relatedness in the same and different enclosures.

All chimpanzees in the study received personality and subjective well-being ratings from at least two raters. Raters were either zoo employees who regularly worked in the chimpanzee enclosure, or volunteers with the ChimpanZoo program of the Jane Goodall Institute who had extensive experience observing chimpanzees during separate projects (for more details, see King & Landau, 2003).

Raters completed the personality and subjective well-being questionnaires at home, and were instructed to base their ratings on the overall impressions they had of the chimpanzees during the time they had been in contact with them. Raters were also instructed not to discuss their ratings with others.

Personality and subjective well-being were defined as they had been in our previous studies (King & Landau, 2003; King et al., 2005; Weiss et al., 2000). For each personality factor, unit-weighted composites were created by summing the mean signed ratings given to adjectives in the factor (see Table

TABLE 19.3. Physical and Social Characteristics of Zoo Enclosures

Zoo	m^2	Males			Females		
		n	Density	M_{age}	n	Density	M_{age}
Dallas	165.864	1	.0060	36.00	3	.0181	23.97
Oakland	296.722	3	.0101	14.40	2	.0067	13.95
Los Angeles	780.360	4	.0051	15.52	7	.0090	15.00
Lowry Park	306.570	3	.0098	20.10	2	.0065	11.90
North Carolina	707.434	3	.0042	17.83	9	.0127	18.66
Sacramento	325.150	2	.0062	38.00	2	.0062	26.30
San Francisco	65.667	1	.0152	15.30	3	.0457	27.63
Sedgewick County	643.332	4	.0062	10.98	4	.0062	20.60
Tulsa Zoo	1040.480	1	.0010	21.30	4	.0038	23.30
Sunset Zoo	627.075	1	.0016	27.70	3	.0048	21.43
Cheyenne Mountain	73.577	4	.0544	10.52	4	.0054	19.52
Taronga Zoo	2340.000	8	.0034	6.12	17	.0073	22.31
Lion Country Safari							
Bashful's Island	1618.690	4	.0025	16.60	2	.0012	17.80
Higgy's Island	1821.030	4	.0022	15.10	6	.0033	28.43
Whitey's Island	809.345	2	.0025	24.80	6	.0074	15.18
Nolan's Island	1616.460	4	.0025	21.82	3	.0019	19.43
Old Man's Island	1416.350	2	.0014	50.30	1	.0007	19.60

Note. Adapted from Weiss (2002), Table 2.3.

TABLE 19.4. Degrees of Relatedness among All Possible Pairs of Chimpanzees

| | *n* pairs | | |
R	Same enclosure	Different enclosures	Total *n*
.000	468	7430	7898
.010–.124	33	2	35
.125–.249	30	11	41
.250–.374	44	26	70
.375–.499	2	1	3
.500–.589	56	25	81
	633	7495	8128

Note. R is Wright's coefficient of relatedness, the proportion of genes on average a pair of individuals have in common. From Weiss, King, and Enns (2002). Copyright 2003 by the American Psychological Association. Adapted by permission.

19.5). Summing the mean ratings on the four subjective well-being items created a unit-weighted subjective well-being score.

The internal-consistency alpha values of these factors were high, ranging from .73 (emotional stability) to .94 (dominance). The internal consistency of subjective well-being was also high (.83) (see King & Landau, 2003, for more details). In addition, the interrater reliabilities of mean ratings (*ICC* [3, *k*]) were high for all five factors and ranged from .73 (agreeableness) to .94 (dominance) (see King & Landau, 2003, for more details, including the reliability of individual raters). The interrater reliability of the mean subjective well-being score was similarly high (.85) (see King & Landau, 2003, for more details).

TABLE 19.5. Chimpanzee Personality Factor Definitions

Factor	Definition
Dominance	+ Dominant + Independent + Decisive + Intelligent + Persistent + Bullying + Stingy – Submissive – Dependent – Fearful – Timid – Cautious
Extraversion	+ Active + Playful + Sociable + Affectionate + Imitative + Friendly – Solitary – Lazy – Depressed
Dependability	+ Predictable – Impulsive – Defiant – Reckless – Erratic – Irritable – Aggressive – Jealous – Disorganized
Agreeableness	+ Sympathetic + Helpful + Sensitive + Protective + Gentle
Emotional Stability	– Excitable + Stable + Unemotional
Openness	+ Inventive + Inquisitive

Note. From Weiss, King, and Figueredo (2000), Table I. Copyright 2000 by Springer Science and Business Media. Adapted by permission.

Because of the multicollinearity among the dependent variables and independent variables, we used a hierarchical general linear model approach described by Gorsuch and Figueredo (1991) to test for the effects of demographic predictors, the physical environment, or the social environment on dominance and subjective well-being. The first hierarchical general linear model had dominance as its dependent variable. The second general hierarchical model was identical to the first, except that the dependent variable was subjective well-being controlled for dominance. This procedure ensured that only direct predictors of subjective well-being (i.e., those independent of dominance) were assessed (Gorsuch & Figueredo, 1991).

The first three effects entered into these models were sex, age, and the sex × age interaction. The second two were measures of how many males and females there were per square meter within an enclosure. The next predictors in the model were the mean male and female ages within the enclosure.

As noted previously, we hypothesized that familial support might contribute to either dominance or subjective well-being in chimpanzees. As with the density and age structure variables, we distinguished between the number of related males and females an individual had within an enclosure. Thus the next variables entered into the equation were male kin density (defined as the mean of the proportion of genes shared with males in the enclosure) and female kin density (defined as the mean of the proportion of genes shared with females in the enclosure). The average male kin density was .116 and the average female kin density was .107, indicating that, on average, other individuals within an enclosure were related at approximately the degree of first cousin to any given target chimpanzee.

The final set of variables that was included in the model assessed whether dominance or subjective well-being were influenced by personality, or the degree to which an individual chimpanzee's personality deviated from that of other chimpanzees in the enclosure. Thus, for predicting dominance, the five factors that were analogous to the human FFM were used. Finally, the effect of deviations of the mean factor score of a chimpanzee from that of its enclosure-mates were assessed by first partialing out the target chimpanzee's scores on the personality domains and then entering the mean factor scores for the enclosure into the model. The original analysis also considered a series of two-, three-, and four-way interactions to test whether different physical and social characteristics of enclosures and characteristics of chimpanzees were predictors of dominance and subjective well-being; these interactions were not significant and will not be described further in this chapter (for more details on these interactions and analyses, see Weiss, 2002).

The main-effects model accounted for more than half of the dominance variance, $R^2 = .58$, $F (19, 108) = 8.01$, $p < .0001$. The significant predictors in this model included age, $\beta = .33$, $F (1, 108) = 31.36$, $p < .0001$, and the age × sex interaction, $\beta = .33$, $F (1, 108) = 10.03$, $p < .01$, indicating that older individuals were rated as being higher in dominance and that this age effect was greater for males than for females. Dominance was also predicted by high extraversion, $\beta = .14$, $F(1, 108) = 13.01$, $p < .001$, and high openness, $\beta = .24$, $F(1, 108) = 8.90$, $p < .01$, as well as by low dependability, $\beta = -.44$, $F(1, 108) = 35.25$, $p < .0001$, and low emotional stability, $\beta = -.36$, $F(1, 108) = 35.82$, $p < .0001$. However, these significant effects were probably the results of using unit weighting to create factor scores, as they were not the original weights used to find an orthogonal solution.

The main-effects model accounted for slightly less than half of the variance in subjective well-being, $R^2 = .48$, $F(20, 107) = 4.89$, $p < .0001$. Dominance accounted for approximately 27% of the variance in subjective well-being, $\beta = .63$, $F(1, 107) = 55.11$, $p < .0001$. Age was negatively related to subjective well-being, $\beta = -.06$, $F(1, 107) = 4.77$, $p < .05$, and both extraversion, $\beta = .28$, $F(1, 107) = 17.08$, $p < .0001$, and dependability, $\beta = .29$, $F(1, 107) = 14.56$, $p < .001$, were positively related to subjective well-being. However, the effects of the physical and social characteristics of the enclosure were not significant.

These analyses suggest that the physical and social characteristics of the zoo, as measured by the degree of crowding, age structure, and kin density within a zoo, did not contribute to individual differences in dominance or subjective well-being. In addition, these domains were not influenced by how similar a chimpanzee's personality was to that of its enclosure-mates. These analyses were not exhaustive, but they were strong tests of potential environmental influences on dominance and subjective well-being.

On the other hand, this research has shown that in these chimpanzees dominance and subjective well-being were largely heritable and correlated because they shared genes in common. These findings also suggested that the remaining variance was due to temporary environmental effects or some other environmental influences. In addition, there was a hint that some heritable trait of chimpanzee mothers may have resulted in happier offspring.

Clearly, the quality and conditions of zoo enclosures can have an effect on the well-being of chimpanzees and other animals; poor housing or group formation, such as that which existed early in the last century, can lead to aberrant behavior (Martin, 2002) or even deadly conflict (Zuckerman, 1932). If such zoos had been included in the current study, it would not be surprising to find significant effects of zoos. However, the range of environments good enough to foster normal development in chimpanzees, humans, and other species is probably large.

Earlier research noted the importance of "contact comfort" and normal social interactions in the typical development of rhesus monkeys (Harlow & Mears, 1979) and chimpanzees (Martin, 2002). Recent research on human subjective well-being suggests that environments of extreme want may lead to populations that are significantly lower in subjective well-being (Myers & Diener, 1995). However, just as a wide range of different sources for social enrichment and other sources of well-being could lead to the typical development of rhesus macaques (and presumably other primates), so a large variety of human societies and parenting techniques could lead to happiness and typical personality development (Diener, Diener, & Diener, 1995; McCrae, 2001), and a large range of different zoos could lead to typical development of chimpanzee personality and happiness.

Several theories about the evolution of individual differences have been proposed. Most of these theories are based on frequency-dependent selection models, though some see personality as being related not to individual fitness but to random variation around some optimal species-specific mean (see Figueredo et al., 2005, for a review). Although there is still debate about the evolution of individual differences in personality, these hypotheses are all plausible explanations and all take into account the major known facts of personality.

Recently, evolutionary psychologists have also proposed a number of theories about the evolution of subjective well-being (Barkow, 1997; Buss, 2000; Nesse, 1990). However, unlike the theories of personality, these hypotheses do not emphasize the fundamental fact about subjective well-being—namely, that it is most closely tied to personality and least tied to situational contexts (Diener, 1996). Instead, they are more often grounded in the older conceptions of subjective well-being as an absence of psychopathology. For example, Buss (2000) remarked that the presence of kin close at hand and the absence of evolutionarily important negative emotions such as sexual jealousy might improve happiness. The current study was unable to test the latter prediction, but it was inconsistent with the former prediction—at least in zoo chimpanzees.

Two findings in particular—the high genetic correlation between dominance and subjective well-being, and the relationships among chimpanzee dominance, reproductive success, and survival—suggest to us that happiness in chimpanzees, and probably in humans, is a sexually selected fitness indicator. Put simply, a chimpanzee's smile is like a peacock's tail.

Subjective well-being in chimpanzees, and probably humans, appears to satisfy two of the major criteria that need to be incorporated in a fitness indicator (see Miller, 2000, for a discussion). First, sexually selected fitness indicators have to be honest, hard-to-fake signals. As subjective well-being is genetically correlated with a fitness-related trait such as dominance, it will be difficult to fake, as only those with genes for dominance will have genes for happiness. If chimpanzees (and possibly humans) were able to fake subjective well-being, and if this feigned subjective well-being were indistinguishable from actual happiness, the genetic correlation between dominance and subjective well-being would be reduced.

Second, sexually selected fitness indicators are easily detectable. There is considerable evidence that happiness is easily detectable both in humans and in our primate cousins. One line of evidence for this is that humans can reliably judge chimpanzee happiness (King & Landau, 2003). Furthermore, happiness is the most easily detectable emotion in humans (Ekman, Friesen, & Ellsworth, 1982).

A third criterion is that the same genes should be responsible for the sexually selected trait within an individual and for a desire for mates that exhibit the sexually selected trait. Although it would be difficult to test this hypothesis in zoo chimpanzees, it certainly would be simple to test this in genetically informative human samples.

LOOKING FORWARD

Apart from methodological and evolutionary considerations, one might be tempted to ask whether these findings offer practical suggestions to the study of personality and happiness in humans. We believe that they do. The study of comorbidity has been a major focus of clinical psychology. We think that the study of positive intercorrelations among positive traits in humans, chimpanzees, and other animals—a phenomenon we call "covitality"—could similarly extend the study of positive psychology. This program of research not only could encompass an examination of whether these positive traits are genetically correlated and whether they operate in ways predicted by evolutionary theory; it could isolate suites of traits that would better enable us to understand important psychological resources contributing to resilience, positive social relationships, and other important outcomes.

ACKNOWLEDGMENTS

The research described in this chapter could not have been completed without the help of Virginia Landau of the ChimpanZoo program of the Jane Goodall Institute, and the raters and caretakers at the zoological parks who rated chimpanzees and provided us with enclosure size information. This research also benefited from the advice of A. J. Figueredo, W. Jake Jacobs, Lee Sechrest, David C. Rowe, and R. Mark Enns. We also would like to thank Jeff McCrae and Antonio Terracciano for their comments on an earlier version of this chapter.

REFERENCES

Akaike, H. (1987). Factor analysis and AIC. *Psychometrika, 52,* 317–332.

Arnold, K., & Whiten, A. (2003). Grooming interactions among the chimpanzees of the Budongo forest, Uganda: Tests of five explanatory models. *Behaviour, 140,* 519–552.

Baker, K. C., & Aureli, F. (1997). Behavioural indicators of anxiety: An empirical test in chimpanzees. *Behaviour, 134,* 1031–1050.

Bard, K. A., & Gardner, K. H. (1996). Influences on development in infant chimpanzees: Enculturation, temperament, and cognition. In A. E. Russon & K. A. Bard (Eds.), *Reaching into thought: The minds of great apes* (pp. 235–256). Cambridge, UK: Cambridge University Press.

Barkow, J. H. (1997). Happiness in evolutionary perspective. In N. L. Segal, G. Weisfeld, & C. C. Weisfeld (Eds.), *Uniting psychology and biology: Integrative perspectives on human development* (pp. 397–418). Washington, DC: American Psychological Association.

Boldman, K. G., Kriese, L. A., Van Vleck, L. D., Van Tassell, C. P., & Kachman, S. D. (1995). *A manual for use of MTDFREML: A set of programs to obtain estimates of variances and covariances.* Unpublished manuscript.

Bouchard, T. J., Jr., & Loehlin, J. C. (2001). Genes, evolution, and personality. *Behavior Genetics, 31,* 243–271.

Buirski, P., & Plutchik, R. (1991). Measurement of deviant behavior in a Gombe chimpanzee: Relation to later behavior. *Primates, 32,* 207–211.

Buss, D. M. (2000). The evolution of happiness. *American Psychologist, 55,* 15–23.

Costa, P. T., Jr., & McCrae, R. R. (1995). Theories of personality and psychopathology: Approaches derived from philosophy and psychology. In H. I. Kaplan & B. J. Sadock (Eds.), *Comprehensive textbook of psychiatry* (6th ed., Vol. 1, pp. 507–519). Baltimore: Williams & Wilkins.

Chapmin, C. A., White, F. J., & Wrangham, R. W. (1993). Defining group size in fission–fusion societies. *Folia Primatologica, 61,* 31–34.

Darwin, C. (1998). *The expression of the emotions in man and animals* (3rd ed.). New York: Oxford University Press. (Original work published 1872)

de Waal, F. B. M. (1996). *Good natured: The origins of right and wrong in humans and other animals.* Cambridge, MA: Harvard University Press.

de Waal, F. B. M. (2000). *Chimpanzee politics: Power and sex among apes* (rev. ed.). Baltimore: Johns Hopkins University Press.

Diener, E. (1996). Traits can be powerful, but are not enough: Lessons from subjective well-being. *Journal of Research in Personality, 30,* 389–399.

Diener, E. (1998). Subjective well-being and personality. In D. F. Barone, M. Herson, & V. B. van Hasselt (Eds.), *Advanced personality* (pp. 311–334). New York: Plenum Press.

Diener, E., Diener, M., & Diener, C. (1995). Factors predicting the subjective well-being of nations. *Journal of Personality and Social Psychology, 69,* 851–864.

Eid, M., & Diener, E. (2004). Global judgements of subjective well-being: Situational variability and long-term stability. *Social Indicators Research, 65,* 245–277.

Ekman, P., Friesen, W. V., & Ellsworth, P. (1982). Does the face provide accurate information? In P. Ekman (Ed.), *Emotion in the human face* (2nd ed., pp. 56–110). Hillsdale, NJ: Erlbaum.

Figueredo, A. J., Sefcek, J. A., Vasquez, G., Hagenah, B. J., King, J. E., & Jacobs, W. J. (2005). Evolutionary personality psychology. In D. M. Buss (Ed.), *Handbook of evolutionary psychology* (pp. 851–877). New York: Wiley.

Furnham, A., & Cheng, H. (2000). Perceived parental behavior, self-esteem, and happiness. *Social Psychiatry and Psychiatric Epidemiology, 35,* 463–470.

Gold, K. C., & Maple, T. L. (1994). Personality assessment in the gorilla and its utility as a measurement tool. *Zoo Biology, 13,* 509–522.

Golden, B. L., Snelling, W. M., & Mallinckrodt, C. H. (1992). *Animal Breeder's Toolkit: User's guide and reference manual* (Technical Bulletin No. LTB92-2). Fort Collins: Colorado State University Agricultural Experiment Station.

Goodall, J. (1968). Behavior of free-living chimpanzees of the Gombe Stream area. *Animal Behavior Monographs, 1,* 163–311.

Goodall, J. (1986). *The chimpanzees of Gombe: Patterns of behavior.* Cambridge, MA: Harvard University Press.

Gorsuch, R. L., & Figueredo, A. J. (1991). *Sequential canonical analysis as an exploratory form of path analysis.* Paper presented at the annual conference of the American Evaluation Association, Chicago.

Gosling, S. D. (2001). From mice to men: What can we learn about personality from animal research? *Psychological Bulletin, 127,* 45–86.

Gosling, S. D., & John, O. P. (1999). Personality dimensions in nonhuman animals: A cross-species review. *Current Directions in Psychological Science, 8,* 69–75.

Gosling, S. D., Ko, S. J., Mannarelli, T., & Morris, M. E. (2002). A room with a cue: Judgments of personality based on offices and bedrooms. *Journal of Personality and Social Psychology, 82,* 379–398.

Grimes, L. W., & Harvey, W. R. (1980). Estimation of genetic variances and covariances using symmetric differences squared. *Journal of Animal Science, 50,* 632–644.

Hamilton, W. D. (1964). The evolution of social behavior. *Journal of Theoretical Biology, 7,* 1–52.

Hare, B., Call, J., & Tomasello, M. (2001). Do chimpanzees know what conspecifics know? *Animal Behavior, 61,* 139–151.

Harlow, H. F., & Mears, C. E. (1979). *The human model: Primate perspectives.* Washington, DC: V. H. Winston.

Johnson, L. D., Petto, A. J., & Sehgal, P. K. (1991). Survival and reproduction as measures of psychological well-being in cotton top tamarins (*Saguinus oedipus*). In M. A. Novak & A. J. Petto (Eds.), *Through the looking glass: Issues of psychological well-being in captive nonhuman primates* (pp. 93–102). Washington, DC: American Psychological Association.

King, J. E., & Figueredo, A. J. (1997). The five-factor model plus dominance in chimpanzee personality. *Journal of Research in Personality, 31,* 257–271.

King, J. E., & Landau, V. I. (2003). Can chimpanzee (*Pan troglodytes*) happiness be estimated by human raters? *Journal of Research in Personality, 37,* 1–15.

King, J. E., Weiss, A., & Farmer, K. H. (2005). A chimpanzee (*Pan troglodytes*) analogue of cross-national generalization of personality structure: Zoological parks and an African sanctuary. *Journal of Personality, 73,* 389–410.

Köhler, W. (1925). *The mentality of apes* (E. Winter, Trans.) New York: Harcourt, Brace. (Original work published 1924)

Lykken, D. T., & Tellegen, A. (1996). Happiness is a stochastic phenomenon. *Psychological Science, 7,* 186–189.

Martin, J. E. (2002). Early life experiences: Activity levels and abnormal behaviours in resocialised chimpanzees. *Animal Welfare, 11,* 419–436.

McCrae, R. R. (2001). Trait psychology and culture: Exploring intercultural comparisons. *Journal of Personality, 69,* 819–846.

McCrae, R. R., & Costa, P. T., Jr. (2003). *Personality in adulthood: A five-factor theory perspective* (2nd ed.). New York: Guilford Press.

Miller, G. F. (2000). *The mating mind: How sexual choice shaped the evolution of human nature.* New York: Doubleday.

Moskowitz, D. S., & Cotes, S. (1995). Do interpersonal traits predict affect?: A comparison of three models. *Journal of Personality and Social Psychology, 69,* 915–924.

Myers, D. G. (2000). The funds, friends, and faith of happy people. *American Psychologist, 55,* 56–67.

Myers, D. G., & Diener, E. (1995). Who is happy? *Psychological Science, 6,* 10–19.

Nesse, R. M. (1990). Evolutionary explanations of emotions. *Human Nature, 1,* 261–289.

Nieuwenhuijsen, K., & de Waal, F. B. (1982). Effects of spatial crowding on social behavior in a chimpanzee colony. *Zoo Biology, 1,* 5–28.

Pederson, A. L., King, J. E., & Landau, V. I. (in press). Chimpanzee (*Pan troglodytes*) personality predicts behavior. *Journal of Research in Personality.*

Purvis, A. (1995). A composite estimate of primate phylogeny. *Philosophical Transactions of the Royal Society of London, Series B, 348,* 405–421.

Pusey, A. I. (2001). Of genes and apes: Chimpanzee social organization and reproduction. In F. B. M. de Waal (Ed.), *Tree of origin: What primate behavior can tell us about human social evolution* (pp. 11–37). Cambridge, MA: Harvard University Press.

Pusey, A., Williams, J., & Goodall, J. (1999). The influence of dominance rank on the reproductive success of female chimpanzees. *Science, 277,* 828–831.

Rosenblum, L. A. (1991). Subjective and objective factors in assessing psychological well-being in nonhuman primates. In M. A. Novak & A. J. Petto (Eds.), *Through the looking glass: Issues of psychological well-being in captive nonhuman primates* (pp. 43–49). Washington, DC: American Psychological Association.

Rowe, D. C. (1994). *The limits of family influence.* New York: Guilford Press.

Rumbaugh, D. M., & Savage-Rumbaugh, E. S. (1994). Language in comparative perspective. In N. J. Mackintosh (Ed.), *Animal learning and cognition* (pp. 307–333). San Diego, CA: Academic Press.

Sarich, V. M., & Wilson, A. C. (1967). Immunological time scale for hominid evolution. *Science, 158,* 1200–1203.

Scarr, S., & McCartney, K. (1983). How people make their own environments: A theory of genotype–environmental effects. *Child Development, 54,* 424–435.

Schopenhauer, A. (1969). *The world as will and representation* (3rd ed., Vol. 1) (E. F. J. Payne, Trans.). New York: Dover. (Original work published 1859)

Seligman, M. E. P. (2002). Positive psychology, positive prevention, and positive therapy. In C. R. Snyder & S. J. Lopez (Eds.), *Handbook of positive psychology* (pp. 3–9). New York: Oxford University Press.

Trivers, R. L. (1971). The evolution of reciprocal altruism. *Quarterly Review of Biology, 46,* 35–57.

Watts, D. P. (2002). Reciprocity and interchange in the social relationships of wild male chimpanzees. *Behaviour, 139,* 343–370.

Weiss, A. (2002). *Genetic and environmental contributions to dominance and subjective well-being in chimpanzees* (Pan troglodytes). Unpublished doctoral dissertation, University of Arizona.

Weiss, A., King, J. E., & Enns, R. M. (2002). Subjective well-being is heritable and genetically correlated with dominance in chimpanzees (*Pan troglodytes*). *Journal of Personality and Social Psychology, 83,* 1141–1149.

Weiss, A., King, J. E., & Figueredo, A. J. (2000). The heritability of personality factors in chimpanzees (*Pan troglodytes*). *Behavior Genetics, 30,* 213–221.

Whiten, A. (1997). The Machiavellian mindreader. In A. Whiten & R. W. Byrne (Eds.), *Machiavellian intelligence II: Extensions and evaluations* (pp. 144–173). New York: Cambridge University Press.

Whiten, A., Goodall, J., McGrew, W. C., Nishida, T., Reynolds, V., Sugiyama, Y., et al. (1999). Cultures in chimpanzees. *Nature, 399,* 682–685.

Willham, R. L. (1972). The role of maternal effects in animal breeding: III. Biometrical aspects of maternal effects in animals. *Journal of Animal Science, 35,* 1288–1293.

Wilson, A. C., & Sarich, V. M. (1969). A molecular time scale for human evolution. *Proceedings of the National Academy of Sciences USA, 63,* 1088–1093.

Wrangham, R. W., & Peterson, D. (1996). *Demonic males: Apes and the origins of human violence.* Boston: Houghton Mifflin.

Yerkes, R, M. (1925). *Almost human.* New York: Century.

Yerkes, R. M. (1929). *The great apes: A study of anthropoid life.* New Haven, CT: Yale University Press.

Yerkes, R. M. (1939). The life history and personality of the chimpanzee. *American Naturalist, 73,* 97–112.

Yerkes, R. M. (1943). *Chimpanzee: A laboratory colony.* New Haven, CT: Yale University Press.

Zuckerman, S. (1932). *The social life of monkeys and apes.* New York: Harcourt, Brace.

How Can Animal Studies Contribute to Research on the Biological Bases of Personality?

Pranjal H. Mehta and Samuel D. Gosling

In his text entitled *The Physical Basis of Personality*, Charles Stockard (1931) used a frontispiece composed of three pairs of photographs. Each pair included two faces side by side, one depicting a dog and the other a human, to illustrate some striking similarities in physical features between the dogs and humans. Stockard suggested that certain morphological features are associated with certain personality traits in both dogs and humans; he argued that the links between morphology and personality common to the two species may be driven by similar underlying biological mechanisms.

Seventy-five years later, there is no question that personality traits have a biological basis. The important questions that remain concern the nature of this basis, in terms of the biological substrates and processes that underlie traits. Many different methods can be used in the service of addressing these questions. Animal studies constitute one such method.

Stockard was not alone in believing that comparative research could illuminate the biological bases of personality. In the 1935 *A Handbook of Social Psychology* (Murchison, 1935), more than a quarter of the 23 chapters focused on nonhuman subjects. In the 1954 handbook, the number of chapters on animals had diminished, but the usefulness of comparative research was still being championed; in one chapter, Hebb and Thomson argued that social psychology will "be dangerously myopic if it restricts itself to the human literature" (p. 532). Unfortunately, this warning was not heeded:

None of the chapters in the latest edition of this handbook (Gilbert, Fiske, & Lindzey, 1998) focused on nonhuman animals, and comparative research has virtually disappeared from social psychology.

Yet animal studies have continued to contribute to many other areas of psychology (Domjan & Purdy, 1995). Here we argue that animal studies still have an important contribution to make to personality psychology, especially studies of the biological bases of personality (Gosling & Mollaghan, in press; Vazire & Gosling, 2003). Indeed, with the emergence of new methods in genomics, neuroscience, physiology, and phylogenetics, the potential contributions to be made by animal research are greater than ever. And with recent progress in the measurement of personality in animals and in identifying cross-species generalities in personality traits, the assessment of personality in animals also stands on increasingly solid ground.

In this chapter, we explore the ways in which animal studies can help shed light on the biological underpinnings of personality. In the first part of the chapter, we offer a brief review of recent advances in the field of animal personality. We evaluate the evidence that personality exists and can be measured in nonhuman animals. We also review and summarize the major traits that have been identified. The second part of the chapter uses two related personality traits—dominance and aggression—to illustrate some of the ways in which animal studies can elucidate the connections between biology and personality.

REVIEW OF RECENT RESEARCH ON ANIMAL PERSONALITY

If comparative research is to help us understand the biological bases of personality, the first steps are (1) to show that personality does indeed exist in animals, (2) to show that it can be measured, and (3) to assess the degree to which personality traits generalize across species.

Does Personality Exist in Animals?

To anyone who has worked with animals or who even owns a pet, it seems preposterous to even question whether personality exists in animals. However, the question cannot simply be dismissed. After all, there was a period in the 1970s when a substantial body of psychologists seriously questioned the idea that personality exists in humans, and concerns that personality descriptions are mere anthropomorphic projections continue to be raised.

To address such issues, Gosling, Lilienfeld, and Marino (2003; see also Gosling & Vazire, 2002) recently evaluated the evidence pertaining to the existence of personality in animals. Explicitly drawing on the lessons learned from the debates surrounding the existence of personality in humans (Kenrick

& Funder, 1988), Gosling, Lilienfield, and Marino considered three major criteria that must be met to establish the existence of personality traits: (1) Assessments by independent observers must agree with one another; (2) these assessments must predict behaviors and real-world outcomes; and (3) observer ratings must be shown to reflect genuine attributes of the individuals rated, not merely the observers' implicit theories about how personality traits covary. On all three criteria, animal personality research met the standards expected of human personality research, providing strong evidence that personality does exist in animals.

Can Personality be Measured in Animals?

Having shown that it is meaningful to refer to personality in animals, we must next determine whether it can be measured. One study examined this question directly in a side-by-side comparison of the accuracy of personality ratings of dogs versus humans (Gosling, Kwan, & John, 2003). Parallel procedures and instruments were used to compare personality judgments of 78 dogs and their owners in terms of three accuracy criteria: internal consistency, consensus, and correspondence. On all three criteria, judgments of dogs were as accurate as judgments of humans, again suggesting that personality differences do exist and demonstrating that personality traits can be measured in animals.

Establishing Cross-Species Equivalence of Personality Traits

For cross-species comparisons to be useful, it is crucial to establish the cross-species generality of traits. For example, we must be confident that fearfulness in rats and fearfulness in humans are essentially the same thing. One response to the challenge of establishing cross-species equivalences in traits is to avoid making cross-species comparisons at the trait level, and instead to focus on the common biological underpinnings of traits that have already been identified in humans. For example, in a phylogenetic analysis conducted across a range of mammals, including tree shrews, rhesus monkeys, chimpanzees, and humans, Lesch and colleagues (1997) focused not on anxiety itself but on a gene sequence associated with anxiety (the serotonin transporter gene-linked polymorphic region, known as *5-HTTLPR*).

Another solution for determining the cross-species equivalence of personality traits is to take some of the principles established in cross-cultural research and apply them in the cross-species context. Consider the issue facing cross-cultural researchers when they go to an entirely new culture and encounter a facial expression that resembles the facial expression ordinarily associated with fear in the researchers' own culture. How can these researchers determine whether the expression that to them resembles fear actually *is* associated with the emotion of fear in this new culture? The solution is to look for similarities across the cultures in terms of the physiological underpinnings, antecedents, and consequences. Thus, if this fear-like expression is associated with physiological responses similar to those associated with known cases of fear, if it follows conditions that logically should induce fear (e.g., discovering a dangerous snake in one's bed), and if it produces reactions that logically should follow fear (e.g., fleeing from the snake), then a strong argument can be made that the fear expression is equivalent in both cultures.

Similarly, if an animal expressing a trait such as fearfulness meets these conditions (similar physiology, antecedents, and consequences), it is reasonable to treat the traits as equivalent across species. Of course, all of these conditions will rarely be formally tested in most cases; instead, it can reasonably be assumed that humans who have become familiar with a species in terms of its ecology and behavioral repertoire can probably recognize the expression of personality traits in that species. Therefore, studies that use personality ratings almost always rely on judges familiar with the target species.

A Review of Cross-Species Evidence for Personality Traits

A large number of personality traits have been identified in animals, but are there any that show particularly strong cross-species generality? Most empirical studies of animal personality focus on just a single species, so cross-species commonalities must be identified by reviews that combine studies. One review summarized the evidence for cross-species commonalities in personality in 19 factor-analytic studies, representing 12 different species (Gosling & John, 1999). The findings were organized in terms of the human five-factor model plus dominance and activity.

The dimensions of extraversion, neuroticism, and agreeableness showed considerable generality across the 12 species included in the review. Of the 19 studies, 17 identified a factor closely related to extraversion, capturing dimensions ranging from sociability in pigs, dogs, and rhesus monkeys to a dimension contrasting bold approach versus avoidance in octopuses. Factors related to neuroticism appeared almost as frequently, capturing dimensions such as fearfulness, emotional reactivity, excitability, and low nerve stability. Factors related to agreeableness appeared in 14 studies, with affability, affection, and social closeness representing the high pole, and aggression, hostility, and fighting representing the low pole. Factors related to openness were identified in all but 4 of the 12 species; the two major components defining this dimension were curiosity/exploration and playfulness. Chimpanzees were the only species with a separate conscientiousness factor; this factor included the lack of attention and goal-directedness and the erratic, unpredictable, and disorganized behavior typical of the low pole of conscientiousness in humans. Dominance emerged as a clear separate factor in 7 of the 19 studies, and a separate activity dimension was identified in two of the studies.

DOMINANCE AND AGGRESSION
AS PERSONALITY TRAITS

In our selective review of animal studies below, we focus on two traits that have enjoyed considerable cross-species support, and that can be applied without controversy to both humans and nonhumans: dominance and aggression.

Dominance has been considered a trait in several systems of personality developed in the human domain (e.g., Wiggins, 1979). In addition, many socially living animal species show individual differences related to status in the dominance hierarchy, so it is no surprise that dominance was identified in multiple studies reviewed by Gosling and John (1999). Further evidence has recently emerged, most notably in chimpanzees, to suggest that dominance can be considered a separate personality trait (e.g., King, Weiss, & Farmer, 2005).

Another trait expressed in humans and many other species is aggression, appearing several times in the Gosling and John (1999) review and in numerous other studies (see Gosling, 2001). It should be noted that many of the animal studies do not discriminate aggression from dominance; they often use aggressive behavior as a proxy for dominance. The purpose of the present chapter is to show how animal studies might inform human research, not to quibble about the ways traits have been conceptualized or operationalized. Therefore, for the purposes of this chapter we draw on studies from both the dominance and aggression domains, without focusing on the inconsistent distinctions maintained between these traits.

THE BENEFITS OF ANIMAL RESEARCH

Although animal research should not replace human research, studies in animals have already enriched our understanding of the biological bases of human personality, and it appears that they will continue to do so. In particular, we suggest that animal research affords five essential benefits to the study of personality: (1) greater experimental control, (2) a greater ability to measure physiological parameters, (3) greater opportunities for naturalistic observations, (4) a shorter life span, and (5) greater opportunities to examine personality–health relationships. In this section, we explore these benefits, illustrating each one with animal studies of aggression and dominance. These studies are summarized in Table 20.1.

Benefit 1: Greater Experimental Control

Animal studies permit experimental manipulations that are not possible in humans. As a result, animal models have yielded new discoveries about the hormones, neurotransmitters, genes, and environments associated with personality traits such as aggression and dominance.

TABLE 20.1. Animal Studies on the Biological Bases of Aggression and Dominance, Categorized According to Benefit

Study	Animal species and gender	Main findings	Significance for personality psychology	Primary benefit	Secondary benefit(s)
Berthold (1849/1944)	Male chickens	Castrated chickens developed into nonaggressive capons, but castrated chickens reimplanted with testes in the abdomen developed into normal roosters.	Shows that the testes facilitate aggression.	Hormone manipulation (1a)	Naturalistic observation (3)
Briganti et al. (2003)	Male rabbits	Testosterone injections only increased aggression in high-ranking rabbits.	Shows a testosterone × social rank interaction in aggression.	Hormone manipulation (1a)	Naturalistic observation (3)
Veiga et al. (2004)	Female starlings	Testosterone-treated females hatched more sons; in addition, these females gained and maintained high social rank.	Shows that testosterone influences social rank in females.	Hormone manipulation (1a)	Naturalistic observation (3)
Ferris & Delville (1994)	Adult male hamsters	Hamsters injected with a vasopressin antagonist into the anterior hypothalamus decreased in aggression.	Shows that vasopressin is associated with aggression.	Pharmacological manipulation (1b)	
Delville et al. (1996a)	Adult male hamsters	Castrated and testosterone-treated animals administered serotonin and vasopressin agonists in the ventrolateral hypothalamus were less aggressive than animals not administered the serotonin agonist.	Shows interaction between serotonin and vasopressin in aggression.	Pharmacological manipulation (1b)	Hormone manipulation (1a)
Nelson et al. (1995)	Adult male mice	Mice lacking gene for neuronal nitric oxide synthase (nNOS-) were more aggressive than wild-type mice.	Identifies a gene associated with aggression.	Genetic manipulation (1c)	
Chiavegatto et al. (2001)	Adult male mice	The aggressiveness observed in nNOS- mice was caused by reduced serotonin turnover and impaired serotonin receptors.	Shows biological mechanism by which a particular gene influences aggression.	Genetic manipulation (1c)	Pharmacological manipulation (1b)

432

Citation	Subject	Findings	Interpretation	Method	Method
Nomura et al. (2002)	Pubertal, young adult, and adult male mice	Male mice lacking the gene for estrogen receptor beta were more aggressive than wild-type mice as adolescents and young adults, but not as adults.	Shows gene × age interaction affecting aggression.	Genetic manipulation (1c)	Hormone manipulation (1a)
Ogawa et al. (1997)	Adult male mice	Male mice lacking the gene for estrogen receptor alpha were less aggressive than wild-type mice, despite having average testosterone levels.	Identifies gene associated with aggression, and suggests that the mechanism of action is not testosterone-dependent.	Genetic manipulation (1c)	Hormone measurement (2c)
De Jonge et al. (1996)	Female piglets, babies to adults	Piglets raised in a poor environment were more aggressive as adults than piglets raised in an enriched environment.	Shows that early environmental conditions influence adult aggression.	Environmental manipulation (1d)	Longitudinal study (4)
Newman et al. (2005)	Male rhesus monkeys (3–5 years old)	Monkeys with low activity of the monoamine oxidase A (MAO-A) gene that were mother-reared were more aggressive.	Shows a genotype × early rearing environment interaction in aggression.	Environmental manipulation (1d)	Gene promoter sequence variation (2c)
Oliveira et al. (2001)	Adult male cichlid fish	Fish watching a fight rose in testosterone, relative to those that did not watch a fight.	Shows an environmental influence on testosterone levels, which in turn may influence dominance and aggression.	Environmental manipulation (1d)	Hormone measurement (2c)
Delville et al. (1996b)	Adult male hamsters	Vasopressin receptor binding in the ventrolateral hypothalamus disappeared in castrated animals, but not in testosterone-treated animals; vasopressin microinjections did not increase aggression in castrated animals, but did increase aggression in testosterone-treated animals.	Suggests a vasopressin-receptor-dependent mechanism by which testosterone influences aggression.	Hormone receptor binding measurement (2a)	Hormone manipulation (1a)
DeLeon et al. (2002)	Adolescent male hamsters	Anabolic–androgenic steroid treatment during adolescence increased vasopressin binding and aggression.	Suggests a vasopressin-receptor-dependent mechanism by which anabolic steroids influence aggression.	Hormone receptor binding measurement (2a)	Hormone manipulation (1a)

(continued)

TABLE 20.1. (continued)

Study	Animal species and gender	Main findings	Significance for personality psychology	Primary benefit	Secondary benefit(s)
Filipenko et al. (2002)	Adult male mice	Social defeat resulted in greater expression of serotonin transporter (SERT) and MAO-A messenger RNA (mRNA).	Shows an environmental influence on gene expression, which may in turn influence aggression.	Gene expression measurement (2b)	Environmental manipulation (1d)
Pinna et al. (2005)	Female mice	Testosterone therapy increased aggression and decreased mRNA expression for 5-alpha reductase type 1.	Suggests that testosterone influences gene expression and aggression.	Gene expression measurement (2b)	Hormone, pharmacological, and environmental manipulations (1a,1b,1d)
Wingfield et al. (1990)	Birds	Testosterone rose to facilitate intermale competition.	Shows that natural increases in testosterone facilitate aggression only during social instability.	Naturalistic observation (3)	Hormone measurement (2c)
Virgin & Sapolsky (1997)	Male baboons	Subordinate individuals that were aggressive after losing a fight had lower cortisol levels than subordinates that were not aggressive after losing a fight.	Shows a relationship between cortisol levels and aggression.	Naturalistic observation (3)	Hormone measurement (2c), personality and health (5)
Muller & Wrangham (2004)	Adult male chimpanzees	Testosterone levels and aggression were higher in dominant individuals.	Shows a relationship between testosterone levels and aggression, as well as between testosterone levels and social rank.	Naturalistic observation (3)	Hormone measurement (2c)
Muehlenbein et al. (2004)	Adult male chimpanzees	Testosterone levels were correlated with social rank.	Shows a relationship between testosterone levels and social rank.	Naturalistic observation (3)	Hormone measurement (2c)
Holekamp & Smale (1998)	Adult male hyenas	Testosterone levels were higher in immigrant than in natal males; testosterone levels correlated with social rank among immigrant males.	Shows a relationship between testosterone levels and social rank.	Naturalistic observation (3)	Hormone measurement (2c)

Study	Species	Primary benefit	Secondary benefit(s)		
Adkins-Regan (1999)	Female zebra finches	Neonatal estradiol plus adult testosterone treatment increased aggression.	Shows that neonatal and adult hormone exposure influence adult aggression.	Longitudinal study (4)	Hormone manipulation (1a)
Wommack et al. (2003)	Male hamsters	Social subjugation during adolescence accelerated the development of aggression.	Shows an environmental influence during adolescence on the development of aggression.	Longitudinal study (4)	Environmental manipulation (1d)
Wommack & Delville (2003)	Male hamsters	Individual differences in coping response during social subjugation in adolescence predicted the development of aggression.	Shows an individual difference × social environment interaction in the development of aggression.	Longitudinal study (4)	Environmental manipulation (1d), hormone measurement (2c)
Mejia et al. (2002)	Male and female mice	A prenatal pharmacological inhibition of MAO increased aggression in adulthood.	Shows a relationship between prenatal biological environment and adult aggression.	Longitudinal study (4)	Pharmacological manipulation (1b)
Granger et al. (2001)	Male mice	High-aggression mice exposed to a postnatal immune stressor were less aggressive as adults.	Shows an early temperament × biological environment influence on adult aggression.	Longitudinal study (4)	Environmental manipulation (1d), personality and health (5)
Tuchscherer et al. (1998)	Male and female pigs	Socially dominant pigs had better immune function than socially subordinate pigs.	Shows a relationship between social dominance and immune function.	Personality and health (5)	Naturalistic observation (3)
Veenema et al. (2004)	Young adult male mice	Long-attack-latency mice had higher stress responsivity than short-attack-latency mice.	Shows a relationship between aggression and stress reactivity.	Personality and health (5)	Environmental manipulation (1d), gene expression measurement (2b)

Note. The numbers and letters in the "Primary benefit" and "Secondary benefit(s)" columns refer to the numbers and letters of subheads in the text section "The Benefits of Animal Research."

a. Hormone Manipulation

The ability to manipulate the presence or absence of hormones in animals has existed for a long time. The first formal endocrinology experiment was conducted in roosters by Arnold Berthold (1849/1944). Berthold found that when chickens were castrated during development, they developed into docile capons instead of normal roosters. These capons refrained from fighting with other males and failed to exhibit mating behavior. However, if the castrated capons were implanted with testes from other birds, they developed into normal roosters. Berthold had discovered the effect of the hormone we now know as testosterone on aggression and sexual behavior.

Hormone manipulations continue to be used today. Through techniques such as castration, injection, or capsule implantation, researchers are able to systematically study the relationships among hormones, biological processes, and behavior. In one recent study, rabbits were injected with subcutaneous testosterone propionate or a control substance (Briganti, Seta, Fontani, Lodi, & Lupo, 2003). All testosterone-treated rabbits increased in marking, digging, and defensive behaviors, but only the highest-ranking rabbits in each social group increased in aggressive behavior. This study showed that testosterone has an effect on aggression in rabbits, but that the effect is moderated by social rank.

In another study, female starlings were implanted with testosterone and placed back in their natural setting (Veiga, Vinuela, Cordero, Aparicio, & Polo, 2004). The testosterone-implanted females hatched more sons than the control females for up to 3 years after the treatment. In addition, the testosterone-treated females seemed to gain and maintain high social rank. These results suggest that the testosterone level of the mother has a direct impact on sex differentiation in offspring. In addition, testosterone may influence dominance among female starlings.

b. Pharmacological Manipulation

Advances in pharmacology have allowed scientists to develop synthetic chemicals that can either enhance (agonists) or block (antagonists) the functioning of neurotransmitters (e.g., serotonin) and hormones (e.g., testosterone) in animals. Such drugs have helped researchers examine the specific mechanisms by which neurotransmitters and hormones affect aggression and dominance.

In one study, hamsters injected with a vasopressin antagonist into the anterior hypothalamus decreased in aggression (Ferris & Delville, 1994), suggesting that vasopressin plays a role in the expression of aggressive behavior. In a follow-up study, researchers castrated hamsters and treated half of them with testosterone (Delville, Mansour, & Ferris, 1996a). Next, the researchers injected fluoxetine (a serotonin agonist) or vehicle (a control substance) into the testosterone-treated hamsters. Finally, vasopressin was injected into all testosterone-treated animals. The researchers found that fluoxetine inhibited the effects of vasopressin on aggression, indicating that serotonin may inhibit aggression by blocking vasopressin functioning.

Such studies demonstrate how pharmacological manipulations can be used to understand the biological mechanisms underlying individual differences in aggression and dominance. Moreover, the second study (Delville et al., 1996a) shows how a pharmacological manipulation (the serotonin agonist fluoxetine) can be combined with hormone manipulations (testosterone and vasopressin manipulations) to examine the interplay between neurotransmitters and hormones. Future research in animals is likely to combine multiple methodologies (e.g., genetic, hormone, and pharmacological manipulations) to test complex models of the relationships among genes, neurotransmitters, hormones, and environments. Personality psychologists can profit from such powerful methodologies.

c. Genetic Manipulation

Technological advances in molecular biology allow animal researchers to remove particular genes from, or insert them into, an animal's DNA. At this time the genetics of laboratory mice are relatively well understood, making them the primary target of genetic manipulation studies. Both knockout mice (those missing a specific gene) and transgenic mice (those in which a gene has been inserted) have been used to investigate the effects of genes on personality traits.

In one study, knockout mice lacking the gene for neuronal nitric oxide synthase (nNOS- mice) were more aggressive than wild-type (normal) mice (Nelson et al., 1995). This result suggests that nNOS is important for inhibiting aggression. A subsequent knockout study using nNOS- mice found that the increased aggression in the knockout mice could be attributed to disrupted serotonin functioning (Chiavegatto et al., 2001), suggesting that the effects of nitrous oxide on aggression was mediated by an impairment in serotonin.

In another study, researchers were interested in examining the effects of the estrogen receptor alpha gene on aggression (Ogawa, Lubah, Korach, & Pfaff, 1997). Previous research in mice had discovered that one pathway by which testosterone leads to aggression is through conversion into the hormone estradiol via the enzyme aromatase (e.g., Bowden & Brain, 1978). To find out which specific estrogen genes were involved, the scientists compared knockout mice lacking the gene for estrogen alpha receptors to wild-type mice. The knockout mice had average testosterone levels, but were less aggressive than the wild-type mice (Ogawa et al., 1997). These results suggest that the reduction in aggression was not due to reductions in testosterone, but rather to a disruption in estrogen receptor alpha functioning.

Together, these two studies show how discoveries regarding the relationships between genes and personality traits can be made by using knockout mice models. Such genetic manipulation studies suggest that the genes for nNOS and estrogen receptor alpha, along with several others (e.g., the monoamine oxidase A [MAO-A] gene, Cases et al., 1995; the serotonin 1B [5-HT$_{1B}$] receptor gene, Saudou et al., 1994) play a role in aggression. Because genes cannot be manipulated in humans, animal models afford unique opportunities to illuminate the genetic underpinnings of personality.

d. Environmental Manipulation

Relative to human researchers, animal researchers are able to exercise greater control over the environments of their subjects. Thus animal studies provide excellent opportunities to examine the role of environmental factors, such as rearing practice, in personality development. For example, in a study of female piglets, those individuals raised in poor environments (an indoor farrowing crate) were more aggressive as adults than individuals raised in enriching environments (an outdoor pasture with a half-open farrowing crate; De Jonge, Bokkers, Schouten, & Helmond, 1996). In a study of rhesus macaques, mother-reared individuals had higher social ranks as adults than peer-reared individuals (Bastian, Sponberg, Sponberg, Suomi, & Higley, 2003). Such experimental animal studies may inform our understanding of how early environments affect personality development in humans (whose rearing environments cannot be manipulated experimentally).

Benefit 2: Greater Ability to Measure Physiological Parameters

Animal studies afford unique opportunities to measure the physiological parameters that may underlie personality. This is because many of the techniques used to examine the biological events that lead to the expression of personality traits require decapitation and examination of brain areas, which are not possible in humans.

a. Measuring Hormone Receptor Density

Autoradiographic technology can be employed in animals to examine the density of hormone receptors in various parts of the brain. High densities in particular brain regions indicate important sites of action for the particular hormone under investigation. Using receptor binding density as an outcome variable, researchers can investigate how various hormones interact to influence personality.

In one study, Delville, Mansour and Ferris (1996b) castrated golden hamsters and implanted half of them with testosterone capsules. Vasopressin and testosterone had been previously linked to aggression, so the researchers decided to examine the effects of testosterone on vasopressin receptor binding. After sacrificing the animals, the researchers performed *in vitro* autoradiography. They found that castrated animals had a very low density of vasopressin receptor binding in the ventrolateral hypothalamus area of the brain. In addition, microinjections of vasopressin failed to increase aggression in castrated males. The authors concluded that testosterone may influence aggression by activating vasopressin receptors within the ventrolateral hypothalamus. Consistent with this result, DeLeon, Grimes, and Melloni (2002) found that anabolic–androgenic steroid treatment in adolescent male hamsters led to increased vasopressin receptor binding in the ventrolateral hypothalamus. In addition, these steroid-treated animals were more aggressive.

Without the ability to measure hormone receptor binding via autoradiography in animals, it would have been much more difficult to examine the testosterone–vasopressin receptor relationship in aggression. Furthermore, this research provides an excellent candidate model for how anabolic steroids may influence aggression in human adolescents through their effects on vasopressin receptors in key areas of the brain.

b. Measuring Gene Expression

The notion that genes and the environment exert independent effects on behavior is now considered simplistic and obsolete. Scientists now know that gene expression itself is influenced by both heredity and the environment (Hamer, 2002; Robinson, 2004). Variation in gene expression affects protein activity, brain processes, and ultimately behavior. Through the development of new genomic techniques using animal models, investigators can measure gene expression by quantifying the amount of messenger RNA (mRNA) produced by a particular gene. The ability to measure gene expression through mRNA allows researchers to consider complex, dynamic models of gene–behavior relationships. Not only can scientists investigate how environmental and hereditary factors interact to influence gene expression, but gene expression variation can also be examined as a predictor of subsequent brain processes and behavior (Gosling & Mollaghan, in press). Thanks to research conducted in animals, psychologists have begun to understand the interplay between hereditary and environmental influences on genetic activity and individual differences.

As an example, consider the animal research examining the effects of social defeat on aggression and the expression of serotonin genes. Social defeat and subordination have been associated with increased serotonin (Blanchard, Sakai, McEwen, Weiss, & Blanchard, 1993) and with decreased aggression (Huhman et al., 2003). Two substances, serotonin transporter (SERT) and MAO-A, are involved in the inactivation of serotonin (Filipenko, Beilana, Alekseyenko, Dolgov, & Kudryavtseva, 2002). Thus the effects of social defeat on SERT and MAO-A gene expression may provide clues about the genetic and biological processes that precede aggression. In one study, repeated exposure of adult male mice to social defeat resulted in greater expression of SERT and MAO-A mRNA than in either mice exposed to social victories or control mice (Filipenko et al., 2002). Thus it seems that social defeat induces the activation of the SERT and MAO-A genes. These findings suggest that the effects of social experiences (social defeats or victories) on aggression may be mediated by differential expression of various genes (SERT and MAO-A) within the serotonin system.

In other animal research, the effects of anabolic androgenic steroids on aggression have been linked to impaired functioning of the neurotransmitter gamma-aminobutyric acid (GABA) and its related genes (e.g., Miczek, Fish, & De Bold, 2003). When female mice underwent long-term testosterone therapy, they increased in aggression but decreased in mRNA expression for 5-alpha reductase type 1, a protein involved in GABA's functioning (Pinna, Costa, & Guidotti, 2005). This result suggests that testosterone treatment causes changes in gene expression, which in turn facilitate a disruption in the GABA neurotransmitter system and lead to increased aggression.

c. Other Opportunities for Physiological Measurement

In addition, animal studies offer several other opportunities for physiological measurement. For example, new imaging techniques allow animal researchers to measure neuronal activity in response to particular stimuli with a greater degree of precision than is possible in human functional magnetic resonance imaging (fMRI) studies (e.g., Whitlow, Freedland, & Porrino, 2002). Consequently, researchers can observe the specific brain areas and neurons involved in a particular biological process or behavior. Another advantage of animal studies is the ease with which neurotransmitter or hormone concentrations can be measured, because these data are normally collected through intrusive access to cerebrospinal fluid, blood, or specific brain areas.

Benefit 3: Greater Opportunities for Naturalistic Observations

The observational opportunities afforded by animal research are far greater than those available in human research. Relative to humans, animals can be observed for greater periods of time, in more detail, and in more contexts. These greater observational benefits are particularly true of captive animals, which can be closely monitored in some cases from conception until death. However, scientists can also observe wild animals living in natural habitats and collect voluminous behavioral and physiological data. Consequently, questions about how behavior and physiology change over time, across seasons, or in response to environmental triggers can be addressed. Equivalent opportunities for detailed and extensive naturalistic observations are rarer in human research. The relative ease with which naturalistic observations can be performed in animals means that more clues can be collected about the biological correlates and environmental factors that influence personality traits.

Research by Wingfield, Hegner, Dufty, and Ball (1990) in a variety of bird species illustrates the benefits of naturalistic observations of animals. These investigators recorded data on testosterone levels as well as aggressive and paternal behaviors in a wide variety of monogamous and polygynous bird species. Wingfield and colleagues proposed the "challenge hypothesis" to account for the relationship between testosterone levels and aggressive behavior in birds. The challenge hypothesis posits that fluctuations in testosterone levels during the breeding season are more closely related to aggressive behavior than to sexual behavior. Specifically, testosterone levels seem to rise as the mating season commences but peak during periods of intermale competition, suggesting that the increases in testosterone levels facilitate aggression. In addition, this theory suggests that testosterone only relates to aggression when there is competition over mates or territory. Thanks to Wingfield and colleagues' research in birds, the challenge hypothesis has been studied and validated in other animal species (e.g., male chimpanzees; Muller & Wrangham, 2004). Unfortunately, this hypothesis has been overwhelmingly overlooked by human researchers of testosterone and dominance (e.g., Mazur & Booth, 1998).

Other researchers have also profited from the naturalistic observational opportunities afforded by animal studies. By studying freely roaming baboons living in the Masai Mara National Reserve in Kenya, Virgin and Sapolsky (1997) uncovered links among testosterone levels, glucocorticoid levels, social status, and aggression. These researchers found that when the status hierarchy was stable, subordinate baboons had elevated glucocorticoid levels and suppressed testosterone levels, relative to dominant baboons. However, they also found individual differences in aggressive behavior and stress responses among subordinate baboons. The subordinate baboons that aggressed against other baboons after losing a fight had higher testosterone levels and lower glucocorticoid levels than did the ones that did not aggress after losing. This finding suggests that individual differences in aggression affect stress responses (Virgin & Sapolsky, 1997). These naturalistic observations shed light on the relationships between endocrinological patterns and individual differences in aggression. Moreover, the finding that displaced aggression is related to lower stress hormone levels suggests that social status and variations in aggression may have health implications for humans.

Benefit 4: Shorter Life Span of Animals

Longitudinal studies in humans bear heavy financial costs, can have high dropout rates, and may require waiting years or decades to answer the research questions of interest. Due to the shorter life span of many animal species, it is possible to conduct longitudinal studies that yield important insights in a timely manner and at a fraction of the cost of equally comprehensive human studies. Combined with the other benefits mentioned above, researchers can use animal studies to examine how genes, physiological variables, and the environment influence the development of personality.

For example, one longitudinal study examined how estradiol and testosterone hormone treatments influenced adult aggression in female zebra finches (Adkins-Regan, 1999). Half of the subjects were treated with estradiol for the first 14 days of life. As adults (just 100 days after hatching), the subjects were implanted with testosterone or an empty implant. The females that received neonatal estradiol treatment coupled with adult testosterone treatment were the most aggressive. These results indicate that adult aggression is increased by early-life estradiol treatment and is activated later in life with adult testosterone treatment. Moreover, the researchers were able to conduct this study in a matter of months, whereas an analogous study in humans would have taken years (even in the unlikely event that it had been approved by an institutional review board).

Other research has examined the effects of social subjugation in adolescent hamsters on the development of aggression. To induce social subjugation, male hamsters were exposed to an aggressive adult for several days during adolescence and were tested for aggressive behavior in later stages of development (Wommack, Taravosh-Lahn, David, & Delville, 2003). This form of social subjugation during adolescence was found to accelerate the development of aggressive behaviors. In another study, those hamsters that displayed fewer submissive behaviors during social subjugation in adolescence became aggressive relatively early in life (Wommack & Delville, 2003). These findings reveal that the ontogeny of aggression is influenced by experiences of social subjugation in adolescence.

In yet another study, prenatal pharmacological manipulations were conducted to assess their influence on the expression of aggressive behavior of male and female mice. The researchers found that a prenatal pharmacological inhibition of MAO increased aggressive behavior in adulthood (Mejia, Ervin, Baker, & Palmour, 2002). These results are consistent with other studies linking MAO to aggression and suggest that perinatal MAO exposure may have an impact on the organization of the nervous system, which in turn influences aggression (Mejia et al., 2002).

Benefit 5: Greater Opportunity to Examine Personality–Health Relationships

One important application of research in personality is to understand the role of personality traits in health. Animal research is particularly well suited for investigating personality–health links, because of the greater experimental control (Benefit 1) and the greater opportunities to measure physiological parameters (Benefit 2) it affords. Not only can animal models reveal relationships between personality traits and health factors, but they can also detail the psychobiological mechanisms and developmental processes that underlie these relationships (e.g., Capitanio, Mendoza, & Baroncelli, 1999). Moreover, animal research can help investigators devise and test preliminary intervention programs that may improve health and well-being for at-risk individuals.

In one study, researchers investigated the relationship between aggression and three biological processes related to stress adaptation. Two lines of mice, a high-aggression line and a low-aggression line, were bred and tested for hypothalamic–pituitary–adrenal (HPA) axis functioning, hippocampal cell proliferation, and serotonin system functioning under typical and stressful conditions (Veenema, Koolhaas, & de Kloet, 2004). HPA axis functioning in response to an acute stressor (forced swimming for 5 minutes) became hyperactive in low-aggression mice, but not in high-aggression mice. In addition, low-aggression mice experienced a 50% reduction in hippocampal cell proliferation after the acute stressor, as well as a reduced increase in serotonin metabolism. Finally, exposure to a chronic stressor led to long-term rises in corticosterone levels in low-aggression individuals, but not in high-aggression individuals. These findings suggest that low-aggression mice have higher stress reactivity than high-aggression mice. In light of these results, the authors concluded that low aggression is predictive of a maladaptive coping style in mice, which may have implications for mood disorders in humans (Veenema et al., 2004).

A second study examined the effects of social status and aggression on immunity in pigs. Groups of pigs were placed together with unfamiliar pigs and tested for aggressive behavior and social dominance (Tuchscherer, Birger, Tuchscherer, & Kanitz, 1998). The results showed that socially dominant pigs had higher lymphocyte proliferation than subordinate pigs, suggesting that social dominance is associated with enhanced immune function.

Summary of the Benefits of Animal Research

In this section, we have argued that studies in animals afford five major benefits to personality researchers. First, the greater experimental control available in animal methodologies allows scientists to examine the genes, hormones, neurotransmitters, brain processes, and environments that influence traits. Second, the greater ability to measure physiological parameters in animals can yield insights into the biological processes that influence trait expression. Third, naturalistic observational studies of animals may inform us about the physiological correlates as well as the environmental conditions that are related to individual-difference variables. Fourth, the shorter life span of animals enables researchers to conduct relatively efficient longitudinal studies. Fifth, animal research affords greater opportunities to study the relationship between personality and health.

Thanks to these advantages, we believe that animal research can contribute greatly to our knowledge about human personality, particularly about the biological underpinnings of personality traits. We have illustrated this point with animal studies of aggression and dominance, but researchers interested in other traits are equally likely to profit from animal research.

ANIMAL AND HUMAN PERSONALITY RESEARCH: A TWO-WAY STREET

The focus of this chapter has been on what human researchers can learn from animal studies. However, this should not be taken to suggest that this process is a one-way street with all the useful information going from animal studies to human studies. The greatest progress will be made only if each field continues to draw on the lessons emerging from the other field.

There are many lessons emerging from the literature on human personality that can be usefully translated to the animal domain. For example, the principles of personality measurement are much more fully developed in human research, so animal studies can benefit from the hard-won lessons learned in that field. These include drawing on the effectiveness of rating (vs. coding) methods and the importance of attending to basic psychometric principles, such as construct validity (Cronbach & Meehl, 1955); for example, one review of the literature on dog temperament showed that studies of dogs often attended to convergent validity, but rarely paid attention to discriminant validity (Jones & Gosling, in press).

Another way animal researchers might profitably benefit from human research is in the overall approach taken to individual differences. In many of the studies reviewed here, the animal researchers examined the links between various biological factors and personality traits by changing the traits via environmental or biological manipulations. At the same time, the researchers paid less attention to natural variation in traits, which could also have informed their studies. This emphasis on manipulated differences reflects the standard perspective in the experimental animal literature, but there is no reason why these very same researchers could not shift their focus slightly to also draw on the naturally existing differences among animals. Such a shift in perspective would also broaden the range of studies on the biological bases of personality to include the many animal studies that do not use experimental designs.

LOOKING FORWARD

Seventy-five years ago, Charles Stockard (1931) argued that animal research would help illuminate common biological systems underlying human and animal personality. Today, we know that human and animal personality traits do have common biological underpinnings, as Stockard believed. Furthermore, thanks to modern technological advances, the opportunities to examine these commonalities are greater than ever. With so much knowledge to be gained, it is time to rediscover the long-neglected bridges between personality psychology and animal behavior.

ACKNOWLEDGMENTS

Preparation of this chapter was supported by National Science Foundation Grant No. BCS0423405. We are grateful to Simine Vazire, Amanda Jones, and Yvon Delville for their helpful comments.

REFERENCES

Adkins-Regan, E. (1999). Testosterone increases singing and aggression but not male-typical sexual partner preference in early estrogen treated female zebra finches. *Hormones and Behavior, 35,* 63–70.

Bastian, M. L., Sponberg, A. C., Sponberg, A. C., Suomi, S. J., & Higley, J. D. (2003). Long-term effects of infant rearing condition on the acquisition of dominance rank in juvenile and adult rhesus macaques (*Macaca mulatta*). *Developmental Psychobiology, 42,* 44–51.

Berthold, A. A. (1944). Transplantation of testes. (D. P. Quiring, Trans.). *Bulletin of the History of Medicine, 16,* 42–46. (Original work published 1849)

Blanchard, D. C., Sakai, R. R., McEwen, B., Weiss, S. M., & Blanchard, R. J. (1993). Subordination stress: Behavioural, brain, and neuroendocrine correlates. *Behavioural Brain Research, 58,* 113–121.

Bowden, N. J., & Brain, P. F. (1978). Blockade of testosterone-maintained intermale fighting in albino laboratory mice by an aromatization inhibitor. *Physiology and Behavior, 20,* 543–546.

Briganti, F., Seta, D., Fontani, G., Lodi, L., & Lupo, C. (2003). Behavioral effects of testosterone in relation to social rank in the male rabbit. *Aggressive Behavior, 29,* 269–278.

Capitanio, J. P., Mendoza, S. P., & Baroncelli, S. (1999). The relationship of personality dimensions in adult male rhesus macaques to progression of simian immuno-deficiency virus disease. *Brain, Behavior, and Immunity, 13,* 138–154.

Cases, O., Seif, I., Grimsby, J., Gaspar, P., Chen, K., Pournin, S., et al. (1995). Aggressive behavior and altered amounts of brain serotonin and norepinephrine in mice lacking MAOA. *Science, 262,* 1763–1766.

Chiavegatto, S., Dawson, V. L., Mamounas, L. A., Koliatsos, V. E., Dawson, T. M., & Nelson, R. J. (2001). Brain serotonin dysfunction accounts for aggression in male mice lacking neuronal nitric oxide synthase. *Proceedings of the National Academy of Sciences USA, 98,* 1277–1281.

Cronbach, L. J., & Meehl, P. E. (1955). Construct validity in psychological tests. *Psychological Bulletin, 52,* 281–302.

De Jonge, F. H., Bokkers, E. A., Schouten, W. G., & Helmond, F. A. (1996). Rearing piglets in a poor environment: Developmental aspects of social stress in pigs. *Physiology and Behavior, 60,* 389–396.

DeLeon, K. R., Grimes, J. M., & Melloni, R. H., Jr. (2002). Repeated anabolic–androgenic steroid treatment during adolescence increases vasopressin V(1A) receptor binding in Syrian hamsters: correlation with offensive aggression. *Hormones and Behavior, 42,* 182–191.

Delville, Y., Mansour, K. M., & Ferris, C. F. (1996a). Serotonin blocks vasopressin-facilitated offensive aggression: Interactions within the ventrolateral hypothalamus of golden hamsters. *Physiology and Behavior, 59,* 813–816.

Delville, Y., Mansour, K. M., & Ferris, C. F. (1996b). Testosterone facilitates aggression by modulating vasopressin receptors in the hypothalamus. *Physiology and Behavior, 60,* 25–29.

Domjan, M., & Purdy, J. E. (1995). Animal research in psychology: More than meets the eye of the general psychology student. *American Psychologist, 50,* 496–503.

Ferris, C. F., & Delville, Y. (1994). Vasopressin and serotonin interactions in the control of agonistic behavior. *Psychoneuroendocrinology, 19,* 593–601.

Filipenko, M. L., Beilina, A. G., Alekseyenko, O. V., Dolgov, V. V., & Kudryavtseva, N. N. (2002). Repeated experience of social defeats increases serotonin transporter and monoamine oxidase A mRNA levels in raphe nuclei of male mice. *Neuroscience Letters, 321,* 25–28.

Gilbert, D. T., Fiske, S. T., & Lindzey, G. (1998). *The handbook of social psychology* (4th ed.). Oxford: Oxford University Press.

Gosling, S. D. (2001). From mice to men: What can we learn about personality from animal research? *Psychological Bulletin, 127,* 45–86.

Gosling, S. D., & John, O. P. (1999). Personality dimensions in non-human animals: A cross-species review. *Current Directions in Psychological Science, 8,* 69–75.

Gosling, S. D., Kwan, V. S. Y., & John, O. P. (2003). A dog's got personality: A cross-species comparative approach to evaluating personality judgments. *Journal of Personality and Social Psychology, 85,* 1161–1169.

Gosling, S. D., Lilienfeld, S. O., & Marino, L. (2003). Personality. In D. Maestripieri (Ed.), *Primate psychology: The mind and behavior of human and nonhuman primates* (pp. 254–288). Cambridge, MA: Harvard University Press.

Gosling, S. D., & Mollaghan, D. M. (in press). Animal research in social psychology: A bridge to functional genomics and other unique research opportunities. In P. A. M. van Lange (Ed.), *Bridging social psychology: Benefits of trans-disciplinary approaches.* Mahwah NJ: Erlbaum.

Gosling, S. D., & Vazire, S. (2002). Are we barking up the right tree?: Evaluating a comparative approach to personality. *Journal of Research in Personality, 36,* 607–614.

Granger, D. A., Hood, K. E., Dreschel, N. A., Sergeant, E., & Likos, A. (2001). Developmental effects of early immune stress on aggressive, socially reactive, and inhibited behaviors. *Development and Psychopathology, 13,* 599–610.

Hamer, D. (2002). Genetics: Rethinking behavior genetics. *Science, 298,* 71–72.

Hebb, D. O., & Thompson, R. W. (1954). The social significance of animals studies. In G. Lindzey (Ed.), *Handbook of social psychology* (pp. 532–561). Cambridge, MA: Addison-Wesley.

Holekamp, K. E., & Smale, L. (1998). Dispersal status influences hormones and behavior in the male spotted hyena. *Hormones and Behavior, 33,* 205–216.

Huhman, K. L., Solomon, M. B., Janicki, M., Harmon, A. C., Lin, S. M., Israel, J. E., et al. (2003). Conditioned defeat in male and female Syrian hamsters. *Hormones and Behavior, 44,* 293–299.

Jones, A. C., & Gosling, S. D. (in press). Temperament and personality in dogs (*Canis familiaris*): A review and evaluation of past research. *Applied Animal Behavior Science.*

Kenrick, D. T., & Funder, D. C. (1988). Profiting from controversy: Lessons from the person–situation debate. *American Psychologist, 43,* 23–34.

King, J. E., Weiss, A., & Farmer, K. H. (2005). A chimpanzee (*Pan troglodytes*) analogue of cross-national generalization of personality structure: Zoological parks and an African sanctuary. *Journal of Personality, 73,* 389–410.

Lesch, K. P., Meyer, J., Glatz, K., Flügge, G., Hinney, A., Hebebrand, J., et al. (1997). The 5–HT transporter gene-linked polymorphic region (5–HTTLPR) in evolutionary perspective: Alternative biallelic variation in rhesus monkeys. *Journal of Neural Transmission, 104,* 1259–1266.

Mazur, A., & Booth, A. (1998). Testosterone and dominance in men. *Behavioral and Brain Sciences, 21,* 353–397.

Mejia, J. M., Ervin, F. R., Baker, G. B., & Palmour, R. M. (2002). Monoamine oxidase inhibition during brain development induces pathological aggressive behavior in mice. *Biological Psychiatry, 52,* 811–821.

Miczek, K. A., Fish, E. W., & De Bold, J. F. (2003). Neurosteroids, GABA$_A$ receptors, and escalated aggressive behavior. *Hormones and Behavior, 44,* 242–257.

Muehlenbein, M. P., Watts, D. P., & Whitten, P. L. (2004). Dominance rank and fecal testosterone levels in adult male chimpanzees (*Pan troglodytes schweinfurthii*) at Ngogo, Kibale National Park, Uganda. *American Journal of Primatology, 64,* 71–82.

Muller, M. N., & Wrangham, R. W. (2004). Dominance, aggression and testosterone in wild chimpanzees: A test of the "challenge hypothesis." *Animal Behaviour, 67,* 113–123.

Murchison, C. (1935). *A handbook of social psychology.* Worcester, MA: Clark University Press.

Nelson, R. J., Demas, G. E., Huang, P. L., Fishman, M. C., Dawson, V. L., Dawson, T. M., et al. (1995). Behavioural abnormalities in male mice lacking neuronal nitric oxide synthase. *Nature, 378,* 383–386.

Newman, T. K., Syagailo, Y. V., Barr, C. S., Wendland, J. R., Champoux, M., Graessle, M., et al. (2005). Monoamine oxidase A gene promoter variation and rearing experience influences aggressive behavior in rhesus monkeys. *Biological Psychiatry, 57,* 167–172.

Nomura, M., Durbak, L., Chan, J., Smithies, O., Gustafsson, J. A., Korach, K. S., et al. (2002). Genotype/age interactions on aggressive behavior in gonadally intact estrogen receptor beta knockout (betaERKO) male mice. *Hormones and Behavior, 41,* 288–296.

Ogawa, S., Lubahn, D. B., Korach, K. S., & Pfaff, D. W. (1997). Behavioral effects of estrogen receptor gene disruption in male mice. *Proceedings of the National Academy of Sciences USA, 94,* 1476–1481.

Oliveira, R. F., Lopes, M., Carneiro, L. A., & Canario, A. V. (2001). Watching fights raises fish hormone levels. *Nature, 409,* 475.

Pinna, G., Costa, E., & Guidotti, A. (2005). Changes in brain testosterone and allopregnanolone biosynthesis elicit aggressive behavior. *Proceedings of the National Academy of Sciences USA, 102,* 2135–2140.

Robinson, G. E. (2004). Genomics: Beyond nature and nurture. *Science, 304,* 397–399.

Saudou, F., Amara, D. A., Dierich, A., LeMeur, M., Ramboz, S., Segu, L., et al. (1994). Enhanced aggressive behavior in mice lacking 5–HT1B receptor. *Science, 265,* 1875–1878.

Stockard, C. R. (1931). *The physical basis of personality.* New York: Norton.

Tuchscherer, M., Birger, P., Tuchscherer, A., & Kanitz, E. (1998). Effects of social status after mixing on immune, metabolic, and endocrine responses in pigs. *Physiology and Behavior, 64,* 353–360.

Vazire, S., & Gosling, S. D. (2003). Bridging psychology and biology with animal research. *American Psychologist, 5,* 407–408.

Veenema, A. H., Koolhaas, J. M., & de Kloet, E. R. (2004). Basal and stress-induced differences in HPA axis, 5–HT responsiveness, and hippocampal cell proliferation in two mouse lines. *Annals of the New York Academy of Sciences, 1018,* 255–265.

Veiga, J. P., Vinuela, J., Cordero, P. J., Aparicio, J. M., & Polo, V. (2004). Experimentally increased testosterone affects social rank and primary sex ratio in the spotless starling. *Hormones and Behavior, 46,* 47–53.

Virgin, C. E., Jr., & Sapolsky, R. M. (1997). Styles of male social behavior and endocrine correlates among low-ranking baboons. *American Journal of Primatology, 42,* 25–39.

Whitlow, C. T., Freedland, C. S., & Porrino, L. J. (2002). Metabolic mapping of the time-dependent effects of delta 9–tetrahydrocannabinol administration in the rat. *Psychopharmacology, 161,* 129–136.

Wiggins, J. S. (1979). A psychological taxonomy of trait-descriptive terms: The interpersonal domain. *Journal of Personality and Social Psychology, 37,* 395–412.

Wingfield, J. C., Hegner, R. E., Dufty, A. M., Jr., & Ball, G. F. (1990). The "challenge hypothesis": Theoretical implications for patterns of testosterone secretion, mating systems, and breeding strategies. *American Naturalist, 136,* 829–846.

Wommack, J. C., & Delville, Y. (2003). Repeated social stress and the development of agonistic behavior: Individual differences in coping responses in male golden hamsters. *Physiology and Behavior, 80,* 303–308.

Wommack, J. C., Taravosh-Lahn, K., David, J. T., & Delville, Y. (2003). Repeated exposure to social stress alters the development of agonistic behavior in male golden hamsters. *Hormones and Behavior, 43,* 229–236.

Index

Addiction
    molecular genetic correlates, 42
    neurophysiology, 24
Adenyl cyclase, 273, 274
Adrenocorticotropic hormone
    5-HT receptor action, 285
    stress response, 203–204
Affiliation
    appetitive phase, 64
    individual differences, 70, 72–74
    mu-opiate mediation, 82–85
    neurobehavioral systems, 63–66
    neurobiology, 68–70
    personality model, 61–62
Agency
    goal acquisition and, 63
    incentive motivation and, 64
    individual differences, 70
    neurobehavioral systems, 63–66
    personality model, 61–63
Aggressive behavior
    animal studies, 386–398, 409–410,
        431, 437–438, 439–441, 442
    brain-derived neurotrophic factor in,
        397
    classification, 386
    clinical conceptualization, 385
    dominance behavior and, 431
    emotional component, 386
    genetic studies, 389–390, 392–397
    hormonal function, 436, 438–439,
        440, 441, 442

maternal, 386, 389
measurement, 387–389
neural cell adhesion molecule in, 397
nitric oxide and, 392–396, 437
opportunities for research, 398
predatory, 386
purpose, 385
serotonergic system in, 390–392, 396,
    397
social defeat and, 439–440, 442
stress response and, 443
submissive behavior and, 385
territorial, 386
See also Antisocial behavior
Aging
    cognitive changes, 159, 160
    emotional functioning and, 160, 161,
        162, 164, 165, 166, 173–175
    frontal cortical functions and, 160
    memory processes and, 168–171
    normal neurophysiological changes,
        159–160, 162
    threat response and, 171–172
Agoraphobia
    depression and, 278–279
    personality trait predictors of, 233–
        234, 266
Amygdala
    aging effects, 162
    anatomy, 162
    in anxiety, 20–21, 22–23
    in behavioral inhibition system, 18–23

Amygdala *(cont.)*
in depression, 366, 367–368
in emotion processing, 96, 98–100,
    162, 163, 167–168, 173, 174, 209,
    299–300, 302–307
5-HTTLPR reactivity, 302–307
in memory encoding, 167–168
in orgasm, 197–198
prefrontal cortex interactions, 300,
    307
in psychopathy, 329
self-stimulation behavior and, 119
in serotonergic system, 299–300
sex differences in, 197, 198, 209
in sexual responding, 187, 192, 195–
    197
stress response, 207, 305
threat response, 162, 300
Anger, 135
Animal studies, 3
aggression, 386–398, 431, 437–438,
    439–441, 442
cross-species trait commonalities,
    429–430
environmental factors, 438
evoked potentials augmenting and
    reducing patterns, 45–46, 47
future prospects, 444–445
genetic manipulation, 437–438, 439–
    440
Gray's research, 7–8
hormone manipulation, 436
individual differences research, 444
mouse model, 386, 437
naturalistic observation, 440–441
personality research, 25, 428–430
pharmacological manipulation, 436–437
rationale, 427–428, 431, 436–444
trends, 427–428
See also Chimpanzee behavior and
    personality
Anterior cingulate cortex
activation of, as indication of
    personality trait, 100–101
in attentional processing, 96
in avoidance behaviors, 20
in depression, 366, 367, 373
in emotion processing, 163, 166, 173
in extraversion neurobiology, 97
in sexual responding, 189
stress response, 211–212

Anticipation
extraversion and, 125–128
gain size and, 123–124
of loss vs. gain, 123, 125–127
neurophysiology, 119–124, 125–128
Antidepressant drugs
5-HT receptor regulation of effects,
    280, 282–283
*See also specific drug; specific drug
    type*
Antisocial behavior
assessment, 318–319
environmental etiology, 324, 326,
    327–328
genetic studies, 319–327
opportunities for research, 327–330
in psychopathy, 317–318
therapeutic interventions, 330
See also Aggressive behavior; Conduct
    problems
Antisocial personality disorder, 47
clinical features, 317
sex differences in risk of, 205
Anxiety, 2–3
amygdala role in, 20–21, 22–23
anxiety sensitivity, 346–347
behavioral inhibition system and, 11–
    14, 18–19, 28
brain activity patterns, 133, 134–135,
    141–142
clinical conceptualization, 7
depression and, 134–135, 238–239,
    253–254
developmental significance, 335
epidemiology, 225–227, 335
extraversion and, 252–268
fear and, 15, 19
gene–environment correlations, 339–
    340, 342
gene–environment interactions, 340–
    344
genetic epidemiology, 236–237, 240
genetic factors, 259–264, 267, 268,
    275, 335–338, 348–349
Gray's research, 7–23
5-HT receptor regulation in, 274,
    276–279, 281–283
neuroticism and, 228–229, 252–268
personality trait predictors of, 232–
    234, 251–268
psychopathy and, 28–29

sensation seeking and, 252, 254
sex differences, 204–205, 267–268
state and trait associations, 347
See also Generalized anxiety
Anxiety stimuli, 16–17
Anxiolytic drugs
behavioral inhibition model, 9–11,
21
in defining anxiety, 7
genetic factors in action of, 279–281
Gray's research, 7, 8–11
neurophysiology, 11, 12–13, 14–16,
21, 274
reward–punishment model, 8–9
Appetitive motivation in sexual
responding, 196–197
Appetitive phase of goal acquisition, 63,
64, 66, 70, 120
Approach behaviors
approach–avoidance model of
personality, 136–137
behavioral activation/approach
system, 23–24, 26–27
brain activity patterns, 135, 136–139,
140–141, 150–151
Arousal
in emotional experience, 161
in emotional memory encoding, 167–
168
in models of extraversion, 118–119,
127–128
in models of neuroticism, 118–119
neurophysiology, 122–124
sensation seeking psychophysiology,
42–43
sex differences in sexual responding,
185–197
Associative learning, 74–75
Attentional processes
emotional functioning and, 171, 172,
175
extraversion and, 97–98
neurobiology, 96
Stroop task assessment, 95–96
Attention-deficit/hyperactivity disorder,
47
gene–sex interactions, 106
Attributional style, depression and, 344–
345
Autonomic nervous system in
neuroticism, 229–230

Avoidance behaviors
in behavioral inhibition system, 10–11
brain activity patterns, 135, 136–139,
140–141, 150–151
defensive direction, 17, 19–20
model of anxiolytic drug effects, 8–9
models of personality, 136–137, 230–
231
neurophysiology, 20, 42

B

Basal ganglia in emotion processing, 208
Behavioral activation/approach system,
23–24
neurobiology, 67
personality theory and, 26–27
Behavioral facilitation system, 24
Behavioral inhibition system
fight–flight response and, 17, 20
goal conflict in, 17, 18, 21, 22
inputs and outputs, 16–17, 22
model of anxiolytic drug effects, 9–
11, 21
neurophysiology, 11–14, 17–23
parallel distributed systems in, 21–22,
23
personality theory, 25–27, 117, 230
psychopathy and, 28–29
trait anxiety and, 28
Behavioral systems, 63–66
Benzodiazepines, 13, 15, 21
Bipolar disorder, sensation seeking and,
48
Borderline personality disorder, 47
sex differences in risk of, 205
Brain-derived neurotrophic factor, 397
Brainstem in emotional processing, 208
Buspirone, 15

C

Callous–unemotional traits
assessment, 318–319
conduct problems and, 325–327
genetic studies, 322–327
neurophysiology, 329
in psychopathy, 317–318
research needs, 327–330

Cardiovascular function in emotional
    experience, 162
Cerebellum
  in emotional processing, 208
  sex differences, 207
Children and adolescents, 3
  cognitive processes in depression,
    360–362
  depression risk, 354, 355–357, 361–
    362, 365–366, 368
  early manifestations of antisocial
    behavior, 317–318
  emotional disorders in, 335
  neurophysiology of depression, 364–366
  psychopathy assessment, 318–319
Chimpanzee behavior and personality
  dominance behaviors, 413, 414, 415–
    422, 416–422, 430, 431
  environmental factors, 411–412, 414,
    415–422
  genetic research, 410–415, 420, 421–
    422
  happiness research, 410, 414–422
  human relevance, 407, 422
  research approach, 408–410, 430
  social structure and interaction, 407–
    408
  territorial defense, 407–408
Cingulate cortex
  in emotion processing, 208
  sex differences, 207, 208, 214
  stress response, 211–213, 214
Circumplex model of psychopathology,
    134
Cocaine, 213
Cognitive functioning
  in depression, 359–362, 370
  emotional functioning and, 160, 163–
    164, 344
  normal aging, 159, 160
  psychopathy and, 329
  temperament-based brain activation
    patterns, 138–139
Conditioning
  contextual facilitation, 79
  model of anxiolytic drug effects, 8–9
  role of emotion in, 116–117
Conduct problems
  assessment, 318–319
  callous–unemotional traits and, 325–
    327

clinical features of conduct disorder,
    317
  neurophysiology, 329
  in psychopathy, 317
  research needs, 327–330
  See also Antisocial behavior
Consummatory phase of goal
    acquisition, 63, 64–66, 70
Coronary artery disease, 209
Cortical evoked potentials
  augmenting and reducing patterns,
    44–45
  biochemical correlates, 50
  sensation seeking and, 44–47, 50, 52–
    53
Corticotropin-releasing factor in stress
    response, 46
Cortisol
  in depression, 359, 362–366, 370
  5-HT receptor action, 285
  in sensation seeking
    psychophysiology, 51, 52
  stress response, 203–204, 363
Cultural influences
  determinants of sexual behavior,
    186
  in personality, 39
Cyclic adenosine monophosphate, 104

D

DAT gene, 105–106
Defensive direction, 17, 19–20
Dehydroepiandrosterone, 365
Depression
  among children and adolescents, 354,
    355–357
  anxiety and, 134–135, 238–239, 253–
    254
  attributional style and, 344–345
  clinical features, 354–355
  cognitive functioning in, 359–362,
    370
  comorbidity, 253–254, 278–279
  developmental significance, 335
  early-onset, 354
  emotion regulation and, 357–358
  epidemiology, 225–227, 335, 354
  gene–environment correlations, 339–
    340, 342

gene–environment interactions, 340–344

genetic epidemiology, 234–236

genetic factors, 106, 240, 259–264, 267, 268, 275, 335–338, 348–349

genetic modulation of treatment effects, 279–281

5-HT receptor regulation in, 276–279, 281, 283

intergenerational transmission, 356–357

neurophysiology, 133, 134–135, 141–142, 206, 358, 359, 362–369, 370–374

in parents, 355–357, 361–362, 365, 369–370

personality trait predictors of, 232–233, 251–268

research needs, 374–375

risk factors, 355–368

sensation seeking and, 252, 254

sex differences, 206, 267–268, 368–374

See also Major depressive disorder

Diathesis–stress model of depression, 357, 363

Dihydroxyphenylacetic acid, 47

Dominance behaviors, 61, 413, 414, 415, 416–422, 430, 431

Dopaminergic system

in behavioral approach system, 24

in extraverted behavior, 74–82, 103–104

in incentive motivation, 67, 75, 119–121

individual differences, 70–72

monoamine oxidase and, 48

normal aging, 160

opiate reward system, 68–69, 70–72

in positive arousal, 122

self-stimulation behavior and, 119

sensation seeking and, 42, 46–47, 47, 48, 49–50, 52

stress response, 46

substance use and, 24, 67

Dorsal ascending noradrenergic bundle, 13

Dorsal striatum in stress response, 207

Dorsolateral prefrontal cortex

in depression, 367–368

lateralization of brain activity in

emotional processing, 142–143, 147, 148–150

normal aging, 160, 164

DRD4 gene, 42, 52

extraversion and, 101–102, 103–104

impulsivity and, 105–106

orienting behavior and, 104–105

Dysthymia, 266

personality trait predictors of, 233–234

E

Electroencephalography

hemodynamic imaging and, 142–143

lateralized brain activity, 133, 141–144

Eltoprazine, 391

Emotional functioning

in aggression, 386

approach–avoidance model of personality, 137–138

approach–avoidance motivation and, 135

assessment, 161

attentional processes in, 171, 172, 175

brain activation patterns, 133, 134–135, 141–143, 147–150, 207

cardiovascular function and, 162

changes in aging, 160, 161, 162, 164, 165, 166, 173–175

cognitive functioning and, 160, 163–164, 344

components, 161

in conditioning, 116–117

definition of emotions, 161

depression model, 357–358

evolutionary theory, 171

extraversion and, 94, 96–97, 118–119, 252

facial expression response, 98–100, 103–104, 162, 171–174, 300

hemodynamic studies, 143–144

5-HT in, 298, 343–344

imaging genomics, 302–307

in incentive motivation, 67

memory and, 166–171, 175, 209

neurophysiology, 119, 142–143, 160, 161, 162–164, 165–166, 176, 299–300

Emotional functioning *(cont.)*
    neuroticism and, 118, 119, 229–230,
        252
    obstacles to genetic research, 298–
        299
    personality theory, 25
    reappraisal in, 165
    regulation, 164–166
    research needs, 175–176
    sex differences in brain activation
        patterns, 207–209, 213–216
    sexual responding and, 194
    stress response, 164–165, 206, 213–
        216
    substance abuse relapse risk and,
        210–213
    suppression of emotions, 165
Estradiol, sensation seeking and, 51
Estrogen, 437–438
Evolutionary theory, 37
    of behavioral systems, 63
    of emotional functioning, 171
    of individual differences, 421
    of individual subjective well-being,
        421–422
    of sex differences in sexual behavior,
        185–186, 188
    of territorial defense, 407–408
Expectancies
    in behavioral inhibition system, 10–
        11
    See also Anticipation
Extraversion, 2, 3
    animal studies, 430
    anticipation and, 125–128
    assessment instruments, 117, 118
    attentional processing and, 97–98
    behavioral inhibition system and, 25–
        26
    brain activity patterns, 139–140
    clinical conceptualization, 251
    contextual facilitation, 79–82
    cortical arousal theory, 117
    emotional functioning in, 94, 96–97,
        118–119, 252
    genetic epidemiology, 237–238
    genomic variation, 101–104
    individual differences, 72–74, 124–
        127
    interpersonal nature, 61
    models of personality, 60–63

    mood and anxiety disorders and,
        252–268
    neurobehavioral model, 74–82, 103–106
    neuroimaging studies, 94–100, 103–
        104, 124–127
    neuroticism and, 229, 230–231
    as predictor of psychological distress,
        232–233
    psychological elements, 94–95
    sensation seeking and, 252

F

Fear
    amygdala role in, 299–300
    anxiety and, 15, 19, 346–347
    neurophysiology, 18, 98
    psychopathy and, 29
Fight–flight(–freeze) system
    behavioral inhibition system and, 17,
        20
    Gray's model, 23
    neurophysiology, 16
    panic disorder and, 15
    psychoticism and, 26, 27
    sex differences and, 204
Flibanserin, 280
Fluvoxamine, 280
Frontal brain asymmetries
    approach–avoidance model of
        personality, 135, 136–139, 140–
        141, 150–151
    clinical significance, 141
    cognitive functions, 138–139
    current understanding, 134–141
    in emotional processing, 133, 134,
        141–142, 147–150
    extraversion–neuroticism model of
        personality, 139–140
    hemodynamic imaging and analysis,
        133, 141, 142, 144–150
    opportunities for research, 150–151
    personality correlates, 133, 134, 135–
        136, 150–151
    in psychopathology, 133, 134–135,
        141, 142
    sex differences in emotional
        processing, 208
Fusiform gyrus in extraversion
    neurobiology, 98

G

Gambling, 47
  dopaminergic system and, 42, 50
Gamma-aminobutyric acid, 216
  in aggression, 440
  in anxiolytic drug action, 15, 21
Generalized anxiety
  anxiolytic drug action, 15
  biosocial approach, 37–39
  genetic epidemiology, 236–237
  personality trait predictors of, 233–234
Genetics
  aggression studies, 389–390, 392–397
  allelic variation of 5-HT receptor function, 275, 280
  allelic variation of 5-HT transporter function, 283–285, 343
  animal research rationale, 437–438, 439–440
  antisocial behavior studies, 319–327
  anxiety epidemiology, 236–237
  anxiety sensitivity, 346–347
  applications of personality research, 107
  attributional style and depression, 344–345
  brain function modulation, 96
  candidate gene association research, 296–297
  chimpanzee personality research, 410–415, 420, 421–422
  continuous-liability model of individual differences, 227–228
  depression epidemiology, 234–236
  endophenotype approach, 102–103
  environmental/experiential correlations, 339–340
  environmental/experiential interaction, 107, 340–344
  extraversion variation, 101–104
  of happiness, 410, 414–415
  individual differences and, 101–102, 227, 295–296, 297
  intermediate phenotype studies, 344
  molecular heterosis, 288
  mood and anxiety disorders, 3, 259–264, 268, 275, 277, 335–349
  mu-opiate reward process, 70, 71–72

panic disorders, 278–279
  personality epidemiology, 237–238
  personality models, 231
  pharmacogenetics of 5-HT receptors, 279–281
  quantitative trait loci, 328
  research needs, 239–240
  risk markers, 343
  sensation seeking heritability, 39–41, 42
  stress response, sex differences in, 217
  therapeutic significance, 329–330
  theta-driving curve and, 13–14
  twin study methodology, 320, 336–338, 341
  See also Imaging genomics
Genomic mapping, 2
Gepirone, 274
Globus pallidus, sex differences in, 207
Glucocorticoid, 441
  5-HT receptor regulation, 277
Glucose metabolism, 367
Goal acquisition
  anticipatory phase neurobiology, 70
  emotional goals, 171, 174, 175
  incentive motivation, 63–66
  neurobehavioral systems, 63
Goal conflict, 17, 18, 21
Gray, Jeffrey, 2
  accomplishments of, 29–31
  anxiolytic drug studies, 7, 8–11
  behavioral approach system, 23–24, 117
  personality theory, 24–27, 230–231
  psychopathology theory, 28–29

H

Happiness, 410, 414–422
Harm avoidance, 230, 231
  clinical conceptualization, 251–252
  genetic epidemiology, 238
  neurophysiology, 303–305, 307
  as predictor of psychological distress, 233
Health status, personality and, 442–443
Hemodynamic imaging
  electroencephalography and, 142–143
  of emotional processing, 143–144

Hemodynamic imaging (cont.)
 lateralized brain activity, 133, 141,
  142, 147–150
 measurement and analytical
  techniques, 144–147, 150
Hippocampus
 in behavioral inhibition system, 11–
  13, 14–16, 17–18, 19, 21
 in depression, 366–367
 in emotional processing, 167–168
 5-HT receptor action in, 277, 280,
  282, 283, 284–285
 in memory, 16, 167–168
 stress response, 207, 211–212, 443
 theta patterns, 11–16, 21
Homovanillic acid, sensation seeking
 and, 48–49
Hormones
 aggression and, 436, 438–439, 440,
  441, 442
 animal studies, 436, 438–439
 sensation seeking and, 51, 52
 in sexual behavior, 198–200
 in stress response, 204, 216
HTR1A, 3, 284
 allelic variation of 5-HT receptor
  function, 275
 brain activation patterns, 287–288
 in emotional processing, 287
 mood and anxiety disorders and, 277
 panic disorder and, 278–279
 pharmacogenetics, 280
 research needs, 288
5-HTTLPR, 3, 103
 amygdala reactivity, 302–307
 cortical evoked potentials and, 50
 depression and anxiety disorders and,
  240, 284, 301–302
 in emotional functioning, 96, 301–
  307, 343–344
 in harm avoidance behaviors, 303–
  305, 307
 5-HT regulation, 300–301
 imaging genomics, 302–303
 personality correlates, 42, 52, 104–
  106
Hullian theory, 10
8-Hydroxy-2-(di-n-propylamino)
 tetralin, 274
5-Hydroxyindoleacetic acid, 301, 396
 sensation seeking and, 48–49, 50

5-Hydroxytryptamine and receptors
 activation and regulation, 273–274
 in aggression, 390–392, 397
 allelic variation of function, 275,
  300–302
 in anxiety disorders and depression,
  276–279, 281–284, 301–302
 distribution, 391
 drug action, 13, 15, 274, 276
 in emotional behavior, 298, 299–300,
  301–302
 knockout mice, 281–283, 391–392
 nitric oxide metabolism and, 396
 obstacles to behavioral research, 298–299
 in panic disorder, 278–279
 pharmacogenetics, 279–281
 presynaptic/postsynaptic signaling,
  273, 274, 275, 276, 281–283, 284–
  285, 391–392
 sensation seeking and, 48, 49
 therapeutic significance, 273, 274
 transporter function, 283–285, 300–
  302, 392
 See also 5-HTTLPR; Serotonergic
  system
Hypothalamic–pituitary–adrenocortical
 axis
 depression and, 358, 362–366, 369,
  370
 stress response, 46, 51, 203–204, 206,
  443
Hypothalamus
 in aggression, 438–439
 in behavioral approach system, 24
 in escape response, 20
 5-HT receptor action in, 284
 sex differences, 207
 in sexual responding, 187–188, 189–
  190, 192, 198

I

Imaging genomics
 advantages, 297–298
 conceptual basis, 297
 role of, 296, 297, 300, 307–308
Imipramine, 15
Impulsivity
 associated gene polymorphism, 105–106
 behavioral inhibition system and, 27

neurophysiology, 42
sex differences, 204–205
Incentive processing, 63–64
contextual facilitation, 82
individual differences, 70–71
neurophysiology, 119–122
in sexual responding, 196–197
Individual differences, generally
animal studies, 444
emotional reactivity, 94
evolutionary theory, 421
in extraversion neurophysiology, 124–127
genetic research, 101–103, 295–296, 297
incentive motivation, 70–71
mu-opiate reward process, 71–72
neurobehavioral model, 72–74, 75
neuroimaging research, 93–94
Information processing theory of depression, 359–362
Insular cortex in sexual responding, 189
International Affective Picture System, 161
Interpersonal relationships
affiliative reward in, 64–66
models of personality, 60–63
neurobehavioral systems, 63–66
sensation seeking as basis for mating attraction, 41
See also Social interaction
Introversion, behavioral inhibition system and, 25–26
In vivo cyclic voltammetry, 120
Ipsapirone, 274, 285

K

Klüver–Bucy syndrome, 187

L

Lateralized brain activity. See Frontal brain asymmetries
Learned helplessness, 344
Learning theory, 26
Life-course-persistent antisocial behavior, 317–318

Limbic system
neuroticism and, 251
pain processing, 210
stress response, 207, 211–212, 213
See also specific anatomical component
Locus coeruleus in behavior inhibition, 13

M

Major depressive disorder
clinical features, 353
course, 353–354
early-onset, 354
epidemiology, 353
social costs, 353
See also Depression
Maternal aggression, 386, 389
Mate selection, 75
neurobehavioral systems in, 64–66
sensation seeking traits as basis for, 41
Medial caudate in incentive processing, 121
Medial prefrontal cortex, 119
in incentive processing, 120, 121–122
in stress response, 207, 211–212
Medial temporal lobe
in emotional memory encoding, 167
in emotion processing, 173
5-HT receptor action in, 275, 276
Memory
changes in aging, 168–171
contextual facilitation, 79, 82
in depression, 360, 361
emotional, 166–171, 175, 209
hippocampus role, 16
visuospatial, 79
Mesolimbic system, 24
Molecular heterosis, 288
Monoamine oxidase
in aggressive behavior, 439–440
in sensation seeking psychophysiology, 47–48, 50, 52
Mood disorders, 2–3
epidemiology, 225–227, 335
neuroticism and, 228–229

Mood disorders *(cont.)*
  personality trait predictors of, 232–
    234
  sex differences in risk of, 205–206
  See also specific disorder

N

Naltrexone, 83
Nefadozone, 280
Neural cell adhesion molecule, 397
Neuroimaging
  emotion regulation, 165–166
  extraversion studies, 94–101, 103–
    104
  future prospects, 54, 129, 150
  HTR1A variation effects, 287–288
  incentive processing, 120–122
  individual differences research, 93–94
  lateralized brain activity and, 133,
    141, 142, 143–150
  orgasm, 197–198
  sexual responding, 186–197
  stress response, 209–210, 211
  See also Hemodynamic imaging;
    Imaging genomics
Neurophysiology
  affiliative reward, 68–70
  of aggression, 390–392
  anxiolytic drug action, 11, 12–13,
    14–16
  arousal during gain anticipation, 127–
    128
  avoidance responses, 20
  behavioral approach system, 24
  behavioral inhibition system, 11–14,
    17–23
  benefits of animal research, 438–440
  elicitation of behavioral process, 72–
    74
  of emotional functioning, 119, 161,
    162–164, 165–166, 173–174, 176,
    362–369, 370–374
  emotional memory, 167–171
  incentive motivation, 67, 119–121
  mood disorders, 133
  of neuroticism, 229–230
  normal aging, 159–160
  personality theory, 27, 85, 106–107

of psychopathy, 329
  sensation seeking behaviors and, 42–
    51, 52–53, 53, 54
  stress response, 363
  stress response, sex differences in,
    203–205, 206–207, 210–217
  threat response, 173–174
  See also Frontal brain asymmetries;
    Neuroimaging
Neuroticism, 3
  allelic variation of 5-HT receptor
    function and, 275
  animal studies, 430
  behavioral inhibition system and, 25–
    26
  brain activity patterns, 139–140
  clinical conceptualization, 228–229,
    251
  emotional functioning in, 118, 119,
    252
  extraversion and, 229
  genetic epidemiology, 237–238
  mood and anxiety disorders and,
    228–229, 252–268
  personality trait correlates, 230–231
  as predictor of psychological distress,
    232–234
  psychobiology of, 229–230
  sensation seeking and, 252
  subcortical arousal theory, 117
  symptom covariance with mood
    disorders, 238
Nitric oxide, aggressive behavior and,
    392–396, 437
Noradrenergic system in behavior
  inhibition, 12–13, 15–16
Norepinephrine in sensation seeking
  behavior, 47, 49, 51
Novel stimuli, response to, 43–44, 52
Novelty seeking, 230–231
Nucleus accumbens
  in extraversion, 124–127
  in incentive motivation, 67, 120, 121–
    122
  in positive arousal, 122–124
  self-stimulation behavior and, 119
  in sensation seeking behavior, 47
  stress response, sex differences in, 210
  substance use and, 67, 69
NUDR/DEAF-1, 275

O

Obsessive–compulsive disorder
  genetic epidemiology, 236–237
  personality trait predictors of, 233–234
Occipito-temporal cortex in sexual responding, 189
Opiates, endogenous
  in affiliative behavior and reward, 68, 82–85
  individual differences in, 71
  mu OR reward process, 68–72
  in stress response, sex differences in, 209–210
Orbito-frontal cortex
  in depression, 367
  in emotion processing, 163
  sex differences, 214
  in sexual responding, 189
  stress response, 207, 214
Orgasm, 197–198
Orienting behavior, 43–44, 104–105

P

Pain response
  brain activation patterns, 210
  research needs, 216
  sex differences in, 210
Panic disorder
  anxiolytic drug action, 15
  attack precipitants, 277–278
  clinical features, 277
  generalized anxiety and, 15
  genetic epidemiology, 236–237
  genetic factors, 278–279
  personality trait predictors of, 233–234, 266
Parachlorophenylalanine, 13, 391
Parietal cortex in emotional processing, 208
Parkinson's disease, sensation seeking and, 50
Partial reinforcement acquisition effect, 10
Partial reinforcement extinction effect, 10, 11–12
Passive avoidance, 9

Periaqueductal gray, 20
Personality
  allelic variation of 5-HT receptor function and, 275
  animal research findings, 428–430
  animal research rationale, 427
  animal research trends, 427–428
  approach–avoidance model, 136–137, 230–231
  behavioral inhibition system in, 23–27
  biological basis, 27, 106–107, 427
  biosocial approach, 37–39, 51–52
  classification systems, 136, 227–228, 230–231
  frontal brain asymmetries and, 133, 134, 135–136, 150–151
  genetic epidemiology, 237–238
  harm avoidance and, 230
  health and, 442–443
  higher-order traits models, 60, 106, 230, 408, 409, 414
  interpersonal domain, 60–63
  mood state effects in trait research, 100–101
  neurobehavioral systems, 63, 85
  neuroimaging studies, 54
  pharmacological studies, 436–437
  predictors of psychological distress, 232–234, 251–268
  research needs, 85
  sex differences, 204–205
  See also Chimpanzee behavior and personality; Extraversion; Neuroticism
Personality disorders, sex differences in risk of, 205
Phobias
  genetic epidemiology, 236–237
  See also specific phobia
Posttraumatic stress disorder, sex differences in risk of, 206
Prefrontal cortex
  aggressive behavior and, 390
  amygdala interactions, 300, 307
  in depression, 366
  in emotion processing, 163–164, 165–166, 168, 173, 176, 300
  in memory encoding, 168
  normal aging, 159, 160, 164
  in sensation seeking behavior, 46–47

Prefrontal cortex *(cont.)*
  in stress response, 207, 214
  subregions, 160, 164
Psychiatric disorders
  continuous-liability model, 227–228
  genetic research methodologies, 295–
    297
  personality trait predictors, 232, 251–
    255
  sex differences in epidemiology, 205–
    206
  taxonomies, 227
  See also specific disorder
Psychopathy
  assessment, 318–319
  behavioral inhibition system and, 28–
    29
  callous–unemotional traits in, 317,
    318
  clinical features, 317
  early manifestations of antisocial
    behavior, 317–318
  genetic studies, 320–322
  neurophysiology, 329
  social costs, 318
Psychoticism, behavioral inhibition
  system and, 26, 27
Putamen
  in orgasm, 198
  sex differences, 207
  stress response, 211–212

Q

Quantitative trait loci, 328

R

Raphe nucleus
  in behavioral inhibition system, 15,
    16
  5-HT receptor action in, 275, 276,
    282, 283, 284
Religious home environment, sensation
  seeking behavior and, 40
Reticular activating system, 251
Reticular formation in anxiolytic drug
  action, 14–15

Revised NEO Personality Inventory,
  118
Reward–punishment systems
  affiliative reward, 64–66, 67
  appetitive phase of goal acquisition,
    63, 64
  associative learning model, 74–75
  behavioral approach system, 23–24
  consummatory phase of goal
    acquisition, 63, 64
  contextual cues, 75, 78
  model of anxiolytic drug behavioral
    effects, 8–9
  neurophysiology, 119–120, 121–122,
    128, 163, 372–373
  opiate reward process, 68–72
  See also Behavioral inhibition
    system

S

Schemas, 359, 362
Schizophrenia, 279
  monoamine oxidase and, 47–48
Screening, depression, 354
Selective serotonin reuptake inhibitors,
  genetic factors in action of, 279–
  281
Sensation seeking, 2, 3
  associated psychopathology, 47–48
  assortative mating and, 41
  behavioral inhibition system and, 27
  biosocial model, 52–53
  clinical conceptualization, 252
  cortical evoked potentials in, 44–47,
    50, 52–53
  cultural differences, 39
  family studies, 40–41
  hormonal correlates, 51
  human correlational studies, 47–50
  molecular genetic findings, 42, 54
  mood and anxiety disorders and, 252,
    254–268
  optimal levels of arousal and, 42–43
  orienting and defensive reflexes in,
    43–44
  parenting factors in child behavior,
    41
  twin studies, 39–40

Septo-hippocampal system, 17–18, 20, 22
Serotonergic system
  in antisocial and violent behavior, 328, 443
  in behavioral inhibition system, 12, 13, 15–16
  in mood and anxiety disorders, 3, 240, 274
  neurobehavioral model, 72–73
  sensation seeking and, 42, 49, 52
  in social defeat and aggression, 439–440
  stress response, 46
  See also 5-Hydroxytryptamine and receptors
Sex differences, 2
  aggressive behavior, 389
  amygdala size, 197, 198
  anxiety disorder risk, 225, 267–268
  brain anatomy, 217
  depression in girls, 368–374
  emotional processing, 207–209
  gene–sex interactions in attention-deficit/hyperactivity disorder, 106
  mood disorder risk, 225, 267–268
  neural correlates of orgasm, 197–198
  neuroticism, 267–268
  pain processing, 210
  personality traits, 204–205
  psychiatric disorder epidemiology, 205–206
  research needs, 199–200
  response to sexual stimulus, 186–197
  sexual behavior, 184–186
  stress response, 203–217
Sexual behavior
  hormonal system in, 198–200, 441
  neural correlates of orgasm, 197–198
  neurophysiology of sexual responding, 186–197
  research needs, 199–200
  response to visual stimuli, 185–186, 188–196, 199
  sensation seeking behaviors, 51
  sex differences in, 184–200
  socialization effects, 186

Social interaction
  biosocial models of personality, 37–39
  chimpanzee behavior, 407–408, 416, 420
  happiness and, 416
  sensation seeking and social dominance, 50
  social hierarchies, 408
  See also Interpersonal relationships
Social phobia, 233–234, 266
Socioemotional selectivity, 161, 175
Startle response, 19
  psychopathy and, 29
State anxiety, 347
Stress response
  aggression and, 443
  brain activation patterns, 207–216
  clinical conceptualization, 203
  depression model, 357–359, 363, 364–365
  emotion regulation, 164–165, 206
  genomic variation, 106
  5-HT receptor regulation of, 282
  intermediate phenotype studies, 344
  neurophysiology, 46, 51, 203–205, 206–207, 210–217, 363, 443
  research needs, 216–217
  sex differences, 203–217
Striatum
  normal aging, 160
  stress response, 211–212
Stroop task, 95–96, 100, 147, 287, 360
Subcortical arousal, 119
  neuroticism and, 117
  in orgasm, 198
Subiculum, 17
Submissive behavior, 385, 439–440
Substance abuse
  brain activation patterns, 213
  dopaminergic system in, 24
  emotional stress and relapse risk, 210–213
  genetic factors, 71
  molecular genetic correlates, 42
  monoamine oxidase and, 47–48
  neurobiology, 67, 69, 71
  sex differences in risk of, 205
Suicidal behavior/ideation, 276, 283–284, 364

T

Temporal lobe, sex differences in, 207
Testosterone
    aggression and, 436, 437, 438–439,
        440, 441, 442
    sensation seeking and, 51
Thalamus
    in emotional processing, 208
    in incentive processing, 121
    in sexual responding, 189
    stress response, 206–207, 211–212
Threat response
    aggression and submission, 385
    attentional processes, 171–172
    behavioral inhibition system and, 16–17
    changes in aging, 171–172
    neurophysiology, 162, 173–174, 300
Touch, sensory processing, 64–66
Trait anxiety, 347
Trauma experience, sex differences in
    response to, 206

V

Valence in emotional experience, 161
Vasopressin, 438–439
Ventral pallidum, 198
Ventral striatum
    in behavioral approach system, 24
    in sexual responding, 189, 194
    in stress response, 207
Ventral tegmental area
    in behavioral approach system, 24,
        67
    in incentive motivation, 67, 70, 75,
        82
    opiate reward system, 69–70
    self-stimulation behavior and, 119
Ventrolateral prefrontal cortex, normal
    aging, 160
Ventromedial prefrontal cortex
    lateralization of brain activity in
        emotional processing, 147, 151
    normal aging, 164